£39.99

Handbook of Clinical
Neuropsychology

**This book is to be returned on or before
the last date stamped below.**

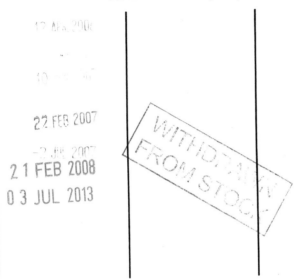

Preface

The past 25 years have seen the field of clinical neuropsychology grow to become an influential discipline within mainstream clinical psychology and an established component of most professional courses therein. Today, it is an essential resource found in most modern clinical departments of neurology, neurosurgery, psychiatry and neuro-rehabilitation where its practitioners are concerned with the psychological assessment, management and rehabilitation of neurological and psychological dysfunction. In fact, the contribution of neuropsychology extends much further than these established areas and includes sub-specialities in developmental, paediatric, neuropsychiatric, geriatric, psychopharmacological and forensic fields.

Creating a handbook of clinical neuropsychology at the beginning of the 21st century offered an opportunity to integrate relevant developments in cognitive neuropsychology, clinical psychology, cognitive neuroscience and neuro-rehabilitation. Given the exponential growth of these fields, we saw the need for a handbook which could serve both as a comprehensive textbook and as a handbook for rapid consultation, available to every clinician. Editing this handbook also provided a challenge to predict and explore future growth areas in clinical neuropsychology. Nonetheless, our main intention was to produce a practical, readable and affordable volume that was relevant to current clinical practice and the diversity of professional applications that is now clinical neuropsychology.

The text is divided into 10 parts. Part 1 provides the necessary historical context, while Part 2 deals with methodological and conceptual issues. Part 3 consists of 18 chapters, each of which deals with the assessment and treatment of specific breakdowns in cognitive ability. Part 4 focuses on the important areas of developmental and paediatric neuropsychology. Part 5 gives prominence to the often neglected field of neuropsychopharmacology. Part 6 concerns the clinical presentation of neuropsychological symptoms within different medical conditions. Part 7 highlights the growing relevance and contribution of neuropsychiatry for clinical neuropsychology. Part 8 is concerned with forensic issues, while Part 9 reviews the functional neuroanatomy underlying disorders of attention, memory, language and executive processes. Finally, in Part 10, resources relevant to clinical neuropsychology are reviewed, including a brief overview of how the internet may contribute to clinical practice.

As with so many large multi-authored volumes, the current book took longer than anticipated to produce and involved changes to both the editorial team and the format. The remit for commissioned contributors was to integrate academic and practical aspects of neuropsychology while using their seasoned judgement to outline for newcomers and less experienced practitioners what they believe constitutes best practice.

Originally planned as a short medical-style handbook characterized by brief, pithy statements, minimal referencing and the avoidance of unnecessary theoretical or technical detail, it soon became clear that this format was ill-suited to clinical neuropsychology. Accordingly, most chapters aim to strike a balance between critical overview (with selective rather than more comprehensive referencing) and practical guide. Where possible, each chapter employs summary paragraphs and 'bullet points' to highlight the main 'take home' message. The result is a more elaborate but structured chapter format which should enable readers from different specialities to acquire relatively painlessly knowledge of the many basic facts, tests and methods currently employed in the field. In addition, chapters, where appropriate, are firmly located within contemporary neuroscience (e.g. functional neuro-imaging, cognitive psychology, cognitive neuropsychology, neuropsychiatry and cognitive rehabilitation) and related to relevant medical investigations.

Writing chapters for large handbooks (or indeed editing them) are not routes to fortune (or fame) and hence it goes without saying that this handbook would not have been possible had it not been for the tolerance, good will and generous time given by busy colleagues. To all of them we extend our sincere gratitude. Special thanks are also due to Professor Graham Beaumont who was involved from the outset and whose experience with large publishing projects benefited the early development of the handbook. Unfortunately, Graham had to drop out of the project early on due to pressure of work and other commitments. We are grateful to Richard Marley, Carol Maxwell and Kate Martin at OUP for their assistance and guidance at different crucial stages of production. We are indebted to the secretarial support provided by Kath Little and Sue Dentten (Cardiff) and the inspiration and technical assistance provided by Lorraine Awcock in helping to design the handbook cover.

Cardiff	P.W.H.
Oxford	U.K.
Oxford	J.C.M.
May 2003	

Contents

Part 10 **Clinical context and resources**

Contributors

Nicole D. Anderson
Kunin-Lunenfeld Applied Research Unit
Baycrest Centre for Geriatric Care
Toronto, Ontario M6A 2E1, Canada,
and Departments of Psychiatry and
Psychology, University of Toronto

Peter A. Arnett
Psychology Department, Pennsylvania
State University, University Park,
Pennsylvania 16802-3105, USA

Claudius Bartels
Department of Neurology,
Otto-von-Guericke-University,
39120 Magdeburg, Germany

Pelagie M. Beeson
National Center for Neurogenic
Communication Disorders and
Department of Speech and Hearing
Sciences and Department of Neurology
University of Arizona, Tucson,
Arizona 85721-0071, USA

Vaughan Bell
School of Psychology, Cardiff University,
Cardiff CF10 3YG, UK

Gerhard Blanken
Department of Neurology, Otto-von-
Guericke University, 39120 Magdeburg,
Germany

François Boller
INSERM U 549, Centre Paul Broca,
75014 Paris, France

Gabriella Bottini
Dipartimento di Psicologia,
Università degli Studi di Pavia,
Piazza Botta, Pavia, Italy

Veronica Bradley
Hurstwood Park Neurological Centre,
Haywards Heath, West Sussex
RH15 4EX UK

C.M. Bradshaw
Psychopharmacology Section, Division
of Psychiatry, Queen's Medical Centre,
University of Nottingham, Nottingham
NG7 2UH, UK

Paul W. Burgess
Institute of Cognitive Neuroscience,
University College London,
London WC1N 3AR, UK

L. Cipolotti
Department of Neuropsychology,
National Hospital for Neurology and
Neurosurgery, London
WC1N 3BG, UK

Meryl Dahlitz
University Department of Psychiatry
and Psychology, Guy's, King's, and
St Thomas' School of Medicine,
St Thomas' Campus, Lambeth Palace
Road, London SE1 7EH, UK

David M. Erlanger
Department of Neurology, Albert
Einstein College of Medicine, Bronx,
New York, Department of Neuroscience
and Education, Columbia University,
New York, New York, and HeadMinder,
Incorporated, New York,
New York, USA

Jonathan J. Evans
Oliver Zangwill Centre, Princess of
Wales Hospital, Ely, Cambridgeshire
CB6 1DN, UK

Joaquín M. Fuster
Neuropsychiatric Institute and Brain
Research Institute, University of
California, Los Angeles,
California 90095-1759, USA

Guido Gainotti
Institute of Neurology, Catholic
University of Rome, 00168
Rome, Italy

Georg Goldenberg
Neuropsychological Department,
Krankenhaus München Bogenhausen,
D-81925 Munich, Germany

Laura H. Goldstein
Department of Psychology, Institute of
Psychiatry, De Crespigny Park, London
SE5 8AF and The Lishman Unit, The
Maudsley Hospital, South London and
Maudsley NHS Trust, Denmark Hill,
London SE5 8AZ, UK

Jennifer M. Gurd
Neuropsychology Unit, University
Department of Clinical Neurology,
Radcliffe Infirmary, Oxford OX2 6HE, UK

J. Richard Hanley
Department of Psychology, University of
Essex, Colchester CO4 3SQ, UK

Eli Jaldow
University Department of Psychiatry
and Psychology, Guy's, King's, and St
Thomas' School of Medicine,
St Thomas' Campus, Lambeth Palace
Road, London SE1 7EH, UK

Helga Johannsen-Horbach
School of Speech and Language Therapy,
79100 Freiburg, Germany

Narinder Kapur
Wessex Neurological Centre,
Southampton General Hospital SO16
6YD and Department of Psychology,
University of Southampton,
Southampton SO17 1BJ, UK

L.D. Kartsounis
Essex Neurosciences Centre,
Department of Neurology,
Oldchurch Hospital, Romford,
Essex RM7 0BE, UK

Janice Kay
Department of Psychology, University
of Exeter, Exeter EX4 4QG, UK

Georg Kerkhoff
EKN—Clinical Neuropsychology
Research Group, Neuropsychological
Department, Bogenhausen Hospital,
D-80992 Munich, Germany

Nigel S. King
Community Head Injury Service,
The Camborne Centre, Jansel Square,
Aylesbury, Buckinghamshire HP21 7ET,
and Oxford Doctoral Course in
Clinical Psychology, Isis Education
Centre, Warneford Hospital,
Oxford OX3 7JX, UK

Udo Kischka
Rivermead Research Centre, Oxford
Centre for Enablement,
Oxford OX3 7LD, UK

Michael D. Kopelman
University Department of Psychiatry and
Psychology, Guy's, King's, and
St Thomas' School of Medicine,
St Thomas' Campus, Lambeth Palace
Road, London SE1 7EH, UK

Tom Manly
MRC Cognition and Brain Sciences Unit,
Box 58 Addenbrookes' Hospital,
Cambridge CB2 2QQ, UK

Lilianne Manning
Laboratoire de Neurosciences
Comportementales et Cognitives (CNRS
UMR 7521) and Faculty of Psychology,
University Louis Pasteur,
67000 Strasbourg, France

Hans J. Markowitsch
Department of Physiological Psychology,
University of Bielefeld, 33501 Bielefeld,
Germany

Jane Marshall
Department of Language and
Communication Science, City University,
Northampton Square,
London EC1V OHB, UK

John C. Marshall
Neuropsychology Unit, University
Department of Clinical Neurology,
Radcliffe Infirmary,
Oxford OX2 6HE, UK

Michaela McGowan
Case Management Services Ltd, Balerno,
Edinburgh EH14 7EQ, UK

William W. McKinlay
Case Management Services Ltd, Balerno,
Edinburgh EH14 7EQ, UK

Robin G. Morris
Department of Psychology,
Institute of Psychiatry,
De Crespigny Park,
London SE5 8AF, UK

Ronan O'Carroll
Department of Psychology, University of
Stirling, Scotland, FK9 4LA

Heather Palmer
Rotman Research Institute
Baycrest Centre for Geriatric Care
Toronto, Ontario M6A 2E1, Canada

Eraldo Paulesu
Psychology Department, University of
Milan-Bicocca, 20126 Milan, Italy

George P. Prigatano
Barrow Neurological Institute,
St. Joseph's Hospital and Medical Center,
Phoenix, Arizona 85013, USA

Steven Z. Rapcsak
Department of Neurology, University of
Arizona, and Neurology Section,
Southern Arizona VA Healthcare System,
Tucson, Arizona 85724, USA

Ian H. Robertson
Department of Psychology, Trinity
College, Dublin 2, Ireland

Bjørn Rishovd Rund
Institute of Psychology, University of
Oslo, N-0317 Oslo, Norway

Carlo Semenza
Department of Psychology,
University of Trieste, 34123 Trieste, Italy

Clive Skilbeck
School of Psychology,
University of Tasmania,
Sandy Bay, Hobart,
Tasmania 7001, Australia

Joke Spikman
Neuropsychology Unit, Department of
Neurology, University Hospital,
Groningen 9700 RB, The Netherlands

Sandra Suarez
Centre de Neurosciences de la
Cognition, Montréal,
Quebec H3C 3P8, Canada

Christine M. Temple
Developmental Neuropsychology Unit,
Department of Psychology,
University of Essex, Wivenhoe Park,
Colchester CO4 3SQ, UK

Pamela J. Thompson
Psychological Services, National Society
for Epilepsy, Chalfont St Peter,
Buckinghamshire SL9 ORJ,
National Hospital for Neurology and
Neurosurgery, Queen Square, London
WClN 3BG, and Department of Clinical
and Experimental Epilepsy, Institute of
Neurology, University College London,
London, UK

Andy Tyerman
Community Head Injury Service,
The Camborne Centre, Jansel Square,
Aylesbury, Buckinghamshire
HP21 7ET, UK

N.J. van Harskamp
Department of Neuropsychology,
National Hospital for Neurology and
Neurosurgery, London
WC1N 3BG, UK

Ed van Zomeren
Neuropsychology Unit, Department of
Neurology, University Hospital,
Groningen 9700 RB, The Netherlands

Derick T. Wade
Rivermead Research Centre, Oxford
Centre for Enablement, Oxford
OX3 7LD, UK

Claus-W. Wallesch
Department of Neurology,
Otto-von-Guericke-University, 39120
Magdeburg, Germany

Stephen Whitfield
David Lewis Centre, Warford,
Nr Alderley Edge, Cheshire SK9
7UD, UK

Klaus Willmes
Section Neuropsychology,
Department of Neurology,
Medical Faculty, RWTH Aachen,
D52074 Aachen, Germany

Barbara A. Wilson
MRC Cognition and Brain Sciences Unit,
Addenbrooke's Hospital, Cambridge
CB2 2QQ and Oliver Zangwill Centre
for Neuropsychological Rehabilitation,
Ely, Cambridgeshire, UK

Gordon Winocur
Rotman Research Institute, Baycrest
Centre for Geriatric Care, Toronto,
Ontario M6A 2E1, Canada,
Department of Psychology,
Trent University, and Departments of
Psychology and Psychiatry,
University of Toronto

Claire L. Worsley
Department of Psychology
Institute of Psychiatry,
De Crespigny Park,
London SE5 8AF, UK

Andrew D. Worthington
Brain Injury Rehabilitation Trust,
West Heath House,
54 Ivghouse Road, West Heath,
Birmingham B38 8JW UK

Abbreviations

5-HT	5-hydroxytryptamine (serotonin)
AAC	alternative and augmentative communication
AAN	American Academy of Neurology
AAT	Aachen Aphasia Test
ACA	anterior communicating artery
AChI	acetylcholinesterase inhibitor
ACTH	adrenocorticotrophin hormone
AD	Alzheimer's disease
ADC	(HIV-1)-associated dementia complex
ADHD	attention deficit hyperactivity disorder
ADL	activities of daily living
ADT	Auditory Discrimination Test
AED	antiepileptic drug
AI	androgen insensitivity
AIDS	acquired immune deficiency syndrome
ALS	amyotrophic lateral sclerosis
ALS	articulatory loop system (in working memory)
AMI	Autobiographical Memory Interview
AMIPB	Adult Memory and Information Processing Battery
AMP	adenosine monophosphate (adenosine 5'-phosphate)
AMPA	DL-α-amino-3-hydroxy-5-methyl-isoxazole proprionate
ANELT	Amsterdam-Nijmegen Everyday Language Test
APM	Advanced (Raven's) Progressive Matrices
ATP	adenosine 5'-triphosphate
AVM	arteriovenous malformation
BA	Brodmann area
BADS	Behavioural Assessment of the Dysexecutive Syndrome
BAER	brainstem auditory evoked responses
BAI	Beck Anxiety Inventory
BAS	British Ability Scales
BBB	blood–brain barrier
BDI	Beck Depression Inventory
BINS	Bayley Infant Neurodevelopmental Screener
BIT	Behavioural Inattention Test
BORB	Birmingham Object Recognition Battery
BPRS	Brief Psychiatric Rating Scale
BPVS	British Picture Vocabulary Scale
BRB	Brief Repeatable Battery (of Neuropsychological Tests in Multiple Sclerosis)
BVRT-R	Benton's Visual Retention Test—Revised
CADASIL	cerebral autosomal dominant arteriopathy with subcortical infarcts and leukoencephalopathy
CAH	congenital adrenal hyperplasia
CANTAB	Cambridge Neuropsychological Test Automated Battery
CBT	cognitive behavioural therapy
CCAP	Centre for Child and Adolescent Psychiatry (Oslo)
CCC	Children's Communication Checklist
CCST	California Card Sorting Test
CDC	Centers for Disease Control (USA)
CELF	Clinical Evaluation of Language Fundamentals
CES	Central executive system
CFQ	Cognitive Failures Questionnaire
CH	congenital hypothyroidism
CICA	Criminal Injuries Compensation Authority (UK)
CJD	Creutzfeldt–Jakob disease
CMDI	Chicago Multiscale Depression Inventory
CMS	Children's Memory Scale
CMV	cytomegalovirus
CN-REP	Children's Test of Non-Word Repetition
CNS	Central nervous system
CNV	contingent negative variation

COWA	Controlled Oral Word Association (test)	FIRDA	frontal intermittent rhythmic delta activity
CPM	Coloured (Raven's) Progressive Matrices	FIS	Fatigue Impact Scale
CPM	Central pontine myelinolysis	FLD	frontal lobe degeneration of non-Alzheimer type
CPR	(Lord Woolf's) Civil Procedure Rules (England)	fMRI	functional MRI
CPT	(Connors) Continuous Performance Test	FSH	follicle-stimulating hormone
		FSS	Fatigue Severity Scale
CRH	corticotrophin-releasing hormone	FTD	frontotemporal dementia
CS	contrast sensitivity	GABA	γ-aminobutyric acid
CSF	cerebrospinal fluid	GAS	Global Assessment Scale
CT	computerized tomography	GCS	Glasgow Coma Scale
CVA	cerebrovascular accident	GDA	Graded Difficulty Arithmetic (test)
CVLT	California Verbal Learning Test	GH	growth hormone
CVS	caloric vestibular stimulation	GnRF	gonadotrophin-releasing factor
DA	discriminant analysis	GPI	general paresis of the insane
DAT	dementia of the Alzheimer's type	HAART	highly active antiretroviral therapy
DEX	Dysexecutive Questionnaire	HADS	Hospital Anxiety and Depression Scale
DHEA	dehydroepiandrosterone	HIV	human immunodeficiency virus
DHEA-S	dehydroepiandrosterone sulfate	HPT	hypothalamic–pituitary–thyroid (axis)
D-KEFS	Delis–Kaplan Executive System (battery)	HRT	hormone replacement therapy
DLBD	diffuse Lewy body disease	IADLs	instrumental activities of daily living
DNET	dysembryoplastic neuroepithelial tumour	IAP	intracarotid amytal procedure
		ICC	item characteristic curve
DSM-IV	*Diagnostic and statistical manual (of mental disorders)* (American Psychiatric Association)	ICD-10	International Classification of Disease (WHO)
		ICIDH	International Classification of Impairments, Disabilities, and Handicaps (WHO)
DSS	double simultaneous stimulation	IDDM	insulin-dependent diabetes mellitus (type I diabetes)
DST	dexamethasone suppression test		
DTVP	Developmental Test of Visual Perception	IES	Impact of Event Scale
EDSS	(Kurtzke's) Expanded Disability Status Scale	IHH	idiopathic hypogonadotrophic hypogonadism
EPS	extrapyramidal side-effect	IM	intramuscular
ERPs	event-related potentials	IPT	integrated psychological therapy (for schizophrenia)
ERT	oestrogen replacement therapy	IV	intravenous
ESES	electrical status epilepticus during slow-wave sleep	K-ABC	Kaufman Assessment Battery for Children
FAS	Fluency Controlled Oral Word Association	LBD	left brain damage
FEEST	Facial Expressions of Emotion Stimuli Test	LBL	letter-by-letter (reading)
		L-dopa	laevodopa
FEFs	frontal eye-fields	LH	luteinizing hormone
FIQ	full intelligence quotient	LIP	lateral intraparietal (sulcus)

LIPS-R	Leiter International Performance Scale—Revised
LPC	lateral prefrontal cortex
LSD	lysergic acid diethylamide
LTD	long-term depression
LTP	long-term potentiation
MAO	monoamine oxidase
MAOI	monoamine oxidase inhibitor
MDMA	methylenedioxymeth-amphetamine ('ecstasy')
MEG	magnetoencephalography
MEP	motor evoked potentials
MET	Multiple Errands Test
MID	multi-infarct dementia
MIT	Melodic Intonation Therapy
MMPI	Minnesota Multiphasic Personality Inventory
MMSE	Mini-mental State Examination
MND	Motor neuron disease
MOR	multiple oral re-reading
MRI	magnetic resonance imaging
MS	multiple sclerosis
NADDs	non-Alzheimer degenerative dementias
NARA	Neale Analysis of Reading
NARI	noradrenaline re-uptake inhibitor
NART	National Adult Reading Test
NEAD	non-epileptic attack disorder
NEPSY	Neuropsychological Assessment of Children
NFTs	neurofibrillary tangles
NIDDM	Non-insulin-dependent diabetes (type II diabetes)
NINDS	National Institute of Neurological Disorders and Stroke (USA)
NMDA	N-methyl-D-aspartate
NPH	normal pressure hydrocephalus
NV	neck muscle mechanical vibration
NVLD	nonverbal learning disability
OCD	obsessive–compulsive disorder
OKS	optokinetic stimulation
PALPA	Psycholinguistic Assessment of Language Processing in Aphasia
PASAT	Paced Auditory Serial Addition Task
PAT	Phonological Abilities Test

PCP	phencyclidine
PCRS	Patient Competency Rating Scale
PCS	post-concussion symptoms
PD	Parkinson's disease
PET	positron emission tomography
PFND	progressive focal neuropsychological deficits
PhAB	Phonological Assessment Battery
PIQ	performance IQ
PML	progressive multifocal leukoencephalopathy
PMS	peripheral magnetic stimulation
PMS	premenstrual syndrome
PPC	posterior parietal cortex
PPVT	Peabody Picture Vocabulary Test
PR	percentile rank
PROMPT	Prompts for Restructuring Oral Muscular Targets
PSD	poststroke depression
PSP	progressive supranuclear palsy
PST	Problem Solving Training
PTA	posttraumatic amnesia
PTS	Posttraumatic stress
PTSD	Posttraumatic stress disorder
RA	retrograde amnesia
RAVLT	Rey Auditory Verbal Learning Test
RBD	right brain damage
RBMT	Rivermead Behavioural Memory Test
RBMT-C	Rivermead Behavioural Memory Test for Children
RBMT-E	Rivermead Behavioural Memory Test—Extended Version
rCBF	regional cerebral blood flow
rCMR	regional cerebral metabolic rate
RDLS	Reynell Developmental Language Scales
RFs	receptive fields (of neurons)
RIMA	reversible inhibitor of MAO-A
RPAB	Rivermead Perceptual Assessment Battery
RR	relapsing–remitting (course type for MS)
RSAB	Rating Scale of Attentional Behaviour
RT	reaction time
RTA	road traffic accident

SAH	subarachnoid haemorrhage		TPM	Time Pressure Management (training)
SART	Sustained Attention for Response Test		TRH	thyrotrophin-releasing hormone
SAS	Supervisory attentional system		TROG	Test for the Reception of Grammar
SCOLP	Speed and Capacity of Language Processing		TSH	thyroid-stimulating hormone
SET	Six Elements Test		VER	Visual evoked responses
SMA	supplementary motor area		VFD	Visual field disorders
SMT	Self-monitoring Training		VIQ	verbal IQ
SNRI	serotonin–noradrenaline re-uptake inhibitors		VMI	Visual-Motor Integration (test)
SPECT	single-photon emission computerized tomography		VOSP	Visual Object and Space Perception
SpLDs	specific learning difficulties		VSSP	visuospatial scratchpad
SPM	Standard (Raven's) Progressive Matrices		WAIS	Wechsler Adult Intelligence Scale
SSER	somatosensory evoked responses		WASI	Wechsler Abbreviated Scale of Intelligence
SSRI	selective serotonin re-uptake inhibitors		WCST	Wisconsin Card Sorting Task
T_3	triiodothyronine		WIPPSI	Wechsler Preschool and Primary Scale of Intelligence
T_4	thyroxine		WISC	Wechsler Intelligence Scale for Children
TAP	Test for Attentional Performance		WMS	Wechsler Memory Scale
TBI	traumatic brain injury		WMTB-C	Working Memory Test Battery for Children
TCA	tricyclic antidepressant			
TCI	transitory cognitive impairments		WOND	Wechsler Objective Numerical Dimensions (Test)
TE	toxoplasma encephalitis		WORD	Wechsler Objective Reading Dimension
TEA	Test of Everyday Attention			
TEA-Ch	Test of Everyday Attention for Children		WRAML	Wide Range Assessment of Memory and Learning
THC	δ^9-tetrahydrocannabinol		WRAT3	Wide Range Achievement Test (3rd edn)
TIA	transient ischaemic attack			
TLE	temporal lobe epilepsy		WRMB	Warrington's Recognition Memory Battery
TMS	transcranial magnetic stimulation			
TOTs	time-on-task effects		WS	William's syndrome
TOWK	Test of Word Knowledge			

Part 1

Historical context

Chapter 1

Neuropsychology: past, present, and future

John C. Marshall and Jennifer M. Gurd

1 Past

Just how far back one might wish to trace the prehistory of neuropsychology is a moot point. Evidence of trepanning of living 'patients' in the Mesolithic period (Lillie 1998) suggests, although it does not prove, that early modern man had some idea of the importance of that cold grey mass within the skull. But we must wait for the Egyptians before hard evidence becomes available. Egyptian surgeons certainly knew that brain and behaviour are related: The Edwin Smith surgical papyrus, which dates from 1700 BCE, describes language disorder consequent on brain damage after head injury. And over a millennium later the Hippocratic corpus (circa 425 BCE) states unambiguously that *all* mental functions have their seat in the brain:

> It ought to be generally known that the source of our pleasure, merriment, laughter, and amuse-ment, as of our grief, pain, anxiety, and tears, is none other than the brain. It is specially the organ which enables us to think, see, and hear, and to distinguish the ugly and the beautiful, the bad and the good, pleasant and unpleasant . . . It is the brain too which is the seat of madness and delirium, of the fears and frights which assail us, often by night, but sometimes even by day; it is there where lies the cause of insomnia and sleep-walking, of thoughts that will not come, forgotten duties, and eccentricities.

Aristotle (384–322 BCE), who believed that the brain merely cools the blood, had clearly not been keeping up with the literature.

Nonetheless, it was another two millennia before relatively reliable associations were discovered between the locus of brain damage (established at autopsy) and the nature of the mental impairment (aphasia, agnosia, apraxia, amnesia, etc.) that in life had resulted therefrom. The ground had been prepared by the Viennese physician Franz Joseph Gall (1758–1828) who conjectured that the brain consists of many 'mental organs', each dedicated to a particular cognitive, conative, or affective function. Many of the organs in Gall's classificatory scheme proved to be valid psychobiological modules that could, to a first approximation, be independently impaired by brain damage. The Gallist organs of form, size, weight, colour, arithmetic calculation, locality (topographic learning and memory), eventuality (memory for facts), time, music, and language are still of intense interest to neuropsychologists. In one instance, that of language, Gall even managed to get the (frontal) localization correct.

Inspired by Gall's achievements, the first golden age of neuropsychology, as practised by behavioural neurologists and neuropsychiatrists from 1861 to 1914, was associated with significant advances in the fractionation of the aphasias (Bastian, Broca, Wernicke), the agnosias (Lissauer), the apraxias (Liepmann), and the alexias (Déjerine), along with the relevant autopsy-confirmed anatomoclinical correlations. Jackson (who first suggested that the right hemisphere was 'leading for spatial cognition') and Balint began to elucidate a wide range of spatial disorders, and Bianchi explored the role of the frontal lobes in reasoning and planning. The study of neurodegenerative diseases that could lead to different types of dementia was also inaugurated by Alzheimer, Korsakoff, and Pick. It is of interest that the early aphasiologists made serious attempts to retrain language skills, often deploying many of the same pedagogical techniques that were currently used to teach children. In Paris, Paul Broca himself attempted to remediate language and reading problems, but noted that the time a busy clinician could devote to speech and language therapy was ridiculously brief. Although employing traditional teaching methods, Broca nonetheless thought it probable that 'the adult and the child will follow different procedures to attain the same end' (Howard and Hatfield 1987). He also conjectured that recovery from aphasia involved training the right hemisphere homologue of (what became known as) Broca's area to take over the functions of the damaged frontal language region in the left hemisphere.

For the most part, classical neuropsychology was based upon patients who had suffered cerebrovascular accidents (and patients with progressive or degenerative conditions, including neurosyphilis). But the period from 1914 to 1956 saw two world wars and the Korean war (and their medical aftermaths). In contrast to previous patients who had typically been elderly and sick, neurologists were now also dealing with the behavioural sequelae of focal lesions caused by high-velocity projectile injury to the brains of young, previously healthy men (and, more rarely, women). Many of the seminal contributions of Gordon Holmes to the understanding of visual and visuospatial deficits were made while he was on active service as a consultant neurologist in France during World War I. Likewise, the neurologist Pierre Marie spent the war studying 'les aphasies de guerre' after gun-shot and shrapnel injuries. Such wounds are often self-sterilizing consequent upon the heat generated by the transit of the missile: As a result there were often fewer medical complications than might initially have been anticipated. Accordingly, the necessity of cognitive rehabilitation became far more pressing as patients who recovered medically from their injuries could often look forward to another 30, 40, or even 50 years of life. This period also saw the development of more formal testing procedures (to ensure the comparability of observations made on different patients). The desirability of using standardized tests and test-batteries (with appropriate norms) for the assessment of language, memory, praxis, and visuospatial skill was reinforced by the earlier success of Alfred Binet in devising intelligence tests for Parisian children (see Weisenburg and McBride 1935). When, in Cologne,

Poppelreuter (1917/1990) was studying impairments of visual attention in brain-injured soldiers, he noted that 'only a result that lies below the normal range should be judged to be definitely pathological'. Poppelreuter's (1917/1990) monograph, *Disturbances of lower and higher visual capacities caused by occipital damage*, is subtitled 'with special reference to the psychopathological, pedagogical, industrial, and social implications', which reflects the concerns of the time. Poppelreuter, a neurologist who had also trained in psychology (with Carl Stumpf in Berlin), was well placed to address these concerns. Rehabilitation was also stressed in the Berlin clinic of Hermann Gutzmann where psychologists and speech therapists treated both organic and functional disorders of language, speech, and voice in the casualties of trench warfare on the Western Front.

Classical neuropsychology had also taken an interest in affective disorders as well as cognitive impairments. The Hippocratic corpus incorporated a humoural theory of the emotions with different temperaments being associated with a preponderance of black bile, phlegm, blood, or yellow bile. Much later, Otto Loewi discovered (in 1924) that synaptic transmission from the vagus nerve to the heart muscle was chemically controlled: The first of many neurotransmitter substances (acetylcholine) had been found. A long and tortuous journey then led to the conjecture that too much or too little of various neurotransmitters was implicated in many neurological and psychiatric conditions (cf. Parkinson's disease, schizophrenia, and bipolar disorder).

The further integration of psychology (and psychologists) into medical teams concerned with acquired cognitive and affective disorders can be illustrated from the career of Kurt Goldstein (1878–1965). Shortly after the outbreak of World War I, Goldstein was appointed medical director of the Frankfurt Hospital and Research Institute for the study of brain-injured soldiers. The institute rapidly developed into a major clinical centre for the diagnosis, treatment, and rehabilitation of military casualties suffering from neurological and psychiatric impairments. Goldstein insisted on treating 'the whole person' and, to that end, involved psychologists in all the work of the Institute: Adhémar Gelb, with whom Goldstein investigated reasoning after brain damage, and Egon Weigl, whose main interest was in the aphasias, were two of the more notable of Goldstein's psychologist collaborators. By one of those fierce ironies of European history, when Goldstein (1942) wrote *Aftereffects of brain injuries in war, their evaluation and treatment*, the United States had entered World War II and Goldstein was working in New York, an exile since 1933 from the Third Reich. But in America too, Goldstein stressed the crucial contributions that psychologists made to the assessment of cognitive impairments: He worked with Martin Scheerer on devising tests of abstract and concrete behaviour, and with Marianne Simmel on acquired disorders of reading. The latter work was an important precursor of current interest in the nature of paralexic errors. Goldstein's concept of 'biological intelligence' as a function of the frontal lobes has similarly been echoed in more recent work on 'fluid' intelligence (Duncan *et al.* 1995).

2 **Present**

By the end of the 1950s, psychologists had a secure role in all aspects of the assessment and rehabilitation of patients with cognitive disorders. Alexander Romanovitch Luria in Moscow, Oliver Zangwill in Edinburgh and then Cambridge, and Hans-Lukas Teuber in New York and Boston stand out among those who pioneered modern testing methods and laid the foundations of modern neuropsychology. Furthermore, physicians such as Norman Geschwind in Boston, Henri Hécaen in Paris, and Ennio De Renzi in Milan, sometimes in collaboration with psychologists, were instrumental in vitalizing post-war behavioural neurology.

Building upon the achievements of these seminal figures, the chapters that follow present an extensive and detailed overview of current knowledge relevant to clinical neuropsychology and best practice therein. This section can accordingly be fairly brief. Nonetheless, it may be useful to highlight some of the innovations that took place between Scoville and Milner's 1957 paper on the memory impairments of the patient H.M. and the consolidation and widespread adoption of functional neuroimaging to study both the healthy and the damaged brain in 2003. We also note some continuities with previous work, e.g. the involvement of psychologists in the study of traumatic brain injury (TBI). But nowadays—in the Western world at least—such injuries result more frequently from the impact of large projectiles (motor vehicles) than from small ones (bullets and shrapnel).

Clinical neuropsychology is now a recognized profession with most practitioners working with patients in hospitals and rehabilitation centres, or in private practice. By contrast, experimental neuropsychologists, typically university-based, have often worked with healthy participants in the laboratory, devising and testing theories of normal relationships between the brain and mental life. The distinction, however, has become increasingly blurred as experimental psychologists began seeing patients for research purposes and clinical neuropsychologists began to take a more lively interest in the theoretical foundations of their practice. This erosion of professional boundaries accelerated when the widespread revival of cognitive psychology in the 1960s gave renewed impetus to all manner of questions that had previously seemed of dubious propriety. The death of behaviourism, the birth of transformational grammar, and the inspiration of information theory and computer science renewed interest in the 'mind' as programmed software that 'ran' on the computer hardware (or more accurately, wetware) of the brain. Experimental psychologists were encouraged to propose and test models of cognitive competence and performance that allowed as many 'mental computations' as the tasks required and the empirical data would support.

Cognitive neuropsychology also underwent a renaissance in the 1960s and 1970s, driven by many of the same factors that had revitalized experimental psychology. The revival of commissurotomy (in the hands of Joe Bogen) for the relief of otherwise intractable epilepsy also drove an intense interest in the cerebral lateralization of cognitive functions (Sperry *et al.* 1969). The overall aim of the discipline was seen as effecting the integration of clinical neuropsychology (the principled description of disorders consequent, for the most part, upon demonstrable brain pathology) and normal cognitive psychology (the construction and empirical validation of general models of complex mental functions). The distinctive character of *cognitive neuropsychology* lies in the explicit endeavour to interpret disorders of cognition in relation to formal information-processing models of normal (brain/mind) systems.

Seen in this light, the study of pathologies of cognition serves a threefold purpose.

◆ Neuropathological fractionations of cognition impose strong constraints upon theories of the normal system. The striking dissociations of impaired and preserved performance seen after brain damage indicate which overt behavioural abilities must *not* be analysed together as manifestations of a single underlying function.

◆ The interpretation of pathological performance by reference to normal theory allows the investigator to move beyond the mere description of overt symptomatology to accounts of the underlying processes that are impaired.

◆ In any complex system, identical *overt* failures and errors can arise from malfunction of different underlying components. Such ambiguities must be resolved by linking the patterns of impaired and preserved performance to specified (and justified) information-processing components.

The relevance of this framework to the practical concerns of clinical neuropsychologists is clear. The obtaining of standardized scores on standardized tests may be a necessary step in examining the patient, but is not a sufficient one. One needs to know why this particular patient shows this particular pattern of vitiated and intact skills. One needs to understand the underlying impairments, not just to describe the overt signs and symptoms of cognitive breakdown. Initially, observations made within this framework were systematized by 'box-and-arrow' diagrams that would have seemed entirely familiar to late nineteenth-century behavioural neurologists (compare, for example, Lichtheim 1885 and Marshall and Newcombe 1973). More recently, such models have been implemented in a computationally more rigorous form (Coltheart *et al.* 1993; Plaut and Shallice 1993).

Progress was first made in the description and interpretation of reading disorders (Marshall and Newcombe 1966) and verbal short-term memory (Warrington and Shallice 1969). But the approach characteristic of cognitive neuropsychology progressively colonized all the traditional domains of behavioural neurology: disorders of language (Caplan and Hildebrandt 1988); object- and face-recognition (Farah 1990; Young 1992); calculation (Butterworth 1999); spatial cognition (Robertson and Marshall 1993); praxis (Rothi *et al.* 1997); episodic memory (Schacter 1996); and planning and executive control (Rabbitt 1997). Eventually, it even became possible to admit to an interest in the neurobiology of consciousness, although the most striking results to date seem to concern what the mind/brain can achieve without conscious awareness (Weiskrantz 1997).

Early work that mapped the performance of individual patients on to (normal) models of the impaired domain quickly showed that the habitual symptom complexes of behavioural neurology (Broca's aphasia, dyslexia with dysgraphia, retrograde amnesia, associative agnosia, ideational apraxia, etc.) fractioned into a wide variety of clinically distinct (and theoretically meaningful) forms. Furthermore, in some domains, knowledge of lesion locus (the traditional correlate of behavioural syndromes) was judged to be irrelevant to the description of pathology-induced cognitive breakdown. The contribution of psychologists to the work of neurosurgical teams concerned with the relief of epilepsy by cortical ablation constitutes the most notable exception to this latter generalization (Scoville and Milner 1957), although it was the horrendous memory impairment of *one* patient, H.M., that first showed the importance of this work. The success of 'radical' cognitive neuropsychology soon became apparent from the insights it gave into the structure of impaired mental functions, and the way in which it drove justified changes to models of *normal* cognition.

Current work has to a large extent preserved a keen distrust of syndromes (except as clinical shorthand), and single-case studies continue to play a supreme role in theoretical innovation and in the evidential support and disconfirmation of cognitive models. In this respect, contemporary studies greatly resemble those of the first golden age (Marshall and Newcombe 1984). Nevertheless, the importance of group studies is now recognized when, for example, effect sizes are small or when correlational analysis of patterns of impaired and preserved performance is demanded (Gurd 2000; Newcombe and Marshall 1988). In some instances, large samples become interesting in their own right. For example, in a major follow-up of World War II veterans, Newcombe (1969) showed that, although selective impairments were frequent after missile injury to the brain, 'no generalized intellectual deterioration was detected in these men as a group'. Interest in neuroanatomical and neurophysiological localization has also grown, driven in the first place by the widespread availability of computerized tomography (CT) and magnetic resonance imaging (MRI) and, more recently, by advances in functional brain imaging using such techniques as positron emission tomography (PET), functional MRI, and magnetoencephalography (MEG) (Frackowiak *et al.* 1997; Cabeza and Kingstone 2001).

With respect to rehabilitation, the 1970s and 80s saw the revival of efforts to produce rational therapies and (even more importantly) rational evaluations of efficacy. An important randomized UK trial of speech therapy for aphasia gave somewhat mixed results: David *et al.* (1982) found that patients seen by professional speech therapists and by untrained volunteers seemed to recover at much the same rate and that patients who started treatment late made as much progress as those who started earlier. Such results suggested that therapies might be more effective if explicitly tailored to the strengths and weaknesses of the individual patient as assessed by a detailed neuropsychological examination.

This single-case approach to therapy for cognitive impairments drew heavily upon arguments that had previously been advanced as to why the description and interpretation of neuropsychological symptoms should be based upon the performance of individual patients and case-series. The polytypic syndromes characteristic of behavioural neurology may not be an appropriate knowledge-base on which to plan therapy. What is required in the first place are longitudinal single-subject experimental designs that can evaluate the efficacy of treatment in the individual. Potentially effective treatments can then be tested on larger samples in a case-by-case fashion. A number of such protocols are now available, including reversal and withdrawal designs, multiple baseline designs, and crossover treatment designs (see Willmes and Deloche 1997). Preliminary results from the new theoretically motivated therapies can be found in Riddoch and Humphreys (1994) and Berndt and Mitchum (1995).

It is not yet clear whether long-term, generalized gains actually accrue from such behavioural retraining of cognitive deficit or attempted substitution of alternative strategies that bypass the deficit (Shallice 2000). Knowing what is wrong does not automatically lead to knowing what should be done to ameliorate the problem.

3 Future

Predicting the future and extrapolating current trends are enterprises that have somewhat different risks attached. It is the latter that we will essay here. What can confidently be predicted, however, is that clinical neuropsychologists will not be short of work in the foreseeable future (see Denes and Pizzamiglio 1999).

Populations (in the developed world at least) are growing ever more elderly and hence suffering more and more from neurodegenerative diseases that have a potentially disastrous impact on cognitive functions and quality of life. When better cognition-enhancing drugs (and transplants) become available, it will be necessary to measure their true efficacy, to distinguish any pharmacological amelioration of performance from placebo effects, and to check for unforeseen side-effects. In younger populations, autoimmune deficiency syndrome (AIDS)-related cognitive impairments are analogous to those associated with neurosyphilis in the nineteenth century, with drug-resistant strains of human immunodeficiency virus (HIV) becoming more and more common. As with the diseases of ageing, significant work will be required to assess the efficacy of new drugs upon cognitive decline in AIDS. The impact of the Human Genome Project will no doubt increase substantially as more knowledge becomes available about neurological and psychiatric conditions whose onset is multiply determined by genetic susceptibility, developmental conditions, and environmental stressors.

The paradigms characteristic of cognitive neuropsychology will undoubtedly make further inroads into our understanding of psychiatric and other 'functional' disorders (Frith 1992). In this context, we note with alarm the high proportion of seemingly 'neurological' conditions for which no organic disorder can be found that would explain the patient's hemiparesis, somatosensory loss, visual field constriction, etc.

(Halligan *et al.* 2001). We are already seeing a significant revival of interest in the neuro-biology of the emotions (LeDoux 1992) and greater concern with how mood and affect interact with problem-solving and decision-making (Damasio 1999). The study of grossly disturbed reasoning and delusion formation should also yield major advances in the relatively near future. It is perhaps in the domain of psychiatric dis-orders that functional neuroimaging techniques and analysis procedures will have one of their most important clinical applications. Advances in the calculation of functional or effective connectivity between brain regions will help imaging techniques to address more directly the functional architecture of cognition, praxis, and affect and their dis-orders. Nonetheless, we must stress that there is no substitute for the controlled obser-vation of the patient's behavioural strengths and weaknesses. Brain imaging is not an alternative to neuropsychological practice and, in some instances, the neuropsycho-logical examination may even be a better guide to the anatomical localization of deficit.

We can also look forward to further insights into the social brain in its natural habitat (Brothers 1997; Cacioppo *et al.* 2002). Too often in the past clinicians have regarded the individual patient and his or her test scores as the primary 'object' of neuropsycho-logical practice. Without in any way wishing to deny the importance of the individual, we emphasize that the 'subject' of our discipline is the person in his or her social and environmental setting. At the moment, it could be embarrassing to inquire too deeply into the ecological validity of many of our neuropsychological measures and rehabil-itation programmes. In too many instances we only pay lip service to the distinctions between impairment (abnormality of function), disability (the effects of impairment on ability), and handicap (the effects of disability in interaction with the patient's physical and social environment). A future in which we paid more attention to how our patients (or are we now only allowed to say 'clients'?) functioned in the kitchen, the department store, the office, the bingo club, and the dinner party would be 'a consum-mation devoutly to be wished' (but see Foundas *et al.* 1995).

Acknowledgements

The work of J.C.M. and J.M.G. is supported by the UK Medical Research Council. We are grateful to Graham Beaumont for allowing us to use suggestions from his unpub-lished manuscript on the history of clinical neuropsychology.

Selective references

Berndt, R.S. and Mitchum, C.C. (eds.) (1995). *Cognitive neuropsychological approaches to treatment of language disorders.* Lawrence Erlbaum Associates, Hove, East Sussex.

Brothers, L. (1997). *Friday's footprint: how society shapes the human mind.* Oxford University Press, New York.

Butterworth, B. (1999). *The mathematical brain.* Macmillan, London.

Cabeza, R. and Kingstone, A. (eds.) (2001). *Handbook of functional neuroimaging of cognition.* MIT Press, Cambridge, Massachusetts.

Cacioppo, J.T., Berntson, G.G., and Adolphs, R. (eds.) (2002). *Foundations in social neuroscience.* MIT Press, Cambridge, Massachusetts.

Caplan, D. and Hildebrandt, N. (1988). *Disorders of syntactic comprehension.* MIT Press, Cambridge, Massachusetts.

Coltheart, M., Curtis, B., Atkins, P., and Haller, M. (1993). Models of reading aloud: dual-route and parallel-distributed-processing approaches. *Psychol. Rev.* **100**, 589–608.

Damasio, A.R. (1999). *The feeling of what happens: body and emotion in the making of consciousness.* Harcourt Brace, New York.

David, R., Enderby, P., and Bainton, D. (1982). Treatment of acquired aphasia: speech therapists and volunteers compared. *J. Neurol., Neurosurg., Psychiatry* **45**, 957–61.

Denes, G. and Pizzamiglio, L. (eds.) (1999). *Handbook of clinical and experimental neuropsychology.* Psychology Press, Hove, East Sussex.

Duncan, J., Burgess, P.W., and Emslie, H. (1995). Fluid intelligence after frontal lobe lesions. *Neuropsychologia* **33**, 261–8.

Farah, M. (1990). *Visual agnosia.* MIT Press, Cambridge, Massachusetts.

Foundas, A.L., Macauley, B.L., Ramer, A.M., Maher, L.M., Heilman, K.M., and Rothi, L.J.G. (1995). Ecological implications of limb apraxia: evidence from mealtime behavior. *J. Int. Neuropsychol. Soc.* **1**, 62–6.

Frackowiak, R.S.J., Friston, K.J., Frith, C.D., Dolan, R.J., and Mazziotta, J.C. (1997). *Human brain function.* Academic Press, San Diego.

Frith, C.D. (1992). *The cognitive neuropsychology of schizophrenia.* Lawrence Erlbaum Associates, Hove, East Sussex.

Goldstein, K. (1942). *After effects of brain injuries in war.* Heinemann, London.

Gurd, J.M. (2000). Verbal fluency deficits in Parkinson's disease: individual differences in underlying cognitive mechanisms. *J. Neurolinguistics* **13**, 47–55.

Halligan, P.W., Bass, C., and Marshall, J.C. (eds.) (2001). *Contemporary approaches to the study of hysteria: clinical and theoretical perspectives.* Oxford University Press, Oxford.

Howard, D. and Hatfield, F.M. (1987). *Aphasia therapy: historical and contemporary issues.* Lawrence Erlbaum Associates, Hove, East Sussex.

LeDoux, J.E. (1992). *The emotional brain.* Simon and Schuster, New York.

Lichtheim, L. (1885). On aphasia. *Brain* **7**, 433–84.

Lillie, M.C. (1998). Cranial surgery dated back to Mesolithic. *Nature* **391**, 354.

Marshall, J.C. and Newcombe, F. (1966). Syntactic and semantic errors in paralexia. *Neuropsychologia* **4**, 169–76.

Marshall, J.C. and Newcombe, F. (1973). Patterns of paralexia: a psycholinguistic approach. *Journal of Psycholinguistic Research* **2**, 175–199.

Marshall, J.C. and Newcombe, F. (1984). Putative problems and pure progress in neuropsychological single case studies. *J. Clin. Neuropsychol.* **6**, 65–70.

Newcombe, F. (1969). *Missile wounds of the brain: a study of psychological deficits.* Oxford University Press, Oxford.

Newcombe, F. and Marshall, J.C. (1988). Idealization meets psychometrics: the case for the right groups and the right individuals. *Cogn. Neuropsychol.* **5**, 549–64.

Plaut, D.C. and Shallice, T. (1993). Deep dyslexia: a case study of connectionist neuropsychology. *Cogn. Neuropsychol.* **10**, 377–500.

Poppelreuter, W. (1917/1990). *Disturbances of lower and higher visual capacities caused by occipital damage.* Clarendon Press, Oxford.

Rabbitt, P. (ed.) (1997). *Methodology of frontal and executive function.* Psychology Press, Hove, East Sussex.

Riddoch, M.J. and Humphreys, G.W. (eds.) (1994). *Cognitive neuropsychology and cognitive rehabilitation.* Lawrence Erlbaum Associates, Hove, East Sussex.

Robertson, I.H. and Marshall, J.C. (eds.) (1993). *Unilateral neglect: clinical and experimental studies.* Lawrence Erlbaum Associates, Hove, East Sussex.

Rothi, L.J.G., Ochipa, C., and Heilman, K.M. (1997). *A cognitive neuropsychological model of limb praxia and apraxia.* Psychology Press, Hove, East Sussex.

Schacter, D.L. (1996). *Searching for memory: the brain, the mind, and the past.* Basic Books, New York.

Scoville, W.B. and Milner, B. (1957). Loss of recent memory after bilateral hippocampal lesions. *J. Neurol., Neurosurg., Psychiatry* **20**, 11–21.

Shallice, T. (2000). Cognitive neuropsychology and rehabilitation: is pessimism justified? *Neuropsychol. Rehabil.* **10**, 209–17.

Sperry, R.W., Gazzaniga, M.S., and Bogen, J.E. (1969). Interhemispheric relationships: the neocortical commissures; syndromes of hemisphere disconnection. In *Handbook of clinical neurology,* Vol. 4 (eds. P.J. Vinken and G.W. Bruyn), pp. 273–90. Elsevier, Amsterdam.

Warrington, E.K. and Shallice, T. (1969). The selective impairment of auditory verbal short-term memory. *Brain* **92**, 885–96.

Weisenberg, T. and McBride, K.E. (1935). *Aphasia: a clinical and psychological study.* The Commonwealth Fund, New York.

Weiskrantz, L. (1997). *Consciousness lost and found: a neuropsychological exploration.* Oxford University Press, Oxford.

Willmes, K. and Deloche, G. (eds.) (1997). *Methodological issues in neuropsychological assessment and rehabilitation.* Psychology Press, Hove, East Sussex.

Young, A.W. (1992). Face recognition impairments. *Phil. Trans. R. Soc. Lond. B* **335**, 47–54.

Part 2

Methodological issues

Chapter 2

Basic concepts and principles of neuropsychological assessment

Jonathan J. Evans

1 Assessment objectives

Neuropsychological assessment is concerned with identifying the cognitive, emotional, and behavioural consequences of brain dysfunction. This type of assessment is used to address a number of different questions.

1.1 Is there evidence of organic brain dysfunction?

Despite considerable technological advances, it is not always possible to diagnose brain dysfunction purely on the basis of evidence from brain imaging, neurophysiological assessment, or other physical tests. In some cases, cognitive impairment is the only indicator of a pathological process. The most common situation of this sort involves identifying whether someone who complains of a memory problem is suffering from an organic brain disease such as dementia of the Alzheimer's type or a mood disorder such as depression. A question that occurs frequently in medicolegal cases is whether someone who has experienced a mild head injury or whiplash has suffered a brain injury sufficient to affect cognitive processing.

1.2 What is the nature and extent of cognitive impairment?

In some cases, the existence of brain dysfunction is not in dispute, but the nature and extent of any cognitive impairment needs to be clarified through more detailed neuropsychological assessment.

1.3 What are the practical consequences of cognitive impairment?

A comprehensive neuropsychological assessment should address the practical or functional consequences of cognitive impairment for the individual in terms of the disabilities caused and the likely handicapping effect of those disabilities in relation to activities of daily living, work, education, leisure, and social relationships. In some circumstances the main question for the assessment is simply whether or not a person is suffering with some form of brain dysfunction, but it is always useful to consider what practical impact particular cognitive, emotional, or behavioural problems might have on the individual's life. For this purpose the use of questionnaires such as symptom checklists or rating scales relating to the performance of everyday tasks are often helpful. It is helpful to observe the patient in practical situations. Although this inevitably produces only qualitative information, if used in combination with standardized test data it is likely to produce more accurate predictions about the practical consequences of brain injury.

1.4 How are an individual's mood and behaviour affected by brain dysfunction?

Although the central focus of neuropsychological assessment is cognition, the neuropsychologist should also examine the impact of brain dysfunction on mood, personality, and behaviour. There are two major reasons why an assessment of mood is essential.

- ◆ The presence of a mood disorder, caused directly or indirectly by brain injury, is an important area of psychological assessment in its own right.
- ◆ A mood disorder may have a significant impact on performance on cognitive tests and therefore must be taken into account when interpreting test results.

1.5 Does cognitive performance change over time?

A further use for neuropsychological assessment is in measuring change over time. This might involve charting the process of decline in cognitive functioning associated with progressive disorders such as Alzheimer's disease or the process of recovery from head injury or stroke. One problem with the use of neuropsychological tests for monitoring change is that many tests are vulnerable to practice effects. A practice effect occurs when the patient who is tested for a second, third, or fourth time on the same test improves simply because of increased familiarity with the test materials and test demands, rather than as a result of any real change in the underlying cognitive skill. This is particularly the case if tests are repeated within a matter of a few weeks, but practice effects may last a lot longer. One solution is to use parallel versions of tests on each occasion, though the number of neuropsychological tests with multiple parallel tests remains very small.

1.6 What are the implications of the pattern of cognitive strengths and weaknesses for the rehabilitation process?

Information about cognitive strengths and weaknesses is used in planning rehabilitation interventions. The presence of severe impairments in some areas of cognition will have implications for the types of intervention that are possible or the way in which patients learn new information or skills. Information about areas of retained cognitive strength can help to plan how to compensate for deficits. The best example of this occurs when an individual has intact visual memory and impaired verbal memory, or vice versa. Rehabilitation efforts may then involve helping the individual to develop compensatory strategies using the intact system. Performance on cognitive tests, however, is not the best way of measuring the impact of rehabilitation, at least not in the post-acute stages. Rehabilitation at this stage is primarily concerned with helping individuals to cope with or compensate for cognitive deficits and improve practical performance in everyday life. In other words, the aim is usually to reduce the disability or the handicapping effect of a disability, rather than reducing the impairment. Using a measure of impairment is therefore unlikely to reflect functional gains made in rehabilitation.

1.7 How might cognitive function be affected by neurosurgery?

One specialist role for neuropsychological assessment is in examining the potential impact on cognitive functioning of surgery carried out, e.g. for the relief of epilepsy. The Wada assessment involves temporarily shutting down each cerebral hemisphere by an injection of sodium amobarbital. The effect on cognitive processes, particularly language and memory, can then be assessed and the information used to inform clinical decision-making about the appropriateness of a surgical intervention.

2 Approaches to assessment—behavioural neurology and neuropsychology

In the behavioural neurology approach observable signs or symptoms are used as indices of brain pathology. However, whilst some patterns of behaviour are clearly absent in the person with no neurological condition and only occur in the context of brain lesions, many forms of cognitive impairment do not fit this dichotomy. For most cognitive skills, there is a continuum of performance in the non-neurological population. Nevertheless, the skilled observer can determine a large amount of information from relatively short interactions with the patient. By spending time talking with or observing the patient, it is possible to identify deficits in a number of cognitive domains. Short bedside tests can also be useful in highlighting the presence of some disorders. However, qualitative observation is usually not sufficient to judge the severity of impairment and may not detect certain forms of more subtle cognitive dysfunction at all.

2.1 The standardized test

The main tool of the neuropsychological assessment is the standardized, or psychometric test. Psychometric tests are tasks that have been designed to assess specified cognitive functions and are administered in a standardized fashion defined in a test manual. Such tests have been given to a normative sample group in order that the performance of the patient can be compared with that of a representative reference or 'normal control group', i.e. individuals who have not suffered any form of neurological condition. The typical scores of the normal control group are used to produce 'norms'. The statistical properties and issues of validation of such tests are considered in Chapter 3. Suffice it to say here that a test is considered to have 'good norms' if the reference group is representative of the general population in terms of all factors likely to influence test performance (e.g. age, level of education, gender). Sometimes, if a particular factor is likely to have a large influence on test performance, separate sets of norms are provided for each category of that factor (e.g. different age bands). With norms available, the performance of the patient can be compared with the average performance of individuals of a similar age, taking into account how much variability there is in 'normal' performance. Test scores are expressed in terms of a 'standard score' or a percentile. A standard score is a measure of the distance of the patient's score from the average of the reference group, taking into account the amount of variability in the scores of the reference group. A percentile is the percentage of the reference group who score the same as, or less than, the patient.

Standardized tests are the most effective tools for quantifying impairments. However, whenever possible, it is also useful to use information from observation of the patient carrying out practical or functional tasks. Some areas of cognitive function are relatively poorly assessed by standardized tests. For example, many of the formal, structured, and time-limited standardized tests may be insensitive to problems of initiation, problem-solving, and sustained attention associated with executive functioning. Although more sensitive, ecologically valid standardized tests are emerging, the qualitative information gained from a task such as planning and preparing an unfamiliar meal can help formulate the patient's impairments. Furthermore, given that one task of the neuropsychologist is to identify the practical or functional consequences of brain injury, supporting evidence from functional situations makes this process a lot easier, and more valid.

3 Assessment prerequisites

Before proceeding with a neuropsychological assessment involving the administration of standardized tests, a number of prerequisites must be checked.

3.1 Concentration

The patient must be able to concentrate for at least the time needed to administer any one test. Most full neuropsychological assessments take several hours to complete, although testing is usually carried out over several shorter sessions. However long the assessment session, it is always necessary for the examiner to be attentive to how well the patient is able to concentrate on task instructions and on carrying out the test. An injury-related impairment in attention might make the patient distractable and unable to sustain attention to the task in hand. Pain, particularly headaches, will impair concentration. Preoccupation with worrying thoughts associated with anxiety or depression can be distracting. Simple fatigue is also a common problem after brain injury and cognitively demanding tests may cause the patient to fatigue rapidly. Poor sleep may mean that the patient is fatigued even before an assessment has begun. Therefore, when testing is likely to proceed over a long time period, it is necessary to ensure that adequate breaks are taken.

3.2 Comprehension

The patient must also be able to comprehend the task instructions for any test given. This does not mean that some tests cannot be given to a person with verbal comprehension difficulties since, of course, the administration of language tests is one means of identifying the presence of receptive dysphasia. Nevertheless, if a test is given to a patient who cannot understand what he or she is required to do, then the results of that test will be invalid. These issues highlight the fact that there are no pure tests of any one cognitive function. For example, verbal memory tests are dependent upon adequate language skills so that, if a memory test involves remembering a short story and the patient does not understand the content of the story, the test results will reflect the patient's language deficits rather than testing memory functioning. Similarly, visual memory tests are dependent upon adequate perceptual skills so there is little point testing a person's memory for a complex design by asking the patient to draw the design from memory if the person cannot adequately copy the design.

3.3 Motivation

A further issue is the motivation of the patient to engage in the assessment process. Brain injury can cause motivational problems directly when the centres in the brain responsible for drive and initiation of activity are damaged. In more extreme forms of this disorder the patient may experience an inability to initiate action unless prompted at every stage. In less extreme forms, the patient may simply not apply him or herself to the task in the same way that it is reasonable to assume that most normative subjects would have done. Once again, therefore, this would result in test results reflecting the motivation problem more than the cognitive skill under scrutiny.

Alternatively, motivation problems may be a result of a mood disorder. The patient who is depressed may not feel able to make an effort during testing and the results of the patient's performance may overestimate the level of impairment. Whilst this issue can affect performance on almost any cognitive test, certain tests are more vulnerable to the effects of motivational problems. For example, tests of memory such as story recall may be more sensitive to motivation problems than tests that use recognition of information as the means of assessing whether information is remembered.

3.3.1 Motivation by hopes of secondary gain

Sometimes a patient is motivated by secondary gain to perform more poorly than determined by the level of impairment that actually exists. This is most likely to occur in the context of medicolegal assessments when the level of a patient's compensation award is dependent upon the severity of the impairment. In this situation the patient may be very compliant with the assessment process, but may attempt to 'fake bad'. This might be in the context of the patient actually having no cognitive deficit at all or, more probably, in the context where the patient is attempting to exaggerate the severity of a genuine impairment. While examples of this sort of malingering are quite rare, it is necessary to consider this as a possibility in any assessment, particularly in any medicolegal assessment (see Halligan, Bass & Oakley 2003).

This issue can be addressed in several ways. First, the examiner needs to be attentive to the situation where the severity of the complaints of the patient appears to be inconsistent with the severity of the injury. However, it is not possible to rely on this type of comparison alone since the relationship between injury severity indicators, such as length of coma or posttraumatic amnesia, and cognitive or functional impairments is not straightforward. For this reason, it can be helpful to use some of the tests that have been specifically designed to identify the patient who is faking bad. Most tests of this sort rely on the assumption that such patients will have a limited knowledge of the typical consequences of brain injury on cognitive functioning or have a poor knowledge of test procedures. As a result of this test naivety the patient may produce a performance that is worse than that of most genuinely impaired patients. For example, on a two-choice recognition memory test, even the most severely amnesic patient would not be expected to score much less than 50% correct simply by guessing. A performance below 'chance' levels (i.e. that which would be obtained from simply guessing) should therefore alert the examiner that further investigation of this issue is needed. For further discussion of this issue see Rogers (1997).

4 Contra-indicators to assessment validity

Even when the assessment prerequisites have been checked, several other factors can significantly affect a patient's performance on neuropsychological tests. Groth-Marnat (2000, p. 95) lists 18 factors that could render the results of neuropsychological tests invalid.

- For example, physical problems may affect performance. In addition to pain, which will affect concentration, sensory or motor disturbances are likely to affect performance speed. Intoxication with alcohol or recreational drugs may impair cognition, as will some prescription medications (see Lezak 1995, p. 311).
- Current or pre-existing psychiatric disorder or learning disability will affect results.
- Congenital or pre-existing neurological conditions including prior brain injury, insult, or epilepsy are also relevant factors.
- People for whom the language in which they are tested is not their first language may be disadvantaged.
- Some tests are considered to be culturally biased, which will compromise the results of someone whose cultural background is different.

- The performance of patients may vary from one testing session to another for a variety of reasons and therefore the neuropsychologist must be cautious in interpreting the results from just one session.

It is critical therefore that the neuropsychologist assesses for the presence of any of these factors and considers carefully their potential impact on each individual assessment.

5 The assessment process

5.1 Review of information provided by the referrer

The assessment process begins with a review of the information provided by the referrer. Sometimes a great deal of information is available, including a detailed clinical history, brain imaging data, and results of neurological evaluation. At other times, the only information may be that the patient is complaining of a particular problem (e.g. difficulty in remembering names or appointments), or that the patient has experienced a particular incident, e.g. a mild head injury.

5.2 Interviewing the patient and his/her relative or carer

Upon arrival the patient should be helped to feel at ease. Neuropsychological assessment is often a lengthy process, which can be upsetting for people who may be faced with difficulties of which they are only partially aware. Thus, the need to maintain their cooperation is vital. An initial interview is used to establish the patient's perspective on the problems, the history, and the impact of the problems on daily living. In addition to the patient, it is usually necessary to interview a relative or carer who knows the patient well. Whilst it is important to obtain the patient's view of the problems, difficulties with insight or memory may mean that this personal account may be inaccurate. Many clinicians will use a semi-structured interview format for this clinical interview. Symptom checklists are also useful in prompting patients and relatives to report problems that may otherwise be forgotten or unstated. It is helpful to interview the patient's relative without the patient being present, so that the relative has the opportunity to express concerns that would otherwise not be discussed through embarrassment or protecting the feelings of the patient.

5.3 Administration of standardized tests

The assessment then proceeds with the administration of standardized tests designed to assess particular cognitive functions. There is no universally agreed set of tests used for neuropsychological assessment. It has been argued that there are two distinct approaches to test selection, the comprehensive or 'big battery' approach and the individualized, hypothesis-testing approach (see Miller 1992; Lezak 1995; Groth-Marnat 2000).

5.3.1 The 'big battery' versus the individualized hypothesis-testing approach

The big battery approach uses, as the name implies, a battery of tasks that is designed to assess most types of cognitive skill on the premise that, if a deficit is present, the battery will detect it. The main disadvantage of this approach is that it can be too time-consuming and may not assess some types of cognitive skill in sufficient detail to fully formulate the impairment.

By contrast, the individualized, hypothesis-testing approach is based on the particular question posed in the assessment. Information available prior to and during the assessment about the patient's strengths and weaknesses is used to select tests to assess in detail particular areas of deficit. For example, the main question in some assessments is whether or not brain damage is present. In this case the clinician will try to select those tests that are most sensitive to any form of brain injury. However, these tests are often not the best ones for making predictions concerning the functional impact of cognitive impairment. If predicting everyday problems and guiding rehabilitation are the main issues, then other tests may be selected. The main disadvantage of the hypothesis-testing approach is that the clinician is vulnerable to failing to assess a particular cognitive skill because a deficit is not readily apparent.

In practice, most clinicians probably use a combination of these approaches, by selecting a broad set of tasks designed to screen most areas of cognitive skill, and incorporating other tests as needed on the basis of test performance, the complaints of the patient or others, or the particular assessment question.

5.3.2 The importance of good normative data

A further issue for test selection is the importance of using well standardized tests that therefore have good normative data. Although the importance of accompanying functional information has been emphasized, the standardized test provides objective evidence of the nature and extent of cognitive impairment. Certain groups are not well represented in most normative samples for cognitive tests, e.g. people with low premorbid intellectual ability or very old people. In such cases the neuropsychologist must be cautious in test interpretation.

6 Cerebral organization and laterality

The brain is not cognitively symmetrical. While some cognitive processes are represented in both cerebral hemispheres, others are more localized to one or other hemisphere or to particular areas within a hemisphere. This is consistent with the currently prevailing view that many cognitive functions are modular in nature and that different cognitive modules rely on different brain regions.

The asymmetry of cerebral organization is most strikingly illustrated with language skills, which for most people are localized to the left hemisphere. It is also illustrated by the phenomenon of handedness, whereby one hand is 'dominant' in terms of being used for tasks requiring higher levels of fine motor skill. Handedness is typically assessed through questions about which hand or foot is used for various tasks or by asking the patient to perform or mime tasks such as writing or throwing and kicking a ball.

The relationship between handedness and localization of cognitive functions such as language is strong, but not complete. The majority of right-handed people have language skills in the left hemisphere, but the picture is more complex for left-handers, with some having language on the left, some on the right, and some with language represented bilaterally. The identification of the speech dominant hemisphere is most critical when surgical procedures are planned, but for these purposes laboratory assessments such as the Wada technique are used.

With the advent of more sophisticated imaging techniques, the usefulness of assessing handedness, in combination with cognitive test performance, for the purposes of lesion location has diminished. Although there are reported group differences in cognitive strengths between left- and right-handers, such differences are at best modest and are unlikely to be helpful when accounting for patterns of performance on an individualized basis. The assessment of cerebral dominance can, however, help with the interpretation of patterns of neuropsychological test results. The assessment of handedness becomes most relevant when an unexpected pattern of performance on cognitive tests is shown, e.g. when a patient with a right hemisphere lesion demonstrates significant language disorder.

7 Specific cognitive skills examined during the neuropsychological assessment

The following sections describe in brief the cognitive skills that are the subject of neuropsychological assessment. More detailed accounts of the assessment process in each cognitive domain are provided in the following chapters. Some of these areas are not assessed in detail unless there are indications of possible problems, though the clinician should be attentive for examples to difficulties that require more detailed examination. The section begins with a discussion of the issue of the importance of assessing premorbid functioning.

7.1 Premorbid functioning

In the neurologically normal population there is a wide range of ability in almost all forms of cognitive skill. Brain injury *can* lead to a performance on a cognitive test that is worse than that of almost any person who has not suffered a brain injury. However, it is also possible for a person who premorbidly functioned at a high level of ability to suffer an impairment, while his or her test score remains within a normal range. While the score is not abnormal in relation to the general population, it is abnormal for that individual. When evaluating a patient's scores on any cognitive test, it is therefore necessary to consider what the patient's score would have been expected to be *before* the brain injury.

Most people will not have had any form of cognitive assessment premorbidly and therefore pre-injury performance has to be estimated. The three most common ways of doing this are to use:

◆ general demographic information (age, years of education, social class);

◆ the individual's best performance on any of the cognitive tests presented;

◆ a test that is usually resistant to the general effects of brain injury.

In the UK, the most common test for estimating premorbid ability is the National Adult Reading Test, 2nd edition (Nelson and Willison 1994). This test has been shown to correlate highly with performance on the Wechsler Adult Intelligence Scale— Revised (Wechsler 1981) in a normative sample and so can be used to estimate pre-morbid intellectual level, except where there is evidence of a pre- or postmorbid dyslexia. An alternative test of this sort is the Spot the Word subtest, from the Speed and Capacity of Language Processing Test (Baddeley *et al.* 1992). Spot the Word is a lexical decision task in which pairs of words are presented, only one of which is real, with the task being to identify the real word.

7.2 Current intellectual functioning

Most clinicians will administer a test, or battery of tests, designed to capture an individual's general level of intellectual functioning. The Wechsler Adult Intelligence Scale (WAIS; now in its third edition) is the most widely used tool for this purpose. The main aims of using such a battery are to provide a means of identifying whether an individual is likely to have suffered a deterioration in cognitive performance in relation to estimates of premorbid functioning and to highlight particular areas of deficit that may need further investigation.

It is worth noting that neither the WAIS nor its subsequent incarnations were designed as neuropsychological assessment tools and poor performance on any one subtest cannot be used to diagnose a deficit in a particular cognitive domain. A formu-lation of a patient's impairments must be developed by careful analysis of the pattern of performance over a range of tests. While the WAIS can be used to determine an intelligence quotient (IQ) score (which is compared with estimates of premorbid IQ in the identification of brain dysfunction), in the neuropsychological context one must be cautious in expressing performance on a range of tests in terms of an IQ score. This is because a cognitive deficit in just one domain may lead to an extremely poor per-formance on a small number of subtests, while performance on other tests remains entirely normal. The averaging process used to calculate the IQ score could therefore mask a severe impairment in just one domain. For this reason it is more important to pay attention to the individual subtest scores.

7.3 **Memory**

A range of different types of memory function must be assessed. (See Chapters 9 and 10.)

7.4 **Attention and concentration**

The terms attention and concentration are used interchangeably to refer to the ability to focus upon a particular stimulus and to maintain that stimulus in mind, sometimes over an extended period of time. (See Chapters 5 and 6.)

7.5 **Speech, language, and communication skills**

Although speech, language, and communication skills are often the domain of the speech therapist/pathologist, in the clinical setting it is necessary for the neuropsychologist to have a good knowledge of the nature of aphasic (language) disorders and dysarthia (impaired articulation), since these problems will impact on performance on other tests and be relevant to considerations of the functional impact of cognitive impairments. (See Chapters 13 and 14.)

7.6 **Visuospatial and constructional skills**

Brain injury may cause visual field disorders, problems with visual acuity, spatial contrast sensitivity, visual (light and dark) adaptation, colour perception, figure–ground separation, or movement perception. Some of these problems can be addressed in opthalmological or neurological examinations and, if such problems are suspected to be present, then appropriate referral should be made. (See Chapter 7 and 11.)

7.7 **Executive functioning**

Executive functioning refers to the ability to plan and problem-solve, self-monitor, and regulate behaviour and is considered in Chapters 17 and 18.

7.8 **Mood, personality, and behaviour**

Direct consequences of brain injury may arise when the regions of the brain responsible for emotional processing or emotional control have been damaged. Indirect consequences arise from the stress of adjusting to losses of cognitive or physical functioning, role, or relationships.

Emotional lability is a common consequence of brain injury. Irritability and anger control are major problems for many patients. Although diagnostically controversial, some people with brain injury suffer from posttraumatic stress syndrome. While they do not usually remember the accident or injury, a small number of individuals suffer flashbacks to isolated memory fragments (islands of memory) of the event or perhaps waking in hospital, which for some is itself traumatic.

Attributions made by relatives concerning changes in personality are often related to changes in levels of inhibitory control and initiative. Those people who are disinhibited, more impulsive, and emotionally labile, or those who are unable to initiate activity in the same way, are those who are most commonly described as having changed in personality.

8 Conclusion

There are no pure tests of any single cognitive skill. The formulation of a patient's pattern of cognitive strengths and weaknesses is a complex task involving the assimilation of information from a wide range of different sources including the detailed history of the client's presenting problems and premorbid functioning, results from standardized tests and functional observation, and an assessment of the mood and motivation of the patient. Many problems experienced after brain injury or illness are very obvious from a short conversation with the patient. Some problems may be revealed by brief cognitive screening tools, but others are much more subtle, albeit no less disabling, and require much more detailed assessment.

Selective references

Baddeley, A.D., Emslie, H., and Nimmo-Smith, I. (1992). *The speed and capacity of language processing test.* Thames Valley Test Company, Flempton.

Groth-Marnat, G. (2000). *Neuropsychological assessment in clinical practice.* John Wiley and Sons Inc, New York.

Halligan, P.W., Bass, C. and Oakley, D. (2003). *Malingering and illness deception.* Oxford University Press, Oxford.

Lezak, M.D. (1995). *Neuropsychological assessment*, 3rd edn. Oxford University Press, Oxford.

Miller, E. (1992). Some basic principles of neuropsychological assessment. In *A handbook of neuropsychological assessment* (ed. J.R. Crawford, D.M. Parker, and W.W. McKinlay), pp. 10–11. Lawrence Erlbaum Associates, Hove, East Sussex.

Nelson, H. and Willison, J. (1994). *National adult reading test*, 2nd edn. NFER, Windsor.

Rogers, R. (1997). *Clinical assessment of malingering and deception*, 2nd edn. Guilford Press, New York.

Wechsler, D. (1981). *Wechsler adult intelligence scale—Revised.* Psychological Corporation, New York.

Chapter 3

The methodological and statistical foundations of neuropsychological assessment

Klaus Willmes

1 Basic psychometric considerations

Neuropsychological tests are not different from psychological tests in general, as far as psychometric aspects are concerned. *Psychometrics* is a specific domain of measurement in psychology concerned with the assignment of numerals to one (or several) property of objects or events according to fixed rules. Measurement proper (or a scaling process) occurs when a quantitative value is assigned to the sample of behaviour collected with a test from which test users draw inferences about the amount or extent of the theoretical construct (trait) that is taken to be characteristic of a person.

◆ Unlike physical attributes, psychological attributes of a person cannot be measured directly.

◆ Psychological attributes are constructs or hypothetical concepts, the existence of which can never be confirmed in an absolute way, nor is there universal acceptance as to how to measure any construct.

◆ The degree or extent to which some psychological construct is characteristic of a person can only be inferred from limited samples of that person's behaviour.

◆ Before any measurement of a construct can be made, one has to establish an operational definition, i.e. a rule of correspondence between the theoretical construct and observable behaviours that may be considered indicators of the construct.

◆ Any measurement obtained is always subject to error.

◆ The units of measurement on the measurement scales are not well-defined *per se*.

◆ The measurements on one construct must also have demonstrated relationships to other constructs within a theoretical system.

In psychology, a *test* is a standard procedure for obtaining a sample of behaviour from some specific domain. One can furthermore make a distinction between:

- (aptitude, achievement, proficiency) tests, with which one can obtain a behavioural sample of a person's *optimal* performance;
- questionnaires or inventories collecting a person's *typical* performance;
- sampling typical performance with a standard schedule and list of behaviours in a naturalistic setting (e.g. observation checklists).

2 The classical test theory model

Test theory is concerned with methods for estimating the extent to which the specifics of assessment of psychological functions influence the measurements in a given situation and with methods for minimizing these problems.

2.1 Basic properties

Most neuropsychological tests—as most psychological tests in general—are constructed along the rationale of the *classical test theory model* or *classical true score model* (Gulliksen 1987; Lord and Novick 1968) with a subject's observed score assumed to be additively composed of a true performance level and a random error (see box below).

Basic properties and principles of the classical test theory model

- The *observed score* random variable X_{ij} (denoting the hypothetical distribution of potential scores) for subject i in test j is composed additively of the subject's true score T_{ij} for test j and the error random variable E_{ij}:

$$X_{ij} = T_{ij} + E_{ij}.$$

- The *true score* can be interpreted as the average of observed scores obtained over an infinite number of repeated test administrations (i.e. the expected value) with the same test.
- The test score of a different examinee represents another random variable with a potentially different true score.
- The expected value of the error variable E_{ij} is zero.
- In a population of examinees the expected error is zero, as well as the correlation between true scores and error scores.

2.2 Reliability

In order to obtain information about how closely related observed and true scores are for some examinee in a given test (dropping the index j for the moment) we have to make use of the *reliability coefficient* ρ. The higher the reliability, the better the observed score represents the true score. The reliability coefficient is defined as the ratio of true score variance $\sigma^2(T)$ to observed score variance $\sigma^2(X)$ in the population of examinees:

$$\rho = \sigma^2(T)/\sigma^2(X); \quad 0 \leq \rho \leq 1.$$

The reliability coefficient ρ is the square of the *reliability index* ρ_{XT} which denotes the correlation between true and observed score. The above expression does not have practical value because true scores are not directly observable. Different approaches to actually assessing reliability are parallel test, split-half, and retest reliability, as well as measures of consistency (see box below).

Different approaches to determining reliability

Parallel test reliability

This is the correlation between parallel tests. In classical true score theory two tests A and A′ are defined as *parallel* when:

♦ each examinee has the same true score on both forms of the test

♦ the error variances for the two forms are identical

(Due to these properties, parallel tests also have identical observed score means and variances. The more general assumption of *essential τ-equivalence*, i.e. that the true scores may only differ by a fixed constant across all subjects, is also sufficient.)

With the additional assumption of uncorrelated error variables for the two separate tests the reliability coefficient is identical to the correlation between both observed variables X, X':

$$\rho_{XX'} = \text{corr}(X, X') = \rho^2_{XT}.$$

Retest reliability

This is a measure of the correlation between two administrations of the same test. It may only be interpreted as a reliability coefficient, if the assumptions of parallel tests are satisfied. In particular, the identity (except for an interindividually constant term in essentially τ-equivalent measures) of true scores across the two measurement occasions for each person may be problematic. It calls for the absolute stability of interindividual differences (with respect to the theoretical (true score) variable of interest.

Different approaches to determining reliability *(continued)*

Split-half reliability

This measure of the correlation of the item totals of a test split into two halves may only be interpreted as a reliability coefficient if the assumptions of parallel (more general: essentially τ-equivalent) tests are satisfied for both test halves. Since there is only half of the items in each part, reliability will be underestimated. The reliability coefficient ρ^* of the full-length test is:

$$\rho^* = 2\,\rho/(1 + \rho), \quad \text{e.g. if } \rho = 0.80, \text{ then } \rho^* = 1.60/1.80 = 0.89.$$

There are many ways to split a test (e.g. odd versus even items, first versus second half, etc.). The last formula represents a special case of the general *Spearman–Brown (prophecy) formula* for modifying the number of items in a test by a factor K ($K = 2$ in the split-half case). The reliability coefficient ρ^* for the modified length test is:

$$\rho^* = K\rho/(1 + (K - 1)\,\rho).$$

Standardized item alpha reliability coefficient

This measures the average correlation ave(ρ) between all $K(K - 1)/2$ pairs of *parallel* items scaled to a test of length K:

$$\rho^* = K\,\text{ave}(\rho)/(1 + (K - 1)\,\text{ave}(\rho)).$$

Cronbach alpha coefficient of consistency

This is a lower bound to standardized item alpha ρ^* for non-parallel items:

$$\alpha = (K/(K - 1))\,(1 - \Sigma\sigma_I^2/\sigma_X^2),$$

where σ_I^2 is the variance of the Ith item and σ_X^2 the variance of the total score. In case of parallel (more generally: essentially τ-equivalent items), the right-hand side in the last formula is identical to $\rho_{XX'}$ with X denoting the total score (or arithmetic mean) of the K items. In case of dichotomous items, Cronbach alpha equals Kuder–Richardson formula-20 (KR-20). (For more details, see Crocker and Algina 1986 and Suen 1990.)

Reliability of difference score

Let $D = X - Y$. Assuming uncorrelated errors among X and Y,

$$\rho_{DD'} = (\rho_{XX'}\,\sigma_X^2 + \rho_{YY'}\,\sigma_Y^2 - 2\rho_{XY}\,\sigma_X\,\sigma_Y)/(\sigma_X^2 + \sigma_Y^2 - 2\rho_{XY}\,\sigma_X\,\sigma_Y).$$

In case of parallel measures, $\rho_{DD'} = 0$.

Example (with identical variances): $\rho_{XX'} = 0.90$, $\rho_{YY'} = 0.95$, and $\rho_{XY} = 0.70$ leads to $\rho_{DD'} = 0.75$ only; but a low correlation $\rho_{XY} = 0.30$ would yield a higher $\rho_{DD'} = 0.89$.

The *reliability of a difference score* may be of particular interest when diagnostic decisions have to be based on the difference $D = X - Y$ between two measures. Often, the reliability of the difference score is less than that of both original measures. Rather reliable difference scores will result when one chooses measures that are both highly reliable, but are not highly correlated. In case of correlated error variables or a correlation of X and $X - Y$, the reliability of the difference score may be higher than for either of the two measures.

The techniques for assessing reliability described so far cannot capture all relevant aspects of reliability estimation. Most restrictive is the assumption of just one non-differentiated error component (or, respectively, one undifferentiated source of unreliability) in the classical true score model. *Generalizability theory*, as a generalization of reliability theory, allows for the introduction of several sources of unreliability (for details see Crocker and Algina 1986, Chapter 8).

2.3 Standard error of measurement and standard error of estimate

One important diagnostic question is how measurement errors can influence the interpretation of an individual person's scores. The exact extent of error in a given score cannot be determined, but classical test theory allows for computing the expected variation of an individual subject's observed score around the true score, the *standard error of measurement*, i.e. the square root σ_E of the error variance (see box below). If one additionally assumes that the error variable E follows a normal distribution, a person's

---

Standard error of measurement and standard error of estimate

- The *standard error of measurement* is related to observed score variance and reliability coefficient:

$$\sigma_E = \sigma_X \sqrt{(1 - \rho_{XX'})}.$$

Often, the 95%-confidence interval for the true score around the observed score X is reported for a test. It is computed as:

$$X \pm 1.96\, \sigma_E.$$

Example: with $\sigma_X = 10$ and $\rho_{XX'} = 0.91$, the standard error is $\sigma_E = 10\sqrt{(1 - 0.91)} = 3$.

- The *standard error of estimate* is:

$$\sigma_{XX'} = \sigma_X \sqrt{(1 - \rho_{XX'}^2)}.$$

The standard error of measurement is less than the standard error of estimate except for the case of perfect or zero reliability; in the example $\sigma_{XX'} = 4.15$.

true score lies within the confidence limits of $X - \sigma_E$ and $X + \sigma_E$ with a probability of about 68%. The standard error of measurement will not be identical for all examinees and σ_E expresses the average of all examinees' individual standard errors. Thus the standard error of measurement provides an interval for the average examinee. Furthermore, the confidence interval has the same width irrespective of the value of X, i.e. the uncertainty about the exact value of the true score is assumed to be the same for poor, medium, and good performance.

Another relevant error, the *standard error of estimate*, is defined as the discrepancy between an examinee's observed score on one test and the predicted score on a parallel form of that test (see the box).

2.4 Normative data, standardization

An examinee's raw score usually cannot lead to useful interpretations or inferences. For example, with 40 items in a visual discrimination test composed of 50 items answered correctly, a statement about visual discrimination ability depends on the difficulty of the test and/or the performance of other similar examinees.

♦ The use of *norms*, i.e. an external reference, helps to enhance interpretability of scores (see box below).

Norms

♦ The *percentile rank* of a raw score k is defined as:

$$PR(k) = 100\% \text{ (cum } f_k + f_k/2)/N,$$

where cum f_k is the cumulative frequency for all scores less than the score of interest, f_k the frequency of the score of interest, and N the normative sample size. Usually, the PR is rounded to the nearest integer number.

♦ *Normalized z-scale* (mean zero, standard deviation one): a certain PR is identified with the corresponding quantile of the standard normal distribution, i.e. with that z-score below which PR per cent of a normally distributed trait are to be found.

♦ *Linear z-score and standard norms*: linear transformation of raw score x_i in normative sample:

$$z_i = \text{(raw score } x_i - \text{mean raw score)/standard deviation of raw scores.}$$

For better interpretability, linear transformation $L + Kz$ into a standard norm with mean L and standard deviation K:

$T = 50 + 10z$ (T-score) $W = 10 + 3z$ (Wechsler scaled score)

$Z = 100 + 10z$ (Standard score) $C = 5 + 2z$ (Centile score)

$IQ = 100 + 15z$ (Deviation IQ)

◆ A *normative score* provides information about an examinee's performance in comparison to the (total) score distribution of some reference group or norm sample representing a well-defined population. It is required to describe the normative sample with respect to demographic characteristics (gender, age, educational background). One also has to decide on the normative sample size, since it determines how adequately the normative sample represents the reference population.

◆ The *percentile rank* (PR) is one common type of normative score (see the box p. 32), denoting the percentage of examinees in the norm sample scoring below or identical to a given raw score. Although the PR is easy to interpret, one has to consider that the PR scale is a nonlinear transformation of the raw score scale with the same gain in raw scores possibly indicating a varying gain in PR scores at different locations on the raw score scale.

◆ A *normalized z-scale* (see the box p. 32) is often constructed in case of a nonnormal raw score distribution by identifying a certain PR with the corresponding quantile of the standard normal distribution. In case of more marked deviations from a normal raw score distribution, this procedure will introduce substantial distortion often at the lower and/or upper end of the raw score scale.

◆ *Linear z-scores* (see the box p. 32) are derived from raw scores in the case of their distribution being normal and they are further transformed into *standard norms* with means and standard deviations that lend themselves to an easy interpretation.

In case of dependence of test performance on age or education (school grade) separate norms for different age or education subpopulations or grade and age equivalents are determined. Another approach is to determine the (linear) regression of age on the raw score for the whole standardization sample and compute a correction score.

2.5 Validity

◆ *Validity* is the potential of the true score to reflect what a test intends to assess—in most cases this is an unobservable trait or psychological construct. Validity has always been regarded as the most fundamental and important property of psychometric instruments. The validity of a test is the extent to which it measures what it purports to measure. Generally, the chosen measure and its related true score only quantify some relevant aspect of a construct—it can never be fully captured by one or a few measures. A measure cannot simply be classified as being valid or invalid in an absolute fashion. Rather validity is a relative property always to be considered with respect to some intended purpose. Validity is an overall evaluative judgement, founded on empirical evidence and theoretical rationales, of the adequacy and appropriateness of inferences and actions based on test scores (Messick in Wainer and Braun 1988, p. 33).

◆ *Validation* describes the process by which a test developer collects evidence to support the types of inferences that are to be drawn from test scores.

Changes in emphasis and orientation towards validity have taken place in the history of psychometrics with an emphasis on the concept of construct validity in more recent times. Key validity issues are the interpretability, relevance, and utility of test scores.

Three main aspects of validity are generally discerned.

◆ *Construct validity* refers to a mutual verification of a measurement instrument and the theory of the construct it is intended to measure by way of testable hypotheses. There are several approaches to *construct validation*. Most of them are related to looking at the pattern and size of correlations implied by consequences from the theoretical conceptions or to looking at the differentiation between groups in terms of theoretically implied expected differences (cf. Crocker and Algina 1986, pp. 232–4).

◆ *Criterion-related* (or criterion) *validity* refers to (cor-)relating one measure of a construct to another measure of the same construct or some 'gold standard', if available (also see the box below on validity coefficient). The criterion can take several forms.

—*Concurrent* validity is looked for in case of another measure of accepted validity.

—*Predictive* validity captures the relation of a measure with some aspect of the expected future, a major aspect of screening and prognostic measures.

◆ *Content validity*—often employed with achievement tests—refers to how well one can draw inferences from an examinee's test score to a larger item domain similar to those belonging to the actual test instrument. Content validation is often based on expert ratings about how well the generation of items from some performance domain has been specified and how well the actual items reflect that domain. Several indices have been proposed to quantitatively summarize expert decisions about item adequacy (cf. Crocker and Algina 1986, pp. 221–2).

Validity coefficient

The validity coefficient ρ is the correlation between the true score of a test and the true score of a second variable (e.g. a criterion variable):

$$\rho(T_X, T_Y) = \rho(X, Y)/\sqrt{\rho_{XX'}}\sqrt{\rho_{YY'}}.$$

This equation is also called the *correction for attenuation*. It also follows that

$$\rho(X, Y) < \sqrt{\rho_{XX'}}\sqrt{\rho_{YY'}},$$

indicating that only reliable measures can present with a high validity coefficient.

3 Criterion-referenced measurement

In cognitive neuropsychological single-case studies with specifically tailored assessment procedures for some cognitive functions, another type of testing approach, criterion-referenced testing, is employed at least implicitly. A *criterion-referenced test* ascertains a person's status with respect to a well-defined behavioural domain (Berk 1980). The principal concern is to obtain rigorous and precise domain specifications to maximize the validity and interpretability of a person's domain score (e.g. test of simple arithmetic: visually presented addition tasks '$a + b = ?$' requiring a written number as the answer; explicitly state the range of numbers to be employed, whether carrying is required, etc.). In tests constructed according to the classical test theory model, less rigorous specifications are the rule and item selection is dominated by empirical aspects, e.g. item difficulty and item discriminability, i.e. its correlation with the total score.

3.1 Basic concepts

- *Content validity* is taken to be the major criterion for item generation and item selection. A test is called *content valid* if it (completely) contains or represents a universe (domain) of items.
- A *domain* is defined either by exhaustive enumeration of its elements or, more often, by stating its properties via generation rules that an item from that particular domain has to fulfil.
- A *representative* item sample from that domain constitutes an actual test.
- A domain is usually *stratified* (structured) according to one or more aspects in a hierarchical or completely crossed fashion with representative item samples drawn from each stratum (subdomain) or combination of strata.

Every test author must decide which of these parameters he/she wants to vary systematically and which he/she is willing to ignore or control for by allocating items with these properties at random to the strata or strata combinations. Representativeness can often be obtained by drawing a random sample of prespecified size from the subset.

- *Content valid parallel tests* can be generated by drawing distinct representative samples from the domain of interest.
- For a specified domain, the *degree of competence* (achievement, proficiency, ability) for a subject i can be defined as the probability p_i of correctly answering items from that domain. Empirically, the level of competence is estimated from a representative sample of items from that domain. The properties of the ability estimate are dependent on the particular test model used (e.g. the binomial model; see Section 3.2).
- Persons can also be characterized according to their *mastery/non-mastery* with respect to a domain. Mastery can operationally be defined to hold if the competence level p_i is no less than some (lower-bound) *criterion probability* p_c, often fixed at some high value of $p_c = 0.90$ or 0.95.

Mastery and criterion-referenced testing thus relate a person's test performance to an *absolute* level of competence, not to a relative distribution of scores across some reference population, as in the classical true score model.

3.2 **The binomial test model**

- The *binomial distribution* gives the probability for the number of x critical events in n independent replications ($0 \leq x \leq n$) of the same chance experiment with a constant probability p for the critical event to happen (e.g. critical event 'head up' in n tosses of a regular coin).

- The *binomial model* is invoked implicitly when the competence level is estimated from dichotomous score items using the relative frequency of items solved correctly as its estimate. But even for very homogeneous domains it is unrealistic to assume identical item difficulties.

- The '*sampling model*' version of the binomial model is more adequate. With a new random sample of items drawn from a domain to assess a new subject, the total score correctly follows a binomial distribution across subjects even for items with varying difficulty. With PC-based item generation facilities there is no limitation in principle to proceeding in this way. The assumption of (local) stochastical independence among items (independent replications of the same chance experiment) cannot be tested in a single subject. Nevertheless, care can be taken not to choose a sequence of items that provokes practice, fatigue, or learning effects.

- The most simple *mastery decision* is based on the exact $(1 - \alpha)$-confidence interval around the observed relative frequency of items scored correct: if upper confidence limit $>p_c$, then the individual competence level p_i is compatible with mastery. More complicated decision rules also taking into account the error of falsely declaring non-mastery have been proposed as well.

  —Example: $n = 80$ items, $x = 72$ correct for person i; competence level estimate = $72/80 = 0.9$; exact 95%-confidence interval (0.8124, 0.9558), computed using StatXact (Mehta and Patel 1999); decision of mastery, since $p_c = 0.95$ is covered by the confidence interval.

3.3 **Operational definition of performance dissociation**

- The concept of mastery can be employed to empirically demonstrate the intactness of some processing components and/or routes in a cognitive neuropsychological model.

- The criterion-referenced measurement approach, utilizing the binomial model in combination with exact statistical tests for dichotomous scores (Fisher's exact test for 2 × 2 tables; exact version of the McNemar test), can be employed to give an operational definition and a procedure to detect (double) dissociation of performance in individual patients, also distinguishing *classical, strong,* and *trend* dissociation as proposed by Shallice (1988, Chapter 10).

Table 3.1 Operational definition of different levels of dissociation using two tasks A (impaired performance) and B (better preserved performance) with dichotomous items (employing the exact Fisher test)

| | Dissociation | | |
	Classical	Strong (robust)	Trend
Requirement	For the better preserved competence p_B in task B ($p_B = p_c$)		
Normal performance at ceiling	$p_c = 0.99$	$p_c = 0.80$ (definitely below normal performance)	p_c definitely below normal performance
Normal performance with variability	p_c related to e.g. 25%-quantile of normal performance, if known	p_c below e.g. 5%-quantile of normal performance or completely below the normal range	p_c definitely below normal performance

Requirement For the poorer competence $p_A < p_B$ in task A; determination of number of items such that effect size h can be attained with test power $1 - \beta$ for type-I error $\alpha = 0.05$ one-tailed

Planned effect size*	Large: $h = 0.8$	Large: $h = 0.8$	Medium: $h = 0.5$
Planned test power	$1 - \beta = 0.95$	$1 - \beta = 0.95$	$1 - \beta = 0.80–0.95$
Empirical effect size	Large	Large	Medium

* $h = 2\arcsin\sqrt{p_B} - 2\arcsin\sqrt{p_A}$; standards for high and medium proposed by Cohen (1988).

◆ *Classical* dissociation: performance in some task A well below the normal range and much inferior to task B within the normal range (possibly close to the premorbid level).

  —For tasks with almost no variability in normal subjects, adopt a very high level of mastery ($p_c = 0.99$) for task B. For tasks with more variability in competence among healthy controls, p_c to be equated with some low quantile in the score distribution of normal subjects (cf. Table 3.1).

  —Much lower competence level for task A, e.g. compatible with chance level for multiple-choice items, definitely significantly lower than task B (e.g. using Fisher's exact test).

  —Moreover, a large effect size (transformed difference h between p_B and p_A) to be actually observed to warrant adequate statistical power (e.g. $1 - \beta = 0.95$; Cohen 1988).

◆ *Strong* dissociation: performance in some task A well below the normal range and much inferior to task B also below the normal range.

  —Standards for effect size the same as for a classical dissociation.

◆ *Trend* dissociation: degree of competence for both tasks well below mastery levels.

  —Number of items large enough for good statistical power in comparison of competence levels

  —Effect size less than for the other types of dissociations, e.g. medium.

◆ *Double dissociation*: two complementary dissociations in two different patients (pt.). For exclusion of resource artefacts falsely indicating a double dissociation, reject 4 null hypotheses such that:

  (i)   within pt. 1: competence task B > task A;

  (ii) within pt. 2: task A > task B as well as

  (iii) for task A: pt. 2 > pt. 1;

  (iv) for task B: pt. 1 > pt. 2.

A worked-out example can be found in Deloche and Willmes (2000).

3.4 Reliability

The reliability of a criterion-referenced test comprises two aspects: reliability of domain score estimation and reliability (consistency) of mastery classification, which is of more interest when a test is primarily used for mastery classification(s) (cf. Crocker and Algina 1986, pp. 197–212, for details).

4 Probabilistic test models

4.1 Basic considerations

There are three attitudes towards the construction of measurement instruments (Rost 1988).

◆ The test score of a measurement instrument is chosen to be the sum total of the item scores and granted interval scale properties per fiat taken to be justified empirically if it provides a powerful predictor for some relevant criterion measure (*'validity pragmatism'*).

◆ The use of total scores is justified via deriving standardized or normative scores for some reference population (*'norm pragmatism'*).

◆ Every assignment of numbers to persons requires a formal model stating testable assumptions and properties for that assignment (*'model priority'*).

Almost all tests and scales in neuropsychological assessment lack a firm measurement basis (cf. Wade 1992, Chapter 2), e.g. for the Barthel Index (cf. Wade 1992) the differential weighting of items and use of different numbers of scale points per item has not been justified psychometrically, nor has it been shown that total score expresses a position on a *unidimensional* (latent psychological) continuum. As a contrasting example, the Glasgow Coma Scale has been shown to lack unidimensionality (Koziol and Hacke 1990).

Since the ground-breaking publication of the probabilistic test theory model (latent trait model) for dichotomous item scores by Rasch (1960, 1980) and its several extensions to polytomous items (cf. Wright and Masters 1982; Rost and Langeheine 1997) there is no excuse in principle for skipping the stage of analysing the measurement properties, in particular the unidimensionality, of a new test or scale. Otherwise, assigning a total score over items to some patient may provide invalid information about her/his level of ability. Willmes (1997) has shown that the *partial credit model*, a very general model for polytomously scored items (Masters 1982), holds within each of the different item groups making up the subtest written language of the Aachen Aphasia Test (AAT) with a ($m=$) 4-point graded item scoring.

4.2 The dichotomous Rasch model

In item response theory a mathematical model specifies how examinees at different ability levels respond to an item. The *item characteristic curve* (ICC) reveals how the probability $P(+)$ of responding correctly to an item depends on the latent unidimensional trait θ that is assumed to underlie performance in the dichotomous items constituting a test.

- For the Rasch model one has the following (logistic) ICC (see Fig. 3.1):

$$P(+, \theta) = \exp(\theta - \sigma_i)/(1 + \exp(\theta - \sigma_i))$$

The *ability* β_n of a person n and the *difficulty* σ_i of an item i are measured on the same unidimensional (interval) scale θ. The item difficulty is the point on the latent dimension where $P(+, \theta) = 0.5$.

- In a *unidimensional* test, statistical dependence among items can be accounted for by a single latent trait: For a specified θ—characterizing a homogeneous subpopulation of examinees with that extent or amount of the latent trait—items are statistically independent (*local stochastical independence* property).

- If the above model holds, estimation of β_n only requires the *number* of items scored correctly irrespective of the actual pattern of items solved correctly.

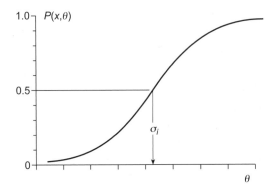

Fig. 3.1 Logistic item characteristic curve (ICC) for the Rasch model with dichotomous item scores. Item difficulty σ_i is the point on the latent dimension for which $P(+, \theta) = 0.5$.

Likewise, estimation of item difficulty σ_i requires only the number of examinees with a correct solution for item i.

◆ In case of model adequacy, item difficulty can be estimated in a *specifically objective* way, i.e. the item difficulty estimate (resp. person ability estimate) is independent of the distribution of person ability estimates (resp. distribution of item difficulty estimates) in the sample.

(For details on estimation procedures and a discussion of the concept of specific objectivity, see Wright and Masters 1982.)

A practical restriction to the use of the Rasch model is the rather substantial number of subjects (usually $n > 100$) to be examined for sufficiently precise parameter estimation and testing of model adequacy. For a demonstration of the unidimensionality and application of the Rasch model to the Token Test see Willmes (1981).

5 Individual case classification

Classification procedures allocate a single subject to a certain prespecified group. The most common questions in clinical neuropsychological diagnostic examinations are these.

◆ How is a patient doing in relation to a normative sample of healthy subjects, possibly after adjustment for age and/or educational level?

◆ To which group does a patient belong among a set of explicitly stated populations?

Soundness of classification is important in clinical work when providing a nosological label or a statement about the normality status. Preferably, the assignment to a population is qualified with a probability statement. It is also reasonable to include a 'non-classifiable' alternative.

5.1 Normality judgement

Normality can be approached from the perspective of:

◆ *mastery*, with the level of performance judged in relation to some task-inherent standard;

◆ *statistical normality*, with performance judged in relation to a group of similar subjects:

—Separate norms for different combinations of demographic variables are rare. A viable way is to work with one fixed norm but adjust an original raw score X_i of patient i by means of a (multiple linear regression) model equation specifying the influence of demographic variables:

adjusted $X_i = X_i + b_1(\text{age}_i - \text{mean age}) + b_2(\text{yrs school}_i - \text{mean yrs school})$.

—The adjusted score is then related to the norm data from the healthy reference population.

There are several ways to reach a decision about (statistical) normality, including the use of *tolerance limits*, i.e. limits within which a given percentage (e.g. 95%) of the population is expected to be observed, together with control of the inferential risk involved because only a limited standardization sample from the population is considered.

- ◆ *Outer tolerance limit*. If the subject's score falls outside the limits, a decision with a controlled risk about non-normality can be made. In neuropsychology, often a unidirectional tolerance limit is required. Non-normality is only related to the region of poor performance.
- ◆ *Inner tolerance limit*. If the subject's score falls inside the limits, the decision is 'normal'.

For scores in the gap between both limits no control of the inferential risk is possible.

- ◆ *Parametric* tolerance limits require the true distribution of original scores to be known or to be estimable from a big sample. After correction for the influence of demographic variables, scale properties of adjusted scores degenerate for scales with fixed upper and lower scores.
- ◆ *Nonparametric* (one-sided) tolerance limits specify that, above the value of the rth ranked observation in the standardization sample, there is at least a prespecified proportion of the population with a prior error risk (cf. Capitani and Laiacona 2000), e.g. the 10th ranked score for a sample of $n = 321$ equals the one-sided outer tolerance limit for the lowest 5% of the population with a risk of 5% that a larger proportion of normal subjects performs below the limit. This way of specifying tolerance limits also works with the ranks of adjusted scores.

There are also ways to set bi- or multi-variate (non-)parametric tolerance limits. The decision about normality can also be reached by operationally declaring a PR or standard norm score to constitute the (one-sided) cut-off between normality and non-normality, e.g. PR = 1, 5, or 10 or norm scores 2, 2.5, or 3 standard deviations below the mean norm score. In cognitive neuropsychology, a cut-off is even determined from a small normative sample simply taking the mean − 2, 2.5, or 3 standard deviations as a cut-off.

5.2 Classification based on discriminant analysis

Discriminant analysis (DA) methods use an allocation rule, determined with previous samples from explicitly specified populations, that optimizes the classification of examinees to either one of a set of populations, preferably with a probability statement. It is desirable to also have a 'non-classifiable' statement when the allocation probability to any of the populations considered falls below some operationally set cut-off value. The allocation rule may be based on *parametric* (linear or quadratic) discriminant functions assuming the data to be (multivariate) normal in the different populations or on *nonparametric* techniques, which estimate the true distributions from the sample data and use a general Bayes theorem for the computation of the allocation probabilities (for an example, see Willmes 1985).

5.3 Deficit measurement

The notion of *deficit* presupposes some ideal, normal, or premorbid level of performance against which the actual functioning of a patient may be compared.

♦ Both normative standards and individual comparison standards are used.

♦ *Direct methods* of individual comparison standards presuppose premorbid test scores, school grades, or other data to be available, but they are often non-existent or very difficult to obtain.

♦ *Indirect methods* aim at estimating the original ability level based on historical and observational data. This provides only shaky evidence in most cases.

♦ Consequently, different approaches to estimate the missing information from the test scores actually obtained have been used, e.g. premorbid intellectual ability level estimated from a vocabulary score or reading performance, but they all have substantial problems as discussed by Lezak (1995, pp. 102–5).

6 Psychometric single-case analysis

A comprehensive inferential statistical approach was suggested by Huber (1973) for:

♦ comparison of performances within an individual subject's profile of standardized test scores;

♦ comparison of two individual performance profiles, e.g. before and after some intervention (see Willmes 1985, for an application; a free PC-program CASE123 for psychometric single-case analysis is available from willmes@neuropsych. rwth-aachen.de).

6.1 Basic concepts

6.1.1 Roots

Zubin's postulates (1950) for the statistical treatment of intraindividual observations are as follows.

♦ Each single individual, in particular if not from the healthy population, has to be treated as an independent 'universe' and not be classified prematurely into one patient group.

♦ Each subject is characterized by a given level and degree of variability of performance.

♦ Internal or external causes (spontaneous recovery, disease progression, or therapeutic interventions) may affect either level or scatter of performances or both.

6.1.2 Principal idea

Treat diagnostic hypotheses about a person's identity of *true* scores (true performance levels) in two (sub-)tests like other statistical hypotheses, e.g. those about the identity of parameters of distributions (e.g. *t*-test: identity of means from two normal distributions).

6.1.3 Connection to classical test theory model

The observed score X_{ij} of subject i in test j is considered a one-element random sample from the distribution of potentially observable scores. It is assumed to be additively composed of the person's true score T_{ij} (individual true performance level) and error E_{ij} (about that true level). An individual diagnostic examination cannot provide information concerning variability and repetitive testing is also not feasible.

6.1.4 Fundamental homogeneity assumption

Identity of the test-specific error variance σ_{ij}^2 is assumed to hold across all subjects i of the reference population for which normative data and reliability information have been obtained; in this case, the test-specific error variance is identical to the square of the standard error of measurement, i.e. $\sigma_{ij}^2 = \sigma^2(X_{.j})(1 - \rho_{jj})$, for the particular test j with $\sigma^2(X_{.j})$ the raw score variance in the reference population and ρ_{jj} a reliability coefficient (internal consistency, split-half, or parallel test reliability) for test j. Both are regularly available in a test manual. Normative data must be available for the general normal (healthy) population and/or for some (well defined) patient population(s).

6.1.5 Concept of τ-standardization

For a comparison of performances across subtests, only standard scores can be employed, since different subtests will usually show differences in difficulty. Diagnostic hypotheses are concerned with the identity of true scores, e.g. $T_{ij} = T_{ih}$. But identity of true raw scores only implies identity of true standardized scores if the reliability of both tests is identical (see Huber 1973). In case of differences between subtest reliabilities an additional transformation, the so-called τ-standardization, has to be carried out on the standardized score Y_{ij}^x (x denoting observed score standardization), which provides the best estimate Y_{ij}^τ of true standardized performance:

$$Y_{ij}^\tau = Y_{ij}^x/\sqrt{\rho_{jj}} + L(1 - 1/\sqrt{\rho_{jj}}).$$

The higher a test's reliability the smaller is the difference between both types of standardized scores. In case of identical reliabilities, ordinary x-standardized scores, as described above, will suffice and the same (average) reliability estimate ρ from the subtests involved is considered.

6.1.6 Choice of error probabilities

When deciding on diagnostic null hypotheses about true standardized scores by means of inferential statistical procedures, type-I and type-II errors occur just as with any statistical test. In the case of diagnostic hypotheses, commitment of type-II errors, i.e. overlooking some difference in true performance levels, may have more detrimental consequences for a patient than committing type-I errors, i.e. falsely declaring an observed difference in standardized scores to be indicative of a true difference in performance. Therefore, a more liberal default type-I error level of $\alpha = 10\%$ is recommended.

6.1.7 Practical requirements

Good reliability estimates for all (sub)tests in the profile (>0.85 approximately) and normative data from a large standardization sample ($n > 400$–500) are needed.

There are two aspects to consider when testing for differences in performance:

- *Reliability aspect.* Is a performance difference unlikely due to errors of measurement alone?

- *Aspect of diagnostic validity.* In case of a reliable difference, what is the probability of observing a still larger difference in the reference population?

If the probability is <20%, this difference is taken to be *diagnostically valid*, i.e. potentially indicative of some relevant piece of diagnostic information (e.g. *dissociation*; see Section 6.4).

6.2 Individual profile analysis

When analysing a performance profile of m subtests, level, scatter, and shape can be discerned.

- *Profile level*: weighted mean h_i^τ of τ-standardized subtest scores with higher reliability implying more weight.

- *Profile scatter*: overall differences among m subtest performances are assessed via the sum of reliability-weighted squared differences between subtest scores and profile level. In case of significant profile scatter (value >90%-quantile of χ^2_{m-1}-distribution), the profile is *real*.

- *Profile shape*: to be analysed in more detail for a real profile under the reliability aspect.

  —Without a specific (neuro-)psychological hypothesis concerning relations of subtest performances, all $M = m(m-1)/2$ *pairwise comparisons* of subtests (j, h) are carried out with individual type-I error adjustment such that, overall, the type-I error <10% (Holm 1979).

  —A *linear contrast* of two non-overlapping groups of subtests, I with m_1 (≥ 1) and II with m_2 (≥ 1) ($m_1 + m_2 \leq m$) may be diagnostically more interesting (e.g. comparing verbal and nonverbal subtests in an intelligence test battery or expressive and receptive subtests in some aphasia test). Technically, the profile level h_{iI}^τ and h_{iII}^τ for subgroups I and II, respectively, is computed and the linear contrast $\psi_i^\tau = h_{iI}^\tau - h_{iII}^\tau$ determined.

  —Profile shape may additionally be analysed under the diagnostic validity aspect.

6.3 Intra-individual profile comparison

Psychometric single-case analysis also offers a way of comparing two profiles of the same subject or patient examined twice in the course of some neurological condition, possibly before and after some phase of therapy or training, or perhaps in a follow-up examination some time after an intervention, in order to find out whether performance has improved, stabilized, or deteriorated again. Three steps of analysis may be discerned.

6.3.1 Global profile comparison

- *Profile identity*: identity—both in level and shape—of two profiles for the same test battery are assessed via the sum of reliability-weighted squared subtest differences between examinations 1 and 2. In the case of significant deviation from identity (value $> 90\%$-quantile of χ^2_m-distribution), one proceeds to profile comparisons of level and shape.

- *Identity of profile levels*: the difference of both profile levels is tested for deviation from zero. Depending on the diagnostic hypothesis, this test is one-sided (improvement after therapy or due to expected spontaneous recovery or, respectively, deterioration after some progressive disorder) or two-sided (e.g. stability at follow-up).

- *Identity of profile shapes*: for a pure comparison of profile shapes, the sum of level-difference-adjusted squared subtest differences between examinations 1 and 2 is assessed. In case of a significant shape difference (value $> 90\%$-quantile of χ^2_{m-1}-distribution), additional comparisons serve to study these differences in profile scatter in more detail.

6.3.2 Specific comparisons for profile shape differences

- Without a specific (neuro-)psychological hypothesis a change of the relation in performance between a pair (j, h) of subtests from examination 1 to examination 2 is carried out for all $M = m(m - 1)/2$ pairs of subtests, applying Holm's adjustment for multiple testing.

- If a specific change in the performance pattern can be expected as a consequence of some intervention or disease progress, the same linear contrast ψ_i^τ may be compared between both examinations 1 and 2, i.e. $\delta_i^\tau = \psi_{i1}^\tau - \psi_{i2}^\tau$ is tested for a deviation from zero.

6.3.3 Comparison of all profile components

A more conventional comparison between two profiles—in case of no identity—that does not involve relations between profile components simply asks whether true subtest performance has changed between two examinations. Again, these comparisons may be one- or two-sided and adjustment for multiple testing using Holm's procedure is required.

6.4 Specific applications in neuropsychology

- *Performance dissociation*. In order to back up a selective sparing/impairment of some cognitive function one can examine whether true performance in that specific subtest *s* is reliably *and* diagnostically validly above/below all or a subset of all other subtests. One computes all $m - 1$ (or a smaller subset) pairwise differences $Y^{\tau}_{ij} - Y^{\tau}_{is}$, which all must be reliable (one-tailed) using Holm's procedure and have diagnostic validity probabilities $p_{js} < 20\%/(m - 1)$.

- *Specific therapy effects*: test for a predicted change of some specific (set of) linear contrast(s) after an intervention period by carrying out one (or several) specific profile comparisons. For example, this approach has been chosen to substantiate the assumed presence of primary progressive aphasia (Poeck and Luzzatti 1988). Besides language impairments revealed in an aphasia test it was shown that a linear contrast comparing language-bound subtests of the Leistungsprüfsystem (LPS) with non-language-bound ones was reliable and diagnostically valid at initial clinical testing. But in the course of disease progression the strong discrepancy between both subtest groups became significantly smaller at an overall lower performance level.

- *Definition of responders*: The profile comparison methods may be used to generate operational criteria for identifying responders to some specific intervention, a more promising approach than only looking for significant group differences.

Neuropsychological assessment has not always kept up with methodological developments in psychological diagnostics in general. Employment of some of the more recent advances in psychometrics—comprising e.g. more refined probabilistic test models and application of more strict criteria for the inferential statistical analysis of single-case data will help to improve the state of neuropsychological assessment.

Selective references

Berk, R.A. (ed.) (1980). *Criterion-referenced measurement*. The Johns Hopkins University Press, Baltimore.

Capitani, E. and Laiacona, M. (2000). Classification and modelling in neuropsychology: from groups to single cases. In *Handbook of neuropsychology*, 2nd edn, Vol. 1 (ed. F. Boller, J. Grafman, and G. Rizzolatti), pp. 53–76. Elsevier, Lisse.

Cohen, J. (1988). *Statistical power analysis for the behavioral sciences*, 2nd edn. Lawrence Erlbaum Associates, Hillsdale, New Jersey.

Crocker, L. and Algina, J. (1986). *Introduction to classical and modern test theory*. Harcourt Brace Jovanovich College Publishers, Fort Worth, Texas.

Deloche, G. and Willmes, K. (2000). Cognitive neuropsychological models of adult calculation and number processing: the role of the surface format of numbers. *Eur. Child Adolesc. Psychiatry* 9 (suppl. 2, II), 27–40.

Gulliksen, H. (1987). *Theory of mental tests*. Lawrence Erlbaum Associates, Hillsdale, New Jersey.

Holm, S. (1979). A simple sequentially rejective multiple test procedure. *Scand. J. Statistics* 6, 65–70.

Huber, H.P. (1973). *Psychometrische Einzelfalldiagnostik*. Beltz, Weinheim.

Koziol, J.A. and Hacke, W. (1990). Multivariate data reduction by principal components with application to neurological scoring instruments. *J. Neurology* 237, 461–4.

Lezak, M.D. (1995). *Neuropsychological assessment*, 3rd edn. Oxford University Press, New York.

Lord, F.M. and Novick, M.R. (1968). *Statistical theories of mental tests scores*. Addison-Wesley, Reading, Massachusetts.

Masters, G.N. (1982). A Rasch model for partial credit scoring. *Psychometrika* 47, 149–74.

Mehta, C. and Patel, N. (1999). *StatXact4 for Windows—user manual*. CYTEL Software Corporation, Cambridge, Massachusetts.

Poeck, K. and Luzzatti, C. (1988). Slowly progressive aphasia in three patients. The problem of accompanying neurological deficit. *Brain* 111, 151–68.

Rasch, G. (1960, 1980). *Probabilistic models for some intelligence and attainment tests*. Nielsen & Lydiche, Copenhagen (2nd edn, University of Chicago Press, Chicago).

Rost, J. (1988). *Quantitative und qualitative probabilistische Testtheorie*. Huber, Bern.

Rost, J. and Langeheine, R. (eds.) (1997). *Applications of latent trait and latent class models in the social sciences*. Waxmann, Muenster.

Shallice, T. (1988). *From neuropsychology to mental structure*. Cambridge University Press, Cambridge.

Suen, H.K. (1990). *Principles of test theories*. Lawrence Erlbaum Associates, Hillsdale, New Jersey.

Wade, D.T. (1992). *Measurement in neurological rehabilitation*. Oxford University Press, Oxford.

Wainer, H. and Braun, H.I. (eds.) (1988). *Test validity*. Lawrence Erlbaum Associates, Hillsdale, New Jersey.

Willmes, K. (1981). A new look at the Token Test using probabilistic test models. *Neuropsychologia* 19, 631–45.

Willmes, K. (1985). An approach to analyzing a single subject's scores obtained in a standardized test with application to the Aachen Aphasia Test (AAT). *J. Clin. Exp. Neuropsychol.* 7, 331–52.

Willmes, K. (1997). Application of polytomous Rasch models to the Subtest Written Language of the Aachen Aphasia Test (AAT). In *Applications of latent trait and latent class models in the social sciences* (ed. J. Rost and R. Langeheine), pp. 127–37. Waxmann, Muenster.

Wright, B.D. and Masters, G.N. (1982). *Rating scale analysis*. Mesa Press, Chicago.

Zubin, J. (1950). Symposium on statistics for the clinician. *J. Clin. Psychol.* 6, 1–6.

Chapter 4

Principles of cognitive rehabilitation

Nicole D. Anderson, Gordon Winocur, and Heather Palmer

1 Overview

Cognitive rehabilitation can be defined as an intervention in which patients and their families work with health professionals to restore or compensate for cognitive deficits, thereby improving the patients' everyday functioning. Three features of this working definition are important.

- Cognitive rehabilitation is a team effort. The patient's awareness of his deficit and his motivation to improve, the family's involvement and support, and the therapists' expertise are all crucial elements for a successful outcome.

- An important theoretical distinction in cognitive rehabilitation is whether the aim is to restore function to its original level, or to compensate for lost functioning. This distinction will be discussed in greater detail in Section 1.2.

- The ultimate goal of cognitive rehabilitation is to facilitate meaningful and measurable improvements in patients' everyday functioning, be it functional, academic, vocational, social, or recreational.

Dixon and Bäckman (1999) argue that the need for rehabilitation ('compensation' in their terms) arises when there is a mismatch between a person's actual performance levels, on the one hand, and environmental demands, on the other hand. A person's skill level can drop, causing such a mismatch, for a number of reasons. Some of these are developmental (e.g. autism, learning disabilities, schizophrenia), some are acquired (e.g. traumatic brain injury (TBI), stroke, neurodegenerative diseases such as Alzheimer's disease), and some occur as part of the normal ageing process. Although there is a need for cognitive rehabilitation in each of these areas, this review will focus on cognitive rehabilitation in adults in the post-acute phase of TBI and stroke. (See Katz and Mills (1999) for an excellent review of the natural history of TBI recovery in the acute phase and Ylvisaker (1998) for reviews of cognitive rehabilitation in children; also see Chapter 24, this volume.) Treating cognitive deficits that are due to neuro-degenerative diseases poses an added challenge in that the deficits are progressive in nature. Hence, rehabilitation goals are often aimed at slowing progression or maintaining functioning for as long as possible. Nevertheless, we do include examples of rehabilitation techniques from studies of these populations. Finally, we later mention that psychological problems (e.g. depression) can cause cognitive deficits. In our view, these should be treated prior to or concurrently with cognitive rehabilitation.

1.1 Impairment, activity limitation, and participation restriction

It is informative to consider the consequences of brain injury in terms of the World Health Organization's (1999) International Classification of Functioning and Disability. In the context of cognitive neuropsychology:

- *impairments* refer to damaged brain structures (e.g. frontal lobe damage) or neuro-psychological functions (e.g. executive dysfunction);
- *activity limitations* refer to changes in an individual's ability to carry out day-to-day behaviours (e.g. multitasking);
- *participation restrictions* refer to changes in an individual's involvement in various life arenas (e.g. work or social engagements).

An individual's impairments and the presence of personality or psychological factors (e.g. depression) can result in activity limitations and/or participation restrictions. In addition, the environment or social setting can contribute to participation restrictions (e.g. barriers to vocational training).

Theorists and practitioners differ in whether their focus is on impairments or activity limitations. Cognitive programmes that emphasize retraining of abilities aim to improve functioning of a damaged structure or underlying process, while those that focus on compensatory mechanisms aim to minimize activity limitations. Cognitive rehabilitation may also focus on participation restrictions insofar as their root is psychological or an environment that does not facilitate effective functioning (e.g. a cluttered workspace). Generally, however, participation is best addressed in practical ways in multidisciplinary settings that include social workers and/or occupational therapists.

The distinction between treating impairments or activity limitations is important on two counts. Treatments of the underlying neuropsychological impairments are often artificial and therefore must demonstrate transfer to 'real-life' situations to be justifiable. Treatments of activity limitations, on the other hand, effectively bypass this step because they focus on the functional consequences of impairments in a reality-based context. The second important difference between impairment- and activity-oriented treatments pertains to their assumptions about the underlying brain mechanisms involved in recovery. Although the cognitive rehabilitation practitioner's level of analysis is the individual's *behaviour* on a given task or in a particular setting, ultimately one must address the relationships between behaviour and *neural mechanisms* (Prigatano *et al.* 1998). This brings us to a discussion of restorative versus compensatory mechanisms of neural repair.

1.2 **Restoration versus compensation**

Cognitive retraining approaches assume that treatment helps to speed up spontaneous neural recovery or promote neural plasticity and/or regeneration, i.e. a restorative process is assumed. By contrast, compensatory approaches assume that treatment helps to induce neural substitution or functional reorganization, whereby undamaged brain regions assume the function of damaged regions in a compensatory manner.

Robertson and Murre (1999) presented a detailed theoretical and computational framework of the role of cognitive rehabilitation in neural repair. The essence of their framework is that the speed and mechanisms of neural repair depend on the size of the lesion, the size of the neural circuit affected by the lesion, the degree of connectivity within the network, and, last but not least, experience. More specifically,

- recovery of function following small lesions that disrupt little connectivity within a larger neural circuit is most likely to occur spontaneously without an added benefit of rehabilitation;
- recovery of function following moderate-sized lesions that disrupt some but not all connectivity within a larger neural circuit can happen through restorative processes such as synaptic turnover and dendritic branching;
- recovery of function following large lesions that disrupt an entire neural circuit can happen only through compensatory processes such as substitution and functional reorganization.

Robertson and Murre emphasize that, although the lesion size and degree of network disruption specify the dominant mechanism by which recovery most probably occurs, restoration and compensation often co-occur.

The notion of experience interacting with neural organization is fundamental to Robertson and Murre's approach. They argue that stimulation can modify restorative and compensatory recovery processes. Stimulation can be 'bottom-up', wherein external stimuli or lower level processes foster recovery of higher-order functions, or 'top-down', wherein higher-order processes facilitate recovery of more basic processes. Stimulation must be appropriate and specific to the deficit to avoid fostering maladaptive connections. Robertson and Murre provide a number of examples of maladaptive recovery in conditions such as phantom limb pain, aphasia, and hemispatial neglect. Another more cognitive example of a maladaptive recovery process might be the compromised learning one sees when memory-impaired individuals are allowed to make errors while trying to recall information (e.g. Baddeley and Wilson 1994).

Robertson and Murre's (1999) framework is theoretical, and is best applied to processes with functionally discrete circuits (e.g. sensorimotor functions). Modifications to their framework may be required in the case of more distributed cognitive networks mediating functions such as memory, attention, and executive skills. Nevertheless, their framework represents an important advance in that it integrates cognitive rehabilitation with neurobiological mechanisms of recovery in a detailed and explicit way. Technology does not exist to assess critical neural processes such as axonal sprouting or dendritic branching *in vivo*. However, one can use functional neuroimaging to help determine whether rehabilitation-assisted recovery is effecting restoration of the original network of brain regions or compensatory recruitment of different brain regions (Grady and Kapur 1999). Merging cognitive rehabilitation with cognitive neuroscience is a relatively new enterprise, but one that is buttressed by the rapid growth in our understanding of the functional neuroanatomy of normal cognition (e.g. Cabeza and Nyberg 2000).

2 Issues in cognitive rehabilitation

2.1 Factors affecting rehabilitation outcome

The following is a brief summary of some of the major factors that affect rehabilitative outcome, as indicated in Table 4.1.

2.1.1 Neurological symptoms

The location, size, and type of lesion are critical determinants of cognitive consequences and the likelihood of recovery. The natural history of TBI recovery depends on whether the head injury is diffuse or focal, with recovery from diffuse injury following a more stereotypic course (coma, posttraumatic amnesia (PTA), post-acute recovery) and recovery from focal injury being more dependent on the lesion location and size (Katz and Mills 1999). Coma severity (typically measured by the Glasgow Coma Scale), coma duration, and PTA duration have been identified as significant predictors of functional outcome from diffuse TBI. Secondary effects of trauma such as oedema, increased intracranial pressure, and haematomas can add variability to recovery prognosis (see Katz and Mills 1999 for a more complete discussion of primary and secondary effects).

2.1.2 Neuropsychological status

A comprehensive neuropsychological evaluation (see Table 4.1) is recommended to determine which skills have been compromised and need to be rehabilitated versus which skills survive and can be recruited to compensate for lost functioning (Caetano and Christensen 1997). Deficits in executive functioning and sustained attention pose particular challenges for the patient's ability to engage in effortful, extended cognitive rehabilitation and to reintegrate in social and vocational activities. Nevertheless, it must be noted that most standard neuropsychological tests assess cognitive impairments rather than disabilities. Hence, they are poor predictors of functional

Table 4.1 Factors affecting rehabilitative outcome

Neurological symptoms
- Location, type, and extent of lesion
- Secondary effects (e.g. oedema, increased intracranial pressure, haematoma)
- Coma severity and duration
- Posttraumatic amnesia duration

Neuropsychological functioning
- Attention
- Memory
- Language functioning
- Visuospatial skills
- Motor skills
- Problem-solving/mental flexibility
- Information-processing speed

Psychosocial factors
- Awareness of deficit
- Motivation
- Coping style
- Anxiety and depression

Background history and supports
- Age
- Personality
- Premorbid level of functioning
- Social supports
- Financial supports

outcome, particularly when neuropsychological functioning is assessed in the post-acute stages of recovery (Dikmen and Machamer 1995). More ecologically valid neuropsychological tests have been devised in recent years that are more predictive of everyday functioning (Burgess *et al.* 1998; Schwartz and McMillan 1989; Wilson 1991). These include the Rivermead Behavioural Memory Test (Wilson *et al.* 1985), the Test for Everyday Attention (Robertson *et al.* 1994), and the Behavioural Assessment of the Dysexecutive Syndrome (Wilson *et al.* 1996). In addition, Wilson (1995) stresses the importance of direct assessments of everyday problems via interviews, questionnaires, observation, and the patient's and family's recording of the difficulties encountered.

2.1.3 Psychosocial factors

It is widely known that psychosocial status and lifestyle affect cognitive function in vulnerable populations and that such factors need to be taken into account in developing treatment programmes. Prigatano (see Prigatano 1999 for a review) has conducted considerable research on the importance of patients' awareness of their functional disabilities and on the relationship between awareness and their ability to benefit from rehabilitation. Poor awareness can lead to passive or resistant behaviour in therapeutic settings. Different approaches have been taken to help improve awareness and/or motivation. These include:

♦ patient and family education about common sequelae of brain injury (Anderson 1996);

♦ records of patients' behaviour (through logs or videotape) to provide the patient with a more objective view of their behaviour (Mateer 1999);

♦ psychotherapy to help patients cope with their disabilities (Ben-Yishay and Diller 1993; Prigatano 1999).

Psychological problems, including anxiety, depression, social withdrawal, and loneliness, and changes in personality are commonly associated with brain injury (Morton and Wehman 1995; Prigatano *et al.* 1998). One could question the causal direction between emotional and cognitive deficits. It is well established that emotional problems negatively affect cognitive functions such as attention, memory, and information-processing speed (e.g. Fields *et al.* 1998), but cognitive deficits have also been shown to relate to social functioning, satisfaction with lifestyle, and optimism (Dawson *et al.* 1999). These and related findings have led to widespread agreement that problems with awareness, motivation, emotion, and personality need to be addressed as part of a comprehensive cognitive rehabilitation programme (e.g. Prigatano 1999; Williams *et al.* 1999; Wilson 1995).

2.1.4 Background history and supports

The patients' background characteristics and social supports play an important role in rehabilitative outcome, yet, with the exception of patients' age (younger individuals have a more positive recovery after brain injury), they are rarely integrated into rehabilitation therapies or outcome evaluations in an objective way. A recent study demonstrating the importance of premorbid patient characteristics found that patients with poor outcome following mild TBI were likely to have had past neurological and psychiatric problems and other life stressors (Ponsford *et al.* 2000). Similarly, a number of studies have documented reductions in patients' social support networks following TBI (Morton and Wehman 1995), reductions that may negatively affect recovery outcome (Lezak 1995). To address these needs, Ruff and Camenzuli (1991) recommended a multi-axial classification system to help identify factors that may influence rehabilitative outcome. This classification system includes premorbid and current emotional, psychological, psychosocial, and vocational status, factors that should be considered prior to establishing outcome goals and expectations.

2.2 Issues in rehabilitation design and outcome assessment

How rehabilitation is designed and how outcomes are assessed are complicated issues and the reader is referred to several excellent reviews on this subject (e.g. Cicerone *et al.*

2000; Ruff and Camenzuli 1991; Sohlberg and Raskin 1996). Here, we limit our discussion to three primary issues.

2.2.1 Individual versus group approaches

There are two issues related to individual versus group approaches. The first is whether to conduct individual or group therapy sessions. Group sessions have the benefit of being more economical, and afford greater development of interpersonal adaptation and acceptance of impairments (Caetano and Christensen 1997; Wilson 1995), but controlled trials examining the efficacy of group therapy are lacking (Wilson and Moffat 1992). Given that patients vary widely in their neurological, cognitive, and emotional status, a strong case can be made for tailoring programmes to meet individual needs (Sohlberg and Raskin 1996; Wilson 1995), but individual programmes suffer the disadvantages of being costly and inefficient, and depriving patients of valuable group support. Also, the evidence regarding outcome is mixed. One recommended solution to this issue is a combination of individual and group rehabilitation, in order to benefit from the strengths of both approaches (e.g. Cicerone *et al.* 2000; Prigatano 1997; Wilson 1997).

The second issue related to individual versus group approaches is how outcome should be assessed. In fact, this decision is independent of whether individual or group therapy is practised, as the efficacy of both approaches can be assessed with either single-subject or group designs. Single-subject designs need not be limited to a sample size of one, as the design can be applied repeatedly to multiple patients to establish generalization across subjects. Some investigators prefer single-subject designs, given the sizeable variability among patients in neurological, psychosocial, and cognitive terms (e.g. Sohlberg and Mateer 1989*a*). However, group designs typically entail more uniform therapy practices across individuals. Once again, a combined individual/group approach that examines both group and individual effects may be advisable.

2.2.2 Control groups

The inclusion of appropriate control groups is essential in order to demonstrate the efficacy of rehabilitation. Park and Ingles's (2001) recent meta-analysis of direct attention retraining studies revealed that, on average, pre- to posttreatment gains were significant only in studies that did not include a control group, indicating that the bulk of the gains reflected practice effects. Only the treatment should differ between the control and treatment groups (Ruff and Camenzuli 1991). Hence, patients who desire treatment should be randomly assigned to treatment and control groups in order to equate motivation levels, and the control group should receive some alternative activity, equal in therapist and interpersonal interaction to the treatment, so that the general effects of being in a therapeutic milieu are equated.

2.2.3 Generalization

The need to show generalization to other similar tasks and to everyday functioning is perhaps the most important issue in cognitive rehabilitation research. With a few exceptions (see Hall and Cope 1995), most studies have not even attempted to show generalization to everyday functional or psychosocial aspects of life, despite the fact that this is the ultimate goal of cognitive rehabilitation. Instead, most studies have examined whether training generalizes to similar but untrained cognitive tasks, and have found transfer only when the training and the target task require very similar underlying processes (Cicerone *et al.* 2000; Park and Ingles 2001). Findings such as this led Park and Ingles (2001) to conclude that retraining methods are beneficial in developing specific skills but not general processes that can be applied to a wide range of tasks and situations.

There are several approaches to the issue of generalization (Stokes and Baer 1977). Historically, investigators have been content to assume, somewhat optimistically, that their treatments will generalize in a meaningful way. Far preferable to this 'train and hope' approach is to build generalization into training from the outset. Following this 'train to generalize' approach, Sohlberg and Raskin (1996) recommend that therapists use everyday stimuli in training and conduct training in a variety of settings in order to facilitate generalization. Ruff and Camenzuli (1991) and High *et al.* (1995) recommended seeking generalization not only to similar activities in everyday life, but also to psychosocial improvements.

3 Approaches to cognitive rehabilitation

There are three primary approaches to cognitive rehabilitation:

- ◆ cognitive retraining;
- ◆ compensatory approaches;
- ◆ holistic approaches.

The goal of each approach is to rehabilitate cognitive functioning over and above that might occur naturally over the passage of time or through generalized practice. We review each approach in turn.

3.1 Cognitive retraining

Retraining programmes usually involve repeated practice of specific cognitive exercises designed to strengthen basic skills (e.g. attention, encoding) that are essential for more complex cognitive function. This approach is continuing to develop and one promising adaptation is a scaffolding approach whereby training begins with basic processes and progresses to more complex skills. This approach is clearly reflected in Sohlberg and Mateer's (1989*a*) 'process-oriented' model in which component processes that are presumed to mediate a particular cognitive skill are trained in a hierarchical order, such that progressively more complex processes are trained as learning occurs. Within each level of training, skills are repetitively practised, under the assumption that repeated practice in a structured setting is a necessary component to strengthen and re-automatize cognitive skills (Mateer 1999).

A specific example of the process-oriented model is Sohlberg and Mateer's Attention Process Training, which includes training in various aspects of attention, including sustained, selective, alternating, and divided attention (Sohlberg and Mateer 1989*a*, 2001; Park *et al.* 1999; and see Gray and Robertson 1989 and Sturm *et al.* 1997 for similar approaches). The efficacy of attention training has been demonstrated in a number of studies showing improvements on independent, untrained tasks that were presumed to tap the same functions (see Mateer 1999 for a review). Subsequent developments of this model (Sohlberg *et al.* 1993) added methods to improve patients' monitoring of their attention performance in order to improve self-control over other cognitive weaknesses.

It may be useful to reconsider cognitive retraining within the framework of Robertson and Murre (1999), who argue that restoration is possible following lesions that disrupt part but not all of a larger neural circuit. One of their principal assumptions is that recovery involves the same mechanisms as normal learning and experience-dependent plasticity processes. As children, we learn how to attend and remember in real-world, contextually rich environments. It is possible that the greatest success in rehabilitation following brain injury has been in the areas of motor, perceptual, and language impairments rather than cognitive impairments because retraining in those fields more frequently relies on practical, everyday functions (e.g. reaching and speaking). Following Robertson and Murre, we suggest that cognitive retraining should be embedded in real-life, everyday contexts, building on residual or already-learned cognitive routines. This suggestion echoes other recommendations for improving generalization beyond the training environment (e.g. Sohlberg and Raskin 1996).

Finally, it should be noted that direct retraining of memory via practice drills has proven ineffective (Sohlberg and Mateer 2001). Indeed, many theorists argue that the ability to learn and remember new events cannot be restored if brain damage affects the hippocampus and associated critical brain structures (e.g. Robertson and Murre 1999), and thus compensatory techniques should be used with these patients.

3.2 Compensatory approaches

Compensatory approaches are based on the principle that individuals can compensate for reduced cognitive abilities by utilizing specific techniques that can help organize information during learning or access stored information for retrieval purposes. Internal strategies can help individuals make the necessary effort to solve a problem. Such techniques place considerable demands on the individual's ability to use them appropriately but, as West (1995) pointed out, an added benefit of this effort is increased attention to the task at hand. With external strategies, the objective is to identify distinctive cues that can be readily associated with to-be-remembered material. The following are some examples of compensatory techniques thought to be of value in cognitive rehabilitation.

3.2.1 Internal strategies

To varying degrees, normal adults depend on well-established internal strategies to support learning and memory. Cognitively impaired patients are less likely to do this, but they can benefit from direct training. Numerous strategies involving verbal and visual aids, organization of information, and executive skills training are available and their usefulness depends partly on the type of information to be remembered.

An example of an internal strategy that makes use of visual aids is used by Yesavage and his colleagues (e.g. 1983, 1990). They successfully trained older adults to use a face-name strategy wherein one identifies a salient facial feature (e.g. a ruddy nose), creates a concrete image transformation of a person's name (e.g. a rose for 'Rosie'), and then forms an interactive visual image of the facial feature and the name transformation (e.g. a rose in place of her nose). While this approach has been used successfully for individuals with mild memory problems, it has been generally less successful for patients with moderate to severe memory impairments (e.g. Gade 1994). The familiar method-of-loci, in which a visual image is associated with each of a series of locations or items on a list, is another example of the use of interactive imagery.

Improved memory performance has also been reported following spaced retrieval training. Sohlberg and Mateer have successfully applied spaced retrieval techniques to train prospective memory—the ability to remember to do things in the future (1989a; Sohlberg et al. 1992a,b). In this technique, individuals are trained to recall information at progressively longer intervals, on the principle that this experience facilitates the spontaneous use of efficient retrieval strategies.

Internal strategies that make use of verbal mediators include forming semantically meaningful associates or easily connected rhymes of material to be remembered. Mediation of this type is thought to be useful in learning people's names, short lists of words, or short sequences (e.g. 'Thirty days hath September . . . .'). For longer lists or more complex material, creating a story can be a useful aid. The idea here is to devise personalized associations to each of the items that can be represented in meaningful and integrated ways and easily accessed at retrieval. Other learning techniques encourage the organization of new information into units of a manageable size or by taxonomic categories. Identifying as many contextual features as possible can also be useful for purposes of registering or encoding new information, and providing effective retrieval cues during recall.

There has been considerable debate over the value of training brain-damaged people to use internal strategies and the extent to which, in the absence of other forms of training, they generalize from the training environment (Prigatano et al. 1998; Wilson 1995). Wilson (1995) emphasizes that relatives, therapists, and teachers can use these strategies to help facilitate memory-impaired individuals' learning. At the same time, there is evidence that severely brain-damaged patients, who have limited potential for recovery, can benefit to some degree from intensive internal-strategy training (e.g. Thoene and Glisky 1995).

Techniques designed to rehabilitate executive skills have been used effectively with patients who have relatively small brain lesions and moderate cognitive impairment. One technique is to help patients regulate their behaviour through self-instruction, wherein one talks his/her way through an activity in order to maintain appropriate attention (Cicerone and Wood 1987; Cicerone and Giacino 1992; Meichenbaum 1977). This technique helps individuals to gain control over thought processes that are needed to plan and regulate behaviour in appropriate ways.

Robertson's (1996) 'Goal Management Training' programme was also designed to reduce executive impairments related to frontal lobe damage. This is a manual-based protocol for helping patients organize their behaviour and execute tasks in a goal-directed manner. Patients are taught that successful task completion requires the implementation of several related strategies:

◆ evaluating the current situation and generating appropriate goals;

◆ selecting goals;

◆ parsing overall goals into subgoals;

◆ learning and retaining the goals and subgoals;

◆ evaluating outcome against the goals.

Goal Management Training is an intensive programme that places considerable demands on patients' residual skills. Nevertheless, there is some evidence that it can be effective. Levine *et al.* (2000) demonstrated the utility of this method in real-life settings. They describe a single-case study of a woman recovering from meningo-encephalitis. Despite normal performance on standard neuropsychological tests of memory and executive functioning, she performed poorly on the more naturalistic tests of everyday attention and memory described earlier in this section, and one of her chief complaints was difficulty in managing meal preparation. After Goal Management Training, there was a significant reduction in the number of cooking errors she made. For example, she was more likely to assemble the necessary ingredients and better able to follow the sequence of the recipe, keep to the task, and get back on track when sidetracked. The primary advantage of this strategy is its applicability to everyday activities that require self-regulated, organized behaviour.

3.2.2 External strategies

External strategies make use of objects in the environment to compensate for cognitive deficits. A simple example is to design environments with built-in cues that reduce disorientation and help navigation. For example, lines painted on floors or ceilings can help guide in-patients to the cafeteria. Labels on cabinets, maps in buildings, and doors painted different colours are other examples of orientation cues. Effective treatments for executive dysfunction have included:

◆ using checklists to facilitate appropriate task sequencing in vocational settings;

◆ providing concurrent verbal feedback to reinforce and shape behaviour (Burke *et al.* 1991);

- cueing to improve self-initiation (Sohlberg *et al.* 1988);
- introducing response cost methods to decrease disinhibited behaviour (Alderman *et al.* 1995).

In the memory domain, external aids include common reminders such as lists, calendars, and alarm clocks, and a 'memory place' in which important objects such as glasses, keys, and wallets are kept (West 1995).

Harris (1978) argued that external aids should meet three criteria.

- They should be active, rather than passive. Passive cues like calendars require one to initiate a checking behaviour, and initiating action is problematic for brain-injured individuals. Active cues, such as those that employ alarms, draw attention to the cue.

- They should be timely. That is, the cue should draw attention at the appropriate time when an action must be performed.

- They should be specific. A string around a finger may remind someone that they need to do something, but it does not specify which activity should be performed.

A very practical external memory aid is a memory book. Memory books often contain sections for personal information (e.g. name, address, phone number), a calendar, daily schedule, and 'things to do' list. Additional sections are added as needed (e.g. medication lists). Sohlberg and Mateer (1989*b*) described a rehabilitation approach to memory book training that involves three stages.

- *Acquisition.* In this phase, patients are taught the name, purpose, and proper use of each section of the memory book.
- *Application.* In this phase, patients practise the use of each section by following the therapist's role-playing instructions.
- *Adaptation.* In this phase, the use of the book is transferred to naturalistic settings.

Sohlberg and Mateer present a case study attesting to the success of this training method (see also Burke *et al.* 1994).

Newer technology has provided increasingly portable and powerful memory aids. Wilson *et al.* (1997) describe the efficacy of an easy-to-use pager system that cues memory-impaired individuals when particular actions must be performed. Palm pilots offer even more flexibility, and will undoubtedly be explored further in future studies (see Kim *et al.* 1999 for a single case study). Technology can have drawbacks, however. Devices such as palm pilots are expensive, and the risk of losing the devices must be considered. In addition, as electronic aids become more flexible, there are greater opportunities for confusion and interference during learning. Investigators and therapists are advised to restrict training to only the essential functions afforded by the devices.

3.2.3 Domain-specific techniques

Domain-specific approaches capitalize on preserved cognitive domains, or systems, to train functions that are normally mediated by other, impaired systems. For example, amnesiacs are severely impaired on tests of explicit memory (e.g. free recall), but perform normally on tests of implicit memory in which no reference is made to a previous event but where past experience nevertheless influences current behaviour (e.g. Schacter and Graf 1986). Specifically, amnesiacs would not be able to recall many words from a previously presented list. However, if provided with the first few letters of each word and asked to complete these 'word stems' with the first word that came to mind, amnesiacs would be as likely as healthy individuals to provide words that had been presented earlier. That is, their implicit memory for the previous event is intact, despite the fact that their explicit memory for past events is severely impaired.

Two approaches are based on these principles.

◆ The method of *vanishing cues* (Glisky *et al.* 1994). Memory-impaired people are provided enough cues to allow successful performance. As learning occurs, cues are gradually withdrawn. This method has been successfully employed to teach amnesiacs new computer skills (Glisky *et al.* 1986*a,b*, 1994).

◆ The *errorless learning procedure*. Baddeley and Wilson (1994) observed that, once a memory-impaired patient makes an error, he or she is more likely to repeat that error, and they reasoned that the preserved implicit memory system is poorly equipped to resolve the interference. Wilson and her colleagues have demonstrated that errorless learning is more effective than standard conditions in which errors are allowed (Baddeley and Wilson 1994; Wilson *et al.* 1994).

3.3 Holistic approaches

In contrast to retraining and compensatory approaches that focus primarily on specific cognitive processes, holistic programmes attempt cognitive rehabilitation in the context of the full range of problems experienced by brain-damaged individuals. The holistic approaches are predicated on several key assumptions.

◆ Cognitive therapies must not be isolated from other (physical, psychological) therapies that are essential to functional rehabilitation.

◆ Cognitive interventions must proceed in sequential fashion from lower levels to more complex functions.

◆ The disorganized and sometimes chaotic nature of thought processes in brain-damaged people necessitates an orderly and structured therapeutic programme.

◆ Because the problems of brain-injured people are highly personalized, treatment must be as individualized as possible (see Ben-Yishay 1996 for a review).

Holistic programmes are multidimensional and attempt to treat cognitive, emotional, and motivational consequences of brain injury in an integrated manner. Individuals participate in a variety of tasks, including simple drills and retraining exercises, as well as learning compensatory techniques. An important feature is to help patients gain insight into their strengths and weaknesses in order to achieve a realistic sense of their potential for improvement. The expectation is that, through heightened awareness and an appreciation of the practical limitations imposed by their brain damage, individuals will be better motivated and equipped to restructure their lives.

Two prominent holistic programmes are those developed by Ben-Yishay (1978), a pioneer in the field, and Prigatano (1986). Ben-Yishay's approach is characterized by the creation of a 'therapeutic community' in which the patients, members of the therapeutic team, as well as family and significant others, work together to promote the rehabilitative process. Prigatano follows a similar approach but one that attaches great importance to the psychosocial consequences of neuropsychological disturbances. Prigatano's programme focuses on residual function and is guided by the philosophy that optimal use of these functions can be achieved if the patient has psychologically adjusted to the injury-induced changes and is coping effectively. While there is continuing need to evaluate the holistic approach, evidence from several studies points to significant benefits to TBI patients in terms of neuropsychological test performance, vocational status, and emotional functioning (see Prigatano *et al.* 1998 for a review).

4 **The Rotman approach**

The preceding review underscores the difficulties inherent in effecting cognitive rehabilitation in individuals suffering brain dysfunction as a result of trauma, disease, or even normal ageing. The problems are compounded further by diverse approaches that emphasize biological, social, or psychological factors to varying degrees. The result is a lack of a coherent strategy for treating symptoms that are common to most cognitively challenged populations. Our review also highlighted limitations in long-term assessment and advised caution in accepting the claims about the efficacy of certain programmes. Apart from limitations already identified, outcome evaluation is hampered frequently by design flaws that include:

◆ inadequate measurement;

◆ poor sampling techniques;

◆ faulty statistical analyses.

These and other concerns have been raised in several excellent reviews (e.g. Chesnut *et al.* 1999; Robertson 1993; Ruff and Camenzuli 1991) to which the reader is referred for more detailed discussion.

To some extent, historical problems in the field of cognitive rehabilitation reflect individual biases and traditions derived from time-honoured practices. An encouraging development in recent years has been the emergence of multidimensional approaches that incorporate the expertise of several disciplines in developing broadly based programmes. The holistic programmes, discussed in Section 3.3, are an example of this trend. An important factor in the shift towards a more integrated model is the growing appreciation of the potential benefits of collaboration between practitioners and basic scientists. Against this background, the Rotman Research Institute, a Toronto-based centre for neurocognitive research, with support from the McDonnell Foundation, assembled a group of clinicians and cognitive scientists to develop a rehabilitation protocol that would form the basis of an effective treatment programme. The programme and progress to date are summarized in this section.

From the outset, the Rotman programme was committed conceptually to the following elements.

- *Comprehensiveness.* Brain-damage is not the only factor that contributes to cognitive deficits, even in patients with extensive damage. In view of a growing literature that points to the importance of non-biological influences, the programme takes into account the impact of psychological, social, and environmental factors.

- *Adaptability.* There are many differences between the various populations that suffer cognitive impairment but there are also common themes, e.g. with respect to attentional and memory problems. A major objective was to exploit those common aspects and develop a versatile programme that could be broadly applied.

- *Evidence-based.* In developing the protocol, accepted procedures in clinical practice were integrated with empirically based theory and knowledge of cognitive processes and cognitive impairment. Several members of the team (e.g. D.T. Stuss, I.H. Robertson, M.P. Alexander, B. Levine, H. Palmer) are actively engaged in rehabilitation research, while others (e.g. F.I.M. Craik, G. Winocur) have well-established research programmes in areas of basic neuropsychology and cognitive science.

- *Outcome evaluation.* The clinical trial includes an assessment component that was designed to withstand scientific scrutiny. The protocol is administered to experimental and control groups under carefully controlled conditions, utilizing a design that allows between- and within-group comparisons over the course of the programme.

- *Cost-effectiveness.* Many programmes are highly individualized and extend for long periods of time. While some are indeed effective, they are labour- and resource-intensive. The Rotman approach was to come up with a group-oriented programme that would cover the essential features in a manageable time period.

4.1 The protocol

The protocol consists of three training components that emphasize cognitive skills, goal management, and psychosocial function.

- *Cognitive skills training* builds on evidence that brain-damaged individuals and older people do not spontaneously use cognitive strategies that normal young adults automatically apply when trying to learn or remember information. Considerable effort is placed on informing participants as to the various external and internal strategies that are available, and how they can be used most effectively. A major objective is to underscore the importance of making the necessary effort in performing cognitive tasks and getting across the idea that, with practice, strategies should eventually become more automatic.

◆ *Goal management.* On the principle that improved test performance in the context of treatment must generalize to real-world situations, the Goal Management Training programme (Levine *et al.* 2000; Robertson 1996), described in Section 3.2.1, was adapted to the protocol. This component focuses on practical tasks (e.g. planning a trip, fixing a small appliance) and emphasizes processes such as task identification, focusing and sustaining attention, and resisting distractions. Participants learn to engage in self-monitoring practices in order to stay on track and develop goal-oriented strategies for meeting task demands.

◆ *Psychosocial training* is based on research by Winocur and Moscovitch (see Dawson *et al.* 1999) that showed a relationship between social, psychological, and lifestyle factors (e.g. personal control, optimism, activity) and cognitive function in normal old people. This component emphasizes the personal rewards to be obtained from successful task performance and the gain in confidence that will help in meeting subsequent challenges. The aim is to add a motivating dimension that will increase the likelihood that participants will apply the techniques acquired in the other components.

The protocol itself is of 12 weeks duration, with 4 weeks devoted to each component. Participants are placed in groups of five or six with careful attention paid to numerous variables including severity of deficit, functional status, and group compatibility. Three-hour sessions are held weekly under the direction of a trained leader. The sessions are conducted in seminar format, which encourages interaction between the leader and participants, as well between the participants. Each session includes practical assignments, some to be completed within the session and others as homework to be reported on in subsequent meetings. In addition, participants meet individually with the group leader on several occasions. The purposes of these meetings are to:

◆ establish personal goals;

◆ monitor progress;

◆ discuss issues that arise;

◆ introduce an individualized component to complement the group format.

A full neuropsychological and psychosocial test battery is administered before the group sessions, immediately after the sessions, and subsequently at 3- and 6-month intervals. At the end of the first and second training components, a mini-test battery is administered to monitor progress and to assess individual effects of each training component.

4.2 Progress

The full trial, conducted on populations of TBI patients and old people, is currently underway and scheduled to be completed by late 2002. The TBI patients are all in the post-acute phase of their recovery, at least 1 year post-injury, and are all under the age of 55, while the older adults are healthy and all over the age of 55. No participant has prior neurological damage, a psychiatric history, or a history of drug or alcohol abuse. It is too early to assess outcome, but the decision to proceed with the trial was based on promising results from a pilot investigation. The pilot study also involved TBI patients and old people and, while sampling criteria were somewhat less stringent than those followed in the full trial, the results clearly indicated benefits following the treatment intervention in both populations. For example, in the condition involving elderly participants, the experimental group exhibited improved performance on tests of free recall, working memory, and prospective memory, as well as on a test of semantic fluency. Of particular interest, a delayed effect was detected at the 3-month follow-up testing. The latter effect was prominent on tests that made substantial demands on frontal-lobe function, raising the possibility that benefits to executive function may become optimal after an extended period of posttreatment consolidation and practice. In addition, improved cognitive performance in the experimental group was accompanied by higher posttreatment scores on the psychosocial tests, indicating an improvement in overall functional status. Similar benefits were observed in TBI patients who underwent the same intervention.

If the full treatment confirms that there are genuine benefits to neuropsychological and psychosocial functioning from our approach, there will be other issues to address, including the following.

◆ Can the protocol can be adapted to other cognitively impaired populations (e.g. focal lesions, neurodegenerative disease)?

◆ Are there differential benefits associated with the three training components and is there an optimal order of presentation?

◆ Can more use be made of family members and other sources of support?

◆ More must be learned about the process of generalization and the practical tasks that are most likely to be sensitive to the intervention.

◆ What are the limits of this approach? This protocol was not intended for all individuals and may be of little value in cases of severe cognitive impairment, or for individuals with coexisting mental health problems. On the other hand, if it proves to be useful for a large proportion of relatively 'uncomplicated' brain-damaged or elderly individuals, it will represent a significant advance and, at the very least, a foundation for developing even more effective cognitive rehabilitation programmes.

5 Conclusions and future directions

Despite the relatively new development of cognitive rehabilitation as a clinical discipline, the studies reviewed in this chapter provide grounds for optimism. The refinement of standard approaches offers more reasons to be optimistic but perhaps the most encouraging development is the growing willingness to combine the best of the various approaches. The result is the emergence of the holistic approaches, which have been associated with positive outcomes, and the development of the promising Rotman approach. Equally encouraging is the broad consensus that cognitive rehabilitation programmes must be evidence-based and must derive from a solid empirical and theoretical basis. The reader is referred to Cicerone *et al.* (2000) who, following a review of evidence-based rehabilitation programmes, reach precisely the same conclusion.

Additional questions remain, however. In this chapter, we have focused primarily on recovery from TBI, but there is considerable overlap among the literatures with other patient and healthy (e.g. normal ageing) populations.

- Which rehabilitation methods generalize across patient populations, and which are more beneficial for some patient populations than others? We argue for the need to train for generalization.

- In what ways can we better collaborate with other professions such as occupational therapy to devise retraining methods that involve everyday activities, yet nevertheless can be standardized and analysed in an empirical manner?

- Finally, with our growing understanding of the functional neuroanatomy of cognition, how best can neuroimaging methods be used to provide neural outcome measures and to improve our understanding of the mechanisms of recovery?

The future of cognitive rehabilitation will be shaped by the answers to these and other questions.

Selective references

Alderman, N., Fry, R.K., and Youngson, H.A. (1995). Improvement of self-monitoring skills, reduction of behaviour disturbance and the dysexecutive syndrome: comparison of response cost and a new programme of self-monitoring training. *Neuropsychol. Rehabil.* 5, 193–221.

Anderson, S.W. (1996). Cognitive rehabilitation in closed head injury. In *Head injury and postconcussive syndrome* (ed. M. Rizzo and D. Tranel), pp. 457–68. Churchill Livingstone, New York.

Baddeley, A. and Wilson, B.A. (1994). When implicit learning fails: amnesia and the problem of error elimination. *Neuropsychologia* 32, 53–68.

Ben-Yishay, Y. (1978). *Working approaches to remediation of cognitive deficits in brain damaged persons*, Rehabilitation Monograph No. 59. New York University Medical Center, New York.

Ben-Yishay, Y. (1996). Reactions on the evolution of the therapeutic milieu concept. *Neuropsychol. Rehabil.* 6, 327–43.

Ben-Yishay, Y. and Diller, L. (1993). Cognitive remediation of traumatic brain injury: update and issues. *Arch. Phys. Med. Rehabil.* 74, 204–13.

Burgess, P.W., Alderman, N., Evans, J., Emslie, H., and Wilson, B.A. (1998). The ecological validity of tests of executive function. *J. Int. Neuropsychol. Soc.* 4, 547–58.

Burke, J.M., Danick, J.A., Bemis, B., and Durgin, C.J. (1994). A process approach to memory book training for neurological patients. *Brain Injury* 8, 71–81.

Burke, W.H., Zencius, A.H., Wesolowski, M.D., and Doubleday, F. (1991). Improving executive function disorders in brain-injured clients. *Brain Injury* 5, 241–52.

Cabeza, R. and Nyberg, L. (2000). Imaging cognition II: An experimental review of 275 PET and fMRI studies. *J. Cogn. Neurosci.* 12, 1–47.

Caetano, C. and Christensen, A.-L. (1997). The design of neuropsychological rehabilitation: the role of neuropsychological assessment. In *Neuropsychological rehabilitation: fundamentals, innovations, and directions* (ed. J. León-Carrion), pp. 63–72. GR/St. Lucie Press, Delray Beach, Florida.

Chesnut, R.M., Carney, N., Maynard, H., Mann, N.C., Patterson, P., and Helfand, M. (1999). Evidence for the effectiveness of rehabilitation for persons with traumatic brain injury. *Head Trauma Rehabil.* 14, 176–88.

Cicerone, K.D. and Giacino, J.C. (1992). Remediation of executive function deficits after traumatic brain injury. *Neurorehabilitation* 2, 12–22.

Cicerone, K. and Wood, J. (1987). Planning disorder after closed head injury: a case study. *Arch. Phys. Med. Rehabil.* 68, 111–15.

Cicerone, K.K., Dahlberg, C., Kalmar, K., Langenbahn, D.M., Malec, J.F., Bergquist, T.F., Felicetti, T., Giacino, J.C., Harley, J.P., Harrington, D.E., Herzog, J., Kneipp, S., Laatsch, L., and Morse, P.A. (2000). Evidence-based cognitive rehabilitation: recommendations for clinical practice. *Arch. Phys. Med. Rehabil.* 81, 1596–615.

Dawson, D., Winocur, G., and Moscovitch, M. (1999). The psychosocial environment and cognitive rehabilitation in the elderly. In *Cognitive neurorehabilitation* (ed. D.T. Stuss, G. Winocur, and I.H. Robertson), pp. 94–108. Cambridge University Press, New York.

Dikmen, S. and Machamer, J.E. (1995). Neurobehavioral outcomes and their determinants. *J. Head Trauma Rehabil.* 10, 74–86.

Dixon, R.A. and Bäckman, L. (1999). Principles of compensation in cognitive neurorehabilitation. In *Cognitive neurorehabilitation* (ed. D T. Stuss, G. Winocur, and I.H. Robertson), pp. 59–72. Cambridge University Press, New York.

Fields, J.A., Norman, S., Straits-Tröster, K.A., and Tröster, A.I. (1998). The impact of depression on memory in neurodegenerative disease. In *Memory in neurodegenerative disease: biological, cognitive, and clinical perspectives* (ed. A.I. Tröster), pp. 314–37. Cambridge University Press, New York.

Gade, A. (1994). Imagery as a mnemonic aid in amnesia patients: effects of amnesia subtype and severity. In *Cognitive neuropsychology and cognitive rehabilitation* (ed. M.J. Riddoch and G.W. Humphreys), pp. 571–89. Erlbaum, Hillsdale, New Jersey.

Glisky, E.L., Schacter, D.L., and Tulving, E. (1986a). Computer learning by memory-impaired patients: acquisition and retention of complex knowledge. *Neuropsychologica* 24, 313–28.

Glisky, E.L., Schacter, D.L., and Tulving, E. (1986b). Learning and retention of computer-related vocabulary in amnesic patients: method of vanishing cues. *J. Clin. Exp. Neuropsychol.* 8, 313–28.

Glisky, E.L., Schacter, D.L., and Butters, M.A. (1994). Domain-specific learning and remediation of memory disorders. In *Cognitive neuropsychology and cognitive rehabilitation* (ed. M.J. Riddoch and G.W. Humphreys), pp. 527–48, Erlbaum, Hillsdale, New Jersey.

Grady, C.L. and Kapur, S. (1999). The use of neuroimaging in neurorehabilitative research. In *Cognitive neurorehabilitation* (ed. D.T. Stuss, G. Winocur, and I.H. Robertson), pp. 47–58. Cambridge University Press, New York.

Gray, J. and Robertson, I. (1989). Remediation of attentional difficulties following brain injury: three experimental single case studies. *Brain Injury* 3, 163–70.

Hall, K.M. and Cope, D.N. (1995). The benefit of rehabilitation in traumatic brain injury: a literature review. *J. Head Trauma Rehabil.* 10, 1–13.

Harris, J.E. (1978). External memory aids. In *Practical aspects of memory* (ed. M.M. Gruneberg, P.E. Morris, and R.N. Sykes), pp. 172–9. Academic Press, London.

High, W.M., Boake, C. and Lehmkuhl, L.D. (1995). Critical analysis of studies evaluating the effectiveness of rehabilitation after traumatic brain injury. *J. Head Trauma Rehabil.* 10, 14–26.

Katz, D.I. and Mills, V.M. (1999). Traumatic brain injury: natural history and efficacy of cognitive rehabilitation. In *Cognitive neurorehabilitation* (ed. D.T. Stuss, G. Winocur, and I.H. Robertson), pp. 279–301. Cambridge University Press, New York.

Kim, H.J., Burke, D., Dowds, M.M., and George, J. (1999). Utility of a microcomputer as an external memory aid for a memory-impaired head injury patient during in-patient rehabilitation. *Brain Injury* 13, 147–50.

Levine, B., Robertson, I., Clare, L., Carter, G., Hong, J., Wilson, B.A., Duncan, J., and Stuss, D.T. (2000). Rehabilitation of executive functioning: an experimental-clinical validation of Goal Management Training. *J. Int. Neuropsychol. Soc.* 6, 299–312.

Lezak, M.D. (1995). *Neuropsychological assessment*, 3rd edn. Oxford University Press, New York.

Mateer, C.A. (1999). The rehabilitation of executive disorders. In *Cognitive neurorehabilitation* (ed. D.T. Stuss, G. Winocur, and I.H. Robertson), pp. 314–32. Cambridge University Press, New York.

Meichenbaum, D. (1977). *Cognitive behavior modification: an integrative approach*. Plenum, New York.

Morton, M.V. and Wehman, P. (1995). Psychosocial and emotional sequelae of individuals with traumatic brain injury: a literature review and recommendations. *Brain Injury* 9, 81–92.

Park, N.W. and Ingles, J.L. (2001). Effectiveness of attention rehabilitation after an acquired brain injury: a meta-analysis. *Neuropsychology* 15, 199–210.

Park, N.W., Proulx, G. and Towers, W. (1999). Evaluation of the Attention Process Training programme. *Neuropsychol. Rehabil.* 9, 135–54.

Ponsford, J., Willmott, C., Rothwell, A., Cameron, P., Kelly, A.-M., Nelms, R., Curran, C., and Ng, K. (2000). Factors influencing outcome following mild traumatic brain injury in adults. *J. Int. Neurol. Soc.* 6, 568–79.

Prigatano, G.P. (1986). Personality and psychosocial consequences of brain injury. In *Neuropsychological rehabilitation after brain injury* (ed. G.P. Prigatano, D.J. Fordyce, H.K. Zeiner, J.R. Roueche, M. Pepping, and B.C. Woods), pp. 29–50. Johns Hopkins University Press, Baltimore.

Prigatano, G.P. (1997). Learning from our successes and failures: reflections and comments on 'Cognitive rehabilitation: how it is and how it might be'. *J. Int. Neuropsychol. Soc.* 3, 497–9.

Prigatano, G.P. (1999). Motivation and awareness in cognitive neurorehabilitation. In *Cognitive neurorehabilitation* (ed. D.T. Stuss, G. Winocur, and I.H. Robertson), pp. 240–51. Cambridge University Press, New York.

Prigatano, G.P., Glisky, E.L., and Klonoff, P.S. (1998). *Cognitive rehabilitation for neuropsychiatric disorders* (ed. P.W. Corrigan and S.C. Yudofsky), pp. 223–42. American Psychiatric Press, Washington, DC.

Robertson, I.H. (1993). Cognitive rehabilitation in neurologic disease. *Curr. Opin. Neurol.* 6, 756–60.

Robertson, I.H. (1996). *Goal management training: a clinical manual*. PsyConsult, Cambridge.

Robertson, I.H. and Murre, J.M.J. (1999). Rehabilitation of brain damage: brain plasticity and principles of guided recovery. *Psychol. Bull.* 125, 544–75.

Robertson, I.H., Ward, A., Ridgeway, V., and Nimmo-Smith, I. (1994). *The Test of Everyday Attention*. Thames Valley Test Corporation, Flempton, UK.

Ruff, R.M. and Camenzuli, L.F. (1991). Research challenges for behavioral rehabilitation: searching for solutions. In *Cognitive rehabilitation for persons with traumatic brain injury: a functional approach* (ed. J.S. Kreutzer and P.H. Wehman), pp. 23–34. Brooks, Baltimore.

Schacter, D.L. and Graf, P. (1986). Preserved learning in amnesic patients: perspectives from research on direct priming. *J. Clin. Exp. Neuropsychol.* **8**, 727–43.

Schwartz, A.F. and McMillan, T.M. (1989). Assessment of everyday memory after severe head injury. *Cortex* **25**, 665–71.

Sohlberg, M.M. and Mateer, C.A. (1989a). Introduction to cognitive rehabilitation: theory and practice. Guilford, New York.

Sohlberg, M.M. and Mateer, C.A. (1989b). Training use of compensatory memory books: A three stage behavioral approach. *J. Clin. Exp. Neuropsychol.* **11**, 871–87.

Sohlberg, M.M. and Mateer, C.A. (2001). *Cognitive rehabilitation: an integrative neuropsychological approach.* Guilford, New York.

Sohlberg, M.M. and Raskin, S.A. (1996). Principles of generalization applied to attention and memory interventions. *J. Head Trauma Rehabil.* **11**, 65–78.

Sohlberg, M.M., Sprunk, H., and Metzelaar, K. (1988). Efficacy of an external cuing system in an individual with severe frontal lobe damage. *Cogn. Rehabil.* **6**, 36–40.

Sohlberg, M.M., White, O., Evans, E., and Mateer, C.A. (1992a). Background and initial case studies into the effects of prospective memory training. *Brain Injury* **5**, 129–38.

Sohlberg, M.M., White, O., Evans, E., and Mateer, C.A. (1992b). An investigation of the effects of prospective memory training. *Brain Injury* **5**, 139–54.

Sohlberg, M.M., Johnson, L., Paule, L., Raskin, S.A., and Mateer, C.A. (1993). *Attention process training II: A program to address attention deficits for persons with mild cognitive dysfunction.* Association for Neuropsychological Research and Development, Puyallup, Washington.

Stokes, T.F. and Baer, D.M. (1977). An implicit technology of generalization. *J. Appl. Behav. Anal.* **10**, 349–67.

Sturm, W., Willmes, K., Orgass, B., and Hartje, W. (1997). Do specific attention deficits need specific training? *Neuropsychol. Rehabil.* **7**, 81–103.

Stuss, D.T., Winocur, G., and Robertson, I.H. (eds.) (1999). *Cognitive neurorehabilitation.* Cambridge University Press, New York.

Thoene, A.I.T. and Glisky, E.L. (1995). Learning of name-face associations in memory impaired patients: a comparison of different training procedures. *J. Int. Neuropsychol. Soc.* **1**, 29–38.

West, R.L. (1995). Compensatory strategies for age-associated memory impairment. In *Handbook of memory disorders* (ed. A.D. Baddeley, B.A. Wilson, and F.N. Watts), pp. 481–500. Wiley, Chicester, UK.

Williams, W.H., Evans, J.J. and Wilson, B.A. (1999). Outcome measures for survivors of acquired brain injury in day and outpatient neurorehabilitation programmes. *Neuropsychol. Rehabil.* **9**, 421–36.

Wilson, B.A. (1991). Long-term prognosis of patients with severe memory disorders. *Neuropsychol. Rehabil.* **1**, 117–34.

Wilson, B.A. (1995). Management and remediation of memory problems in brain-injured adults. In *Handbook of memory disorders* (ed. A.D. Baddeley, B.A. Wilson, and F.N. Watts), pp. 451–79. Wiley, Chicester, UK.

Wilson, B.A. (1997). Cognitive rehabilitation: How it is and how it might be. *J. Int. Neuropsychol. Soc.* **3**, 487–96.

Wilson, B.A. and Moffat, N. (1992). The development of group memory therapy. In *Clinical management of memory problems*, 2nd edn (ed. B.A. Wilson and N. Moffat), pp. 243–73. Chapman and Hall, London.

Wilson, B.A., Cockburn, J., and Baddeley, A.D. (1985). *The Rivermead Behavioural Memory Test.* Thames Valley Test Corporation, Bury St. Edmunds, UK.

Wilson, B.A., Baddeley, A.D., Evans, J.J., and Shiel, A. (1994). Errorless learning in the rehabilitation of memory impaired people. *Neuropsychol. Rehabil.* 4, 307–26.

Wilson, B.A., Alderman, N., Burgess, P., Emslie, H., and Evans, J.J. (1996). *The behavioral assessment of the dysexecutive syndrome.* Thames Valley Test Corporation, Flempton, UK.

Wilson, B.A., Evans, J.J., Emslie, H., and Malinek, V. (1997). Evaluation of NeuroPage: a new memory aid. *J. Neurol., Neurosurg., Psychiatry* 63, 113–15.

World Health Organization (1999). *International classification of functioning and disability* [Beta-2 draft]. WHO, Geneva.

Yesavage, J.A., Rose, T.L. and Bower, G.H. (1983). Interactive imagery and affective judgments improve face-name learning in the elderly. *J. Gerontol.* 38, 197–203.

Yesavage, J.A., Sheikh, J.I., Friedman, L., and Tanke, E. (1990). Learning mnemonics: roles of aging and subtle cognitive impairment. *Psychol. Aging* 5, 133–7.

Ylvisaker, M. (1998). *Traumatic brain injury rehabilitation: children and adolescents.* Butterworth-Heinemann, Woburn, Massachusetts.

Part 3

Neuropsychological impairments

Chapter 5

Assessment of attention

Ed van Zomeren and Joke Spikman

1 Introduction

Attention is a broad concept that has been defined in various ways. In daily language it is often used to refer to concentration, which refers to a person who is selectively looking at or listening to a certain task while spending some effort in the process. Thus, attention has two broad dimensions: *selectivity* and *intensity*. These dimensions are readily visible in the spotlight metaphor: attention can be directed like a spotlight to illuminate a certain object, while the intensity of the light may vary. Attention can be seen as a quality of information-processing: perception, processing, and storing of information is optimal when the system is directed properly and when the required level of intensity is present. Thus, attention can be defined as the state of a processing system that is optimally tuned in terms of selectivity and intensity.

It is important to note that attention, despite this definition, is not a unitary concept. Our definition already distinguishes two dimensions, and when attentional behaviour is described several additional task-related terms will appear, for example when investigators speak of divided attention or sustained attention. In fact, different taxonomies of attention have been proposed, some of them psychological (Mirsky *et al.* 1991; van Zomeren and Brouwer 1994) and others based on neuroanatomy (Mesulam 1985; Posner and Petersen 1990). The existence of these different approaches inspires two caveats.

- General statements about 'the attention' of a patient should be avoided. The situation or the task at hand determine to a large extent which aspects of attention will be essential and whether deficits will become visible. A patient's attention may be adequate for a social chat, but inadequate for driving a car through dense traffic in the rush hour. Thus, statements about the attention of a patient should always be qualified in terms of the specific task and situation.

- The assessment of attention should never be limited to performance on a single test. For example, a recording of simple reaction time can tell us something about the basic speed of processing in a particular patient, but tells us little or nothing about his or her ability to react flexibly in a dual task or to sustain attention over half an hour.

In practice, the clinician will be interested in certain aspects of attention, depending on the type of brain damage involved and the practical questions to be addressed.

In the assessment of epileptic patients transient cognitive impairments may be critical, whereas in stroke patients hemineglect will be most relevant. In head-injured patients the clinician might want to study speed of information-processing. Practical questions may range from fitness to drive, in which divided attention is important, to educational situations in which sustained attention on a task in a noisy environment is essential. Hence, the selection of attention tests should be made in relation to the neurological diagnosis of the patient and those decisions about daily life and occupational risks that are required to be made.

2 Ways of assessing attention

As a mental construct, attention can only be measured indirectly. As noted in Section 1, attention can be defined as a quality in the subject's perception, processing, and storing of information. This implies, that attention has to be measured through other behaviours, e.g. by studying the efficiency of visual search or the speed of visuomotor responses. In this sense one could say, 'There are no tests of attention.' The ideal paradigm for studying the attentional component in a particular activity consists of a task with two conditions, with a variation that taps a certain aspect of attention. For example, focused attention can be tested by presenting the same task twice, i.e. without and with distraction by irrelevant stimuli. The best known paradigm in this regard is found in the Stroop Colour Word Test, where speed of colour naming is measured twice, the second time under distraction by word meaning. Hence, the efficiency of a certain aspect of attention is expressed as a difference between two time scores. Unfortunately, difference scores raise a number of metric and reliability problems, among them decreased reliability (Spikman *et al.* 2000; Zoccolotti and Caracciolo 2002). Although solutions to deal with such problems were presented (Zoccolotti and Caracciolo 2002; Spikman 2001) the clinical usefulness of these methodological contributions is as yet unknown.

A second problem is that most clinical tests available tap more than one aspect of attention. A time score obtained in a visual search task may reflect both the speed of processing of visual information and higher-order aspects of attention such as strategy and flexibility.

2.1 Observation and rating

The oldest approach to the assessment of attention as a psychological construct is *clinical observation*. Observation has obvious advantages: it does not require any equipment and it hardly requires extra time, as it is integrated in the natural contact between clinician and patient. During bedside conversation or an apparent social chat on the way to the neuropsychology department, the psychologist may observe whether the patient is alert and paying attention to his environment and the investigator and whether there are any signs of hemineglect or drifting attention (Stuss and Benson 1986). Technical assistants may note whether patients are distracted by noises from outside during formal assessment and whether they are attending adequately to tests that, in themselves, are not considered as attention tests.

Observation can be standardized by the use of *rating scales*. The Neurobehavioral Rating Scale, devised by Levin *et al.* (1987), contains a few items that are aimed at attention. The scale has satisfactory interjudge reliability and validity. A questionnaire that can be filled out by patients and their relatives is the Cognitive Failures Questionnaire (Broadbent *et al.* 1982). A Rating Scale of Attentional Behaviour (RSAB) was developed by Ponsford and Kinsella (1991). This instrument uses 5-point scales to record the frequency of attentional problems in patients. Its validity and usefulness were demonstrated in a rehabilitation institute where professionals (speech therapists and ergotherapists) rated aspects of attention in head-injured patients. The RSAB has a high interrater reliability (0.91).

2.2 **Categorization of attention tests**

Any review of the available tests used to assess attention is faced with the problem of how to organize them. At first sight, a division of tests in terms of focused attention, divided attention, and sustained attention may seem useful but this turns out to be an unsatisfactory approach. As mentioned before, several taxonomies of attention have been proposed and the choice of a particular one for the organization of assessment methods would always be arbitrary. Also, there is evidence from statistical studies that shows that concepts that seem quite useful for the description of behaviour, such as divided attention or sustained attention, are not supported by factor analyses in the case of a large series of subjects tested on attention tests. Spikman *et al.* (2001) studied the construct validity of well known attentional concepts, listing several statistical studies that showed little agreement about useful factors. It appeared that each investigation produced new factors and hence new constructs. Still, two main factors were noted that seemed to commonly appear, albeit under various names, in most of the statistical studies:

◆ speed or processing capacity;

◆ control or working memory.

Thus, a distinction with an empirical, statistical basis is available. In our own experience, this distinction is quite helpful for the analysis of attention problems in head-injured subjects (Spikman *et al.* 2001). However, it also seems useful for a practical categorization of attention tests. The two concepts of speed and control are not completely independent. It should be realized that control processes occur at a certain speed and that these processes may slow down in case of brain damage. Also, changes in speed of processing may affect control. When speed of processing increases or decreases, this will bring along changes in the amount and nature of control required.

The relative weights of speed and control can vary from task to task. This is partly due to *task characteristics* or task demands. Some tasks are experienced as easy and proceeding almost 'on their own' once they have been started. For example, performance on a finger tapping test is an easy repetitive motor task requiring very little control—the only control necessary is to monitor one's speed of tapping. On the other hand, writing a letter of application requires intensive control while speed is rarely essential. Generally speaking, control is maximal in unstructured tasks that cannot be tackled with routine responses. Control always implies activity of working memory, in which rules for the performance of the task have to be kept activated. A second task characteristic is the time pressure involved.

Another source of variation is found in *subject characteristics*, in particular, learning effects. In general, the amount of control required decreases with the amount of learning of a task. In fact, many well-trained tasks require so little control that we consider them to be automatized and not requiring much effort. Learning to drive is a good example of a task consisting of many subtasks, that requires control and a lot of effort in the first lessons, but that gets automatized to a high degree in the experienced driver. A second important subject characteristic is the individual speed/accuracy trade-off.

Thus, the distinction between speed and control is related to the distinction between time pressure and structure. This allows us to look at attention tests at three levels: the operational level, tactical level and strategic level.

2.2.1 Operational level

At this level, speed is the main factor while control is minimal. Time pressure is high, as patients are instructed to work as quickly as possible, or by presentation of stimuli at a high rate. On the other hand, the task presented to the subject is highly structured, signals and responses are simple, and, through instruction, the subject knows exactly what he or she should do. Attention can be tested here at a basic level, with time as the essential dependent variable. Speed of response is measured, or the number of milliseconds exposure time required before a subject recognizes a picture in a tachistoscope. At this level, the subject can do little other than 'pay attention and try to be fast'. Tasks are relatively simple and highly structured but there is always a considerable time pressure. Performance on these basic tasks may be called stimulus-driven (see Table 5.1).

2.2.2 Tactical level

At this level, both time pressure and structure are intermediate. Tasks are more complicated and being fast is no longer sufficient for optimal performance. A certain amount of control is required, but the nature of this control is specified in instructions to the

Table 5.1 Characteristics of the three levels of attention tests

Level	Time pressure	Structure of task
Operational	High	Highly structured, stimulus-driven
Tactical	Intermediate	Partially structured, memory-driven
Strategic	Low	Unstructured, strategy-driven

subjects. For example, they are told to ignore distracting stimuli, or to divide their attention while reacting to two kinds of symbols. At this level, subjects have to find a personal speed/accuracy trade-off, i.e. a balance between working speed and error rate. Performance on this level can be called memory-driven, as instructions and rules for performance must be kept activated in working memory.

2.2.3 Strategic level

At this level, time pressure is minimal but subjects have to find their own approach to an optimal performance of the task. Hence, instructions do not dictate completely what should be done and, in this sense, these tests of attention offer less structure than the tests that are aimed at the operational and tactical level. Basically, the subject has to apply his own strategy, i.e. performance is strategy-driven.

3 The operational level: speed of information-processing

At this level time scores are essential while errors do not play a role of any importance. An example would be the recording of simple reaction times in response to either visual or auditory stimuli. Neurological patients may be slow on this task, but the signals are clear and the responses are so simple that errors are extremely rare and thus not useful for assessment. What one tries to assess at this level is the basic speed of information-processing. Reaction time recordings, as they feature in many computerized test batteries, are an excellent method for the assessment of basic mental speed. Test–retest reliability is sufficient, e.g. 0.78 for a visual four-choice reaction (van Zomeren 1981). Apart from reaction times, the clinician may use the basic conditions of well known clinical tools such as Trailmaking A and word reading and colour naming in the Stroop Colour Word Test. Test–retest reliability is satisfactory for both tests, ranging from 0.70 to 0.90 for Trailmaking A and from 0.83 to 0.91 for reading and colour naming in the Stroop test (Spreen and Strauss 1991). Also, Digit Symbols from the Wechsler Adult Intelligence Scale (WAIS)-R can be used for the assessment of speed. Visual search tasks can also be useful, as long as they are well-structured; Letter Search, with a simple target to be found in horizontal lines of letters, is a good example.

As noted in Section 1, no attention test ever taps one aspect of attention only. This will be clear from the tests mentioned above: many of them require some visuomotor skill and, in the Letter Search task, the subject will exert some control in an effort to work accurately, not skipping any target. A second important point is that the assessment of speed of processing requires finely graded norms. In particular, age is an important factor. Generally speaking, processing speed decreases with increasing age. For some tasks, gender is also important. For example, men react slightly faster than women to simple signals. Thus, the clinician should take age and sex into account when testing attention in the basic sense of speed of processing.

Theoretically, the question of domain-specific slowness can be raised. In the clinical literature, mental slowness is usually discussed as a global phenomenon that manifests itself in all task domains and all sensory modalities. In practice, this simplification seems justified. In case of diffuse injury to the brain or of (more or less) diffuse degenerative processes such as Alzheimer's disease, the slowness indeed manifests itself in all aspects of behaviour. Even in the case of focal damage such as that caused by stroke or neoplasm, a general mental slowness is often noted and confirmed on subsequent testing. However, it is conceivable that a focal lesion may disrupt or slow down specific processes only, e.g. the manipulation of verbal information in the case of left hemisphere damage in right-handed subjects.

4 The tactical level: focused and divided attention

In tests at this level, subjects are still expected to work as quickly as possible, but more control is required in order to prevent errors. A good example would be Trailmaking B. While in Trailmaking A the instruction is rather straightforward—to connect numbered circles by a pencil line—in Trailmaking B a certain load is placed on working memory in which two sequences have to be kept active, i.e. the alphabet and the numbers from 1 to 13. As the correct response depends on keeping track in both sequences and using them alternately, there is ample opportunity for making errors. As far as visuomotor behaviour is required, Trailmaking B is roughly comparable to Trailmaking A. Hence, the fact that healthy subjects need more than twice the time required for A when doing B reflects the far greater amount of control involved in the latter condition of the test.

On the tactical level, the distinction between tests of *focused* and *divided* attention is useful.

- The concept of focused attention can be applied whenever the subject has to respond selectively, i.e. when irrelevant stimuli are present.

- The concept of divided attention refers to task situations in which subtasks can be distinguished and more than one type of response is required.

4.1 Focused attention

When irrelevant stimuli can act as distractors, subjects have to focus on the relevant ones. Visual search tasks are attention tests that require some selectivity, as all stimuli are irrelevant except the ones designated as targets. In Trailmaking A, all numbered circles are to be regarded as 'noise' except the number that the subject is searching for. An important distinction should be made between structured and unstructured fields of search. Visual search tasks with a structured field are easier, i.e. require less control, than tests with an unstructured field. For example, letter cancellation tasks present letters in horizontal lines, and the d-2 test (Brickenkamp 1981) also presents its stimuli in convenient lines. In contrast, some visual search tasks present quasirandom fields, thus forcing the subjects to scan the field according to their own insight. Trailmaking is a good example, but tests for the detection of hemineglect also make use of unstructured fields (Albert's (1973) test of neglect; Bells test, Gauthier *et al*. 1989). The Test of

Everyday Attention (Robertson *et al.* 1994) contains two visual search tasks with eco-logical validity and satisfactory reliability—Map Search and Telephone Search.

Many visual search tasks allow the clinician to consider the speed/accuracy trade-off in patients, by studying number of errors in relation to speed. For example, in our own laboratory we found that severely head-injured patients were working slowly but accur-ately on the Bourdon dot configuration test (van Zomeren and Brouwer 1994).

In most visual search tasks, all distractors are present simultaneously. A classic test of focused attention, the Continuous Performance Task, presents distractors successively in time, while the subject is on the look-out for the target letter A. This test also has a condition requiring slightly more control by working memory—in the XA condition, the letter A is a target only when it is preceded by an X.

Distractors differ greatly in their distracting power. In the case of visual search, it is usually quite easy to search for a target while processing all other stimuli very superfi-cially only. A good example of a strong distractor is found in the classic Stroop para-digm, where stimuli have two features: a colour and a word meaning that conflicts with the colour. As reading is highly automatized, the instruction to focus on the colours of the words creates a strong response interference that is measured in a slowing of per-formance, compared to that in simple colour naming. For this interference subtask of the Stroop, reliability coefficients of 0.89 and 0.91 have been reported (Spreen and Strauss 1991). Bohnen (1991) devised an ingenious variation of the Colour Words Test that demands an even greater amount of control and effort by the subject. Randomly, one-fifth of all coloured words were marked by boxes, and subjects were instructed to read these marked words. Thus, while trying to concentrate on the colour of words, every now and then they had to switch back to reading—the very response that they had to suppress at all other stimuli. The Bohnen variant in this way also taps flexibility, the ability to change response mode quickly and repeatedly. Bohnen found that his variant had some validity in the study of acute effects of mild head injury.

4.2 Divided attention

The classic paradigm to test divided attention is a dual task, in which a subject is instructed to perform two tasks simultaneously. The complexity of such tasks may vary greatly, depending on the amount of control required in each subtask. Park *et al.* (1999) demonstrated that divided attention is impaired in head-injured subjects when the tasks require controlled processing, but not when the tasks can be carried out relat-ively automatically. Unfortunately, the dual-task paradigm has hardly been used in clinical assessment. The Test of Everyday Attention (TEA, Robertson *et al.* 1994) con-tains the subtest Telephone Search while Counting, in which subjects have to find items in a telephone directory while at the same time counting the number of tones in a tape-recorded series. Reliability of the dual-task decrement effect was satisfactory in two groups of non-brain-damaged subjects (0.59 and 0.61) but somewhat lower in a group of patients with cerebrovascular accidents (0.40).

4.2.1 Paced Auditory Serial Addition Task (PASAT)

A well known instrument in this domain is the Paced Auditory Serial Addition Task (PASAT; Gronwall and Sampson 1974). This presents series of 61 digits to the subject, with the instruction to add the last digit to the preceding one, giving the answer aloud. This task can be seen as a divided attention task, as subjects are dividing their processing capacity over several activities: listening, adding, answering, and keeping track in their working memory. As the series of digits are presented with interstimulus intervals that get progressively shorter (from one digit per 3.2 seconds to one digit per 1.6 seconds), the PASAT is also widely seen as a test of the speed of information-processing. Doing the test requires a considerable effort and patients frequently dislike the faster presentation rates. Several studies have demonstrated the validity of PASAT, i.e. sensitivity to the effects of head injury and factor-analytic evidence of loading on an attention/concentration factor. Gronwall and Sampson claimed that performance on PASAT was not related to arithmetic ability and general intelligence, but this statement has been challenged repeatedly. As Zoccolotti and Caracciolo (2002) put it: 'The overall picture seems to reveal a mild to moderate link between general intellectual abilities and performance on the PASAT. Clinicians should consider this finding and further research might allow for a possible adjustment of normative data based on the general intelligence g factor.'

4.2.2 Test for Attentional Performance (TAP)

In the 1990s, two batteries of attention tests were presented that assess attention mainly at the tactical level. Both of them can be seen as attempts to approach assessment with a firm theoretical basis and well-defined concepts and both of them originated in Europe. Zimmerman and Fimm (1993) devised the *Test for Attentional Performance* or TAP, a computerized battery with unusual psychometric qualities. While each subtest was based on the relevant theoretical literature, the authors have made an effort to make the tasks feasible in a clinical setting, in terms of ease of administration, standardization of instructions, and solid normative data. Among its subtests are tests of Divided Attention, a Go/No go task and Visual Scanning. In addition, the TAP contains original paradigms such as Alertness and Vigilance. In the subtest Alertness, the difference between reaction times with and without warning signal is calculated. The subtest Vigilance presents a classic vigilance task, i.e. a quite boring situation in which the subject is required to watch a monotonously moving line for 15 or 30 minutes, and to push a button whenever an irregularity in this movement occurs. The psychometric characteristics of the TAP are discussed extensively by Zimmermann and Fimm (2002).

4.2.3 Test of Everyday Attention (TEA)

A second useful battery of attention tests was presented in 1994 by Robertson *et al.* The Test of Everyday Attention (TEA) is marked by its attempt to demonstrate ecological validity. Like the TAP, the TEA attempts to assess attention from a sound theoretical background, but its outward appearance is quite different. While the TAP is compu-terized, the TEA requires minimal instrumentation as its visual tasks are paper-and-pencil while the acoustic tasks require a tape recorder for presentation. Ecological validity is created by choosing tasks that closely resemble daily life situations. For example, an aspect called 'selective attention' is assessed by means of two visual search tasks, called Map Search and Telephone Search. In the first of these subtests, the subject is required to search for gas stations or restaurants on part of a real map; in the second the subject has to find certain items in a telephone directory. All subtests have loadings on factors found by factor analyses of normal subject data. These factors (with their subtests) are:

- selective attention (Map Search, Telephone Search);
- working memory (Elevator Counting with Distraction, Elevator Counting with Reversal);
- attentional switching (Visual Elevator);
- sustained attention (Elevator Counting, Telephone Search while Counting, Lottery).

The validity of the TEA has been studied in cerebrovascular accident (CVA) and head-injured patients and can be judged as satisfactory. The reliability of all subtests is good, with the exception of Telephone Search while Counting.

5 The strategic level: supervisory control

Testing attention on the strategic level meets with a paradox: strategy can be deployed only in an unstructured situation, but a test requires standardization and hence struc-ture. As a result of this paradox, it is hard to find paradigms that truly assess the higher aspects of attention, i.e. supervisory attentional control. Still, there are a few instru-ments that can be recommended.

5.1 The Wisconsin Card Sorting Task (WCST)

The oldest of these is the Wisconsin Card Sorting Test (Lezak 1995). In this task, the subject has to change his or her response set on the basis of feedback by the experimenter. That is, while sorting cards according to a principle originally chosen by the subject (e.g. colour of symbols on the cards), from a certain point in the process the experimenter no longer confirms the sortings, now indicating that the subject is sorting cards on the wrong pile. Thus, the subject has to find a new principle (e.g. number of symbols on the cards). This shifting can be seen as requiring flexibility, which links it to attention on the strategic level. There exists an extensive literature on the validity of the WCST and its revised ver-sions. While originally it was believed that the WCST was especially sensitive to frontal brain damage, this view has been criticized with good arguments.

5.2 The Tower of London test

Shallice (1988) devised the Tower of London test. This test, derived from an oriental puzzle game, is closely connected to the theoretical model of the Supervisory

Attentional System as proposed by the same author. Three coloured beads (red, blue, and yellow) have to be arranged on three sticks of increasing length, in order to reach a certain pattern in a prescribed number of moves. There are restrictions in the handling of the beads, e.g. one may handle only one of them at a given time, and they may not be put down on the table. The solving of each puzzle item requires some thinking ahead and practically always a certain bead has to be placed temporarily on a stick that is not its final destination. Thus, subjects have to plan their moves and to suppress impulsive 'solutions', and in this regard it might tap supervisory attentional control. Unfortunately, normative data are lacking and both validity and reliability are unknown.

5.3 The Six Elements Test and the Zoo Test

Thirdly, located within a battery called the Behavioural Assessment of the Dysexecutive Syndrome (BADS; Wilson *et al.* 1996), there is an interesting task called the *Six Elements Test*. In this task, subjects are given 10 minutes to perform six tasks. They are expected to use this limited time wisely and to respect certain shifting rules. For example, the six tasks fall in three categories but the subject is not allowed to shift from task A to B within the same category. The Six Elements Tests is largely unstructured, as it does not tell the subject how to divide the available time over the different tasks. Hence, it offers good opportunity to observe the subject's strategy. In particular, the test has a strong ecological appeal as it enables us to judge whether the subject is paying attention to passing time—there is a little clock on the desk counting down the minutes and seconds.

Finally, the BADS also contains the *Zoo Test*, in which subjects have to visit a number of sites in a certain order, while respecting certain rules. Finding the correct route requires planning and overview in a fairly complex situation, and thus the task taps aspects of supervisory control.

5.4 Testing the strategic level in daily life

Still, these four tests are far removed from essential attentional strategies in daily life. What one would like to test is the subject's ability to attend to highly relevant but unpredictable cues in an unstructured situation. For example, attention for nonverbal cues in the social domain is essential for the maintaining of smooth relationships, both in private life and in professional situations. However, it is hardly possible to devise standardized situations that deserve the name of 'test' and that will yield objective and quantified information on these higher aspects of attention. Spikman *et al.* (2000) attempted to assess executive functioning in head-injured patients in a chronic stage (2–5 years after injury) by observing them when they were trying to find their way through the University Hospital in Groningen. It was recorded how these subjects used available information (signs) and searched for additional information by addressing passers-by and hospital staff. Spikman *et al.* found, among their head-injured subjects, that those with frontal lesions on computerized tomography (CT) or magnetic resonance imaging (MRI) scans needed more time and were less efficient in the search for and use of information. As far as this Executive Route Finding Task assesses 'attention for sources of additional information', it may be viewed as a test of attention on the strategic level.

6 Sustained attention, sustained control

The term 'sustained attention' refers to assessment on a longer timescale than usual, covering intervals from 10 to 30 minutes. A distinction should be made between high event-rate tasks and low event-rate tasks. In the former subjects are kept quite busy, in the latter they are exposed to a boring situation and their main task is to maintain an adequate level of alertness in order to detect rare and subtle stimuli. The former type of task is called a *continuous performance test*; the latter type a *vigilance test.*

Unfortunately, in clinical practice it is often concluded that 'sustained attention is poor' when a patient is performing below standard, for whatever reason, on a lengthy test. In most cases, this will be unjustified. Even when patients are reacting slowly on a continuous reaction time (RT) task or missing many signals in a vigilance task, it may well be that they are sustaining their 'poor' attention quite well. Conclusions about sustained attention should be based on time-on-task effects (TOTs). These are changes in performance over time, and sustained attention may be considered insufficient when a patient shows an abnormal TOT, i.e. abnormally increasing response times or an abnormal increase of missed signals or errors. To detect such deterioration, the duration of the test should be divided in blocks, e.g. of 5 minutes each.

The demands of a sustained attention test depend on whether the task is self-paced or experimenter-paced. In other words, who determines the time pressure? If one uses a prolonged visual search task such as the Bourdon dot configuration test (lasting 12 to 15 minutes) subjects choose their own speed of working. Many well known tests, however, are experimenter-paced, e.g. the Continuous Performance Test. The essential difference, of course, is that time pressure cannot be influenced by the subjects in experimenter-paced tasks.

Another important feature of sustained attention tests is the amount of control required. In our experience, brain-damaged subjects can usually deal with prolonged tasks if these are self-paced and require little control (see Fig. 5.1). On the other hand, head-injured patients very frequently complain of increased mental fatiguability, meaning that they cannot concentrate long on daily-life tasks that require some mental effort. This suggests that prolonged control is the key feature in the question of sustained attention in subjects with brain lesions.

6.1 Tests assessing sustained attention

The classical test for the assessment of sustained attention is the *Continuous Performance Test* (Rosvold *et al.* 1956) in which subjects have to react to the target letter A in a long random series of letters. The TAP battery (Zimmermann and Fimm 1993,

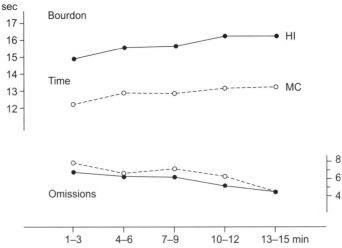

Fig. 5.1 A case of low speed but adequate control. Performance of head-injured patients (HI) in a chronic stage and of matched controls (MC) on a visual search task (Bourdon) lasting 15 minutes. In this self-paced task, subjects have to search for groups of four dots, in lines that contain 25 groups of three, four, and five dots. Patients need about 3 seconds more per line than control subjects, but at this working speed their accuracy is perfectly normal. In fact, curves are strikingly similar and no special time-on-task effects are visible in the head-injured group.

2002) contains a useful *Vigilance Test* in an auditory and a visual format, with adequate norms. The Test of Everyday Attention (Robertson *et al.* 1994) contains three subtests that have a loading on sustained attention. The first of these is *Lottery*, in which subjects have to listen for their 'winning number' that ends in '55'. They are presented with a 10-minute audiotaped list of numbers such as BC 143 and LD 967, and their task is to write down the two letters preceding all 10 target numbers. The two other subtests loading on sustained attention, *Elevator Counting* and *Telephone Search while Counting*, have an unusually short timescale and operationalize the concept in a highly specific way: counting strings of audiotaped tones. The tasks have an interesting link with neuroanatomy, i.e. the right frontal lobe. All three subtests have a satisfactory validity but reliability is low (0.41 to 0.61) for Telephone Search while Counting.

Robertson and Manly (1997) devised a paradigm that is not yet available as a formal test, but might turn out to be quite useful—the *Sustained Attention for Response Test* or SART. This offers a high-event-rate situation, in which subjects have to react continuously to a random series of digits (0 to 9) appearing on a screen. Only the digit 3 is a non-target, i.e. a response to any 3 should be suppressed. As the digits come at a high rate, approximately one per second, the responding quickly gets automatized, with the result that subjects are lured into reacting to the non-target 3 ('Oops!'). Robertson and Manly demonstrated that their paradigm has some validity in the study of head-injured subjects: these patients do not sustain their control as well as healthy subjects.

7 Hemi-inattention

Hemineglect or hemi-inattention differs from other impairments of attention by its basic nature: it is a disturbance in a preconscious aspect, i.e. our normally symmetrical orientation with respect to the outside world. This biological prerequisite is realized by a cortico–limbic–reticular loop and thus it can be disturbed by lesions at different anatomical levels (Mesulam 1985). Hemi-inattention, or neglect of one-half of the outer world, can manifest itself in all sensory domains and also in the motor domain. Clinically most important, however, is visual hemi-inattention. This is seen most frequently after lesions in the right hemisphere, in which case the patient no longer pays attention to stimuli from the left half of the visual field.

7.1 Assessing hemi-inattention

The first method of assessment is *observation*. A patient may bump into furniture on the left side or against the left doorpost. During testing, it can happen that the patient overlooks the first words or coloured stimuli in the Stroop Colour Words Test.

7.1.1 Line bisecting and drawing

For formal testing of neglect a large array of tests is available (Lezak 1995). A classic method of assessment of neglect is *line bisecting*, in which subjects have to mark the centre point of horizontal lines by placing an X on it (Marshall and Halligan 1990). Patients with left-sided neglect tend to deviate to the right pole of the lines, as they are not aware of the complete left half of these lines. Another paper-and-pencil approach of neglect is *drawing*: patients will often leave their drawings of a clock, star, or flower incomplete on the left side (Halligan and Marshall 1997). For obvious reasons, objects that are more or less symmetrical are most suitable for the judgement of hemi-inattention.

7.1.2 Visual search tasks

Next, neglect can be assessed with *visual search tasks* with either structured or unstructured fields. Structured fields consist of lines of stimuli as in Letter Cancellation Tests, while unstructured fields present quasi-random arrays of stimuli such as the Albert's Test and the Bells Test. In the latter, target stimuli are in fact grouped into seven columns and a ratio for neglect can be calculated based on numbers of omissions in 3 columns on the left versus 3 on the right side (Vanier *et al.* 1990).

7.1.3 Reading tests

Visual neglect can also be assessed with reading tests, in which words on the far left are neglected by the subject. A special case is the *Indented Paragraph Reading Test* (Caplan 1987) in which the first word of each line is indented from 0 to 25 spaces. This lay-out precludes the possibility that the neglecting subject could form a compensatory 'spatial set', as each refixation from the end of one line to the beginning of the next requires a separate act of controlled scanning.

7.1.4 The Test of Attentional Performance

In the last decade computerized assessment of neglect has been developed as well. The *Test of Attentional Performance* (Zimmermann and Fimm 2001) contains a subtest in which 3-digits numbers are presented that are distributed randomly over the screen of a personal computer. Among these, there are target numbers that seem to flicker, as their value is changing at a high rate. Subjects have to react to these apparently moving targets. As neglect patients attend predominantly to the non-target stimuli in the ipsilesional visual field, they miss the critical stimuli on the left half of the screen due to extinction.

7.1.5 The Behavioural Inattention Test

For those who want to study neglect extensively, Wilson *et al.* (1987) developed an attractive battery called the *Behavioural Inattention Test*. This test is composed partly of traditional hemineglect tests such as letter cancellation and line bisection, but it also contains tasks with a clear ecological validity, such as telephone dialing, coin sorting, and map navigation. For the set of conventional subtests, reliability is satisfactory ($r = 0.75$) while for the behavioural set it is excellent (test–retest $r = 0.97$).

8 Cognitive rehabilitation of attention

A more detailed review of the cognitive rehabilitation of attention is provided in Chapter 6. However, a few remarks can be made. First, the clinical neuropsychologist can advise his patients on how to cope with their attentional limitations, i.e. coach them in the 'management of slowness' (Spikman 2001). This boils down to supplying general *guidelines* that will be useful in various daily life tasks and situations. In Section 2.2 it was argued that the attentional demands of a given task situation are determined by two task characteristics: time pressure and structure. Thus, several guidelines can be formulated to reduce time pressure and improve the structure of tasks.

◆ Avoid or reduce time pressure.

◆ Create structure.

◆ Keep subtasks separate when possible.

◆ Avoid interruptions.

◆ Determine priorities in advance.

This approach has been formalized and validated by Fasotti *et al.* (2000) who devised a training called *Time Pressure Management* (TPM). This compensatory strategy training TPM teaches patients how to deal with their slowness. It consists of a general self-instruction ('Let me give myself enough time to do the task') followed by four specific steps in the form of questions the patient has to ask himself. These steps are as follows.

1 Anticipate time pressure by analysing stages in the task where two or more things have to be done at the same time.

2 Make a plan for things that can be done before the actual task begins.

3 Make an emergency plan to deal as quickly and effectively as possible with over-whelming time pressure.

4 Make regular use of the anticipatory plan and the emergency plan.

Fasotti *et al.* demonstrated that head-injured patients could learn this strategy and apply it to a new task, which consisted of reproducing the relevant information of a videotaped short story.

As described in Section 2.2, performance on a task is also determined by subject characteristics, in particular learning and *experience*. The history of attention training has shown, that 'attention in general' cannot be trained by stimulation or repetition. Time and again, it was found that training effects do not, or do not sufficiently, gener-alize to attention-demanding tasks in daily life. In contrast, task-specific training can be effective: it is possible to teach subjects to attend to relevant aspects within a given daily life task, even when this effect does not generalize. Hence, for the cognitive rehabilitation of attention, two options seem to exist: strategy training or task-specific training (for an extensive review, see Fasotti and Spikman 2002).

Selective references

Albert, M.L. (1973). A simple test of visual neglect. *Neurology* 23, 658–64.

Bohnen, N.I. (1991). *Mild head injury and postconcussive sequelae*. Doctoral dissertation, Rijksuniversiteit Limburg, Maastricht, the Netherlands.

Brickenkamp, R. (1981). *Test d-2, Aufmerksamkeits-Belastungstest*. Hogrefe Verlag, Göttingen.

Broadbent, D.E., Cooper, P.F., FitzGerald, P., and Parkes, K.R. (1982). The Cognitive Failures Questionnaire (CFQ) and its correlates. *Br. J. Clin. Psychol.* 21, 1–16.

Caplan, B. (1987). Assessment of unilateral neglect: a new reading test. *J. Clin. Exp. Neuropsychol.* 9, 359–64.

Fasotti, L., Kovacs, F., Eling, P.A.T.M., and Brouwer, W.H. (2000). Time pressure management as a compensatory strategy training after closed head injury. *Neuropsychol. Rehabil.* 10, 47–65.

Fasotti, L. and Spikman, J.M. (2002). Cognitive rehabilitation of central executive disorders. In *Neuropsychological rehabilitation: a cognitive approach* (ed. W.H. Brouwer, A.H. van Zomeren, I.J. Berg, J.M. Bouma, and E.H.F. de Haan), pp. 107–23. Boom, Amsterdam.

Gauthier, L., Dehaut, F., and Joannette, Y. (1989). The Bells Test: a quantitative and qualitative test for visual neglect. *Int. J. Clin. Psychol.* 11, 49–54.

Gronwall, D. and Sampson, H. (1974). *The psychological effects of concussion*. Auckland University Press, Auckland.

Halligan, P.W. and Marshall, J.C. (1997). The art of visual neglect. *Lancet* 350, 139–40.

Levin, H.S., High, W.M., and Goethe, K.E. (1987). The neurobehavioral rating scale: assessment of the behavioral sequelae of head injury by the clinician. *J. Neurol., Neurosurg., Psychiatry* 50, 183–93.

Lezak, M.D. (1995). *Neuropsychological assessment*. Oxford University Press, New York.

Marshall, J.C. and Halligan, P.W. (1990). Live bisection in a case of visual neglect: Psychophysical studies with implications for theory. *Cognitive Neuropsychology* 7, 107–30.

Mesulam, M.M. (1985). *Principles of behavioral neurology*. Davis, Philadelphia.

Mirsky, A.F., Anthony, B.J., Duncan, C.C., Ahearn, M.B., and Kellam, S.G. (1991). Analysis of the elements of attention: a neuropsychological approach. *Neuropsychol. Rev.* 2, 109–45.

Park, N.W., Moscovitch, M., and Robertson, I.H. (1999). Divided attention impairments after traumatic brain injury. *Neuropsychologia* 37, 1119–33.

Ponsford, J. and Kinsella, G. (1991). The use of a rating scale of attentional behaviour. *Neuropsychol. Rehabil.* 1, 241–57.

Posner, M.I. and Petersen, S.E. (1990). The attention system of the human brain. *Ann. Rev. Neurosci.* 13, 182–96.

Robertson, I.H. and Manly, T. (1997). *Oops! The Sustained Attention for Response Test, SART.* Neuropsychologia, 35, 747–58.

Robertson, I.H., Ward, T., Ridgeway, V., and Nimmo-Smith, I. (1994). *The Test of Everyday Attention.* Thames Valley Test Company, Bury St. Edmunds.

Rosvold, H.E., Mirsky, A.F., Sarason, I., Bransome, E.D., and Beck, L.H. (1956). A continuous performance test of brain damage. *J. Consult. Psychol.* 20, 343–50.

Shallice, T. (1988). *From neuropsychology to mental structure.* Cambridge University Press, Cambridge.

Spikman, J.M. (2001). *Attention, mental speed and executive control after closed head injury: deficits, recovery and outcome.* Doctoral thesis, University of Groningen.

Spikman, J.M., Deelman, B.G., and van Zomeren, A.H. (2000). Executive functioning, attention and frontal lesions in patients with chronic CHI. *J. Clin. Exp. Neuropsychol.* 22, 325–38.

Spikman, J.M., Kiers, H.A.L., Deelman, B.G. and Van Zomeren, A.H. (2001). Construct validity of concepts of attention in healthy controls and closed head injured patients. *Brain and Cognition* 47, 446–60.

Spreen, O. and Strauss, E. (1991). *A compendium of neuropsychological tests.* Oxford University Press, New York.

Stuss, D.T. and Benson, D.F. (1986). *The frontal lobes.* Raven Press, New York.

Vanier, M., Gauthier, L., and Lambert, J. (1990). Evaluation of left visuospatial neglect: norms and discrimination power of two tests. *Neuropsychology* 4, 87–96.

Wilson, B.A., Cockburn, J., and Halligan, P. (1987). *Behavioural Inattention Test.* Thames Valley Test Company, Titchfield.

Wilson, B.A., Alderman, N., Burgess, P.W., Emslie, H., and Evans, J.J. (1996). *BADS— Behavioural Assessment of the Dysexecutive Syndrome.* Thames Valley Test Company, Bury St. Edmunds.

van Zomeren, A.H. (1981). *Reaction time and attention after closed head injury.* Doctoral dissertation, University of Groningen.

van Zomeren, A.H. and Brouwer, W.H. (1994). *Clinical neuropsychology of attention.* Oxford University Press, New York.

Zimmermann, P. and Fimm, B. (1993). *Testbatterie zür Erfassung von Aufmerksamkeitsstörungen,* Version 1.02. Psytest, Freiburg.

Zimmermann, P. and Fimm, B. (2002). A test battery for attentional performance. In *Applied neuropsychology of attention* (ed. M. Leclercq and P. Zimmermann), pp. 110–51. Psychology Press, London.

Zoccolotti P. and Caracciolo B. (2002). Psychometric characteristics of attention tests in neuropsychological practice. In *Applied neuropsychology of attention* (ed. M. Leclercq and P. Zimmermann), pp. 152–85. *Psychology Press,* London.

Chapter 6

The rehabilitation of attentional deficits

Tom Manly and Ian H. Robertson

1 Overview

Over the last 30 years there have been considerable developments in how we understand attention. Of most relevance to the clinical field is the view that attention is not a single entity but rather a fractionated set of brain processes that are vulnerable to selective damage. (see Chapter 5). With a clearer idea of what we are looking at, the role of attention in influencing clinical outcome—both as a function in its own right and as an essential adjunct to the useful expression of other abilities—is becoming increasingly apparent.

As we will discuss, attention and other 'central' functions cannot be observed directly. The scientific inferential techniques of neuropsychology and clinical neuropsychology are essential in determining how these processes operate (and break down) and in making specific assessments. The contribution of a particular impairment to difficulties faced by patients in daily life is not always clear. In the rehabilitation of attention—as with any other deficit—a broader psychological perspective that takes into account coexisting impairment, premorbid factors, and the psychosocial context of a patient is vital. Pharmacological interventions for attentional disorders, at least for adults with neurological damage, are at a relatively early stage. Although very useful developments may take place in this respect, the role of the neuropsychologist in careful assessment and targeted rehabilitation is likely to remain crucial in fostering positive outcomes.

Here we examine various attempts to enhance the natural recovery of attentional processes—or to better manage the consequences of impairment—following adult brain injury. The results we review give grounds for cautious optimism. However, rehabilitation is—or should be—about working with patients to achieve functional goals in everyday life. If the promising findings showing changes on neuropsychological tests are to usefully filter through to clinical care, the extent to which these translate into meaningful functional improvements must be evaluated.

2 Contemporary views of attention

Improvements in assessment often trigger theoretical advances. In the case of attention, such assessment is inherently difficult. We cannot measure what happens when people attend in the abstract, so we must give them an activity to perform (read a passage, press a button, name colours, etc.). Variations in all the other abilities necessary for this task may well be just as influential as our 'hidden' attention system in determining performance. One way around this problem, and one that has probably underpinned much of the resurgence in scientific interest in attention over the past few decades, is to infer 'its' presence from the systematic variation in performance under different 'attentional conditions'. A simple and highly influential example of this approach can be found in visual cueing paradigms. Here participants are asked to keep their gaze fixated at the centre of a screen and to press a button as soon as they see a target appear. Whilst for the most part they will have no idea where this will be (and therefore should ideally monitor the whole screen), on a few trials they receive a helpful cue as to the most probable location. Such cues, when accurate, result in significant reductions in reaction times and, when inaccurate, in significant increases. As all other aspects of the task remain constant, these differences can be attributed to the participants prioritizing signals from one location—in other words—the movement of spatial attention (Posner 1980). A similar approach focusing on decrement and enhancement underpins many other areas such as the effect of distraction, the effect of time, and the consequences of attempting to perform two tasks simultaneously.

Such methods have led to much clearer accounts of the capacities and limitations of normal human attention and, when combined with the study of brain-damaged patients, neuroimaging, or neurophysiological techniques, to the neural basis of these abilities. Reviewing the area in 1990, Posner and Petersen (p. 26) proposed three key principles of attentional function.

> First . . . the attention system of the brain is anatomically separate from the data processing systems that perform operations on specific inputs even when attention is oriented elsewhere. In this sense, the attention system is like other sensory and motor systems. It interacts with other parts of the brain but maintains its own identity. Second, attention is carried out by a network of anatomical areas. It is neither the property of a single centre, nor a general function of the brain operating as a whole . . . Third, the areas involved in attention carry out different functions and these specific computations can be specified in cognitive terms.

They proposed that these different functions included, as discussed, the capacities:

♦ to prioritize signals from one spatial location (*spatial attention*);

♦ to prioritize some forms of information and to suppress others on the basis of a functional goal or a stored representation of a target (*selective* or *focused attention*);

♦ to self-maintain an alert, ready to respond state (*arousal/sustained attention*).

This and similar taxonomies (e.g. Van Zomeren *et al*. 1984; Mirsky *et al*. 1991; Cohen and Kaplan 1993) are, of course, provisional and vulnerable to further fractionation. The most important clinical implication is that deficits can arise that are exclusively or predominantly attentional in nature and that quite distinct forms of impairment profile (with quite different functional implications) can arise depending on the location and extent of damage. This should influence how we perform assessment and how we go about rehabilitation.

2.1 A note on terminology

There is a great deal of conceptual overlap between the fields of 'attention', 'executive function' (Chapter 18), and aspects of 'working memory' (Chapter 9). Whether one or another term is used often has more to do with terminological or theoretical preference than any imagined hard division. For example, the executive functions of the brain can be seen as resulting from a 'supervisory attentional system' (Norman and Shallice 1980) or attention viewed as the product of a central executive (Baddeley 1993). Certainly for rehabilitation it is often of greater use to specify more clearly what a patient actually has difficulty with (e.g. finds it difficult to follow conversations in noisy environments, fails to follow or adjust plans) than to subsume such problems beneath any of these higher-order theoretical categories.

3 Attention and outcome

As attention, in one form or another, pervades almost all aspects of our cognitive life we would expect far-reaching consequences of serious impairment. As the assessment of attention becomes more widespread, evidence supporting this contention is increasingly apparent. For example, improvements in attention, as indexed by simple reaction time, are one of the earliest predictors of emergence from posttraumatic amnesia following traumatic brain injury, consistent with a general role in 'bootstrapping' the rest of the cognitive system (Wilson *et al.* 1999). Further down the line, persistent problems in attention are associated with poor social and occupational outcome (Brooks and McKinlay 1987; McPherson *et al.* 1997; Woischneck *et al.* 1997).

In learning to cope with the consequences of brain damage, patients need to be aware of experiencing difficulties, to focus on rehabilitation techniques, and, often, to learn new strategies to get around problems. In each stage impairments in attention are likely to undermine progress. In addition to these functional properties there is now evidence that the neural correlates of 'paying attention' may play a more direct role in the recovery and organization of damaged circuits. Attention has been observed to modulate or 'gate' activity in primary sensory areas of the brain (Desimone and Duncan 1995). This has been reported in vision (Moran and Desimone 1985), audition (Woldorff *et al.* 1993), and in somatosensory perception (Drevets *et al.* 1995). The role of such inputs in influencing synaptic connectivity is suggested by animal (Recanzone *et al.* 1993) and now by human studies. Pascual-Leone and colleagues, for example, found that areas of the motor cortex associated with a particular action were enlarged following purely mental practice of this skill (Pascual-Leone *et al.* 1995).

Such factors may explain why the ability to attend and maintain a focus of attention may form a good predictor of recovery in other capacities. To take one example,

Robertson and colleagues found that sustained attention function assessed at 2 months poststroke formed a significant predictor of motor function and ability to perform activities of everyday living 2 years later (Robertson *et al.* 1997*b*; see also Ben-Yishay *et al.* 1968).

One very important reason to target attention deficits, therefore, is that, in addition to any direct effects, their presence may undermine recovery in other capacities and prevent the useful expression of abilities that may be relatively intact.

4 **A note on rehabilitation (see also Chapter 4)**

Clinical neuropsychology largely developed from (or in parallel with) the academic discipline of cognitive neuropsychology. However, the two fields should have very different priorities. In order to constrain models, cognitive psychology requires more and more focused assessments capable of isolating one or other specific capacity. For clinical neuropsychology an important aim is to predict difficulties in everyday life, for which such specific assessments may, at times, be rather ill-suited (see Wilson 1999; Burgess *et al.* 1998). The same difficulty can pervade what is viewed as rehabilitation. For many cognitive psychologists, rehabilitation is most interesting if it helps to constrain a model of the function in question, e.g. that a particular rehabilitative gambit might improve working memory as indexed by digit span performance. In contrast, patients—and therefore clinicians—should be most interested in what improves outcome at the level of functional goals. Having a long digit span might be nice for all sorts of reasons but it doesn't (in itself) get you to the shops.

In this chapter we therefore adopt a broad definition of rehabilitation that encompasses interventions at a number of levels:

- the restitution or enhancement of basic function;
- training in compensatory strategies;
- the use of environmental aids.

While our focus is on research that allows conclusions about specific interventions, it almost goes without saying that for individual patients a combination of approaches directed at achieving *their* particular individual goals is desirable.

5 **Unilateral neglect**

Unilateral neglect (or hemispatial neglect) is one of the most striking and extensively studied forms of attentional impairment (Robertson and Halligan 1999; Karnath, Milner and Vallar 2002). Perhaps not coincidentally, it is also the area where rehabilitation is most advanced. Unilateral neglect refers to a difficulty in detecting, acting on, or even thinking about information from one side of space. Patients may fail to notice food on the left side of their plate, fail to dress or wash the left side of their body, have difficulty in imagining the left side of familiar objects, and, in some cases, even deny ownership of their own left limbs (see the box below for an example). Although classically associated with lesions to the right posterior parietal cortex (Heilman and Watson 1977; Vallar and Perani 1986), neglect has been observed following damage to a variety of brain structures including the right prefrontal cortex and subcortical areas (Damasio *et al.* 1980; Mesulam 1981; Samuelsson *et al.* 1997; Karnath *et al.* 2001).

An example of unilateral neglect

Joan suffered a right hemisphere stroke in July 1999 that left her with quite extensive damage to the right parietal and temporal cortices. After an initial period in which she was very confused, staff at the hospital noted her tendency to keep her trunk, head, and eyes oriented to the right. Often, she would fail to notice people approaching her from the left (unless they were able to attract her attention by raising their voices) and would be unable to locate objects such as her teacup if it was to the left of her bed-table. Although her language and memory appeared relatively unaffected by the stroke, she had great difficulty in making any sense of what she read. Sometimes she appeared very confused, e.g. claiming after she had been moved to a different bed that she was no longer in the same hospital. Although she was capable of making some movements with her left arm, hand, or leg she largely ignored them. When asked by the psychologist to imitate an action with her left hand, she simply performed it with her right. Joan required help with washing and dressing and in navigating her wheelchair around the ward.

Four months after her stroke, Joan's persistent problems with left space were having serious implications for her rehabilitation sessions. The physiotherapists found it very difficult to get her to focus on left-sided movements and the occupational therapists found that many activities that she would have been able to perform without thinking—such as making a sandwich—were now an almost insurmountable ordeal. Unless there was to be a considerable change in these symptoms, the chances of Joan being able to return to an independent life style were slim.

5.1 The natural recovery of neglect

An attentional neglect of contralesional space is seen with approximately equal frequency (up to 50%) in patients with right or left hemisphere lesions in the immediate poststroke period (Stone *et al.* 1991, 1992). However, over the next weeks and months an asymmetry develops. Although the majority of patients with lesions to either hemisphere will spontaneously recover from the salient spatial bias, the remaining small group with persistent difficulties will be almost entirely comprised of right hemisphere patients.

An important question in thinking about rehabilitation is whether the spontaneous improvements in neglect take place primarily because of recovery of the underlying systems (e.g. through a reduction in diaschitic effects) or through the operation of compensatory mechanisms. Goodale *et al.* (1990) studied a group of nine right hemisphere patients 21 weeks after they had experienced a stroke. None of the patients now showed clinically significant signs of neglect and were able to reach for visual targets with the same accuracy as a control group. However, when the reach trajectories were analysed, significant deviations into right space were observed—deviations that were only corrected just before the hand reached the target. In addition, when patients were asked to estimate and reach towards the midpoint between two targets, significant rightward deviations were again apparent. Taken together with the results of Mattingley *et al.* (1994), this suggests that underlying distortions in the representation of space may persist in some or many cases but be masked in most day-to-day activity.

There is some evidence to suggest that these compensatory processes make demands on limited capacity resources. Robertson and Frasca (1992), for example, worked with patients who had apparently recovered from many aspects of neglect. When performing a simple reaction time task to left- and right-sided stimuli, no clear spatial bias was apparent. When, however, they were asked to simultaneously perform another attentionally demanding task, reaction times to left-sided targets were disproportionately compromised. Bartolomeo (2000) recently found that dual-task interference with a spatial task was relatively greater for 'recovered' neglect patients than for patients still showing clinical evidence of the disorder (who, by inference, were not yet using a compensatory strategy). In Section 6 we will return to limitations in *non-spatial* attentional capacity as a marker of persistent neglect.

Spontaneous reductions in neglect therefore occur for the majority of patients without the need for specific intervention, and compensation for a persistent spatial bias appears to be one mechanism underpinning these changes. Many patients who do not show spontaneous improvement are, however, able to become temporarily more aware of left-sided information if cued to do so (e.g. Riddoch and Humphreys 1983; Mattingley *et al.* 1993). The investigation of whether chronic patients can be trained to make compensatory scans has therefore been central to rehabilitation in this area.

5.2 Interventions

5.2.1 Scanning training

Early attempts encouraging leftward scans, such as asking patients to find the left side of a line of text before trying to read it, tended to show significant improvements on the trained materials, but little generalization to other activities (Lawson 1962; Seron *et al.* 1989; Wagenaar *et al.* 1992; Robertson 1990). At times the specificity could be striking, in one case not even transferring between two different editions of the same book (Lawson 1962). Although such failure to generalize does not preclude a useful rehabilitation effect, the need to train in each and every important context that a patient encounters would have clear resource implications.

It is possible that one barrier to generalized improvements in these studies lay not in the methods used *per se*, but in the diversity and duration of training. More recently, Pizzamiglio *et al.* (1992) provided scanning training to 13 patients between 3 and 34 months poststroke. The training, which took place over 40 sessions, included a wide variety of scanning tasks with cues (such as warning tones, flashing lights to the left of the display) being systematically faded as performance improved. Significant improvements were observed on the trained tasks and, most importantly, on untrained measures and life-like structured activities. Subsequent evaluation using a full randomized-controlled design verified the efficacy of these techniques (Antonucci *et al.* 1995).

5.2.2 **Non-volitional leftward scanning methods: optokinetic stimulation, caloric vestibular stimulation, neck muscle vibrations, and prism lenses**

Neglect is known to operate within different spatial frameworks. Patients may, for example, neglect the left side of objects within an array despite the represented (right) side of those objects being to the left of the array as a whole (object-centred neglect; Driver and Halligan 1991), or show dissociation between the degree of spatial bias between near (within arms reach) and far space (Halligan and Marshall 1991). There is also strong evidence of a distortion within egocentric coordinates and, in particular, a displacement of subjective body-midline to the right (Karnath 1994).

We discussed how the spontaneous compensatory strategies adopted by 'recovered' neglect patients appear to use limited capacity resources, which for some patients are a rather scarce commodity. A number of interventions are known, however, to induce distortions in the perception of (egocentric) space within healthy individuals regardless of their intentions. These have been harnessed to provide corrective input to neglect patients.

If healthy individuals watch a unidirectional moving background display, rapid involuntary eye movements and a subjective displacement of the body midline can be induced. If neglect patients are exposed to such displays during the performance of a spatial task, bias can be magnified or minimized according to the direction of movement (Pizzamiglio *et al.* 1990). Similar temporary but dramatic distortions can be induced:

- via the vestibular system by irrigation of the contralesional ear by cold water and/or the ipsilesional ear with warm water (Cappa *et al.* 1987; Rubens 1985);

- by vibration of the posterior neck muscle on the contralesional side (Karnath *et al.* 1993);

- by wearing prism spectacles that bring the contralesional periphery into central vision (Rossi *et al.* 1990).

Although these interventions have been theoretically useful in calibrating the spatial biases of neglect, the generally short-lived effects and requirement for less-than-portable apparatus have led to pessimism about their role in rehabilitation. However, it is possible that they may serve an important role as part of a more general training programme—perhaps particularly where patients have difficulty in exerting even temporary corrective control over neglect (Antonucci *et al.* 1995). Beis *et al.* (1999), for example, used patches to occlude the right visual field as a means of forcing increased awareness of left space. Three months after training the technique was associated with significantly improved eye movements and performance of everyday activities (compared with patching of the entire left eye and a no treatment control).

5.2.3 Limb-activation

Influential views of spatial attention suggest that it is intimately linked with the preparation for action (e.g. Rizzolatti and Camarda 1987; Allport 1992). It is certainly the case that changes in the motor context (e.g. the difference between reaching to point and reaching to pick up) can exert a significant influence on the degree of spatial bias shown by neglect patients (Robertson *et al.* 1995*a*). Halligan and Marshall (1989) reported that, when a patient used his left hand to perform a spatial task, he showed significantly less neglect of left space than when he used his right. Robertson and colleagues systematically examined these effects. In particular, they controlled for the inevitable visual cue formed by the moving hand by asking patients to make movements out of sight whilst performing a spatial task that required only a verbal (naming) response (Robertson and North, 1992, 1993, 1994; Robertson *et al.* 1994).

The results of this series of studies are summarized in (Fig. 6.1). They show that the most significant reductions in left-sided omissions are associated with the left hand moving within left space (defined relative to the patient's midline). Movement of the right hand within left space, or of the left hand within right space produced much less dramatic effects, and simultaneous movements of both hands abolished any benefits of left limb movement.

The important question is whether this striking experimental effect can be extended into improving everyday function. Two recent studies suggest that this is the case.

♦ Robertson and colleagues developed a portable 'neglect alert device' to prompt patients to continue to make left-hand movements (a buzzer sounded if the button was not pressed regularly). Significant improvements in a number of everyday spatial activities (including combing the hair and navigating around a hospital route) coincided with the onset of training (Robertson *et al.* 1998*a*).

♦ Wilson *et al.* (2000) worked with a 62-year-old man whose very strong left neglect (including of his own body) was seriously affecting his ability to take care of himself. To create an ecological measure his morning washing routine was divided into distinct steps (washing both arms, washing both legs, etc.). The measure of his independence was the number of prompts he required to complete each stage (prompts were given if activity stopped for 20 seconds). As shown in (Fig. 6.2), after a 10 day baseline the introduction of limb activation training was associated with a significant increase in his independence. Importantly, as was the case for some patients in Robertson *et al.*'s study, these gains were well maintained even when formal training had stopped.

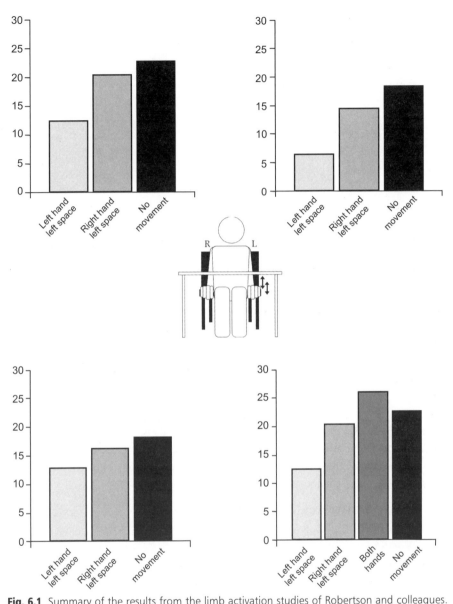

Fig. 6.1 Summary of the results from the limb activation studies of Robertson and colleagues. Unseen movement of the left hand to the left side of the body is associated with a reliable reduction in spatial attention bias. Movement of the left hand on the right, or of the right hand on the left produces less striking effects (units are the number of target omissions made by the patients).

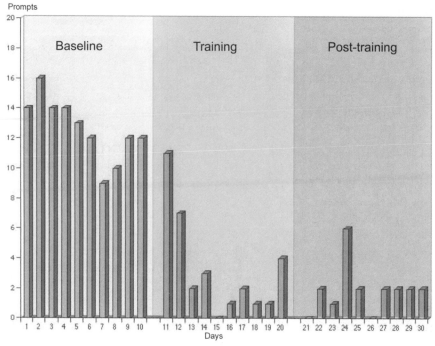

Fig. 6.2 Improvement in independence in a morning self-care programme with the introduction of limb activation training.

It seems possible, therefore, that in some cases the initial encouragement to use the left hand enhances awareness of left space—which in turn leads to greater spontaneous use of the left hand. By this means, a rather positive feedback loop could be established that maintains and enhances the effect.

5.2.4 **Sustained attention training**

Reading the textbooks one might imagine that the only difficulty experienced by patients with unilateral neglect is their curious lack of awareness of left space. This is rarely the case. Clinically, one very noticeable feature of such patients is the immense difficulty they can have in remaining engaged in *any* task—regardless of its spatial content. This impression is supported by research showing that patients with neglect have particularly poor sustained attention—even when compared to other patients with right hemisphere lesions (Robertson *et al.* 1997a; Samuelsson *et al.* 1988).

As with leftward cueing and use of the left hand, experimental evidence that the associated deficits of neglect and poorly maintained alertness are *functionally* connected may inform a different approach to rehabilitation. Such evidence emerged from a study in which patients were occasionally alerted by a loud tone as they performed a spatial task. Although the tone had no predictive value for whether a target would appear on left or right, when presented it completely abolished (and in some cases even reversed) the neglect (Robertson *et al.* 1998*b*).

Robertson *et al.* examined whether longer-term training in self-maintaining an alert, 'ready to respond' state could reduce neglect. In the training patients were asked to perform various nonspatial and rather tedious activities. Every so often (with the patient's prior consent) the therapist would bang the table top—both to cause an involuntary alerting effect and to cue patients to say to themselves 'Wake up!' or 'Attend'. In line with a procedure first described by Meichenbaum and Goodman (1971; see also Meichenbaum and Cameron 1973), the external cueing was progressively faded. In a multiple baseline × patient design (a method of controlling for spontaneous improvements), 1 week of daily training produced significant reductions in neglect on non-trained measures (Robertson *et al.* 1995*b*).

At least three very different approaches have therefore produced significant rehabilitative results with unilateral neglect. Other highly promising therapies, such as prism adaptation (Rossetti *et al.* 1998) and neck muscle vibration (Karnath *et al.* 1993), may also lead to tractable clinical results in due course. Unilateral neglect is a highly fractionated set of symptoms that can arise from damage to a variety of brain areas. More research is needed in clarifying the applicability of these methods to different manifestations of spatial bias and, indeed, in clarifying whether the effects may be additive in some cases.

6 Non-spatial attention

See the box for a case example of deficits in non-spatial attention.

An example of deficits in non-spatial attention

Brian was a well-educated man in his mid 40s. In 1995 he suffered a serious head injury in a road accident that left him in coma for 3 days. In many ways his recovery was remarkable. Over 2 years his performance on tests of reasoning and memory returned to above average levels. Unfortunately, it was only when Brian returned to work that his remaining deficits became apparent. His job required a great deal of flexibility. In order to achieve goals and meet deadlines he would need to keep track of a changing situation, re-prioritize, and switch between one activity and another. It was precisely this level of organization that Brian now found so difficult. He was now highly distractable and would leave jobs unfinished or fail to notice crucial details that he had omitted. At home he found it difficult to complete simple jobs without needing constant reminders and was described by his wife as often drifting into a world of his own. Despite retaining many of his premorbid abilities, Brian was now very frustrated by his inability to harness these effectively in order to achieve goals.

6.1 **Interventions**

6.1.1 A behavioural, goal-based approach

Our discussion of unilateral neglect focused on interventions designed to improve underlying ability, as this can represent a more general solution to the functional problems experienced by the patient. When the underlying problems are less clearly understood, as is currently the case for many forms of non-spatial attention, it can be more appropriate to tackle a specific activity. Wilson and Robertson (1992), for example, worked with a man whose severe head injury had left him with problems in 'keeping his mind' on what he was reading. They adopted a rather behavioural approach. Initially, the man was asked to monitor how many times his attention slipped when he was reading. In training he was initially encouraged to read for only very brief periods. If these were completed without slip the duration of the subsequent session was increased by 10%. Over 160 sessions in 40 days, the goal of reliably reading for 5 minutes without a slip was attained. Most importantly, the number of slips reported when reading material relevant to his job—although not directly trained—had also significantly reduced.

This systematic, shaping approach does not tell us a great deal about the underlying nature of the difficulties experienced by the patient. There was also little evidence that the training produced any improvements in other activities in this case (although this can be very hard to measure). It does show, however, that appropriate reinforcement and learning can modulate the consequences of poor attention and offers a technique that could be easily applied to many situations.

6.1.2 Improving attention through general training

We have seen how the duration of rehabilitation may be crucial. The revolution in computer technology and price over the last 2 decades has made long periods of systematic and reflexive training increasingly possible. For researchers, the use of computers to 'deliver' therapy also means that exposure to treatment can be highly standardized—improving the interpretation of particular factors that can promote performance change.

In a study by Gray et al. (1992), 31 patients with reported attention difficulties were randomly allocated to one of two conditions. One consisted of approximately 15 hours of computerized training including:

- a reaction time task with feedback on speed;
- a task requiring the identification of two identical digit strings from a briefly presented array of 4;
- a digit–symbol translation task;
- a colour-word Stroop task.

The other condition was 15 hours of recreational computing.

Immediately following the 3–9 week training, the experimental group showed significant improvements on two *non-trained* tasks relative to the controls, the Wechsler Adult Intelligence Scale (WAIS)-R Picture Completion subtest, which requires visual search and reasoning, and the Paced Auditory Serial Addition Task (PASAT), widely considered as primarily a measure of processing speed (Gronwall and Sampson 1974). At 6 months follow-up, the benefits on these measures had been maintained and, in addition, further untrained measures were showing training benefit (backward digit span, mental arithmetic, and WAIS-R Block Design).

As the groups were well matched on task performance prior to training, the results suggested both that the training had produced generalized improvements and that a 'sleeper effect' led to continued improvement beyond the training period. While little evidence exists on this, it is possible to speculate that such effects emerge both through consolidation of the learning and from the increased exposure to attentionally demanding situations consequent upon initial improvements.

The results are persuasive in suggesting a specific effect that, thanks to the well matched control group, cannot be interpreted in terms of generalized recovery. The generalization to *functional activities* of everyday life was not, however, examined in this study.

6.1.3 Training specific functions

We have discussed how attention is viewed as a fractionated set of processes. If this is the case then training one form of attention may have minimal consequences for another. Sturm *et al.* (1997) examined this by randomly allocating 38 stroke patients to different training programmes. The programmes, which were made up of separate modules targeting a particular form of attention, differed only in the order in which the modules were presented. If attentional functions were relatively encapsulated, observed improvements should broadly follow the order of training. If they were not, or if the patients were simply showing spontaneous recovery, no particular pattern should emerge.

Each of the exercises was in the form of a computer game that became more challenging as performance improved. Alertness, for example, was trained using a motorbike simulation while selective attention required the patients to 'shoot' one but not another form of target. Improvements were evaluated on an untrained computerized measure (Zimmermann *et al.* 1993). After approximately 56 hours of training the hypothesis was substantially supported. The detection rate for targets in the untrained test battery vigilance task was significantly improved only after vigilance training and not following training in selective or divided attention. Similarly, reaction times in the selective attention test were improved following selective, but not sustained attention training. As might be expected, some cross-over effects were also observed. Performance on the divided attention task, for example, was significantly enhanced following training in selective, as well as divided, forms of attention.

6.2 **Environmental support for attention**

Within specialist clinical settings it is possible to organize the environment in a way that minimizes demands on patients deficient attentional and executive skills (e.g. reducing distraction, having a very set schedule, keeping a written record of an agreed plan, systematic reinforcement of goal-directed behaviour). Such techniques can be useful in helping very severely impaired patients to control inappropriate behaviour and to focus on other important rehabilitation goals (see Alderman and Ward 1991; Alderman and Burgess 1994; Alderman 1996), but are clearly inappropriate for many patients with less severe problems. Recently, we have been examining whether it is possible to introduce 'portable' environmental support for attention that is compatible with (and hopefully enhances) independence. This type of approach is neatly demonstrated in a case study by Evans *et al.* (1998). They describe a patient who had suffered damage to her frontal cortex. Although on many standard IQ and memory tests her function was relatively well preserved, in everyday life she had great difficulty in achieving goals and was highly dependent on the support of others. In particular (as has been described in a number of frontal patients), she appeared to get overly caught up in whatever activity she was currently performing and completely ignored her other essential activities. The patient was given an electronic pager that had originally been designed for amnesic patients—remotely sending messages to cue an important activity (the 'Neuropage' system; Wilson *et al.* 1997). In this case, its introduction significantly improved her capacity to begin goal-directed activity, often without her needing to see the content of the message. It appeared that this environmental intrusion was acting to refocus her attention on her goals and, once this had occurred, her other intact capacities allowed her to achieve them.

To investigate these effects at a group level we (Manly *et al.*, 2002) developed a modification of the Six Elements Test (Shallice and Burgess 1991) in which patients were asked to perform a number of tasks associated with running a hotel (calculating bills, ordering conference labels alphabetically, proof-reading a tourism leaflet, etc.). As with the Six Elements, the key feature was that the total time available for the test (20 minutes) was far less than the time required to fully complete each component task. In order to comply with the goal of trying *some* of *each* activity in the test, patients would therefore need to plan at the outset to switch tasks at a certain frequency and to keep this goal actively in mind throughout the test. As with the patient reported by Evans *et al.*, the key error made by the traumatically brain-injured patients we worked with was to become so engrossed in one activity that this goal was neglected.

The patients were administered two versions of the task in random order 1 week apart. During one session we told the patients that they would periodically hear a rather salient bleeping noise and that this was a reminder to them to think about what they were doing in the task. In this group, not only did the presence of the tone significantly improve their performance, the performance had now become indistinguishable from that of healthy control participants. This result was useful in ruling out a number of other causes of poor performance in the test such as failure to understand the task or remember what the plan was. Most importantly, it suggests that, even if attention can not be directly improved, its functional consequences on complex activities can be minimized. Developments in mobile phone, pager, and palm-top computer technologies make such interventions increasingly possible.

7 Summary

The scientific study of functions that are *specifically* attentional, although at an early stage, has begun to inform improved assessment and rehabilitation for neurological patients. Perhaps the most important development lies in seeing attention not as a single entity but as a set of processes that are vulnerable to separate damage and that can have very different consequences. As assessment has improved, the negative impact that poor attention on recovery and outcome is increasingly clear—evidence that makes interventions designed to enhance natural recovery in these systems a particularly pressing clinical goal.

We have reviewed different approaches to working with attentional deficits:

◆ attempting to improve underlying function;
◆ targeting particular behavioural/functional goals;
◆ using external aids to maximize residual function.

Work with unilateral neglect is by far the most advanced area in this field. Three separate interventions, training patients to make compensatory left-ward scans, encouraging use of the left hand and arm, and teaching self-alerting techniques have all produced generalized improvements—other techniques exploiting new experimental effects may well follow. Although often more loosely defined, work with non-spatial attentional functions has also produced positive results. It has been demonstrated that systematic practice and reinforcement can shape attentive behaviour—perhaps to a much greater degree than has proved possible in the rehabilitation of memory (Wilson 1999). Carefully evaluated computer training packages have produced clear and apparently rather specific improvements in function.

A key feature in a number of the studies we have considered seems to be the duration of training. Whether the processes necessary to enhance basic function are learning new strategies, using different neural pathways to achieve the same ends, or plastic re-organization within damaged areas, effects should not be expected within a few sessions.

For researchers, clinicians, and, most particularly, patients, careful evaluation of interventions is essential. Showing changes on well controlled experimental designs and using targeted neuropsychological measures is essential in understanding the specific relationship between what we do and any improvements, but this is not, in itself, rehabilitation. Many of our operational definitions of attention have been imported from cognitive psychology and the relationships between these entities and everyday difficulties can sometimes be obscure. While it defies belief to argue that we have cognitive capacities that are only tapped by neuropsychological tasks and untouched in daily life, a great deal more work is needed in examining the impact of particular deficits and the functional consequences of any improvements that we might help bring about.

Selective references

Alderman, N. (1996). Central executive deficit and response to operant conditioning methods. *Neuropsychol. Rehabil.* 6 (3), 161–86.

Alderman, N. and Burgess, P.W. (1994). A comparison of treatment methods for behaviour disorder following herpes simplex encephalitis. *Neuropsychol. Rehabil.* 4 (1), 31–46.

Alderman, N. and Ward, A. (1991). Behavioural treatment of the dysexecutive syndrome: reduction in repetitive speech using response cost and cognitive overlearning. *Neuropsychol. Rehabil.* 4 (4), 65–80.

Allport, A. (1992). Attention and control: have we been asking the wrong questions? A critical review of twenty-five years. In *Attention and Performance*, Vol. XIV (ed. D. E. Meyer and S. Kornblum), pp. 183–218. MIT Press, Cambridge, Massachusetts.

Antonucci, G., Guariglia, C., Judica, A., Magnotti, L., Paolucci, S., Pizzamiglio, L., and Zoccolotti, P. (1995). Effectiveness of neglect rehabilitation in a randomized group study. *J. Clin. Exp. Neuropsychol.* 17, 383–9.

Baddeley, A.D. (1993). Working memory or working attention. In *Attention: selection, awareness and control: a tribute to Donald Broadbent* (ed. A.D. Baddeley and L. Weiskrantz), pp. 152–70. Oxford University Press, Oxford.

Bartolomeo, P. (2000). Inhibitory processes and spatial bias after right hemisphere damage. *Neuropsychological Rehabilitation* 10 (5), 511–26.

Beis, J.M., Andre, J.M., Baumgarten, A., and Challier, B. (1999). Eye patching in unilateral spatial neglect: efficacy of two methods. *Archives of Physical Medicine and Rehabilitation* 80, 71–6.

Ben-Yishay, Y., Diller, L., Gerstman, L., and Haas, A. (1968). The relationship between impersistence, intellectual function and outcome of rehabilitation in patients with left hemiplegia. *Neurology* 18, 852–61.

Brooks, D.N. and McKinlay, W. (1987). Return to work within the first seven years of severe head injury. *Brain Injury* 1, 5–15.

Burgess, P.W., Alderman, N., Evans, J., Emslie, H., and Wilson, B.A. (1998). The ecological validity of tests of executive function. *J. Int. Neuropsychol. Soc.* 4, 547–58.

Cappa, S.F., Sterzi, R., Vallar, G., and Bisiach, E. (1987). Remission of hemineglect and anosognosia during vestibular stimulation. *Neuropsychologia* 25, 775–82.

Cohen, R.A. and Kaplan, R.F. (1993). Attention as a multicomponent process—neuropsychological validation. *J. Clin. Exp. Neuropsychol.* 15 (3), 379.

Damasio, A.R., Damasio, H., and Chui, H.C. (1980). Neglect following damage to frontal lobe or basal ganglia. *Neuropsychologia* 18, 123–32.

Desimone, R. and Duncan, J. (1995). Neural mechanisms of selective visual attention. *Annual Review of Neurosci.* 18, 193–221.

Drevets, W.C., Burton, H., Videen, T.O., Snyder, A.Z., Simpson, J.R., and Raichle, M.E. (1995). Blood flow changes in human somatosensory cortex during anticipated stimulation. *Nature* 373, 249–52.

Driver, J. and Halligan, P.W. (1991). Can visual neglect operate in object-centred co-ordinates? An affirmative single-case study. *Cognitive Neuropsychology* 8, 475–96.

Evans, J.J., Emslie, H., and Wilson, B.A. (1998). External cueing systems in the rehabilitation of executive impairments of action. *J. Int. Neuropsychol. Soc.* 4, 399–408.

Karnath, H.-O., Milner, D. and Vallar, G. (2002). The cognitive and neural bases of spatial neglect. Oxford University Press, Oxford.

Goodale, M.A., Milner, A.D., Jakobson, L.S., and Carey, D.P. (1990). Kinematic analysis of limb movements in neuropsychological research: subtle deficits and recovery of function. *Canadian Journal of Psychology*, **44**, 180–95.

Gray, J.M., Robertson, I.H., Pentland, B., and Anderson, S.I. (1992). Microcomputer based cognitive rehabilitation for brain damage: a randomised group controlled trial. *Neuropsychol. Rehabil.* **2**, 97–116.

Gronwall, D.M.A. and Sampson, H. (1974). *The psychological effects of concussion.* Auckland University Press, Auckland.

Halligan, P.W. and Marshall, J.C. (1989). Laterality of motor response in visuo-spatial neglect: a case study. *Neuropsychologia* **27**, 1301–7.

Halligan, P.W. and Marshall, J.C. (1991). Left neglect for near but not far space in man. *Nature* **350**, 498–500.

Heilman, K. M. and Watson, R. T. (1977). The neglect syndrome—a unilateral deficit of the orienting response. In *Lateralisation in the nervous system* (ed. S. Harnad, R. W. Doty, L. Goldstein, J. Jaynes, and G. Krauthamer), pp. 285–302. Academic Press, New York.

Hier, D.B., Mondlock, J., and Caplan, L.R. (1983). Recovery of behavioural abnormalities after right hemisphere stroke. *Neurology* **33**, 345–50.

Karnath, H.O., Christ, K., and Hartje, W. (1993). Decrease of contralateral neglect by neck muscle vibration and spatial orientation of trunk midline. *Brain* **116**, 383–96.

Karnath, H. O. (1994). Subjective body orientation in neglect and the interactive contribution of neck muscle proprioception and vestibular stimulation. *Brain* **117**, 1001–12.

Karnath, H.O., Ferber, S., and Himmelbach, M. (2001). Spatial awareness is a function of the temporal not the posterior parietal lobe. *Nature* **411**, 950–3.

Lawson, I.R. (1962). Visual-spatial neglect in lesions of the right cerebral hemisphere: a study in recovery. *Neurology* **12**, 23–33.

Manly, T., Hawkins, K., Evans, J. J., Woldt, K., & Robertson, I. H. (2002). Rehabilitation of executive function: facilitation of effective goal management on complex tasks using periodic auditory alerts. *Neuropsychologia* **40** (3), 271–81.

Mattingley, J.B., Pierson, J.M., Bradshaw, J.L., Phillips, J.G., and Bradshaw, J.A. (1993). To see or not to see: the effects of visible and invisible over on line bisection judgements unilateral neglect. *Neuropsychologia* **31**, 1201–15.

Mattingley, J.B., Bradshaw, J.L., Bradshaw, J.A., and Nettleton, N.C. (1994). Residual right attentional bias after apparent recovery from right hemisphere damage: implications for a multicomponent model of neglect. *Journal of Neurology, Neurosurgery and Psychiatry* **57**, 597–604.

McPherson, K., Berry, A., and Pentland, B. (1997). Relationships between cognitive impairments and functional performance after brain injury, as measured by the functional assessment measure (FIM+FAM). *Neuropsychological Rehabilitation*, **7** (3), 241–57.

Meichenbaum, D. and Cameron, R. (1973). Training schizophrenics to talk to themselves: a means of developing attentional control. *Behav. Ther.* **4**, 515–34.

Meichenbaum, D. and Goodman, J. (1971). Training impulsive children to talk to themselves: a means of developing self-control. *J. Abnormal Psychol.* **77**, 115–26.

Mesulam, M.M. (1981). A cortical network for directed attention and unilateral neglect. *Ann. Neurol.* **10**, 309–25.

Mirsky, A.F., Anthony, B.J., Duncan, C.C., Ahearn, M.B., and Kellam, S.G. (1991). Analysis of the elements of attention: a neuropsychological approach. *Neuropsychol. Rev.* **2**, 109–45.

Moran, J. and Desimone, R. (1985). Selective attention gates visual processing in the extrastriate cortex. *Science* **229**, 782–4.

Norman, D. A. and Shallice, T. (1980). Attention to action: willed and automatic control of behaviour: Centre for Human Information Processing (Technical Report No. 99).

Pascual-Leone, A., Dang, N., Cohen, L.G., Brasilneto, J.P., Cammarota, A., and Hallett, M. (1995). Modulation of muscle responses evoked by transcranial magnetic stimulation during the acquisition of new fine motor skills. *J. Neurophysiol.* **74**, 1307–45.

Pizzamiglio, L., Frasca, R., Guariglia, C., Incoccia, C., and Antonucci, G. (1990). Effect of optokinetic stimulation in patients with visual neglect. *Cortex* **26**, 535–40.

Pizzamiglio, L., Antonucci, G., Judica, A., Montenero, P., Rrazzano, C., and Zoccolotti, P. (1992). Cognitive rehabilitation of the hemineglect disorder in chronic-patients with unilateral right brain-damage. *J. Clin. Exp. Neuropsychol.* **14** (6), 901–23.

Posner, M.I. (1980). Orientating of attention. *Quart. J. Exp. Psychol.* **32**, 3–25.

Posner, M.I. and Petersen, S.E. (1990). The attention system of the human brain. *Ann. Rev. Neurosci.* **13**, 25–42.

Recanzone, G.H., Schreiner, C.E., and Merzenich, M.M. (1993). Plasticity in the frequency representation of primary auditory cortex. *J. Neurosci.* **13**, 87–103.

Riddoch, M.J. and Humphreys, G.W. (1983). The effect of cueing on unilateral neglect. *Neuropsychologia* **21**, 589–99.

Rizzolatti, G. and Camarda, R. (1987). Neural circuits for spatial attention and unilateral neglect. In *Neurophysiological and neuropsychological aspects of neglect* (ed. M. Jeannerod). North Holland Press, Amsterdam.

Robertson, I. (1990). Does computerized cognitive rehabilitation work? A review. *Aphasiology* **4** (4), 381–405.

Robertson, I.H., and Frasca, R. (1992). Attentional load and visual neglect. International Journal of *Neuroscience*, **62**, 45–56.

Robertson, I.H. and North, N. (1992). Spatio-motor cueing in unilateral neglect: the role of hemispace, hand and motor activation. *Neuropsychologia* **30**, 553–63.

Robertson, I.H. and North, N. (1993). Active and passive activation of left limbs: influence on visual and sensory neglect. *Neuropsychologia* **31**, 293–300.

Robertson, I.H. and North, N. (1994). One hand is better than two: motor extinction of left hand advantage in unilateral neglect. *Neuropsychologia* **32**, 1–11.

Robertson, I.H., Tegnér, R., Goodrich, S.J., and Wilson, C. (1994). Walking trajectory and hand movements in unilateral left neglect: a vestibular hypothesis. *Neuropsychologia* **32** (12), 1495–502.

Robertson, I. H., Nico, D., and Hood, B. (1995). The intention to act improves unilateral neglect: two demonstrations. *Neuroreport* **7**, 246–8.

Robertson, I.H., Tegnér, R., Tham, K., Lo, A., and Nimmo-Smith, I. (1995*b*). Sustained attention training for unilateral neglect: theoretical and rehabilitation implications. *J. Clin. Exp. Neuropsychol.* **17**, 416–30.

Robertson, I.H., Manly, T., Beschin, N., Haeske-Dewick, H., Hömberg, V., Jehkonen, M., Pizzamiglio, L., Shiel, A., Weber, E., and Zimmermann, P. (1997*a*). Auditory sustained attention is a marker of unilateral spatial neglect. *Neuropsychologia* **35**, 1527–32.

Robertson, I.H., Ridgeway, V., Greenfield, E., and Parr, A. (1997*b*). Motor recovery after stroke depends on intact sustained attention: a 2-year follow-up study. *Neuropsychology* **11** (2), 290–5.

Robertson, I.H., Hogg, K., and McMillan, T.M. (1998*a*). Rehabilitation of unilateral neglect: improving function by contralesional limb activation. *Neuropsychol. Rehabil.* **8** (1), 19–29.

Robertson, I.H., Mattingley, J.M., Rorden, C., and Driver, J. (1998*b*). Phasic alerting of neglect patients overcomes their spatial deficit in visual awareness. *Nature* **395**, 169–72.

Robertson, I.H. and Halligan, P.W. (1999). *Spatial neglect: A clinical handbook for diagnosis & treatment.* Erlbaum, Hove, East Sussex.

Rossetti, Y., Rode, G., Pisella, L., Farne, A., Li, L., Boisson, D., and Perenin, M.T. (1998). Prism adaptation to a rightward optical deviation rehabilitates left hemispatial neglect. *Nature* **395**, 166–9.

Rossi, P.W., Kheyfets, S., and Reding, M.J. (1990). Fresnel prisms improve visual perception in stroke patients with homonymous hemianopia or unilateral visual neglect. *Neurology* **40**, 1597–9.

Rubens, A.B. (1985). Caloric stimulation and unilateral visual neglect. *Neurology* **35**, 1019–24.

Samuelsson, H., Hjelmquist, E., Jensen, C., Ekholm, S., and Blomstrand, C. (1988). Nonlateralized attentional deficits: an important component behind persisting visuospatial neglect? *J. Clin. Exp. Psychol.* **20** (1), 73–88.

Samuelsson, H., Jensen, C., Ekholm, S., Naver, H., and Blomstrand, C. (1997). Anatomical and neurological correlates of acute and chronic visuospatial neglect following right hemisphere stroke. *Cortex* **33**, 271–85.

Seron, X., Deloche, G., and Coyette, F. (1989). A retrospective analysis of a single case neglect therapy: a point of theory. In *Cognitive approaches to neuropsychological rehabilitation* (ed. X. Seron and G. Deloche), pp. 236–89. Laurence Erlbaum Associates, Hillsdale, New Jersey.

Shallice, T. and Burgess, P. (1991). Deficit in strategy application following frontal lobe damage in man. *Brain* **114**, 727–41.

Stone, S.P., Wilson, B.A., Wroot, A., Halligan, P.W., Lange, L.S., Marshall, J.C., and Greenwood, R.J. (1991). The assessment of visuo-spatial neglet after acute stroke. *J. Neurol., Neurosurg., Psychiatry* **54**, 345–50.

Stone, S.P., Patel, P., Greenwood, R.J., and Halligan, P.W. (1992). Measuring visual neglect in acute stroke and predicting its recovery: the visual neglect recovery index. *J. Neurol., Neurosurg., Psychiatry* **55**, 431–6.

Sturm, W., Willmes, K., Orgass, B., and Hartje, W. (1997). Do specific attention deficits need specific training? *Neuropsychol. Rehabil.* **7** (2), 81–103.

Vallar, G. and Perani, D. (1986). The anatomy of unilateral neglect after right-hemisphere stroke lesions: a clinical/CT scan correlation study in man. *Neuropsychologia* **24**, 609–22.

Van Zomeren, A.H., Brouwer, W.H., and Deelman, B.G. (1984). Attentional deficits: the riddles of selctivity, speed and alertness. In *Closed head injury. Psychological social and family consequences* (ed. D.N. Brooks). Oxford University Press, Oxford.

Wagenaar, R.C., Wieringen, P.C.W.V., Netelenboss, J.B., Meijer, O.G., and Kuik, D.J. (1992). The transfer of scanning training effects in visual attention after stroke: five single case studies. *Disability Rehabil.* **14**, 51–60.

Wilson, B.A. (1999). *Case studies in neuropsychological rehabilitation.* Oxford University Press, Oxford.

Wilson, B.A., Evans, J.J., Emslie, H., Balleny, H., Watson, P.C., and Baddeley, A.D. (1999). Measuring recovery from post traumatic amnesia. *Brain Injury* **13** (7), 505–20.

Wilson, B.A., Evans, J.J., Emslie, H., and Malinek, V. (1997). Evaluation of NeuroPage: a new memory aid. *J. Neurol., Neurosurg., Psychiatry* **63**, 113–15.

Wilson, C. and Robertson, I.H. (1992). A home-based intervention for attentional slips during reading following head injury: a single case study. *Neuropsychol. Rehabil.* **2**, 193–205.

Wilson, F.C., Manly, T., Coyle, D., and Robertson, I.H. (2000). The effect of contralesional limb activation training and sustained attention training for self-care programmes in unilateral spatial neglect. *Restor. Neurol. Neurosci.* **16** (1), 1–4.

Woischneck, D., Firsching, R., Ruckert, N., Hussein, S., Heissler, H., Aumuller, E., and Dietz, H. (1997). Clinical predictors of the psychosocial long term outcome after brain injury. *Neurological Research*, **19** (3), 305–10.

Woldorff, M.G., Gallen, C.C., Hampson, S.A., Hillyard, S.R., Pantev, C., Sobel, D., and Bloom, F.E. (1993). Modulation of early sensory processing in human auditory cortex during auditory selective attention. *Proc. Natl Acad. Sci. USA* **90**, 8722–6.

Zimmermann, P., North, P., and Fimm, B. (1993). Diagnosis of attentional deficits: theoretical considerations and presentation of a test battery. In *Developments in the assessment and rehabilitation of brain damaged patients* (ed. F. Stachowiak). G. Narr-Verlag, Tübingen.

Chapter 7

Assessment of perceptual disorders

L.D. Kartsounis

1 Sensation and perception

For many centuries philosophers have been asking questions about the validity of human experiences. To understand this issue a distinction should be made between sensation and perception. The senses capture information from the environment in various forms of physical energy (*stimulus*). They accomplish this via specially dedicated receptors of a single cell or a group of cells. The receptors convert this energy into appropriate neural signals (*sensory transduction*). Subsequent elaborations and interpretations of the neural signals in different parts of the brain (broadly referred to as *perceptual processes*) enable one to become aware of external stimulation. It is often forgotten that we do not solely derive our experience of the outside world from our senses.

1.1 Principles of assessment of perceptual disorders

The neural events taking place between sensory stimulation and interpretation are normally experienced as 'automatic'. This 'automaticity' may be lost with brain damage/disease (injury, stroke, tumour, anoxia, degenerative disorder). The affected patient is then unable to analyse environmental stimuli meaningfully. Neurologists, neuropsychologists, and other professionals are asked to identify the deficit(s) responsible for the breakdown—a task often akin to a detective's work.

For the assessment of perceptual impairments the examiner needs to be acquainted with the chain of events between sensory stimulation and awareness of stimuli. It requires sound understanding of both the nature of stimuli as sounds, sights or smells and the abilities of humans to discriminate disparate types of neural signals. Different techniques have been developed for the assessment of perceptual skills as they relate to physical stimuli (*psychophysics*). Some testing procedures have been refined into standardized formal tests. However, from time to time, procedures may need to be invented 'on the spot'. Clearly, these procedures are not in keeping with mental test theory and lack normative data. The implicit assumption in these cases is that there is discontinuity between normal and abnormal performance that can readily and universally be understood.

When perceptual skills are assessed, a range of constitutional, cultural, and other factors ought to be taken into account, including the following.

♦ Individuals may vary in their ability to distinguish different stimulus signals due to primary sensory deficits. Some people have defects in the eyes that prevent them from experiencing the full range of colours. Others have defects in their ears or tongues and are unable to experience aspects of sounds (e.g. pitch) and taste (e.g. bitter).

♦ With advancing age, senses become less sensitive and perceptual experiences become 'bland'.

♦ The state of the perceiver may also influence the perception of a stimulus. The experience of the warmth of water in a basin does not depend on the temperature in the water alone but on the perceiver's own state at the time. If his or her hand had previously been in hot water, the water of the basin would feel cold and vice versa (John Locke).

♦ A patient may be unable to comply with the demands of tests due to deficits in skills different to those being examined, e.g. severe language problems would hinder a patient responding appropriately to tests of tactile sensitivity.

In clinical practice the assessments of perceptual skills are undertaken by different professionals. Neurological examinations include the assessment of sensory organs (eye, ear, nose), perception of pain, touch, etc. in different parts of the body. From a neuropsychological point of view the best known types of perceptual deficits are:

♦ auditory;

♦ tactile;

♦ visual.

A common term, 'agnosia', may be applied to all of them, implying inability to know or interpret sensory experiences.

2 Auditory recognition deficits

This is a group of disorders consisting of impairments in the ability to recognize verbal and nonverbal sounds. A *cortically deaf* patient presents with a range of auditory perceptual deficits, including abnormal pure tone, sound localization, and temporal auditory analysis.

The term '*auditory sound agnosia*' refers to a loss of the ability to recognize common sounds, e.g. bell ringing, dog barking, and train, that is not due to cortical deafness. When asked to identify these sounds the patient makes mistakes, e.g. a telephone ring may be interpreted as a sound of a railroad crossing.

2.1 Word deafness (verbal auditory agnosia)

The term '*pure word deafness*' refers to the impairment in analysing/understanding spoken words in the context of preserved recognition of nonverbal sounds and relative preservation of spontaneous speech, reading, and writing. Unlike patients with primary comprehension problems (transcortical sensory aphasia), those with pure word deafness deficits are impaired on word repetition tasks. Word deafness is associated with bilateral temporal damage. The critical lesions are thought to disconnect Wernicke's areas from auditory input. This is in keeping with observations indicating that the patients are neither deaf nor aphasic.

Despite the adjective 'pure', clinical experience suggests that word deafness may be associated with an impairment in temporal resolution of auditory stimuli or abnormal click-fusion thresholds, although the predominant deficit involves spoken word stimuli. It is critical the clinician establishes the integrity of primary auditory perceptual skills before a diagnosis of word deafness is made. As a first step, ask the patient to discriminate softly spoken words or finger snaps. For proper delineation of a patient's auditory sensory/perceptual skills an audiological assessment is required. This includes measures of pure tone audiometry and speech detection thresholds. Provided significant auditory sensory deficits and aphasia are excluded, the assessment for word deafness may proceed by asking the patient to discriminate whether spoken pairs of words and nonwords are the same or different (house/*house* versus house/*mouse*, pef/*bef*) (e.g. Kay *et al.* 1992). These tests require special care.

- Prevent lip reading.
- Make sure the patient is able to 'hold' in mind and compare two items.
- Stimulus pairs may differ according to the examiner's voice and accent (use a native speaker with clear articulation).
- It may be difficult to convey to the patient the requirements of the test and you will need to use pictorial material to demonstrate the nature of the task.

2.2 Auditory amusia

This refers to a loss of the ability to recognize familiar music (well-known melodies or a particular voice). Both hemispheres contribute to music appreciation and the anatomical correlates of amusia are multiple (underpinning the multifactorial nature of music). Given also the wide range of individual differences in innate ability and musical education/exposure, the assessment of auditory amusia is very difficult. Melody perception, however, may be assessed by various subtests of the Seashore Test of Musical Talent.

3 Tactile recognition deficits

These are impairments in object recognition by touch, in the absence of somatosensory impairment, neglect, aphasia, or dementia. Tactile agnosia as a selective disorder has been the subject of dispute in the past, not least due to lack of precise quantitative measures.

Somaesthetic functions may be divided into basic, intermediate, and complex types (Caselli 1997).

◆ *Basic* somaesthetic impairments include light touch, position sense, vibration, two-point discrimination, pain perception, and temperature (usually assessed by neurologists).

◆ *Intermediate* somaesthetic impairments include texture discrimination and simple form discrimination that is part of *astereognosis* (usually assessed by neurologists, sometimes by neuropsychologists).

◆ *Complex* somaesthetic impairments are disorders of pure forms of tactile agnosia, with preserved basic and intermediate functions. Tactile agnosia is usually associated with damage to parietal operculum.

Somaesthetic deficits are unilateral and the examiner may use a patient's good hand as control. Tactile agnosia may initially be assessed by light touch, position sense, etc. Patients are asked to discriminate texture and basic form by touch (e.g. between different kinds of edges, flat and curved surfaces). If they pass these tests (reflecting basic and intermediate skills), ask them to name objects by touch. Each object (e.g. a cassette tape) is placed randomly in either hand. Tests of tactual memory may be added, e.g. 'Which is smoother an almond or a walnut', to ensure that the deficit is specific to the tactile modality (see Reed *et al.* 1996). If patients are aphasic they will have difficulty in naming objects placed in either hand. When they have a specific difficulty in naming objects palpated with only one hand, tactile agnosia may be inferred.

4 Visual object recognition deficits

Visual object recognition deficits are much more common in clinical neuropsychological practice than in other modalities. They are also much better understood and, hence, in this review, they are presented in more detail.

4.1 Historical background

The first descriptions of visual object recognition disorders can be traced in the nineteenth century. In 1890 Lissauer made a distinction between deficits in the ability to consciously perceive stimuli and those reflecting an inability to ascribe meaning to what is perceived. He referred to them as *aperceptive* and *associative* 'mindblindness', respectively. Similarly, in 1891 Freud made a distinction between deficits of sensation and disorders of '*gnosis*' (knowledge)—hence the term '*agnosia*' (without knowledge). This terminology has largely survived but there is no general agreement as to what the term 'perceptual' (as in aperceptive mindblindness) denotes. For some cognitive neuropsychologists it encapsulates a wide range of deficits ranging from early visual processing to high-level object recognition impairments (e.g. Farah 1990, Humphreys, and Riddoch 1987). For others (including the present author) the term refers to more circumscribed deficits that arise after satisfactory early visual processing is accomplished and before meaning is ascribed to stimuli (see McCarthy and Warrington 1990). This is not just a theoretical point—the distinction between early visual (cortical) deficits and aperceptive deficits corresponds to different anatomical correlates and is therefore of diagnostic significance (Table 7.1). There is a wider ongoing debate regarding the classification of impairments in visual cognition. Unlike cognitive psychologists, visual physiologists and anatomists appear reluctant to accept notions of high-level visual 'agnosic' deficits. Instead, they consider them to signify impairments in integrating sensory information or accessing long-term memory.

4.2 Caveats

The assessment of deficits in object recognition needs to be flexible and adaptable to the individual patient. A patient's performance may be impaired as a result of deficits in other cognitive domains.

- A test involving, say, drawing may primarily be failed due to motor deficits (sensory/motor weaknesses, dyspraxia) or planning (executive) problems.

- Visual object recognition tests may be failed due to sensory deficits, visuospatial neglect, severely restricted visual fields, or impairments in eye movements. The latter include disorders involving subcortical/brainstem structures and frontal eye fields (e.g. Luria 1976).

- Tests dependent on verbal responses may not be appropriate for dysphasic patients.

When multiple deficits are present, you need to validate observations with additional testing (this requires considerable expertise and, at times, inventiveness by the examiner).

Visual object recognition impairments may be due to a variety of deficits, although the outcome is the same. They range from *early visual (cortical) processing disorders* to high-level deficits relating to the structure and identity of objects (*visual agnosias*).

Table 7.1 Object recognition deficits

Early visual processing	Visual agnosias	
	Aperceptive	**Associative**
Acuity	Inability to access structure/spatial properties of visual stimuli	Inability to access meaning of visual stimuli
Eye fixation (visual disorientation)		
Movement (akinetopsia)		
Shape discrimination		
Figure/ground discrimination		
Colour (achromatopsia)		
Texture		
Anatomical correlates		
Posterior brain (occipital lobes)	Right post-Rolandic hemisphere	Inferior left post-Rolandic hemisphere
No hemispheric asymmetry		

4.3 Early visual processing disorders

Early visual processing skills are organized in a modular form. They involve specialized areas of the posterior part of the brain that code different properties, including colour, size, basic shape, and movement. Given their segregation, these skills may be selectively impaired with brain damage/disease in the occipital lobes (*partial cortical blindness*). There is no asymmetry between the two hemispheres at this level of visual processing. Early visual processing deficits are generally assessed with tests measuring physical differences between two or more stimuli.

4.3.1 Acuity

Occipital lobe damage may affect visual acuity similarly to disorders of the eye or optic nerve. There may be effects on the ability to detect the presence or absence of light, different changes in contrast sensitivity, and a target varying in size. A significant impairment in one of these aspects of acuity results in deficits in object recognition by sight. Acuity can be assessed by Snellen charts and other similar ophthalmological instruments.

When assessing visual acuity the ability of the patient to cope with the demands of commonly used acuity charts needs to be considered. Patients with lesions in the posterior areas of the brain may perform poorly for reasons other than poor acuity. They may find it difficult to fixate on or scan visual targets due to *visual disorientation, visuospatial neglect, or simultanagnosia* (inability to perceive more than one stimulus at a time). To exclude such problems, ask the patient to count or point to random arrays of dots (e.g. Counting Dots test, Visual Object and Space Perception (VOSP) battery; Warrington and James 1991) or to pick up small items (e.g. paper clips) from a desk. An alternative way of assessing problems of visual disorientation is to ask the patient to reach with the index finger a visual target in different parts of space. Patients with visual disorientation are very inaccurate when attempting these simple tasks.

The acuity of patients with problems in fixating stimuli or scanning visual arrays (above) may be assessed with a test comprising simple shapes (square, circle, triangle) decreasing in size. Each target stimulus is presented individually and the clinician obtains good visual acuity measures (James *et al.* 2001).

4.3.2 Movement

The ability to locate points in space (Section 4.3.1) dissociates from the ability to detect movement of stimuli in space. A selective impairment in the perception of movement (*akinetopsia*) is very rare and associated with lateral occipitotemporal lesions. The perception of motion is thought to be *retinotopically* organized (confined to one visual field contralateral to the lesion).

Zihl *et al.* (1991) described a female patient who was able to locate targets in space but was unable to detect their movements. Visual scenes appeared to her as a series of static snapshots. She was unable to perceive traffic or to use motion as a cue when attempting to pour liquid.

For the assessment of akinetopsia, record what a patient reports when observing moving objects in space, e.g. vehicles. The patient may report a car in positions A and B but not between these two points. Milder forms of this disorder need to be studied with special equipment in ophthalmological departments.

4.3.3 Size

Some patients may be able to recognize small but not 'large' visual stimuli, e.g. letters of the alphabet (Kartsounis and Warrington 1991). This disorder may be independent of any sensory problems, including restrictions in visual fields.

Assessment of size perception:

◆ Ask the patient to judge whether lines of the same or different lengths are the same or not. Present pairs of lines in random order, one pair at a time. To control for possible visual field defects or inattention, the lines may be printed horizontally, vertically, and in other directions.

◆ Ask the patient to judge whether pairs of simple geometric shapes (e.g. circles) are of the same size or not (Fig. 7.1). Present randomly the same and different pairs of shapes.

4.3.4 Shape/form

Patients may become impaired in form perception due to bilateral occipital lesions. These patients may have good visual acuity and be able to perceive colours, match surface textures, and locate obstacles in space.

Efron (1968) described a patient who was unable to recognize objects and his impairment was attributed to this fundamental deficit. Efron devised a shape discrimination test comprising stimuli of squares and oblongs matched for total surface area and contrast (simplified form of the test in Fig. 7.2). Each test stimulus is presented individually and the patient is asked to indicate whether it is a square or an oblong.

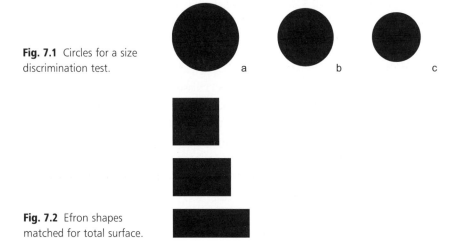

Fig. 7.1 Circles for a size discrimination test.

a   b   c

Fig. 7.2 Efron shapes matched for total surface.

Research has indicated that certain visual skills may support action but not conscious discrimination of stimuli. A patient described by Milner and colleagues performed at chance level in discriminating a square from an oblong pattern of equal area, up to a ratio of 1 : 2. Despite her lack of awareness of shapes, she was able to reach and pick up solid rectangular blocks of different widths without difficulty. Her grip was perfectly precalibrated (aperture between her index finger and thumb) during midreach for a skilled grasp. These observations are consistent with the notion that there are two visual systems, one serving action (dorsal stream) and the other serving visual discrimination and cognition (ventral stream) (Milner 1997).

4.3.5 Figure—ground discrimination

An early visual processing skill involves figure—ground discrimination. This enables the viewer to analyse separately the defining outlines of a stimulus and its background. Impairments of this skill are associated with occipital lesions and may dissociate from form perception deficits (Davidoff and Warrington 1993). A useful test for the assessment of figure—ground discrimination deficits is included in the VOSP (Warrington and James 1991) (Fig. 7.3(a)).

Several other tasks can be used for the assessment of this disorder. Ask the patient to identify line drawings of simple geometric shapes, e.g. a square, circle or triangle, each printed separately on a card. If the patient performs this task satisfactorily, then proceed with overlapping drawings comprising geometric shapes. Patients with figure—ground discrimination impairment may fail to report whole shapes or report parts of them (Fig. 7.3(b)). They may similarly be impaired in perceiving subjective contours (Fig. 7.3(c)).

4.3.6 Colour

Achromatopsia refers to impairment in colour perception. A patient may be unable to see colour at all or perceive colours as lacking in intensity. Impairments in colour perception are associated with occipitotemporal lesions. They may be confined to one visual field contralateral to a lesion (retinotopic).

Assessment of colour perception:

♦ Exclude congenital abnormalities.

♦ Ask the patient to name, match colour patches, or arrange them in a series according to brightness or saturation.

—The *Holmgren Wool Test* consists of pieces of wool that the patient is asked to sort according to their hues.

—The *Farnsworth–Munsell 100-Hue and Dichotomous Test for Color Vision* (Farnsworth 1943) is a more demanding task requiring the patient to arrange in the appropriate sequence coloured small counters (matched for saturation and brightness) according to hue.

—The *Ishihara plates* can also be used for testing colour vision but they may not be sensitive to milder cases of achromatopsia.

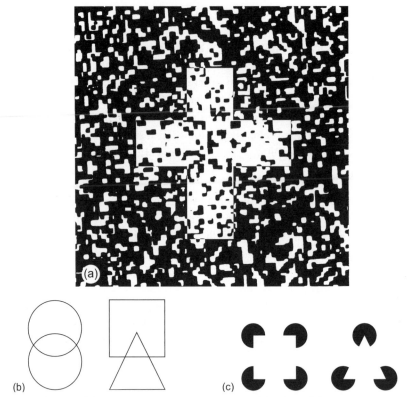

Fig. 7.3 Examples of figure–ground discrimination tests. (a) Adapted from VOSP. (b) Overlapping geometric shapes. (c) Kanizsa type figures.

Unlike patients with retinal coloured blindness, achromatopsic patients are impaired in all sectors of the spectrum, although discrimination of shades of grey may be preserved.

◆ For some patients who are unable to cope with tasks involving a large number of items (above) a new test has been devised. It comprises arrays of a few colour patches of the same hue varying in brightness, including one colour patch of 'medium' brightness but of different hue. The patient is asked to indicate which patch is the odd one out (James *et al.* 2001).

Patients with left posterior lesions may have normal colour vision but are impaired in naming/comprehending colour names. Others may present with a loss of colour knowledge (*colour agnosia*). These patients find it difficult to colour accurately with crayons black and white drawings of objects, fruit, animals (e.g. a frog may be painted blue). These tests require special care—a deficit in object recognition (Section 4.4) may confound results.

4.3.7 Texture

Psychology textbooks refer to different examples of illusory phenomena whereby perspective (impression of depth) influences perceived size (Fig. 7.4(a)). However, surfaces that recede in depth (Fig. 7.4(b)) and have a visible texture, e.g. the grain in wood, may have additional effects. Texture gradients may provide precise information about the distances of surfaces and the sizes of stimuli on these surfaces. Abrupt changes in texture gradient may signal the presence of edges and corners, and strongly influence the perception of stimuli (Gibson 1950). It is possible that texture perception is selectively preserved or impaired in the same way as other early visual processing skills.

Assessment of texture perception:

◆ Ask the patient to describe stimuli with different texture gradients. Impairment is identified when the patient is unable to perceive the effects of texture (analogous deficit to the inability to perceive illusory phenomena).

4.4 Higher visual recognition disorders

These deficits refer to visual agnosias for *objects* or *faces* (*prosopagnosia*). The diagnosis of these disorders presupposes well preserved primary sensory and early visual processing systems (Section 4.3). Higher visual recognition problems are due to a failure in attainment of a coherent structured percept (*structural perception*) or in assignment of meaning to an object or face (*semantic processing*).

4.4.1 Structural perception of objects

In life, objects are encountered in unlimited variations. Normally, we are able to recognize them both in prototypical and a range of unconventional views and lighting conditions. This ability relates to *object constancy*, which may become impaired with right post-Rolandic lesions.

Patients with this disorder (*apperceptive agnosia*) are unable to process the necessary information for the attainment of coherent spatial properties of objects. It is thought that there is stored representation of objects (*object-centred representation*) with information about volume and structure of familiar objects. When this information cannot be

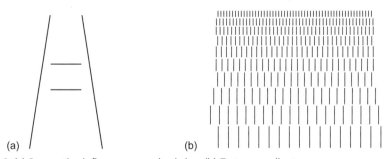

Fig. 7.4 (a) Perspective influences perceived size. (b) Texture gradient.

accessed, the affected patient cannot identify degraded (or rotated) versions of familiar objects. In non-optimal conditions this results in misidentification of objects.

For the assessment of deficits in structural perception ('*visual perceptual deficits*' proper) a variety of test materials can be used, examples of which can be seen in Fig. 7.5. Many perceptual tasks are dependent on the ability of the patient to communicate verbally. The Object Decision test (VOSP) does not require verbal responses and can be used for the assessment of aphasic patients (the patient is simply required to point to target stimuli). Other tests may also be used without requiring the patient to respond verbally—ask patient to match incomplete stimuli, with their complete versions, e.g. incomplete letters, with alternative 'solid' letters.

4.4.2 Semantic processing of objects

Patients with a disorder in semantic processing (*associative visual agnosia*) perform satisfactorily on early visual processing and perceptual tests (Sections 4.3 and 4.4.1). They are able to copy objects and pictures of stimuli but fail to say what they are. Their problem is not a naming deficit. It reflects their inability to provide accurate information about the uses of objects, colour, and size and where they can be found. These patients cannot indicate whether two visually distinct examples of the 'same' object, e.g. two types of glass, have identical function. However, they may be able to identify objects by

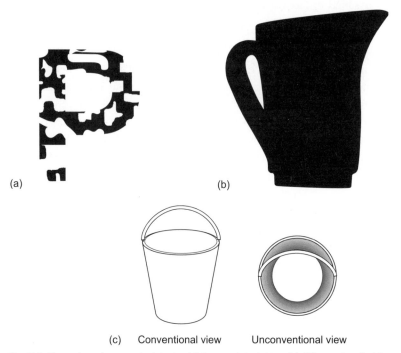

(a)　　　　　　　　　　　　　　　　(b)

(c)　　Conventional view　　　Unconventional view

Fig. 7.5 Examples of perceptual tests. (a) Incomplete letter. (b) Silhouette of object. (c) Conventional view; unconventional view of object.

touch. Associative visual agnosia does not necessarily affect all types of visual stimuli, e.g. face recognition may be spared. Studies in the past suggested that semantic processing deficits are associated with bilateral posterior brain lesions. More recently, single-case studies of agnosic patients with unilateral left posterior (inferotemporal) lesions have superseded the earlier reports (e.g. McCarthy and Warrington 1986). That unilateral left posterior lesions are sufficient to give rise to associative visual agnosia is also indicated from group studies—patients with right posterior hemisphere lesions are impaired on perceptual tasks; patients with left posterior lesions are impaired in matching tasks.

Assessment of associative visual agnosia:

◆ Present patients with pictures or models of animals, tools, or other objects and ask them to name them, ask them about their properties and where they can be found. A naming test that includes different categories of stimuli can be used for this purpose (McKenna 1997).

Be aware. Patients may be unable to identify by name objects due to *optic aphasia*. In this disorder, both visual and verbal semantic knowledge may be preserved but a disconnection between these two cognitive domains prevents the patient from naming an object. Patients with optic aphasia are able to demonstrate by other (nonverbal means) the uses of objects.

◆ Present patients with pictures of a wide range of objects (e.g. kitchen items, tools, sport equipment, animals, means of transport) and ask them to sort them according to use or the category to which they belong.

◆ Real and unreal objects (comprising configurations of features of objects that may or may not be encountered in the real world) can also be used (Riddoch and Humphreys 1993; Fig. 7.6). Ask patients to say whether these items exist in the real world or not.

◆ Ask patients to choose which one of two pictures relates to a target picture (Fig. 7.7). A test using this technique is the *Pyramids and Palms Trees Test* (Howard and Patterson 1992). The distractors in this task are chosen to be similar to the items matched so that the patient would find it difficult to choose simply on the basis of visual similarity.

4.4.3 Structural perception of faces

Impairments in recognition of familiar faces are collectively referred to as prosopagnosia. They are thought to be distinct deficits in visual recognition. The core deficit lies in a selective, faulty perceptual analysis of faces (other types of visual stimuli may be perceived normally). This disorder is associated with lesions in the posterior regions of the right hemisphere.

Assessment of deficits in structural perception of faces:

◆ Patients may be assessed on tasks involving photographs of three or more faces differing in sex or age ('who is the oldest?'), with faces photographed from different viewpoints or with same/different expressions ('is it the same or different person?').

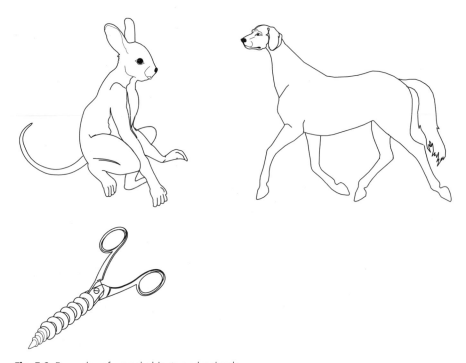

Fig. 7.6 Examples of unreal objects and animals.

Patients affected by structural deficits find it difficult to tackle these tasks or are very slow in their responses, tending to use a feature-by-feature analysis.

◆ More formally, structural disorders in face recognition can be assessed with the *Benton Facial Recognition Test* (Benton *et al.* 1978). Patients are required to find a target face amongst six alternative faces shown in different viewpoints and different lighting conditions.

4.4.4 Semantic processing of faces

Patients with this type of prosopagnosia are capable of passing structural perceptual tasks (Section 4.4.3) but are unable to recognize familiar faces. They may be able to recognize them by other features, including their voices, hairstyles, and clothing. Semantic deficits in face recognition can be assessed using photographs of family members, friends, and well known public figures.

A test for measuring face recognition ability has been devised by Young and colleagues (Ellis *et al.* 1989). It consists of two sets of public figures, one comprising 20 very well known people (e.g. Margaret Thatcher, John Wayne) and another comprising 20 'low-familiarity' faces (e.g. Marlene Dietrich and Max Bygraves). A further set of 20

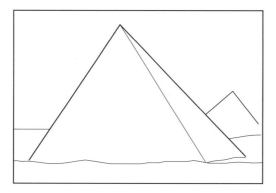

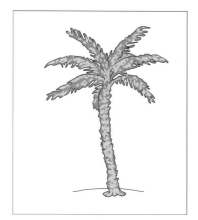 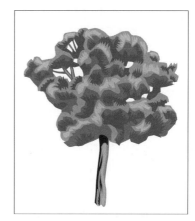

Fig. 7.7 Example of semantic processing task.

comprises unfamiliar faces. The test requires that each face is first rated for familiarity on a 7-point scale ('totally unfamiliar'–'highly familiar'). Then the subject is asked to provide the known person's profession and name. This is a sensitive test, yielding quantitative measures at different levels of familiarity, leading to complete recognition of a face. It is limited by the fact that 'familiar' faces need to be updated. Another potential critical variable that may confound results is the individual patient's media exposure (or lack thereof; e.g. Kapur *et al.* 1999).

Prosopagnosic patients may show covert recognition skills for faces. Although unable to identify faces verbally, they may show differential electrodermal responses to familiar and unfamiliar faces involving correct and incorrect name–face pairings. Prosopagnosic patients may also show different reaction times and memory performance towards familiar and unfamiliar faces. However, these techniques are not readily accessible to a clinical neuropsychologist and are usually used as research tools.

4.4.5 False recognition of faces

A complementary deficit to prosopagnosia may be observed in patients with right frontal lesions, that is, 'recognition' for unfamiliar faces. This type of deficit is considered to be due to the impairment in strategic memory retrieval and monitoring skills of patients with frontal lesions.

4.4.6 Recognition of emotional expressions

The ability to recognize emotional expressions may dissociate from the ability to identify faces. Patients with right hemisphere damage are more impaired than those with left hemisphere damage. They may become impaired in recognizing the emotion of fear (following amygdalectomy) and disgust (presymptomatic patients with Huntington's disease). For the assessment of these disorders clinicians may devise their own stimuli depicting unambiguous emotions. For a greater variety of emotional expressions see e.g. Ekman *et al.* (1972).

5 Conclusion

The implicit assumption in the review above is that visual object recognition skills have a hierarchical and parallel organization (Table 7.1). In ordinary clinical practice, however, object recognition disorders are 'random'. The question arises as to where a clinician should start when assessing a patient with object and/or face recognition problems.

The first consideration must be to obtain information on potential sensory problems, visuospatial neglect, aphasia, etc. that may at least partly account for perceptual/agnosic deficits. As a general rule, clinicians should be alert to the complaints and errors patients make during other tasks involving picture interpretation. They may 'misname' (misperceive) common objects or give 'don't know' answers when asked to name them. Questions about the properties/uses of these stimuli may elicit further information about the underlying impairments—e.g. whether these reflect language or visual recognition deficits. Patients' answers may also suggest the level of the visual recognition deficit.

- If they refer to very limited, basic features of an object when shown a picture (e.g. 'there is a line here and another one there . . .'), it may be assumed that the disorder reflects an early visual processing deficit. Formal tests of early visual processing should then be the starting point (e.g. point localization to exclude visual disorientation, form perception, figure/ground discrimination).

- If patients are able to indicate the basic structural form of a stimulus but fail to identify it correctly, their deficits are more likely to be of a higher order. In these cases the assessment should start with tests of apperceptive agnosia (object decision, incomplete letters tasks, and other degraded stimuli).

- When perceptual skills are found to be well preserved, proceed with tests of associative agnosia (questions about properties of objects, matching tasks, etc.) (Table 7.2).

Table 7.2 Tests of object recognition deficits

Early visual processing	Visual agnosias	
	Aperceptive	**Associative**
◆ *Acuity* Snellen charts, Queen Square*	Incomplete Letters, Object Decision, Silhouettes (VOSP)	Questions *re* names, colour, size, location, functions of objects (pictures/models)
◆ *Visual disorientation* Point Localization, Dot Counting *Size*: see Fig. 7.1	Stimuli shown from unconventional views (BORB)	Sorting of stimuli (pictures/ models) according to category
◆ *Shape*: see Fig. 7.2	*Copying tasks*	Matching objects that are visually dissimilar but have the same function
◆ *Figure/ground* VOSP ◆ *Colour* Holmgren Wool Test, Farnsworth–Munsell 100-Hue Test, Queen Square*, Ishihara		The Pyramids and Palm Trees Test
◆ *Texture*: see Fig. 7.4(b)		

* Queen Square Cortical Vision Screening Test.

Clearly, when a patient is known to be grossly impaired in analysing a wide range of real stimuli, including objects, faces, etc., testing should begin with early visual processing tasks. If the patient fails these tests, there is no need for tests of visual agnosias either of the aperceptive or associative type—any agnosia diagnosed in this context would be 'pseudo-agnosia' (Warrington 1985).

The assessment methods outlined above are adequate for the identification of the main types of impairments in object recognition. Occasionally, and for a more precise definition of a deficit, the clinician may need to devise a series of new tests. In doing so, both the precise nature of a deficit may be delineated and refinement in our knowledge of object recognition may be attained. This knowledge can then be harnessed for the development of more sensitive and accurate methods of assessment.

Selective references

Benton, A.L., Hamsler, K., Varney, N.R., and Spreen, O. (1978). *Contributions to neurological assessment.* Oxford University Press, New York.

Caselli, R.J. (1997). Tactile agnosia and disorders of tactile perception. In *Behavioural neurology and neuropsychology* (eds. T.E. Feinberg and M.J. Farah), pp. 277–88. McGraw-Hill, New York.

Davidoff, J. and Warrington, E.K. (1993). A dissociation of shape discrimination and figure–ground perception in a patient with normal acuity. *Neuropsychologia* 31, 83–93.

Ellis, A.W., Young, A.W., and Critchley, E.M.R. (1989). Loss of memory for people following temporal lobe damage. *Brain* 112, 1469–83.

Farah, M.J. (1990). *Visual agnosia*. MIT Press, Cambridge, MA.

Farnsworth, D. (1943). Farnsworth–Munswell 100-Hue and Dichotomous Test for Color Vision. *J. Opt. Soc. Am.* 33, 568–78.

Gibson, J.J. (1950). *The perception of the visual world*. Houghton-Mifflin, Boston.

Howard, D. and Patterson, K. (1992). *The Pyramids and Palm Trees Test*. Thames Valley Test Company, Bury St Edmunds.

Humphreys, G.W. and Riddoch, M.J. (1987). *To see or not to see: a case study of visual agnosia*. Lawrence Erlbaum, London.

James, M., Plant, G.T., and Warrington, E.K. (2001). *The Queen Square Cortical Vision Screening Test*. Thames Valley Test Company, Bury St Edmunds.

Kapur, N., Thompson, P., Kartsounis, L.D., and Abbott, P. (1999). Retrogade amnesia: clinical and methodological caveats. *Neuropsychologia* 37, 27–30.

Kartsounis, L.D. and Warrington, E.K. (1991). Failure of object recognition due to a breakdown of figure–ground discrimination in a patient with normal acuity. *Neuropsychologia* 29, 969–80.

Kay, J., Lesser, R. and Coltheart, M. (1992). *Psycholinguistic assessments of language processing in aphasia*. Lawrence Erlbaum Associates, Hove, East Sussex.

Luria, A.R. (1976). *The working brain, an introduction to neuropsychology*. Penguin Books, Middlesex.

McCarthy, R.A. and Warrington, E.K. (1986). Visual associative agnosia: a clinico-anatomical study of a single case. *J. Neurol. Neurosurg. Psychiatry* 49, 1233–40.

McCarthy, R.A. and Warrington, E.K. (1990). *Cognitive neuropsychology, a clinical introduction*. Academic Press, London.

McKenna, P. (1997). *The Category-Specific Names Test*. Psychology Press, Hove, East Sussex.

Milner, A.D. (1997). Vision without knowledge. *Phil. Trans. R. Soc. Lond. B, Biol. Sci.* 352, 1249–56.

Reed, C.L., Caselli, R.J., and Farah, M.J. (1996). Tactile agnosia: underlying impairment and implications for normal tactile object recognition. *Brain* 119, 875–88.

Riddoch, M.J. and Humphreys, G.W. (1993). *Birmingham Object Recognition Battery* (*BORB*). Lawrence Erlbaum Associates, Hove, East Sussex.

Warrington, E.K. (1985). Agnosia: the impairment of object recognition. In *Handbook of clinical neurology*, Vol 45 (eds. P.J. Vinken, G.W. Bruyn, and H.L. Klawans), pp. 333–49. Elsevier Science Publishers, Amsterdam.

Warrington, E.K. and James, M. (1991). *Visual Object and Space Perception Battery* (*VOSP*). Thames Valley Test Company, Bury St Edmunds.

Zihl, J., Von Cramon, D., and Schmid, C.H. (1991). Disturbance of movement vision after bilateral posterior brain damage. *Brain* 114, 2235–52.

Chapter 8

Recovery and treatment of sensory perceptual disorders

Georg Kerkhoff

1 Basic principles of perceptual relearning

In a summary of studies about perceptual learning in the three main modalities, Gibson (1953) showed that nearly any sensory or motor ability can be improved considerably by training in healthy subjects. This holds also true for sensory-perceptual relearning after brain damage. However, the capacity for full recovery through training is often limited by several factors, i.e. aetiology, age, and size of lesion, as well as the modality and the sensory ability (see box below).

Principles of treatment in sensory perceptual neurorehabilitation

- **Restitution.** Direct, repetitive training of the impaired function is expected to promote improvements that are important in themselves, but also relevant for other related abilities (e.g. training of basic somatosensory abilities improves this ability, but also has positive effects on motor performance since somatosensory perception is important for motor control (see Section 3.2). The efficacy of restitutive treatments is more limited in 'lower' cortical areas (e.g. primary sensory cortex) than in 'higher cortical areas' (parietal lobe; Buonomano and Merzenich 1998).

- **Compensation.** Utilization of a spared function to compensate for a deficit, e.g. in patients with homonymous scotomata the treatment of visual scanning and reading effectively reduces everyday problems associated with the field cut (bumping into obstacles or persons, slow reading) but has little effect on the field defect itself. Compensation techniques are widely used in sensory perceptual rehabilitation because restitution of elementay sensory deficits is often strictly limited due to the relatively fixed brain topography of primary sensory cortical representations (primary visual, auditory, or somatosensory cortices).

Principles of treatment in sensory perceptual neurorehabilitation *(continued)*

- ◆ **Substitution**. Use of technical/prosthetic devices to compensate for a deficit (e.g. use of special light-absorbing glasses in patients with blinding to reduce the amount of light). Also, environmental changes designed to adapt the patient's environment optimally to the patients's deficits that cannot be cured by restitution nor compensation treatments (e.g. modifying the house of a patient to improve his spatial orientation and reduce falls).

- ◆ **Combination of principles**. In sensory perceptual neurorehabilitation it is often necessary and fruitful to combine two or all three principles listed above to maximize outcome for the patient.

2 Visual disorders

Visual perceptual disorders occur after brain damage in about 30% of the patients with cerebrovascular disorders and some 50% of patients with traumatic brain injury (TBI). Consequently, routine screening of the various types of visual deficits is necessary for rehabilitation planning. Nonneglecting patients can easily be given the questionnaire in Table 8.1 and 95% of the patients make correct indications.

2.1 Visual acuity

Primary and secondary causes of impaired static visual acuity have to be distinguished before initiating treatment.

- ◆ *Primary causes*. Bilateral postchiasmatic lesions (Frisén 1980), which may cause partial up to total loss of visual acuity in both eyes that cannot be corrected by glasses. This is often associated with bilateral visual field defects (Kerkhoff 1999).

- ◆ *Secondary causes*. Disturbed visual exploration, fixation difficulties due to Balint's syndrome, impaired contrast sensitivity, eccentric fixation due to cerebral hypoxia, or nystagmus. Impairments in acuity for moving targets (dynamic acuity) are caused by deficient smooth pursuit eye movements (Haarmeier and Thier 1999).

2.1.1 Recovery

Recovery often occurs in patients with secondary causes but rarely in those with primary causes of disturbed visual acuity. As impaired acuity affects all subsequent visual activities as well as neuropsychological testing, treatment of the secondary causes should be started immediately.

Table 8.1 Schema for the patient history of visual disorders after acquired brain lesions. Insert the questions in the table into the following phrase: 'Did you experience . . . since your brain lesion?' (Based on Kerkhoff *et al.* 1990)

Question	Purpose of question, underlying disorder
1 . . . any changes in vision . . .?	Awareness of deficits? Information about case history?
2 . . . diplopia . . .? Permanent or transient?	Type of gaze palsy? If transient, fusional disorder?
3 . . . reading problems . . .? Syllables/words missing, change of line, reduced reading span?	Hemianopic alexia? differential diagnosis of neglect dyslexia, aphasic alexia or pure alexia
4 . . . problems in estimating depth on a staircase or reaching with your unimpaired hand for a cup, hand, door handle . . .?	Depth perception? Optic ataxia?
5 . . . bumping into obstacles or failure to notice persons . . .? Which side?	Visual exploration deficits in homonymous visual field disorders?
6 . . . blinding after exposure to bright light . . .?	Foveal photopic adaptation?
7 . . . dark vision or that you need more light for reading . . .?	Foveal scotopic adaptation?
8 . . . blurred vision . . .? Transiently or permanently?	Contrast sensitivity? Acuity? Fusion?
9 . . . that colours look darker, paler, less saturated . . .?	Colour hue discrimination? Impaired contrast sensitivity?
10 . . . that faces look darker, paler, unfamiliar . . .?	Face discrimination/recognition disorders?
11 . . . problems in recognizing objects . . .?	Object discrimination/recognition disorders?
12 . . . problems in finding your way in familiar/unfamiliar environments . . .?	Topographic orientation deficits?
13 . . . visual hallucinations (stars, dots, lines, fog,faces, objects, etc.) or illusions (distorted objects, faces) . . .	Simple or complex visual hallucinations, illusions? When? Awareness of their illusory character?

2.1.2 Treatment

The following short recommendations can be given (Kerkhoff 2000).

◆ *Bilateral postchiasmatic lesion.* Use magnification software (for PCs) or screen reading machines for permanent enlargement of printed text, pictures, letters.

◆ *Visual exploration deficit.* Improve visual search by providing the patient with a systematic (horizontal or vertical) saccadic search strategy. Acuity will improve when visual search is more systematic, quicker, and when omissions are reduced (see Section 2.4).

◆ *Nystagmus.* Calm nystagmus with orthoptic (prisms) or pharmacological means (Straube and Kennard 1996).

◆ *Spasmodic fixation* (Balint's syndrome). Test acuity with single-letter charts. Acuity for single letters should be normal. Improving simultaneous perception by repetitive treatment enlarges the useful field of view (Perez *et al.* 1996) and improves activities of daily living.

◆ *Dynamic visual acuity.* Treat smooth pursuit eye movements in the horizontal domain (left, right) for different velocities. The recognition of moving objects is important for vocational tasks (Gur and Ron 1992) and improves in parallel with the increase of the smooth pursuit gain.

2.2 Spatial contrast sensitivity (CS) and foveal photopic and scotopic adaptation

Spatial CS denotes the ability to discriminate between striped patterns (gratings) of differing luminance (contrast) and stripe width (spatial frequency). It is often impaired in posterior brain lesions (80%, Bulens *et al.* 1989).

◆ *Foveal photopic adaptation* is the continuous adaptation to a brighter illumination.

◆ *Scotopic adaptation* is the adaptation to an illumination darker than the present one.

Both processes are dissociable and impaired in some 20% of patients with posterior cerebral artery infarctions or cerebral hypoxia (Zihl and Kerkhoff 1990). Loss of photopic adaptation leads to blinding, loss of scotopic adaptation to data vision.

2.2.1 Recovery

◆ *Contrast sensitivity.* Rapid recovery in the majority of patients; permanent deficits in about 20%.

◆ *Adaptation.* No recovery (even after years) in the patients tested so far (Zihl and Kerkhoff 1990).

2.2.2 Treatment

◆ *Impaired CS.* CS can be trained effectively in normal subjects but this has never been tried in brain-damaged cases. In those 20% with permanent deficits the use of additional, indirect lighting is helpful because it improves contrast.

◆ *Isolated loss of photopic adapation or combined disorder.*
   —Avoid direct lighting, use dimmer to adjust light individually.
   —Avoid flickering neon lights.
   —Use sunglasses outside buildings.
   —Avoid continuously adapting sunglasses (Varilux) because they are expensive and are too slow in readapting inside a building.
   —Car driving at night ('blinding') is not advisable.

◆ *Isolated loss of scotopic adaptation.*
   —Increase indirect lighting by additional light bulbs.
   —Use dimmer to adjust lighting individually.

2.3 Stereopsis and convergent fusion

Local and global stereopsis are reduced in patients with occipital, parietal, or temporal brain lesions and impair manual activities in near space (reaching and grasping, technical work, depth perception), which is relevant for vocational rehabilitation. Convergent fusion is a prerequisite of stereopsis and means the fusion of the left and right eye's image to one combined (fused) picture of the world. Fusion is impaired in some 20% of patients with posterior vascular lesions and about one-third of TBI patients (Kerkhoff 2000). Patients with impaired fusion have severe reading problems after some 10 minutes. They rapidly develop diplopia and are impaired in all near-work activities.

2.3.1 Recovery

The percentage of patients showing recovery is unknown in stereopsis. In TBI patients with fusional disorders three-quarters have persistent disorders for years after their injury (Hart 1969).

2.3.2 Treatment

Fusion and stereopsis can be trained together using simple orthoptic or binocular devices (Kerkhoff and Stögerer 1994) with this treatment plan.

- *Patient history.* Asthenopic disorders (eye pressure, fatigue in reading or PC-work), blurred vision, problems in near-work activities?

- *Therapy.* Improvement of fusion and stereopsis by repetitive display of dichoptic images with increasing disparity angle; 8–20 sessions advisable

- *Outcome.* Favourable in 80% of patients with improvements in reading duration, stereopsis, and fusional range; relief from asthenopia; better functioning in vocational life

- *Exclusion criteria.* Premorbid deficits in binocular integration; permanent diplopia with angle $>15°$.

See the box below for the efficacy of fusional training and the effects on functional activities in daily life.

Efficacy of fusional training in brain-damaged patients (Kerkhoff *et al.* 2000)

- **Efficacy of convergent fusional treatment.** 80% of trained patients show a significant improvement of convergent fusion within 8–12 treatment sessions (hence within 4–6 weeks), which remains stable at a follow-up after several months.

- **Improvements of functional activities in daily life following training.** Less blurred vision, longer reading duration (100 minutes instead of 15 minutes), improved stereopsis, less asthenopic symptoms, and improved sustained attention during PC work. Especially in young victims with closed head injury, fusional training may often be an important requirement before initiating vocational rehabilitation programmes (because these often require at least 1 hour of reading or PC work).

2.4 **Homonymous visual field disorders (VFD)**

VFDs are present in 20–30% of all neurological patients in neurorehabilitation centres. Field sparing is 5° or less in 70% of them (Zihl and von Cramon 1986). VFD patients may present three types of associated deficits: visual exploration deficits; reading disorders; and visuospatial deficits.

- *Visual exploration deficit.* Time-consuming, inefficient visual search due to loss of overview and unsystematic search strategies; numerous, small-amplitude staircase-saccades in blind hemifield; omissions of targets in blind field (Zihl 1995*a*).

- *Hemianopic reading disorder.* Slow reading with few errors in VFDs with field sparing <5°; also present in paracentral scotomas and quadrantanopia. Reading of short, single words is normal (no aphasia or alexia) (Zihl 1995*b*).

- *Visuospatial deficits.* Subjective midline (in line bisection) is shifted towards the blind field (horizontally in left/right VFDs, vertically in altitudinal VFDs) in 90% of the patients (Kerkhoff 1993). This shift is also evident in daily life (walking through doorways, sitting in front of table)

2.4.1 **Recovery**

Field recovery is present in the first 2–3 months postlesion in 10–20% of patients (mean field increase: 2.8° in central vision; 6.3° in peripheral vision beyond 15° eccentricity). After 3 months postlesion, spontaneous recovery is very rare (Zihl and von Cramon 1986).

2.4.2 **Treatment**

Since field recovery is very limited, restorative field training is appropriate only in a small minority of patients detailed below. For the majority of VFD patients (95%) compensatory treatment of the associated disorders is advocated (see Table 8.2).

- Prisms are *not useful* in the treatment of VFDs because the patients get confused. However, short-term prismatic adaptation (30 min exposure) may effectively reduce visual neglect phenomena (in neglect patients with or without VFDs) for up to 72 hours at least (see Chapter 6).

- Compensatory head shifts towards the scotoma (either spontaneously adopted by the patient or instructed by staff) are of *no use* in the rehabiltation of VFDs, because they lead to visual exploration deficits in the ipsilesional visual field and stays of the neck muscles and delay treatment progress in visual scanning training (Kerkhoff *et al.* 1992).

- Training of 'blindsight' in VFDs is probably *not á* useful therapy (Zihl and Kennard 1996) because it does not lead to improved functioning in daily life.

2.5 **Visual hallucinations**

- *Simple formed visual hallucinations* (Lance 1976: light dots, bars, lines, stars, fog, coloured sensations, etc.) are frequently reported by patients (however, only when

Table 8.2 Summary of compensatory approaches* (hemianopic reading and visual exploration training) and restorative treatment† (visual field training) in patients with postchiasmatic scotoma

Hemianopic reading training

Patient history. Change of line, types of errors (omissions, substitutions, problems with long words or numbers), maximum reading duration, asthenopic disorders

Type of treatment. Improvement of oculomotor reading strategies to substitue the lost parafoveal visual field: tachistoscopic reading of single words, moving window technique, floating words, search for words in a text, scanning reading technique, training of numbers with embedded zeros. Variation of physical and linguistic parameters: word length and frequency, position on screen (left, centre, right), number of words, presentation time, complexity of text, variation of instructions

Transfer. Reading of newspaper, book, or own manuscripts; text editing on a PC; increase of maximal reading duration

Outcome and follow-up. Increase in reading speed; 500% reduction in reading errors; partial field recovery (mean 5°) in one-third of patients

Visual exploration training

Patient history. Limited overview, bumping into persons and obstacles, defective orientation in visual space, e.g. crowded situations, traffic

Type of treatment. Increase amplitude and velocity of saccadic eye movements towards scotoma: variation of size, reduction of saccadic reaction time; discourage head movements or compensatory head shifts. Teach systematic, spatially organized (horizontal or vertical) visual search strategy on wide-field displays. Start search in blind field; use visual displays requiring serial and parallel search; possibly combine with other stimulation devices (optokinetic stimulation)

Transfer. Treat orientation in clinic, own urban district, new environments. Management of *visual* activities of daily living: find objects on table or in room, find therapist's room, find objects in supermarket, cross street, use public traffic, find way home

Outcome and follow-up. Reduction of omissions and search time. Partial field recovery (mean: 5–7°) in 34% of patients

Visual field training

Patient history. Residual visual capacities (often movement of a stimulus) in regions of scotoma. Search for amblyopic transition zones, which are most likely candidates for field recovery

Type of treatment. Improvement of saccadic localization at field border or in amblyopic transition zone. Recognition of colour, form, orientation, or luminance of the target. Total length of treatment: 30–500 hours.

Transfer. Improvement in reading und subjective awareness of visual problems

Outcome and follow-up. Mean field increase 5–10°. Stability at follow-up. 70% of patients have a field recovery <5°

* As a rule, compensatory treatments are advisable in 95% of postchiasmatic visual field defects (VFDs).
† Restorative visual field treatment is only promising when lesions are incomplete and a high degree of residual visual capacity (light, motion, form, or colour perception) is present in specific regions of the scotoma (Kerkhoff 2000).

questioned systematically!) with posterior vascular lesions and most often occur after occipital lesions. Typically, they occur shortly before, during, or after the lesion and the patients are aware that they perceive something 'unreal'. Often, patients rub their eyes, change fixation, or move their head to cancel the hallucination. Simple visual hallucinations are typically short (a few seconds), and often confined to a hemianopic field defect.

◆ *Complex visual hallucinations and methamorphopsias* are rare and most often associated with temporal lobe lesions (Kölmel 1984, 1985). Patients report complex visual hallucinations reluctantly (only when forced to describe them!)—these may be complex scenes or faces. Often, but not always, there is a relationship to previously seen objects, persons, or environments (Halligan *et al.* 1994). They can last much longer than simple visual hallucinations (up to minutes or hours) and may irritate the patient considerably.

◆ *Metamorphopsia* denotes geometrical alterations in visual perception due to a brain lesion, retinal disease, or migraine. These may include tilted (often in Wallenberg's syndrome) or even inverted vision (seeing things upside down) which occurs both after cerebellar or frontal lesions. Micropsia (seeing things smaller) and macropsia (seeing things larger) both occur after lateral occipital lesions and lead to the impression that patients misperceive the size of the contralesional hemispace in relation to the ipsilesional hemispace. Often this is clinically evident when looking at faces (including their own face): one-half appears larger, as if turgid. This irritates patients, but rarely impairs face recognition (Young *et al.* 1990). Finally, things may be misperceived as farther away (porropsia) or closer to the observer (pelopsia). These may occur after parieto-occipital lesions. Note that all types of metamorphopsias also occur after acute retinal disease (detachment) without any brain pathology.

◆ *Visual perseveration (palinopsia)* also occurs after (often bilateral) occipital lesions and means transposition of parts of the visual scene to another fixation. For instance, after the patient looks at one person (A), he changes gaze to another person (B)—if he continues to see parts of person A (i.e. the glasses), although he is no longer looking at A, he has visual perseveration. Those patients who are aware of this transposition of parts of the visual scene feel very irritated.

2.5.1 Recovery

The recovery is rapid and complete in 95% of the patients, so that at 6 weeks postlesion the occurrence is quite rare (Kölmel 1984, 1985).

2.5.2 Treatment

As hallucinations and illusions are irritating but mostly transient phenomena, information and reassurance to the patient are important.

◆ *Inform your patient.* Visual hallucinations are a quite normal but *transient* phenomenon after a vascular brain lesion.

- *Calm your patient.* Most patients experiencing simple hallucinations know that they perceive erroneous visual stimuli not present in the outer visual world. Tell the patient that he/she is not going to be mad. If necessary, demonstrate to the patient that hallucinations can be provoked in any person by pressing the eye-ball (pressure phosphenes) or when suddenly rising from a supine position (blood-pressure-related).

- *Complex versus simple hallucinations.* Complex visual scenes have a higher appearance of reality than simple hallucinations, and are therefore more frightening for the patient. These patients are very reluctant to talk about their experience because they fear to be misdiagnosed as a psychiatric case. Note that psychatric patients much more often have *auditory* rather than *visual* hallucinations, while the opposite holds true for patients with organic visual hallucinations after posterior brain lesions. Furthermore, brain-damaged patients very rarely report 'hearing voices', although some report hearing music.

- *Persistent visual hallucinations.* Check if there is an epileptic focus (using electroencephalography (EEG)), the possibility of a new infarction developing, or a psychiatric disease.

2.6 Colour perception

Colour and form perception are typically impaired in two types of disorders—in particular locations of a postchiastmatic VFD, and in central vision in patients with bilateral postchiasmatic lesions of various aetiologies (Meadows 1974; Zeki 1990). The deficit in central vision may range from a subtle deficit of hue discrimination (often in unilateral occipitotemporal lesions) to a nearly total achromatopsia after bilateral lesions.

2.6.1 Recovery

Recovery of colour and form vision within a scotoma is often observed in patients with partial field recovery (Zihl and von Cramon 1985). As a rule, the progression of visual recovery (if there is some!) in VFDs is as follows:

Light detection → light localization → brightness discrimination → form discrimination → colour perception.

Hence, colour vision is the last to recover. In those patients with colour vision deficits in central vision no recovery had been reported over 6 years in one study (Pearlman *et al.* 1979).

2.6.2 Treatment

- *Defective colour vision in visual field regions.* In patients with residual colour perception in a scotoma and incomplete lesions, improvement of colour discrimination can be trained by displaying coloured targets at the field border and having the patient saccade to them and discriminate the colour (as described in Table 8.2, 'Visual field training').

◆ *Defective colour perception in central vision.* Forced disrimination of differently coloured forms is partially effective in cerebral anoxia—however with limited transfer to nontrained colours (Merrill and Kewman 1986). Often, the patients can learn to base their colour judgements on other cues such as the brightness or saturation despite permanently impaired hue discrimination.

2.7 Visual form recognition

Recognition deficits for simple visual forms (rectangle, square, triangle, etc.) without a semantic dimension (such as real objects) are only observed in patients with extensive bilateral or diffuse-disseminated, posterior brain lesions. When present, the patients are unable to discriminate simple geometric forms equated for total luminance (Milner *et al.* 1991). The rarity of the disorder is due to the fact that it occurs most often after extensive anoxic brain damage.

2.7.1 Recovery

Recovery is often incomplete or even absent, possibly due to the bilateral or diffuse-disseminated lesions in cerebral anoxia or carbon monoxide poisoning. The case reported by Sparr *et al.* (1991) showed the disorder for more than 40 years. Recovery may be more likely in patients with cerebrovascular aetiologies and/or unilateral lesions.

2.7.2 Treatment

Visual form recognition can be improved by repetitive discrimination training for simple geometric forms equated for total luminance. Verbal or computerized feedback is essential, and progressive increase in the similarity of the stimuli to be discriminated as well. As a result, visual form discrimination of simple geometric forms but also of line drawings and partially of photographs displaying real objects is improved, along with increased visual acuity and contrast sensitivity. Treatment can be accomplished either with self-constructed paper-made stimuli, or using computerized devices that give detailed quantitiative feedback and allow variations of colours, sizes, and forms (rectangular, oval; Kerkhoff and Marquardt 1998).

2.8 Visual object and face perception

Visual agnosias for objects and faces are rare conditions, occurring probably in less than 1% of all neurological patients (Zihl and Kennard 1996). Both types of agnosia occur most frequently after bilateral occipitotemporal lesions (Farah 1990). In object agnosia, a more perceptual subform (aperceptive agnosia) and a more semantic subform (associative agnosia) are usually distinguished. The former indicates a deficit in perceptual object discrimination and the latter implies loss of semantic knowledge related to visually presented objects (Farah 1990).

2.8.1 Recovery

Detailed case reports about recovery are rare. Partial recovery in the recognition of real-life objects has occasionally been noted, while recognition of photographs of objects or faces rarely improves. Recovery is particularly unlikely in anoxic brain damage, probably due to the widespread diffuse lesions and the additional cognitive impairment impeding the acquisition of compensatory strategies (Sparr *et al.* 1991). Partial recovery is more likely in traumatic or vascular lesions, and in those few cases with unilateral right-sided lesions showing face agnosia (Farah 1990).

2.8.2 Treatment

Controlled treatment studies are rare. Zihl and Kennard (1996) noted improvement of object and face discrimination on photographs and in real life in three patients following an intensive (120 hours) treatment procedure focusing on the specific search for key features of objects or faces. Furthermore, the use of context information (knowledge about objects and faces and the relevant social situation) is advisable and helpful for these patients.

2.9 Visual motion perception

Relative impairments of visual motion perception may occur after focal lesions of the motion centre in the occipitoparietotemporal cortex, but permanent deficits are probably rare, and even in these patients only relative (frequency of relative deficits, 13%; Schenk and Zihl 1997). However, many brain-damaged patients subjectively report problems in estimating the velocity- and position-changes of moving vehicles in traffic situations as a pedestrian or when driving in a car. This may result either from impaired motion perception (linearly or in depth), disturbed visuospatial perception, or a combination of both.

2.9.1 Recovery

Little is known about recovery. In those rare patients with bilateral lesions no recovery has been reported (Zihl *et al.* 1991), while those with unilateral lesions may show recovery. Even the motion-blind patient reported by Zihl *et al.* (1991) readapted to moving stimuli in daily life by certain compensatory techniques, despite her permanent motion deficit under laboratory conditions.

2.9.2 Treatment

Due to the rarity of severe impairments in visual motion processing and probably the multiplicity of cortical and subcortical areas involved in visual motion perception, treatment approaches have not been developed. However, the treatment of an associated ability, smooth pursuit eye movements when tracking a moving target, is useful to improve visual scanning on PC-screens and visual orientation in daily life (Gur and Ron 1992). Treatment can be accomplished through use of a large PC screen, where the subject follows a moving target in different directions with a stabilized head. Target velocity should be adapted so that pursuit eye movements can be performed with relatively few catch-up saccades. In addition, a training of situations in daily life where motion is important (crossing a street, using a moving staircase) can improve orientation and reduce the likelihood of accidents due to reduced motion perception.

Secondary cues may help to code visual motion of vehicles, i.e. by position or size changes, despite a stable impairment in motion processing under laboratory conditions.

3 **Somatosensory disorders**

Somatosensory deficits are present in the majority of hemiplegic patients and in about 30–40% of all stroke patients with unilateral lesions depending on assessment (Winward, Halligan & Wade 2002). In a large sample of 272 brain-damaged patients Hermsdörfer *et al.* (1994) found that 29.8% of all patients had somatosensory disorders, and 37.9% reported subjectively somatosensory hallucinations, metamorphognosia, hypersensitivity, or pain. Of those patients impaired in somatosensory testing, the frequencies of differential deficits were:

- impaired passive movement discrimination of fingers (82.7%), wrist (70.4%), elbow (51.8%), shoulder (48.2%);
- impaired localization of finger parts (55.5%);
- impaired two-point discrimination at the index finger (53.1%);
- astereognosia (37.1%);
- impaired detection of light finger touches (32.1%).

3.1 **Recovery**

Few systematic patient studies about recovery exist. Primate studies suggest substantial recovery of somatosensory dysfunctions spontaneously and after controlled treatment (Jenkins *et al.* 1990).

3.2 **Treatment**

The few controlled treatment studies for patients with tactile deficits all indicate that these can be trained efficiently (Goldman 1966; Zane and Goldman 1966; Yekutiel and Guttman 1993). The following types of treatment are useful and have been evaluated quantitatively.

Retraining of different somatosensory functions Most somatosensory abilities can be trained (location of touch, sense of elbow position, two-point-discrimination, stereognosis) using the following therapeutic principles (Yekutiel and Guttman 1993).

- Improve awareness of sensory dysfunction by allocating attention to it.
- Start treatment with sensory tasks the patient *can do* in order to improve motivation and reduce frustration of the patient.
- Use or develop tasks that are interesting and relevant for the patient in order to involve selective attention because that improves sensory functioning.
- Also use vision and the good hand during training to teach tactics and useful strategies of perception.
- Frequent rests are necessary.

Examples of tasks are:

◆ identification of line orientations, numbers, or positions drawn on the arm or hand of the patient;

◆ discrimination of shape, size, weight, or temperature of objects placed in patient's contralesional hand;

◆ identification of forms drawn with a pencil on the patient's hand/arm from a visually presented multiple-choice display (detailed in Yekutiel and Guttman 1993).

One key feature of this approach is to implement systematic sensory training in relevant functional tasks (also see box below).

Efficacy of somatosensory training in brain-damaged patients (Yekutiel and Guttmann 1993)

◆ **Efficacy of somatosensory treatment.** 80% of trained patients show a significant improvement of somatosensory (hand) functions within 4–6 weeks of treatment; improvements remain stable at a follow-up after several months. A non-treated control group showed no significant improvement during the same time period.

◆ **Transfer of improvements to functional activities in daily life.** Two-point discrimination, sensibility, cold/warm-discrimination.

Tactile extinction training The main idea of this is to improve the patient's attention to double simultaneous stimulation (DSS) of the hand's surface. For this purpose, either light touches on different fingers or positions on the hand or any other body region can be used. Patients are required to direct their attention to the touch on the impaired hand, which should be hidden from direct vision. The improvements obtained with this simple procedure are impressive, reducing tactile extinction of contralesional stimuli considerably (Goldman 1966; Zane and Goldman 1966). A critical therapeutic element is the focusing of attention towards the contralesional tactile stimulus and the relearning of the 'twoness' of the DSS task.

Improvement of tactile functions by peripheral magnetic stimulation (PMS) With this novel method the dorsal palm of the contralesional hand is stimulated magnetically (nonpainfully). After one single (20 minute) stimulation session we found a 27% reduction in tactile extinction for different surfaces delivered to both hands, while a matched control group did not show any improvement (Heldmann *et al.* 2000; Kerkhoff *et al.* 2001*a*). Probably, multiple stimulation sessions lead to stable and greater improvements. Subjectively, the patients report that they feel more in their contralesional arm; this could be especially helpful in patients with tactile neglect and unawareness of their contralesional hand/arm.

Optokinetic stimulation (OKS)   OKS moving to the contralesional hemispace in patients with tactile neglect (Vallar *et al.* 1997) improves the subjective awareness of different angular arm positions (contra- and ipsilesional arm) and reduces tactile extinction (Nico 1999) transiently. Repetitive OKS over several sessions should improve tactile and kinaesthetic functions permanently.

Treatment combinations   Although speculative, the combination of several treatments might be most effective and could improve the patient's self-awareness for the contralesional body side. Furthermore, the use of visual imagery might be helpful for patients with astereognosia, since this process is helpful in tactile object recognition and mediated by the intact visual cortices (Deibert *et al.* 1999).

Conclusion   Obviously, systematic treatments of somatosensory dysfunctions following brain lesions are just developing, despite their frequency and relevance for the patient. Nevertheless, the above-mentioned techniques yield significant improvements.

4 Auditory disorders

Significant alterations of a variety of auditory-perceptual functions have been reported following lesions below as well as beyond the medial geniculate bodies (auditory radiation). Largely, the deficits can be categorized into *audiospatial disorders* and *auditory feature discrimination* deficits, suggesting modular processing in audition (Rauschecker 1998).

4.1 Audiospatial disorders

Among these, the following deficits have been reported with the following lesion sites, and will be reported together with the few findings about recovery and treatment.

4.1.1 Deviation of the subjective straight ahead or midline position

Patients with spatial neglect, often following right parietal lesions, show a significant shift of their subjective auditory midline in azimuth towards the *ipsilesional* side in front space (Bisiach *et al.* 1984) and also in back space (Vallar *et al.* 1995). Patients without neglect, but with homonymous hemianopia show the opposite, *contralesional* deviation (towards the scotoma; Kerkhoff *et al.* 1999).

- ◆ *Recovery.* During recovery from multimodal neglect the ipsilesional auditory midline shift often regresses. Likewise, during improvement of compensatory visual exploration functions in patients with homonymous visual field disorders (see Section 2.4), a reduction of the contralesional auditory midline shift is also observed.

- ◆ *Treatment.* Optokinetic stimulation (OKS) towards the neglected hemispace normalizes the auditory midline shift not only transiently, but also permanently after repetitive treatment (see box; also Kerkhoff *et al.* 2001*b*; Kerkhoff 2003).

Therapeutic effects of repetitive optokinetic stimulation (OKS) on the deviation of the auditory subjective straight ahead in neglect patients (Kerkhoff *et al.* 2001*b*)

♦ Type of optokinetic treatment. Three patients with left-sided spatial (visual and auditory) neglect received 5 sessions of repetitive OKS using small squares ($2 \times 2°$) drifting continuously from the right to the left side of a 17 inch computer screen. The patients were required to follow the squares with their eyes towards the left as far as possible. If possible, they were encouraged to fixate with their eyes for a few seconds the left margin of the screen. Drift speeds (from $5–50°/s$) and layout of the squares displayed varied from trial to trial to engage selective attention throughout the training.

♦ Efficacy of the treatment. No effects during a baseline interval of 14 days without OKS. In this period the auditory straight ahead remained continuously deviated $20°$ towards the right, ipsilesional side (mean). After 5 treatment sessions (40 minutes each) with leftward OKS, all 3 patients showed an improvement in their auditory straight ahead in the horizontal plane into the normal range (range: $-2°$ to $+2°$). Neglect dyslexia improved as well in all 3 patients.

4.1.2 General spatial uncertainty of auditory localization

Patients with visual neglect after right parietal lesions (Pavani *et al.* 2002) often have a general deficit in auditory localization (but not necessarily in detection) in their contralesional hemispace (horizontally and vertically). Patients undergoing cerebral hemispherectomy initially also have large localization errors in their contra-operated hemispace.

♦ *Recovery.* Zatorre *et al.* (1995) reported substantial recovery of auditory localization in the contralesional hemispace in patients with unilateral hemispherectomy, without a hemispheric difference. Obviously, long-term experience can lead to a substantial reorganization of the brain processes responsible for spatial hearing. Clinical experience in neglect patients indicates that localization accuracy improves as general attentional capacities improve (see Chapters 5 and 6).

♦ *Treatment.* No systematic studies are available. As in visuospatial neglect, sustained attention training (see Chapter 6) may reduce the general uncertainty of neglect patients in auditory localization.

4.1.3 Auditory extinction of contralesional stimuli

This occurs after lesions of the auditory pathways in the temporal lobes (De Renzi *et al.* 1984) in small lacunar (Arboix *et al.* 1996) and basal ganglia lesions (Bellmann *et al.* 2001).

♦ *Recovery.* Rapid recovery is found in frontal lobe lesions, while persisting auditory extinction occurs with lesions of the auditory pathways (De Renzi *et al.* 1984).

♦ *Treatment.* No systematic studies available.

4.1.4 Auditory motion processing

The right parietal cortex is involved in horizontal auditory motion perception (Griffiths *et al.* 1998) and, consequently, right parietal cortex lesions impair auditory motion discrimination (Griffiths *et al.* 1996).

- *Recovery.* Unknown.
- *Treatment.* Unknown.

4.1.5 Recognition of speech sound stimuli from different spatial directions

In daily life, speech sounds reach our ears from many different directions in left and right hemispace. Ziegler *et al.* (2001) showed that the recognition of sequentially presented word pairs was relatively impaired in the right (contralateral) hemispace of aphasic patients (without neglect) and in the left (contralateral) hemispace of right-brain-damaged patients with left-sided visual neglect. Furthermore, recognition was more impaired when the two words were heard from different spatial positions than when heard sequentially from the same spatial position. This deficit of switching their auditory focus rapidly to another location in space could be normalized by informing the patients before hearing the stimuli about their location (precueing).

- *Treatment.* Attentional (auditory) cueing might thus be an effective treatment technique for patients with this disorder.

4.2 Deficits in auditory feature discrimination

The following deficits have been reported and will be summarized together with the few findings on recovery and treatment.

4.2.1 Cortical deafness

Cortical deafness is an extremely rare condition resulting either from brainstem lesions, subcortical lesions disrupting the auditory pathways, or from bilateral temporal lesions destroying the primary auditory cortex bilaterally (see review in Polster and Rose 1998). It comprises, as in cerebral blindness, the total or near-total inability to hear any sounds despite preserved afferent pathways up to the primary auditory cortices.

- *Recovery.* some degree of recovery has been noted (Mendez and Geehan 1988). Usually, cortical deafness evolves into auditory agnosia, followed by selective auditory agnosia for certain tasks, pure word deafness and/or amusia, and, finally, a residual disorder of temporal processing.
- *Treatment.* No treatments have been published due to the rareness of permanent deficits.

4.2.2 Auditory agnosia

Auditory agnosia is the inability to recognize auditorily presented sounds independent of any deficit of processing spoken language. This may include the inability to recognize environmental sounds (i.e. different vehicles), human sounds (coughing, baby cries), although perception of these sounds and perceptual discrimination is unimpaired, and peripheral hearing is normal as well. Generally, the disorder is held to be analogous to the two types of object agnosia found after bilateral occipitotemporal lesions in vision (aperceptive and associative agnosia, see Section 2.8). As in vision, a differentiation into a more perceptual deficit, probably most often found after right-hemispheric (temporal) lesions, and a more associative-semantic deficit, most often seen in left-hemispheric lesions, is made (Polster and Rose 1998).

- *Recovery*. Engelien *et al.* (1995) observed recovery in a case with auditory agnosia that was paralleled by activations (assessed with positron emission tomography (PET) in a large bilateral frontal, middle temporal, and inferior parietal network. Further, they noted activation of peri-infarct cortices that may enable recovery from auditory agnosia. In a case with 'deaf-hearing' after bilateral auditory cortex lesions, directing selective attention to sound recognition improved auditory functions considerably and was paralleled by bilateral PET-activations in the lateral prefrontal, middle temporal, and cerebellar cortices (Engelien *et al.* 2000). In summary, selective attention may play a key role in adapting to auditory disorders, and surviving perilesional cortex as well as more widespread cortical networks in both hemispheres may be critical for behavioural recovery.

- *Treatment*. Fechtelpeter *et al.* (1990) described a treatment of environmental sound recognition in a patient with auditory agnosia due to bilateral temporal lesions. The 4-week treatment included the following elements and may be paradigmatic for similar cases.

  —*Sound imitation*. The patient had to imitate or actually perform a typical sound of an object (i.e. telephone) and was then later confronted with the tape-recorded sound of this object and had to decide whether they were the same.

  —*Semantic association*. The patient had to associate a sound to a specific object out of a sample of 10 visually presented objects

  —*Auditory analysis*. The therapist taught the patient acoustic features of specific sounds (a starting car first makes a deep sound and later interrupted sounds according to the different gears).

All treatment techniques effectively reduced the auditory deficits with a significant transfer to daily life in this case. These or similar individually adapted techniques may be used to treat patients with auditory agnosia or more subtle perceptual deficits.

4.2.3 Pure word deafness

This is defined as the inability to process spoken words despite normal hearing thresholds and normal processing of auditory, nonlanguage stimuli.

- *Recovery*. As mentioned above, pure word deafness often evolves into a more subtle auditory-perceptual disorder (Mendez and Geehan 1988).

- *Treatment*. Unknown.

4.2.4 Nonverbal auditory perception and recognition disorders

Among these the following types of deficits have been described.

- *Phonagnosia.* Impaired recognition of familiar voices due to right hemispheric lesions (reviewed in Polster and Rose 1998).

- *Voice discrimination disorders.* Impaired perceptual discrimination of different (unfamiliar) voices occurs after right temporal lesions (reviewed in Polster and Rose 1998)

- *Impaired perception of emotional prosody.* This occurs preferentially in right-hemispheric lesions and denotes the inability to understand affectively intoned speech (Ross 1981).

- *Impaired perception of pitch direction.* This occurs after right temporal lesions (Johnsrude *et al.* 2000).

- *Altered music perception.* This is mostly impaired after right or bilateral temporal lesions (reviewed in Polster and Rose 1998).

- *Nonrecognition of environmental sounds.* This occurs in right temporal lesions (reviewed in Polster and Rose 1998).

- *Temporal processing disorders.* These have been described in unilateral lesions of either hemisphere, but especially the left hemisphere is most critical for short acoustic transients.

- *Hypersensitivity to sounds.* This occurs in TBI patients (Waddell *et al.* 1984) and is often coupled with hypersensitivity to light (blinding) (see Section 2.2). The problem is important in work rehabilitation (avoid noisy workplaces!).

- *Recovery and treatment.* No systematic studies are available.

4.3 Summary

The consequences of auditory-perceptual deficits in daily life are poorly understood. Often it is assumed that most of these deficits can be compensated easily since preserved auditory abilities may be used for compensation or multiple cues are available in daily life. However, this view may be wrong, as many patients do not report spontaneously and therefore fail to realize their auditory deficits. Hence, their consequences for nonverbal communication are likely to be underestimated (e.g. in neglect patients who never complain about their auditory deficits).

Selective references

Arboix, A., Junqué, C., Vendrell, P., and Marti-Vilalta, J.L. (1996). Auditory ear extinction in lacunar syndromes. *Acta Neurol Scand.* **81**, 507–11.

Bellmann, A., Meuli, R., and Clarke, S. (2001) Two types of auditory neglect. *Brain* **124**, 676–87.

Bisiach, E., Cornacchia, R., Sterzi, R., and Vallar, G. (1984). Disorders of perceived auditory lateralization after lesions of the right hemisphere. *Brain* 107, 37–54.

Bulens, C, Meerwaldt, J.D., Van der Wildt, G.J., and Keemink, C.J. (1989). Spatial contrast sensitivity in unilateral cerebral ischaemic lesions involving the posterior visual pathway. *Brain* 112, 507–20.

Buonomano, D.V.I. and Merzenich, M.M. (1998). Cortical plasticity: from synapses to maps. *Ann. Rev. Neurosci.* 21, 149–86.

Deibert, E., Kraut, M., Kremen, S., and Hart, J. (1999). Neural pathways in tactile object recognition. *Neurology* 52, 1413–17.

De Renzi, E., Gentilini, M., and Pattacini, F. (1984). Auditory extinction following hemisphere damage. *Neuropsychologia* 22, 733–44.

Engelien, A., Silbersweig, D., Stern, E., *et al.* (1995). The functional anatomy of recovery from auditory agnosia. A PET study of sound categorization in a neurological patient and normal controls. *Brain* 118, 1395–409.

Engelien, A., Huber, W., Silbersweig, D., *et al.* (2000). The neural correlates of 'deaf-hearing' in man. Conscious sensory awareness enabled by attentional modulation. *Brain* 123, 532–45.

Farah, M. (1990). *Visual agnosia.* MIT Press, Cambridge, Massachesetts.

Fechtelpeter, A., Göddenhenrich, S., Huber, W., and Springer, L. (1990). Ansätze zur Therapie von auditiver Agnosie. *Folia Phoniatrica* 42, 83–97.

Frisén, L. (1980). The neurology of visual acuity. *Brain* 103, 639–70.

Gibson, E.J. (1953). Improvements in perceptual learning as a function of controlled practice or training. *Psychol. Bull.* 50, 401–31.

Goldman, H. (1966). Improvement of double simultaneous stimulation perception in hemiplegic patients. *Arch. Phys. Med. Rehabil.* 63, 681–7.

Griffiths, T.D., Rees, A., Witton, C., *et al.* (1996). Evidence for a sound movement area in the human cerebral cortex. *Nature* 383, 425–7.

Griffiths, T.D., Rees, G., Rees, A., *et al.* (1998). Right parietal cortex is involved in the perception of sound movement in humans. *Nature Neurosci.* 1, 74–9.

Gur, S. and Ron, S. (1992). Training in oculomotor tracking, occupational health aspects. *Israel J. Med. Sci.* 28, 622–628.

Haarmeier, T. and Thier, P. (1999). Impaired analysis of moving objects due to deficient smooth pursuit eye movements. *Brain* 122, 1495–505.

Halligan, P.W., Marshall, J.C., and Ramachandran, U.R. (1994). Ghosts in the machine: a case description of visual and haptic hallucinations after right hemisphere stroke. *Cogn. Neuropsychol.* 11, 459–77.

Hart, C.T. (1969). Disturbances of fusion following head injuries. *Proc. R. Soc. Med.* 62, 704–6.

Heldmann, B., Kerkhoff, G., Struppler, A., and Jahn, Th. (2000). Repetitive peripheral magnetic stimulation alleviates tactile extinction. *NeuroReport* 11, 3193–8.

Hermsdörfer, J., Mai, N., Rudroff, G., and Münssinger, M. (1994). *Untersuchung zerebraler Handfunktionsstörungen.* Borgmann Verlag, Dortmund.

Jenkins, W.M., Merzenich, M.M., Ochs, M.T., *et al.* (1990). Functional reorganization of primary somatosensory cortex in adult owl monkeys after behaviorally controlled tactile stimulation. *J. Neurophysiol.* 63, 82–104.

Johnsrude, I.S., Penhune, V.B., and Zatorre, R.J. (2000). Functional specificity in the right human auditory cortex for perceiving pitch direction. *Brain* 123, 155–63.

Kerkhoff, G. (1993). Displacement of the egocentric visual midline in altitudinal postchiasmatic scotomata. *Neuropsychologia* 31, 261–5.

Kerkhoff, G. (1999). Restorative and compensatory therapy approaches in cerebral blindness—a review. *Restor. Neurol. Neurosc.* 15, 255–71.

Kerkhoff, G. (2000). Neurovisual rehabilitation: recent developments and future directions. *J. Neurol., Neurosurg., Psychiatry* 68, 691–706.

Kerkhoff, G. (2003). Modulation and rehabilitation of spatial neglect by sensory stimulation. In *Progress in Brain Research*, Vol. 142 (ed. C. Prablanc, D. Pélisson, and Y. Rossetti), pp. 257–71. Elsevier Science, Amsterdam.

Kerkhoff, G. and Marquardt, C. (1998). Standardised analysis of visuospatial perception after brain damage. *Neuropsychol. Rehabil.* 8, 171–89.

Kerkhoff, G. and Stögerer, E. (1994). Recovery of fusional convergence after systematic practice. *Brain Injury* 8, 15–22.

Kerkhoff, G., Schaub, J., and Zihl, J. (1990). The anamnesis of cerebral visual disordes after brain damage [in German]. *Nervenarzt* 61, 711–18.

Kerkhoff, G., Münssinger, U., Haaf, E., *et al.* (1992). Rehabilitation of homonymous scotomata in patients with postgeniculate damage of the visual system, saccadic compensation training. *Restor. Neurol. Neurosci.* 4, 245–54.

Kerkhoff, G., Artinger, F., and Ziegler, W. (1999). Contrasting spatial hearing deficits in hemianopia and spatial neglect. *NeuroReport* 10, 3555–60.

Kerkhoff, G., Haaf, E., Eberle-Strauss, G., and Rettinger, E. (2000). Recovery of fusional disorders after systematic treatment in patients with brain damage [abstract]. *Restor. Neurol. Neurosci.* 12, 83.

Kerkhoff, G., Heldmann, B., Struppler, A., Havel, P., and Jahn, T. (2001a). The effects of magnetic stimulation and attentional cueing on tactile extinction. *Cortex* 37, 719–23.

Kerkhoff, G., Marquardt, C., Jonas, M., and Ziegler, W. (2001b). Repetitive optokinetic stimulation for the treatment of visual and auditory neglect—results of a pilot study [in German with an English abstract]. *Neurologie Rehabil.* 7, 179–84.

Kölmel, H.W. (1984). Coloured patterns in hemianopic fields. *Brain* 107, 155–67.

Kölmel, H.W. (1985). Complex visual hallucinations in the hemianopic field. *J. Neurol., Neurosurg., Psychiatry* 48, 29–38.

Lance, J.W. (1976). Simple formed hallucinations confined to the area of a specific visual field defect. *Brain* 99, 719–34.

Meadows, J.C. (1974). Disturbed perception of colours associated with localized cerebral lesions. *Brain* 97, 615–32.

Mendez, M.F. and Geehan, G.R. (1988). Cortical auditory disorders, clinical and psychoacoustic features. *J. Neurol., Neurosurg., Psychiatry* 51, 1–9.

Merrill, M.K. and Kewman, D.G. (1986). Training of color and form identification in cortical blindness, a case study. *Arch. Phys. Med. Rehabil.* 67, 479–83.

Milner, A.D., Perrett. D.I., Johnston, R.S., *et al.* (1991). Perception and action in visual form agnosia. *Brain* 114, 405–28.

Nico, D. (1999). Effectiveness of sensory stimulation in tactile extinction. *Exp. Brain Res.* 127, 175–82.

Pavani, F., Ladavas, E., and Driver, J. (2002). Selective deficit of auditory localisation in patients with visuospatial neglect. *Neuropsychologia* 40, 297–307.

Pearlman, A.L., Birch, J., and Meadows, J.C. (1979). Cerebral color blindness, an acquired defect in hue discrimination. *Ann. Neurol.* 5, 253–61.

Perez, F.M., Tunkel, R.S., Lachmann, E.A., and Nagler, W. (1996). Balint's Syndrome arising from bilateral posterior cortical atrophy or infarction—rehabilitation strategies and their limitation. *Disability Rehabil.* **18**, 300–4.

Polster, M.R. and Rose, S.B. (1998). Disorders of auditory processing, evidence for modularity in audition. *Cortex* **34**, 47–65.

Rauschecker, J.P. (1998). Parallel processing in the auditory cortex of primates. *Audiology NeuroOtology* **3**, 86–103.

Ross, E.D. (1981). The aprosodias. Functional–anatomic organization of the affective components of language in the right hemisphere. *Arch. Neurol.* **38**, 561–9.

Schenk, Th. and Zihl, J. (1997). Visual motion perception after brain damage, I. Deficits in global motion perception. *Neuropsychologia* **35**, 1289–97.

Sparr, S.A., Jay, M., Drislane, F.W., and Venna, N. (1991). A historic case of visual agnosia revisited after 40 years. *Brain* **114**, 789–800.

Straube, A. and Kennard, C. (1996). Ocular motor disorders. In *Neurological disorders. course and treatment* (eds. T. Brandt, L.R. Caplan, J. Dichgans, H.C. Diener, and C. Kennard), pp. 101–11. Academic Press, San Diego.

Vallar, G., Guariglia, C., Nico, D., and Bisiach, E. (1995). Spatial hemineglect in backspace. *Brain* **118**, 467–72.

Vallar, G., Guariglia, C., and Rusconi, M.L. (1997). Modulation of the neglect syndrome by sensory stimulation. In *Parietal lobe contributions to orientation in 3-dimensional space* (eds. P. Thier and H.-O. Karnath), pp. 555–78. Springer, Berlin.

Waddell, P.A. and Gronwall, D.M.A. (1984). Sensitivity to light and sound following minor head injury. *Acta Neurol. Scand.* **69**, 270–6.

Winward, C.E., Halligan. P.W., and Wade, D.T. (2002). The Rivermead Assessment of Somatosensory Performance (RASP): standardization and reliability data. *Clin Rehabil.* **16** (5): 523–33.

Yekutiel, I.M. and Guttman, E. (1993). A controlled trial of the retraining of the sensory function of the hand in stroke patients. *J. Neurol., Neurosurg., Psychiatry* **56**, 241–4.

Young, A.W., De Haan, E.H.F., Newcombe, F., and Hay, D.C. (1990). Facial neglect. *Neuropsychologia* **28**, 391–415.

Zane, M.D. and Goldman, H. (1966). Can response to double simultaneous stimulation be improved in hemiplegic patients? *J. Nerv. Ment. Dis.* **142**, 445–52.

Zatorre, R.J., Ptito, A., and Villemure, J.-G. (1995). Preserved auditory spatial localization following cerebral hemispherectomy. *Brain* **118**, 879–89.

Zeki, S. (1990). A century of cerebral achromatopsia. *Brain* **113**, 1721–77.

Ziegler, W., Kerkhoff, G., ten Cate, D., Artinger, F., and Zierdt, A. (2001). Spatial processing of spoken words in aphasia and in neglect. *Cortex* **37**, 754–6.

Zihl, J. (1995a). Visual scanning behavior in patients with homonymous hemianopia. *Neuropsychologia* **33**, 287–303.

Zihl, J. (1995b). Eye movement patterns in hemianopic dyslexia. *Brain* **118**, 891–912.

Zihl, J. and Kennard, C. (1996). Disorders of higher visual functions. In *Neurological disorders. course and treatment* (eds. T. Brandt, L.R. Caplan, J. Dichgans, H.C. Diener, and C. Kennard), pp. 201–12. Academic Press, San Diego.

Zihl, J. and Kerkhoff, G. (1990). Foveal photopic and scotopic adaptation in patients with brain damage. *Clin. Vision Sci.* **2**, 185–95.

Zihl, J. and von Cramon, D. (1985). Visual field recovery from scotoma in patients with postgeniculate damage. *Brain* **108**, 335–65.

Zihl, J. and von Cramon, D. (1986). Recovery of visual field in patients with postgeniculate damage. In *Neurology* (eds. K. Poeck, H.J. Freund, H. Gänshirt), pp. 188–94. Springer, Heidelberg.

Zihl, J., von Cramon, D., Mai, N., and Schmid, C. (1991). Disturbance of movement vision after bilateral posterior brain damage. Further evidence and follow up observations. *Brain* 114, 2235–51.

Chapter 9

Neuropsychological assessment of memory disorders

Veronica Bradley and Narinder Kapur

1 Introduction

Memory difficulties are often the first and the most prominent sign of insidious or acute cerebral dysfunction, and may also represent the most common, or most notable, disability that remains after initial recovery from brain pathology. It follows that most neuropsychological assessments will include tests of memory, and the clinician will select tests that will enable him/her to answer questions that differ according to the context of the referral. When the main purpose of the assessment is diagnostic, consideration of the pattern of performance on memory tests and the severity of the memory deficit relative to deficits in other areas of cognitive functioning will enable an opinion to be given about the most likely cause of the impairment. For example, memory loss is the hallmark of the majority of presentations of Alzheimer's disease. In the early and middle stages of the illness the memory impairment will be very marked in relation to other cognitive deficits, while in the cortico-subcortical dementias (which accompany, for example, Parkinson's disease, Huntington's disease, and progressive supranuclear palsy) memory impairment will be more subtle and accompanied by characteristic executive deficits and slowing of response. Other questions that should be addressed in the diagnostic assessment are the following.

- To what extent can the patient continue with his/her normal activities?
- What coping strategies can be recommended on the basis of the strengths and weaknesses identified in the assessment?

The information obtained from the assessment may inform the decision to treat. For example, in normal pressure hydrocephalus, the extent to which cognitive impairment affects quality of life will be taken into account when the neurosurgeon discusses with the patient the benefits and risks of insertion of a shunt. Additionally, the presence of a co-occurring disorder will affect the risk–benefit ratio.

A certain amount of information on prognosis can be given on the basis of a single assessment, but repeated assessment will provide additional information. Repeated assessment is essential when the requirement is to monitor the recovery or decline of memory function which occurs naturally or following medical/surgical intervention.

When the assessment is carried out for the purposes of rehabilitation the assessment results will help to identify areas of weakness that may be targeted in the rehabilitation programme, as well as preserved abilities that may help the patient to compensate for deficits. More generally, information about the patient's capacity to learn will always be helpful in determining the most fruitful approach to rehabilitation. For example, if there is relative preservation of learning, repeated instruction or repeated presentation of material may pay off. If there is little capacity to benefit from repeated presentation of material then external cues may need to be provided. Other questions that need to be addressed in this context are the following.

- To what extent can the patient's continue with his/her normal activities, and what is the likelihood that she/he will be able to return to a normal routine in the future?

- What impact has therapeutic intervention had on formal test performance or on perceived disability as measured by rating scales or questionnaires?

The effects of memory disorders on everyday life vary with the severity and nature of the disorder, from mild deficits that can be effectively managed with the help of memory aids (such as a diary or a notebook) to severe difficulties that render independent living impossible. It should, however, be borne in mind that very mild impairments can be extremely disruptive for people whose jobs or personal circumstances require highly efficient memory processing. Kapur and Moakes (1995) describe the devastating effects of post-encephalitic amnesia on a young woman's everyday life. She regained some degree of quality of life, but a return to her job as a teacher was not possible. Household chores could be completed, but only by following a strict routine. Even the preparation of a shopping list was a problem because, as the authors point out, knowing that a particular item is needed requires memory. Different types of memory impairment can give rise to more circumscribed (and more easily managed) difficulties, such as inability to do mental arithmetic resulting from working memory deficit (Campbell and Conway 1995).

2 Memory: theoretical background and terminology

There is now a considerable body of research indicating that human memory is a multi-component system. Theories about different components of the system abound. For clinical purposes, a model developed from studies of dysfunctional memory resulting from neurological illness or insult is appropriate. Such a model also underpins a good deal of experimental work, including investigations of neurologically unimpaired subjects. Some components of the memory system, such as perceptual representation memory, which briefly records a visual or auditory image of a stimulus (termed iconic and echoic memory, respectively), have been investigated quite extensively in experimental studies, but are not readily testable in the clinical setting and will not be discussed here. In recent years, experimental studies using techniques such as positron emission tomography (PET) scanning and functional magnetic resonance imaging (fMRI) have enhanced our understanding of brain activity during both clinical and experimental tests, but these developments have not yet fundamentally changed approaches to the assessment of memory disorders in the clinic, though they may do so in the future (Bigler 2001).

2.1 Terminology (Fig. 9.1)

2.1.1 Short- and long-term memory

A pervasive distinction in clinical and experimental studies of human memory is that between short- and long-term memory. *Short-term memory* is the temporary information store that holds a limited amount of information for a short period of time. The neuropsychologist should be aware that the medical profession, and indeed the general public, may have a rather different understanding of the term 'short-term memory'. They use it to refer to everyday episodic memory settings, covering events over a few hours, days, or weeks, often using it as synonymous with the term 'recent memory'. They contrast this with memory for events that have occurred many years before, which in clinical settings is termed *long-term memory* or 'remote memory'. Most clinical and cognitive psychologists use the term 'short-term memory' or, more commonly, *working memory*, to refer to a set of processes for holding and manipulating in temporary store, over a period of seconds, information that has just been acquired.

2.1.2 Implicit versus explicit memory

Two further broad distinctions, based on testing methodology, have been made in memory research. One distinguishes *implicit* from *explicit* memory. The terms do not describe memory systems as such, and are generally used to refer to varying states of awareness of the individual with respect to stored memories.

- *Implicit memory* is memory that is expressed through behavioural or physiological changes, where the individual has absent or limited conscious awareness of the information that has been stored. It usually includes tasks such as priming, conditioning, and skill learning. An important set of observations that gave rise to the concept of implicit memory indicates that amnesic patients who present with profound explicit memory impairment may be able to acquire new information or learn new skills. An example is the ability to learn to perform a pursuit rotor task

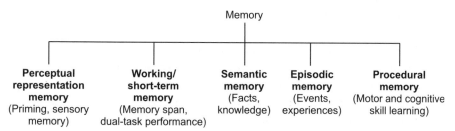

Fig. 9.1 Memory systems and associated components.

where a moving target is tracked by a probe. *Implicit memory* has been extensively investigated experimentally. It is not routinely assessed in the clinical setting but may be detectable in the pattern of performance on certain tests, such as enhanced naming of pictures on repeat testing.

◆ *Explicit memory* is memory that is consciously accessed, and covers most standard memory tasks.

2.1.3 Semantic and episodic memory

A further broad-ranging distinction is between *semantic* and *episodic* memory.

◆ *Semantic memory* refers to an organized body of knowledge about words and concepts, and culturally and educationally acquired facts. It includes general knowledge, and covers a wide range of materials and modalities—familiar faces, language, and knowledge of the world.

◆ *Episodic memory* generally refers to the encoding, storage, and utilization of memory for personally experienced events that can be related to specific spatial and temporal contexts.

2.1.4 Recent and remote memory

As indicated earlier, a clinical distinction is often made between *recent* and *remote* memory.

◆ *Recent memories* are those stored within the last few hours, days, weeks, or even months.

◆ *Remote memories* date from childhood and early adulthood.

There is no clear cut-off point between the two, but the distinction is an important one in clinical neuropsychology, in that many patients with early-stage dementia will describe problems with recent memory in the context of preserved remote memory.

2.1.5 Anterograde and retrograde memory loss

Particularly relevant in clinical settings is the distinction between *anterograde* and *retrograde* memory loss.

◆ *Anterograde amnesia* is characterized by difficulty in acquiring new material and remembering events from the point at which neurological illness or traumatic injury to the brain occurred. Memory for events prior to the illness or injury may be unaffected, even when the anterograde amnesia is severe.

◆ The term *retrograde amnesia* is used when memory for events preceding the onset of brain damage is affected. The retrograde amnesia may cover a relatively short period (e.g. a few minutes or hours preceding a head injury) or can extend over decades. Conditions in which extensive retrograde memory loss can occur include Korsakoff syndrome, viral infections of the brain and late-stage dementia of the Alzheimer type.

2.1.6 Prospective memory

Prospective memory requires interaction between episodic memory and executive functions to enable an individual to remember to do something at a particular time in the future.

2.1.7 Material specificity

Another important concept is that of *material specificity*. Memory for nonverbal and verbal material may be differentially affected by neurological illness or injury. In general, verbal information is dealt with by the left cerebral hemisphere, and nonverbal information by the right.

2.1.8 Recall and recognition

Different techniques for the assessment of memory are available and some patients may appear more or less impaired according to the type of test used. There is an important distinction to be made between *recall* and *recognition*.

♦ *Recall* is uncued retrieval and involves an active search process.

♦ In tests based on a *recognition* paradigm there is thought to be a familiarity and a recall component, since the individual selects from a number of stimuli that include the target.

Recognition is almost always easier than recall, for the neurologically unimpaired as well as the neurologically impaired, and test norms reflect this. In some cases, e.g. certain cortico-subcortical or frontal presentations, recognition memory may be spared relative to recall, with discrepancies evident on standardized test scores, and this difference in performance can be an important diagnostic indicator.

Learning can occur after a single presentation, but the term is usually used in clinical neuropsychology to refer to tests in which there is repeated presentation of material. Retrieval may then be tested by the recall or recognition method.

Recall or recognition is typically tested after a period of roughly 30 minutes (occasionally less) when a delayed trial is included. There are situations in which it would be helpful to assess *long-term anterograde forgetting*. In particular, patients with epilepsy sometimes report 'fading' memory of an event, such as a holiday or social occasion, which a relative or friend has said that they initially remembered quite well. Unfortunately, we do not have well-established norms for retrieval trials over weeks or months. Existing test materials may be used in this way, but interpretation will need to be carried out in the light of experimental studies (e.g. Blake *et al.* 2000).

3 Assessment of memory: the clinical interview

In some types of referral, especially those with a diagnostic component and where the patient may have limited insight and/or memory for his difficulties, the presence of a relative/close friend/carer will be valuable. Two main sets of information should be sought:

- the memory symptoms which the patient or carer offers either spontaneously or in response to direct questioning;
- an indication of the patient's memory functioning gained from general questioning about recent autobiographical and public events.

Once an account of symptoms has been given, specific probes may be made for symptoms such as the following:

- forgetting a message;
- losing track of conversation;
- forgetting to do things;
- forgetting what has been read, or events in TV films/soap operas;
- inability to navigate in familiar places.

The patient may be asked questions relating to his/her medical history (when she/he last saw the doctor, medication prescribed, and, if an in-patient, when she/he was admitted and what investigations have been carried out). Word-finding difficulties that could come under the rubric of semantic memory should also be probed. In the case of public events, it may be worth sampling both memory for famous personalities and memory for discrete events. This can be done by asking about a famous personality who has recently died and indirectly probing whether the patient knows that the personality is dead and how she/he died. In the case of a news event, it may be useful to start with a cue word to see if the patient can provide a news event relating to that word, and then probe for more specific information. Very accurate or very inaccurate responses to questions such as these may give a rough guide as to the direction in which more detailed memory assessment should proceed, although in some cases the responses may be equivocal, e.g. if there is patchy knowledge of recent news events in a patient who has little interest in the news and limited exposure to the news media. To obtain maximal information, this part of the clinical interview and its interpretation must be tailored to the individual patient.

The context in which the memory impairment is occurring is always relevant, and particularly so when assessment is carried out for diagnostic purposes. In some cases relevant information is provided in the letter of referral; in others very little background information is available at the start of the session. Obtain data from direct questioning and observe the patient carefully throughout the assessment. Note whether the patient presents as alert or lethargic and whether there is evidence of affective disorder or test anxiety. Is the patient willing to persevere with difficult tasks or does she/he respond with frequent 'Don't know' or 'Can't remember' responses? The following questions should elicit useful diagnostic information:

- How severe is the memory impairment? To what extent has it necessitated a change in the patient's daily routine?

- Has it affected ability to work or to engage in pastimes?

- Was the onset of the memory impairment sudden or gradual?

- Is the memory impairment consistently present or does it occur only on certain occasions?

- Is the memory impairment constant or are there fluctuations in severity?

- Has it been remarked upon by other members of the family? (Obtain details in a separate interview.)

- Has it progressed over time?

- Is the memory impairment occurring in isolation, or is the patient aware of impairment of other cognitive functions? (Note that many impairments such as dyspraxia or dyscalculia may be experienced by the patient as memory problems—'I can't remember how to do x'; 'I can't remember how to add up'.)

- Are there accompanying physical or mental symptoms (e.g. headache, movement disorder, hallucinations)?

- What is the patient's alcohol consumption? Does she/he take prescribed drugs or use recreational drugs? Has she/he been exposed to toxic chemicals?

Following assessment, the issue of consistency, both in terms of performance on different tests and the extent to which test performance is compatible with reported disruption to daily life, should be considered.

4 Questionnaires and rating scales

With a thorough clinical interview there is seldom a need to use formal questionnaires or rating scales. However, there may be occasions on which these may prove useful. For example, when assessment is carried out in a forensic and/or medicolegal setting, a normed questionnaire or rating scale may be considered more objective than interview data alone.

- The *Neurobehavioral Functioning Inventory*, devised by Kreutzer *et al.* (1999), includes a number of items relating to memory and has the advantage of there being two versions of the form, one for the patient and one for the family to complete. Responses to the items that make up the various scales, which include a Memory/Attention Scale, are summed and can be converted into standardized scores. The standardization sample is composed of pairs of patients and informants, the patients having sustained traumatic brain injury.

- The *Cognitive Symptoms Checklists*, developed by O'Hara *et al.* (1993), include a Memory Checklist, with questions divided according to different potential areas of difficulty, such as 'safety', 'money management', and 'time'. The completed checklist forms the basis for an in-depth clinical interview and has been designed with the setting of rehabilitation goals in mind.

◆ The *Cognitive Behaviour Rating Scales* (Williams 1987) are designed for completion by a relative or carer, and include a Memory Disorder Scale. This scale may be helpful in evaluating the cognitive sequelae of dementia.

In some cases, memory assessment procedures may have to be improvised. For example, in monitoring the effects of memory aids on everyday memory functioning, the clinician may wish to have a carer keep a daily diary of specific everyday memory lapses recorded before and after therapeutic intervention.

5 Memory tests

5.1 Test selection

Issues of validity and reliability apply to the selection of all neuropsychological tests and will not be discussed here. The issue of *ecological validity* is also widely applicable, but can be particularly relevant to memory assessment, as everyday situations in which memory comes into play can be very hard to simulate. The question of ecological validity is particularly relevant when important decisions, e.g. about the patient's capacity to return to work or to live independently, are under consideration. A good understanding of the demands that will be made on the patient in a given setting and an awareness of the way in which the clinic or office differs from real-life settings are important. For example, during assessment the patient will be in a one-to-one situation that is deliberately kept as free from distraction as possible. This should give rise to optimal performance on formal tests but may be very different from a real-life situation in which there is extraneous noise and other competing demands on attention. Memory may need to be assessed sequentially to monitor recovery or rate of progression in degenerative illness. In this case the existence of *parallel forms* of tests is extremely useful. Finally, the severity of memory impairment varies from mild forgetfulness to profound amnesia. Care must be taken to avoid *floor* and *ceiling effects*, which can occur if tests that are, respectively, too difficult or too easy for the patient are used.

Reference is made to specific tests in the sections that follow. The intention is not to supply an exhaustive list of tests suitable for assessing different aspects of memory, but to give examples. Where possible, examples are selected from tests or test batteries that are widely used and are likely to be readily available. In many cases, alternatives exist that will do the job just as well.

5.2 Working memory/short-term memory

This is usually measured by span tasks. The *Wechsler Adult Intelligence Scale-III* (WAIS-III; Wechsler 1998*a*) and the *Wechsler Memory Scale-III* (WMS-III; Wechsler 1998*b*) contain verbal digit span tasks. The WAIS-III also contains a letter–number sequencing task that requires manipulation of material held in short-term store and is slightly more demanding than the 'digits backward' section of the digit span task. As regards visuospatial span, the WMS-III contains a visual span task similar to the *Corsi Block-Tapping Test*, described by Milner (1971).

Since the early 1970s, *dual task* paradigms have been used widely in experimental settings. Only a few tasks requiring dual tasking are available clinically. These are discussed in Chapter 5, this volume.

5.3 Semantic memory

◆ General knowledge is readily assessable using the 'Information' subtest of the WAIS-III. It is advisable to have details of the patient's educational history when interpreting test results as this test is education-related.

◆ Knowledge of word meanings can be assessed using the 'Vocabulary' and 'Similarities' subtests of the WAIS-III.

◆ Verbal semantic breakdown can show up on tests of confrontation object naming, such as the *Graded Naming Test* (McKenna and Warrington 1983; see Warrington 1997 for up-dated norms) or the *Boston Naming Test* (Goodglass and Kaplan 1983). These picture-naming tests are sensitive to anomia (difficulty in naming), which can have a number of underlying causes. One cause is disturbance of comprehension—most research supports the view that, if a patient no longer has a store of semantic information about a visually presented object, she/he will be unable to name it.

All of the above require a spoken response, which may render them inappropriate for use with aphasic patients.

◆ *Pyramids and Palm Trees* (Howard and Patterson 1992) is a useful test of a patient's ability to access detailed semantic representations from words and pictures. It is a matching test that does not require a spoken response. The authors provide normative data from control groups, and a cut-off score. Although the test has been used extensively with clinical populations, norms from these populations are not included in the manual, since it is the pattern of performance, rather than the subject's absolute score, that is felt to be important in understanding semantic impairment.

Throughout the last decade, there has been particular interest in the syndrome termed *semantic dementia*, a condition in which progressive impairment of semantic memory occurs in the absence of more widespread impairment of cognitive function—there is relative sparing of episodic memory. Investigation of the deficits shown by patients with this disorder has enhanced our understanding of the semantic system (Hodges *et al.* 1992; Garrard and Hodges 2000). The tests described so far are (*inter alia*) routinely used in the neuropsychological diagnosis of semantic dementia, whether for clinical or research purposes.

◆ The *Speed and Capacity of Language Processing* (SCOLP) *Test* (Baddeley *et al.* 1992) is designed to provide a holistic measure of the efficiency of language comprehension. It includes the 'Speed of Comprehension Test', which is based on Collins and

Quillian's (1969) 'Silly Sentences'. Simple statements about the world must be judged to be true or false.

◆ The *Autobiographical Memory Interview* (AMI) (Kopelman *et al.* 1990), as its title suggests, takes the form of a structured interview. It encompasses two components. The first is what the authors call 'personal semantic'. It assesses patients' recall of facts about their earlier life. These facts, such as the pre-school address and the names of primary and secondary schools attended, are likely to have been acquired without conscious memory of their acquisition—hence the inclusion of this part of the instrument in this section. The second component, relating to memory for personally experienced events, is discussed in Section 5.4.1.

5.4 Episodic memory

By far the greatest number of memory tests routinely used in the practice of clinical neuropsychology are tests of episodic memory. The majority are tests of recent memory. They require the patient to memorize information and retrieve it immediately after presentation or within half an hour or so. It is more difficult to test remote memory in the clinical setting but an instrument has been devised and will be discussed before looking at the range of tests of recent memory that are available. The examples of tests of recent episodic memory reflect the number and range available and tests mentioned in Section 5.4.2 are summarized in Table 9.1.

5.4.1 Remote episodic memory

The second component of the AMI (see Section 5.3) assesses the patients' recall of specific events in childhood and early adulthood, as well as memory for more recent personal events. A potential problem for a test of this type is the absence of any way of checking the accuracy of the patient's recall. Even if a relative or carer is present she/he may not recall or be aware of certain incidents and events that have occurred in the patient's life. As part of their validation procedure the authors checked the accuracy of recall with relatives of patients in their validation sample. They concluded that the tendency was for patients' responses to be accurate on about 90% of occasions. Responses that are not obviously confabulatory (confabulatory responses may be bizarre and illogical or may not be consistent with other information which the patient has given) are therefore scored as correct and, in theory, therefore, the instrument can be used with patients who are not accompanied by a relative or carer. However, the question of reliability of answers needs to be kept in mind, as well as the possibility that autobiographical memory is present but is not tapped by the particular episodic memory items in the test.

5.4.2 Batteries and sets of tests assessing recent episodic memory

It is almost always necessary to administer a range of memory tests in order to obtain meaningful information. When the purpose of assessment is to obtain a diagnostic

Table 9.1 Tests of episodic memory

Test*	Measure			Delayed recall		Prospective memory	Age range (years)	No. of parallel forms	Ceiling effects possible	Suitable for use in severe deficit	Response required		Ecological validity a feature
	Recognition	Recall	Learning	Short	Long†						Spoken	Complex motor	
AMIPB Design Learning			+	+			18–75	2				+	
AMIPB Figure Recall		+			+		18–75	2				+	
AMIPB List Learning			+	+			18–75	2			+		
AMIPB Story Recall		+			+		18–75	2			+		
California Verbal Learning Test	+		+	+	+		16–89	2			+		
Camden Face Recognition	+						18–85		+	+			
Camden Paired Associate Learning			+				18–85		+	+	+		
Camden Pictorial Recognition	+						18–85		+	+			
Camden Topographical Recognition	+						18–85		+	+			
Camden Word Recognition	+						18–85		+	+			
Doors and People Verbal Recall		+	+		+		16–97		+	+	+		
Doors and People Verbal Recognition	+						16–97			+			
Doors and People Visual Recall		+	+		+		16–97			+		+	

Table 9.1 (Continued)

Test*	Measure — Recognition	Recall	Learning	Delayed recall — Short	Delayed recall — Long†	Prospective memory	Age range (years)	No. of parallel forms	Ceiling effects possible	Suitable for use in severe deficit	Response required — Spoken	Complex motor	Ecological validity a feature
Doors and People Visual Recognition	+						16–97			+			
Rey Auditory Verbal Learning Test	+		+				13–97‡,§	3§			+		
Rey–Osterreith Complex Figure	+ˣ	+			+		6–89‡,§	2§				+	
RBMT Appointment						+	16–96	4	+	+	+¶		+
RBMT-E Appointment						+	16–76	2			+¶		+
RBMT Belonging						+	16–96	4	+	+	+¶		+
RBMT-E Belonging						+	16–76	2			+¶		+
RBMT Faces	+			+			16–96	4	+	+			+
RBMT-E Faces	+			+			16–76	2					+
RBMT Message				+	+	+	16–96	4	+	+			+
RBMT-E Message					+	+	16–76	2					+
RBMT Name		+					16–96	4	+	+	+		+
RBMT-E Name		+					16–76	2			+		+
RBMT Pictures	+						16–96	4	+	+			+
RBMT-E Pictures	+						16–76	2					+
RBMT Route		+		+			16–96	4	+	+			+
RBMT-E Route		+		+			16–76	2					+
RBMT Story		+		+			16–96	4	+	+	+		+
RBMT-E Story		+			+		16–76	2			+		+

Table 9.1 (Continued)

Test*	Measure						Age range (years)	No. of parallel forms	Ceiling effects possible	Suitable for use in severe deficit	Response required		Ecological validity a feature
	Recognition	Recall	Learning	Delayed recall		Prospective memory†					Spoken	Complex motor	
				Short	Long†								
Warrington RMT Faces	+						18–70						
Warrington RMT Words	+						18–70		+				
WMS-III Face Recognition	+				+		16–89						
WMS-III Family Pictures		+			+		16–89				+		
WMS-III List Learning	+	+	+	+	+		16–89				+		
WMS-III Logical Memory	+	+	+||		+		16–89				+		
WMS-III Paired Associate Learning	+		+		+		16–89				+		
WMS-III Visual Reproduction	+	+			+		16–89					+	

* AMIPB, Adult Memory and Information Processing Battery; RBMT, Rivermead Behavioural Memory Test (-E, extended version); WMS, Wechsler Memory Scale.

† In most cases this is a 30-minute delay.

‡ When normative studies are combined; individual studies have narrower ranges.

§ Readily available. Additional parallel forms and normative studies are in existence.

¶ Only a minimal spoken response required; could be used with aphasic patients.

|| One passage is presented twice and a learning slope calculation can be made.

× In the Meyers and Meyers (1995) version only.

ʸ Excluding modified children's versions.

profile, different tests are included to establish whether impairment is generalized or whether there are discrete areas of impairment, occurring in the context of preserved function in other areas.

A number of batteries that sample a range of abilities using different techniques are available. When there is a need to compare performance on different tests, e.g. those using nonverbal and verbal stimuli, it is worth selecting tests from the same set or battery where possible, since they will have been normed on the same population.

The Wechsler Memory Scales The Wechsler Memory Scales (WMS) are probably the best-known and most widely used batteries. They have expanded in scope since the original scale was published in 1945. Revisions in 1987 and 1997/98 were welcome in bringing the tests up to date. The most recent revision, the WMS-III (Wechsler 1998*b*), is described here. The battery contains six primary subtests, used in calculating 'Index Scores' that are directly comparable with WAIS-III IQs.

◆ Two of these, a verbal digit span task and a visual span task, are tests of working memory and have been discussed in Section 5.2.

◆ The *Logical Memory* test comprises two short stories that are read to the patient. Free recall is required immediately after presentation and after a half-hour delay. It is also possible to examine recognition memory for the story.

◆ The other primary test of verbal memory is a paired associate learning task, in which the patient is required to learn novel word associations over a number of trials and to respond with the second word of a pair when presented with the first.

◆ On the nonverbal side, a series of 24 photographs of faces is presented. Memory for these faces is tested through recognition—the patient is asked to pick out the target photographs from a set that includes distractors.

◆ In the *Family Pictures* subtest, a family photograph and a series of scenes are presented. The patient is asked to recall who is in each scene, what they are doing, and where in the picture they are. This new addition to the battery was designed as a visual analogue to the Logical Memory test, but it is not clear that it is entirely a test of visual memory as a certain amount of verbal encoding could improve performance.

All of these tests require immediate and delayed recall. Although a half-hour delay is not particularly significant in terms of models of memory—both trials test recent episodic memory—the inclusion of delayed recall trials is clinically significant. Performance in conditions such as Alzheimer's disease, in which material is lost over a delay, contrasts with performance in, e.g. the subcortical dementias or in anxiety states, in which there may be problems at the encoding stage, while material that is successfully encoded may be retained reasonably well over a delay.

Optional subtests include:

◆ a learning task, in which the patient is asked to recall the contents of a 12-word list presented on four consecutive trials plus delayed recall and recognition trials;

◆ a nonverbal memory task, in which the patient is required to draw from memory a series of five designs, with delayed recall and recognition memory also assessed.

The battery is psychometrically quite complex, and a number of composite scores can be calculated in addition to the Index Scores. Administration of the entire battery to neurologically impaired patients is usually too demanding, but one advantage that this latest revision has over earlier versions is that norms for individual tests are available so that the clinician can select appropriate tests from the battery when time constraints or lack of stamina on the patient's part preclude administration of the entire battery.

One disadvantage that the current revision does have is the absence of a parallel form, which was available for the first WMS. This means that interpretation of the results of repeated presentation within 6 months is complicated by the possibility of a practice effect.

The Rivermead Behavioural Memory Test (RBMT)   The RBMT (Wilson *et al.* 1985) was devised specifically to meet the objection that many memory tests used in the clinical setting are adapted from laboratory-based tests and lack ecological validity. It contains a story recall test and picture and face recognition tests.

It also contains a number of subtests that are rather different from those contained in most other batteries, and that are felt to be closer to the everyday situations in which a patient might experience memory difficulties. One example is an item in which the patient is required to remember and follow a short route within the testing room. A number of tests of prospective memory are included—these are discussed in Section 5.5.

The battery has the advantage of four parallel versions to allow for repeated assessments. It yields two scores, a screening score, based on a pass/fail grading of each item, and a more detailed profile score. There is a children's version (Wilson *et al.* 1991). The tests can be used with patients who have severe memory impairment, but are subject to ceiling effects if used to detect mild memory impairment. The authors have developed an extended version of the test to increase sensitivity to subtle deficit.

The Rivermead Behavioural Memory Test—Extended Version (RBMT-E)   The RBMT-E (Wilson *et al.* 1999) provides longer, and therefore more demanding, subtests. This has been achieved by combining parallel forms. This version of the test, therefore, has two rather than four parallel forms. Although the authors have modified the test to avoid floor effects, this battery is less appropriate than the RBMT for patients with severe memory impairment.

The Adult Memory and Information Processing Battery (AMIPB)   The AMIPB (Coughlan and Hollows 1985) is an easy-to-administer set of four memory tests and two information-processing tests. The memory tests comprise:

◆ story recall;

◆ word-list learning;

◆ figure recall;

◆ design learning.

The design learning task is felt to be a particularly good measure of nonverbal memory since it is very difficult to encode any part of the design verbally. Both learning tests include a delayed recall trial following interference. The tests can be administered individually and norms are provided for each individual test. There is no overall memory quotient or composite score but this is in no way a disadvantage in the clinical neuropsychological setting, where the focus tends to be on relative strengths and weaknesses.

The Doors and People Battery   The Doors and People Battery (Baddeley *et al.* 1994) was designed principally to provide an improved measure of visual episodic memory that would be acceptable to a wide range of subjects. It includes verbal recall and recognition tasks as well as nonverbal recall and recognition tests. Tests are relatively short and the battery is easy to administer. Norms are available for individual tests and an overall score. Scaled scores are also provided for nonverbal–verbal and recall–recognition discrepancies.

The Recognition Memory Test (RMT)   This battery (Warrington 1984) contains only two subtests. The verbal test uses visually presented words and the nonverbal test uses faces. Both are forced-choice recognition memory tests. A discrepancy score can be calculated to assist the evaluation of differences between scores on the tests. Each test contains 50 items and, although they are easy to administer and usually quite pleasant from the patient's point of view, they are less suitable than some of the shorter tests for patients who have very severe impairments of memory or problems with maintaining attention. However, there is the possibility of ceiling effects when the verbal test is used with very mildly impaired patients. As stimuli are visually presented, with a recognition testing format, it is an appropriate measure of memory for patients with certain types of language impairment.

The Camden Memory Tests   This set (Warrington 1996) contains five tests—two verbal and three nonverbal—that are intended to be presented individually and not as a battery. They are all presented visually. Four are forced-choice recognition tests and do not require a spoken response. The fifth is a paired-associate learning test that requires a single-word spoken response. These tests are shorter than the subtests of the Recognition Memory Test and include word and face recognition tests with similar formats. The least demanding is the 'Pictorial Recognition Memory Test' in which stimuli are photographs of London scenes. Selection of the target is made from unrelated distractors. This test is subject to ceiling effects when used with patients with mild or even moderate problems, but it is extremely useful for patients who have severe memory impairments or limited stamina in the early days following neurological insult. In relation to the latter group, all of the tests are easy to administer at the bedside. It may also be helpful in detecting memory loss due to malingering.

5.4.3 Individual tests assessing recent episodic memory

The Rey Auditory Verbal Learning Test (RAVLT)   The RAVLT (Rey 1964) requires recall of an auditorily presented 15-word list over five learning trials. Delayed recall tests, following an interference trial, and a recognition test are provided. A number of parallel forms have been developed since the initial publication of the test. A selection of these can be found in Lezak (1995). The test is not available from a commercial source, and the clinician is free to design his/her own scoresheets for ease of administration. Normative data are provided by Spreen and Strauss (1998) and Schmidt (1996), and discussed by Lezak (1995).

The Rey–Osterreith Complex Figure   This test of visual recall was devised by Rey in 1941 and standardized by Osterreith in 1944 (papers translated by Corwin and Bylsma 1993). Taylor (1979) contributed a parallel form and scoring criteria. Until 1995 the test was not available from a commercial source. Information detailed enough to permit the clinician to design his/her own stimuli and scoresheets are provided by Lezak (1995) and Spreen and Strauss (1998). A version is now commercially available (Meyers and Meyers 1995).

The California Verbal Learning Test (CVLT)   The CVLT (Delis *et al.* 2001) is another word-list learning task, which differs from the RAVLT and AMIPB list learning tasks in that stimuli are semantically related. In each list, items have been selected from a limited number of semantic categories and there are cued recall trials that ask for items within a given category. In the first edition of the test (Delis *et al.* 1987), items that could make up shopping lists were used, with the aim of increasing the test's ecological validity. This aspect of the test has been abandoned in the 2001 edition, in order to improve ease of understanding. Short- and long-delay recall is required and there is a long-delay recognition trial.

Norms are provided for a range of measures, such as vulnerability to interference and learning strategy. Computer-assisted scoring is an option. A children's version is available (Delis *et al.* 1994). The first edition of the test did not have a parallel form, but one was developed and published by Delis *et al.* (1991). The second edition has one parallel form, and this edition also includes a short form that roughly halves administration time.

5.5 Prospective memory

A number of items tapping prospective memory are included in the RBMT and in RBMT-E (Wilson *et al.* 1985, 1999; see Section 5.4.2). The patient must remember to:

- deliver a message;
- ask about his/her next appointment;
- request the return of a belonging at predetermined points.

The timespan over which the patient is required to remember varies for different items. It ranges from a few seconds for the immediate trial of memory for a route that includes remembering to pick up and deliver a message, through a 20-minute time delay for remembering to ask question(s) when a timer rings, while the request for the return of belonging(s) must be made at the end of the session.

5.6 Computerized assessment

Computerized batteries that include tests of memory are available, but these tests have not been included as examples because, in spite of considerable interest in their development and use over the past 3 decades, none have yet come into general use in clinical settings. As mentioned previously, computer-assisted scoring is available for the CVLT, but this simply facilitates response recording and data analysis, and does not change the nature of the test in any way.

It is probable that administration of memory tests will be computer-assisted rather than fully computerized for the foreseeable future. An extremely sophisticated system would be required to capture qualitative data, give encouragement and reassurance, and deal with unexpected hitches in order to replace the clinician. Nevertheless, this may well be a growth area in the coming decade.

At present, the most readily available battery is probably the CANTAB Battery (available from Cambridge Cognition, Vision Park, Histon, Cambridge; see Robbins and Sahakian 1994), which has been developed and researched over many years. It has been designed primarily with applications for therapeutic trials in mind, but has been reported to be useful in some diagnostic settings—some clinical norms are now available. It includes tests of visuospatial and working memory. Like most computerized tests, it can be an expensive option.

5.7 Malingered memory impairment

There are a number of ways in which the neuropsychologist may detect malingering and certain tests can be helpful in checking the validity of a memory complaint. The most frequent indicator of malingering is inconsistency between the patient's day-to-day functioning and performance on memory tests. The latter may show profound impairment, yet the patient is able to answer questions about certain recent events, or to cope independently at home.

Tests, such as *Rey's Memorization of 15 Items* (Rey 1964; full details in Lezak 1995), which are presented as demanding but are, in fact, quite easy for the patient who is not severely impaired, are likely to be failed by the malingering patient. In Rey's test, the need to remember 15 different items is stressed. In fact, the test consists of five sets of three items, which greatly reduces the memory load. Similarly, the forward digit span, a test of short-term memory, may be unexpectedly short. Performance on forced-choice recognition tests, such as the RMT or Camden tests described above, can be revealing in that the malingerer may score well below chance. (see Halligan, Bass, and Oakley 2003)

5.8 Normative data for older adults

A welcome development over the last few years is the extension upwards of norms when new tests are developed or existing tests revised. WMS III norms are now provided for adults up to 89 years. Camden norms go up to 85 years, and the Doors and People standardization sample includes individuals up to 97 years. Testing the older adult is, in this respect, much easier than it was a decade ago when norms were often not available for the over-75s. Mayo's Older Americans Norms (Ivnik *et al.* 1992) have now been largely superseded by revisions of the WAIS and WMS. However, norms up to age 97 for the Rey AVLT are still of value. Lezak (1995) and Spreen and Strauss (1998) give additional test norms that are updated with each revision of their books. If appropriate age norms for a test are not provided in the test manual or in one of these volumes, it is worth checking journals for normative studies. The *Clinical Neuropsychologist* and the *Journal of Clinical and Experimental Neuropsychology* (both published by Swets and Zeitlinger) are good sources.

Selective references

Baddeley, A., Emslie, H., and Nimmo Smith, I. (1992). *The Speed and Capacity of Language-Processing Test.* Thames Valley Test Company, Bury St Edmunds.

Baddeley, A., Emslie, H., and Nimmo Smith, I. (1994). *Doors and People.* Thames Valley Test Company, Bury St Edmunds.

Baddeley, A.D., Wilson, B.A., and Kopelman, M.D. (eds.) (2002). *Handbook of memory disorders,* 2nd edn. Wiley, Chichester.

Berrios, G.E. and Hodges, J.R. (eds.) (2000). *Memory disorders in psychiatric practice.* Cambridge University Press, Cambridge.

Bigler, E.D. (2001). The lesion(s) in traumatic brain injury: implications for clinical neuropsychology. *Arch. Clin. Neuropsychol.* **16**, 95–131.

Blake, R.V., Wroe, S.J., Breen, E.K., and McCarthy, R.A. (2000). Accelerated forgetting in patients with epilepsy: evidence for an impairment in memory consolidation. *Brain* **123**, 472–83.

Campbell, R. and Conway, M. (eds.) (1995). *Broken memories: case studies in memory.* Blackwell Publications, Oxford.

Collins, A.M. and Quillian, M.R. (1969). Retrieval time from semantic memory. *J. Verbal Learning Verbal Behav.* **8**, 240–7.

Corwin, J. and Bylsma, F.W. (1993). Translations of excerpts from Andre Rey's *Psychological examination of traumatic encephalopathy* and P.A. Osterreith's *The Complex Figure Copy Test. Clin. Neuropsychologist* 7, 3–15.

Coughlan, A.K. and Hollows, S.E. (1985). The Adult Memory and Information Processing Battery. A.K. Coughlan, Psychology Department, St James's University Hospital, Leeds.

Delis, D.C., Kramer, J.H., Kaplan, E., and Ober, B.A. (1987). *California Verbal Learning Test* (Version 1). The Psychological Corporation, San Antonio, Texas.

Delis, D.C., Kramer, J.H., Kaplan, E., and Ober, B.A. (1994). *California Verbal Learning Test of Children.* The Psychological Corporation, San Antonio, Texas.

Delis, D.C., Kaplan, E., Kramer, J.H., and Ober, B.A. (2001) *California Verbal Learning Test,* 2nd UK edn. The Psychological Corporation, San Antonio, Texas.

Delis, D.C., McKee, R., Massman, P.J., *et al.* (1991). Alternate form of the California Verbal Learning Test: development and reliability. *Clin. Neuropsychologist* 5, 154–62.

Garrard, P. and Hodges, J.R. (2000). Semantic dementia: clinical, radiological and pathological perspectives. *J. Neurol.* **247**, 409–22.

Goodglass, H. and Kaplan, E. (1983). *Boston Naming Test.* Lea and Febiger, Philadelphia.

Halligan, P.W., Bass and Oakley (2003). *Malingering and illness Deception.* Oxford University Press, Oxford.

Hodges, J.R., Patterson, K., Oxbury, S., and Funnell, E. (1992). Semantic dementia. *Brain* 115, 1783–806.

Howard, D. and Patterson, K. (1992). *The Pyramids and Palm Trees Test.* Thames Valley Test Company, Bury St Edmunds.

Ivnik, R.J., Malec, J.F., Smith, G.E., *et al.* (1992). Mayo's older Americans normative studies: updated AVLT norms for ages 56 to 97. *Clin. Neuropsychologist* 6 (suppl.), 83–104.

Kapur, N. and Moakes, D. (1995). Living with amnesia. In *Broken memories: case studies in memory* (ed. R. Campbell and M. Conway). Blackwell Publications, Oxford, 1–7.

Kopelman, M., Wilson, B., and Baddeley, A. (1990). *The Autobiographical Memory Interview.* Thames Valley Test Company, Bury St Edmunds.

Kreutzer, J.S., Seel, R.T., and Marwitz, J.H. (1999). *Neurobehavioral Functioning Inventory.* The Psychological Corporation, San Antonio, Texas.

Lezak, M.D. (1995). *Neuropsychological assessment*, 3rd edn. Oxford University Press, New York.

McKenna, P. and Warrington, E.K. (1983). *Graded Naming Test.* NFER-Nelson, Windsor, Berkshire.

Meyers, J.E. and Meyers, K.R. (1995). *Rey Complex Figure Test and Recognition Trial.* The Psychological Corporation, San Antonio, Texas.

Milner, B. (1971). Interhemispheric differences in the localisation of psychological processes in man. *Br. Med. Bull.* 27, 272–7.

O'Hara, C., Harrell, M., Bellingrath, E., and Lisicia, K. (1993). *Cognitive Symptom Checklists.* Psychological Assessment Resources Inc, Odessa, Florida.

Rey, A. (1964). *L'examen clinique en psychologie.* Presses Universitaires de France, Paris.

Robbins, T.W. and Sahakian, B.J. (1994). Computer methods of assessment of cognitive function. In *Principles and practice of geriatric psychiatry* (eds. J.R.M. Copeland, M.T. Abou-Saleh, and D.G. Blazer). Wiley, Chichester, 205–9.

Schacter, D.L., Wagner, A.D., and Buckner, R.L. (2000). Memory systems of 1999. In *Oxford handbook of memory* (eds. E. Tulving and F. Craik). Oxford University Press, New York, 627–43.

Schmidt, M. (1996). *Rey Auditory Verbal Learning Test: A handbook.* Western Psychological Services, Los Angeles. Distributed by Thames Valley Test Company, Bury St Edmunds.

Spreen, O. and Strauss, E. (1998). *A compendium of neuropsychological tests*, 2nd edn. Oxford University Press, New York.

Taylor, L.B. (1979). Psychological assessment of neurosurgical patients. In *Functional neurosurgery* (eds. T. Rassmussen and R.Marino). Raven Press, New York, 165–80.

Tulving, E. and Craik, F. (eds.) (2000). *Oxford handbook of memory.* Oxford University Press, New York.

Warrington, E.K. (1984). *Recognition Memory Test.* NFER-Nelson, Windsor, Berkshire.

Warrington, E.K. (1996). *The Camden Memory Tests.* Psychology Press, Hove, East Sussex.

Warrington, E.K. (1997). The Graded Naming Test: a restandardisation. *Neuropsychol. Rehabilitation* 7, 143–6.

Wechsler, D. (1998*a*). *Wechsler Adult Intelligence Scale-III.* The Psychological Corporation, San Antonio, Texas.

Wechsler, D. (1998*b*). *Wechsler Memory Scale-III.* The Psychological Corporation, San Antonio, Texas.

Williams, J.M. (1987). *Cognitive Behaviour Rating Scales. Manual. Research edition.* Psychological Assessment Resources Inc, Odessa, Florida.

Wilson, B.A., Cockburn, J., and Baddeley, A. (1985). *The Rivermead Behavioural Memory Test.* Thames Valley Test Company, Bury St Edmunds.

Wilson, B.A., Ivani-Chalian, R., and Aldrich, F. (1991). *The Rivermead Behavioural Memory Test for Children Aged 5–10 Years.* Thames Valley Test Company, Bury St Edmunds.

Wilson, B.A., Clare, L., Cockburn, J.M., Baddeley, A.D., Tate, R., and Watson, P. (1999). *The Rivermead Behavioural memory Test—Extended Version.* Thames Valley Test Company, Bury St Edmunds.

Chapter 10

The natural recovery and treatment of learning and memory disorders

Barbara A. Wilson

1 People with memory and learning disorders

This chapter focuses on people who have memory problems resulting from a neurological condition such as traumatic head injury, stroke, encephalitis, and hypoxic brain damage. It is not concerned with those who have developmental learning difficulties. Because learning is, to a large extent, dependent on memory, people with memory problems have difficulty learning new information. People with progressive neurological conditions such as Alzheimer's disease and multiple sclerosis also experience memory and learning difficulties and, although it is possible to reduce the everyday problems faced by these people (e.g., Clare *et al.* 1999, 2000; Clare and Woods 2001), they will not be discussed here because they are not expected to recover or improve their functioning.

The typical person with memory and learning difficulties will have:

♦ a normal or nearly normal immediate memory when this is measured by forward digit span;

♦ difficulty learning and retaining most new information;

♦ a period of retrograde amnesia, i.e. a memory gap for a period preceding the insult.

Some will have normal functioning of other cognitive abilities and are said to have a pure amnesic syndrome. The majority will have additional cognitive deficits such as poor attention, word-finding difficulties, impaired problem-solving, and slowed information-processing.

2 What do we mean by recovery?

Recovery can be understood in several different ways. Finger and Almli (1988) see recovery as a complete regaining of the identical functions that were lost or impaired after brain injury. Few people with memory and learning disorders achieve recovery in this sense. Jennett and Bond (1975) regard recovery as resumption of normal life even though there may be minor neurological and psychological deficits. This is sometimes achievable for those with organic memory problems. Marshall (1985) defines recovery as the diminution of impairments in behavioural or physiological functions over time. Probably most people who sustain memory and learning deficits following non-progressive brain injury will show some diminution of their impairments over the first few days, weeks, or months. Kolb (1995) suggests that recovery typically involves partial recovery of function together with substitution of function. Wilson (1998, p. 281) defined recovery operationally as 'complete or partial resolution of deficits incurred as a result of an insult to the brain'.

The most common cause of brain damage (and memory impairment) in people under the age of 25 years is traumatic head injury. People incurring such injury usually undergo some, and often considerable, recovery. This is likely to be fairly rapid in the early weeks and months postinjury, followed by a slower recovery that can continue for many years. A similar pattern may be seen following other kinds of non-progressive injury such as hypoxia, encephalitis, and cerebrovascular accident. In these latter cases, however, the recovery process may last months rather than years.

3 Factors affecting recovery

A number of factors influence the extent of recovery, some of which we can do nothing about once the damage has occurred. These include the age of the person at the time of insult, the severity of damage, the location of damage, the status of undamaged areas of the brain, and the premorbid cognitive status of the brain. Other factors such as motivation, emotions, and the quality of rehabilitation available can be manipulated.

3.1 Age

Age, often thought to be an important factor, is less clear-cut than many believe. There would appear to be a general belief that younger people recover better from injury to the brain than older people. This is known as the 'Kennard principle' after Kennard (1940) who showed that young primates with lesions in the motor and premotor cortex exhibited sparing and partial recovery of motor function. Even Kennard, however, recognized that such sparing did not always occur and that some problems became worse over time. Reeder *et al.* (1996) found that, once severity, aetiology, and other demographic factors are taken into account, age is not always predictive of good outcome. Thomsen (1984) also showed that younger people sustaining severe head injury often do worse than older people in terms of behavioural problems and social deficits. A review of the evidence that younger people show better recovery than older people can be found in Wilson *et al.* (1991).

Age, then, is just one factor in the recovery process that has to be considered alongside other perhaps more important factors, e.g.:

- whether the lesion is focal or diffuse;
- the severity of the insult;
- the time since acquisition of the function under consideration (e.g. someone who has just learned to read at the time of the insult is more likely to show reading deficits than someone who learned to read many years before).

3.2 **Cognitive reserve**

Stern *et al.* (1995) and Kapur (1997) discuss the possibility of 'cognitive reserve', i.e. people with more education and high intelligence may show less impairment than those with poor education and low intelligence. Stern (2000) says that most clinicians are aware of the fact that any insult of the same severity can produce profound damage in one patient and minimal damage in another. The concept of cognitive reserve has been used in studies of HIV infection (Stern *et al.* 1996) and Alzheimer's disease (Stern *et al.* 1995). This concept may prove useful in understanding recovery from non-progressive brain injury. As Symonds (1937, p. 1092) said in an often quoted remark, 'It is not only the kind of head injury that matters but the kind of head.' Basso and Farabola (1997) provide support for the idea of cognitive reserve. They show that severity of aphasia and site of lesion are not unfailing predictors of improvement. Max *et al.* (1997) also hinted at cognitive reserve when they described a 15-year-old boy who sustained right frontal and amygdala damage from a gunshot wound and yet showed remarkably few deficits.

Stern (2000) suggests that individuals with high intelligence may process tasks in a more efficient way. Consequently, in cases of Alzheimer's disease, task impairment manifests itself later in the disease in people with such cognitive reserve. One piece of evidence to back this up came from a study published by Stern *et al.* (1995) showing that more educated people died sooner than less educated people, matched for severity. This suggests that those with more intelligence were coping for longer before the disease manifested itself.

4 **Mechanisms of recovery (see also Chapter 4)**

The process of recovery is not well understood and probably involves different biological processes (Ponsford 1995). Changes seen in the first few minutes (e.g. after a mild head injury) presumably reflect the resolution of temporary dysfunction without accompanying structural damage. This is akin to what Robertson and Murre (1999) refer to when they say that plastic reorganization may occur because of a rapidly occurring alteration in synaptic activity taking place over seconds or minutes. Recovery after several days is more likely to be due to resolution of temporary structural abnormalities such as oedema or vascular disruption (Jennett 1990), or to the depression of metabolic enzyme activity (Whyte 1990).

Recovery after months or years is even less well understood. Finger and Stein (1982) suggest several ways in which this might be achieved including regeneration, diaschisis, and plasticity.

4.1 **Regeneration**

Regeneration in the central nervous system (CNS) can occur in adults (Eriksson *et al.* 1998; Kolb 1995; Ramachandran *et al.* 1992) but is more likely to occur early in life (e.g. Farmer *et al.* 1991; Vargha-Khadem *et al.* 1997). Thus, the view held for many years that cerebral plasticity is severely restricted in the adult human brain is no longer credible. As McMillan *et al.* (1999) stated, 'the limits of neurorehabilitation have been significantly influenced by the basic premise that brain cells can never regenerate'. This is now known to be false and our horizons may well be extended. What is less clear, however, is the extent to which regeneration can lead to functional gains in coping with real-life problems.

4.2 **Diaschisis**

Diaschisis is a term coined by von Monakow (1914, translated by Pribram, 1969). It assumes that damage to a specific area of the brain can result in neural shock or disruption elsewhere in the brain. The secondary neural shock can be adjacent to the site of the primary insult or much further away (Miller 1984). In either case, the shock follows a particular neural route. Similar to this, but not identical, is Luria's (1963) theory of inhibition. In inhibition, however, the shock is more diffuse and affects the brain as a whole. Robertson and Murre (1999, p. 547) interpret diaschisis as 'a weakening of synaptic connections between the damaged and undamaged sites, contingent on the reduced level of activity in the lesioned area'. Because cells in the two areas are no longer firing together, synaptic connectivity between them is weakened and this results in the depression of functioning in the undamaged but partly disconnected remote site.

4.3 **Plasticity**

Plasticity implies anatomical reorganization based on the idea that undamaged areas of the brain can take on the functions subserved by a damaged area (Nirkko *et al.* 1997). Until recently, this idea was discredited as an explanation for recovery in adults, although views are now changing. Robertson and Murre (1999), in a thought-provoking paper, suggest that plastic reorganization may occur because of:

◆ a rapidly occurring alteration in synaptic activity taking place over seconds or minutes;

◆ structural changes taking place over days and weeks.

The authors focus in particular on people who are likely to show recovery provided they have assistance and rehabilitation.

According to Robertson and Murre:

◆ there are some individuals who show autonomous recovery;

◆ others show very little recovery, even over a period of years;

◆ still others show reasonably good recovery provided they receive rehabilitation.

They refer to this as a triage of spontaneous recovery, assisted recovery, and no recovery. Robertson and Murre argue that the spontaneous recovery group do not need rehabilitation as they will get better anyway. They suggest that the strategy of choice for people in the no-recovery group is to teach compensatory approaches. Consequently, they focus on the assisted recovery group to address issues concerning brain plasticity. They also believe that the severity of the lesion maps on to this triage, with:

- mild lesions resulting in spontaneous recovery;
- moderate lesions benefiting from assisted recovery;
- severe lesions necessitating the compensatory approach.

Although heuristically useful, this idea may be too simplistic. For example, people with mild lesions in the frontal lobes could be more disadvantaged in terms of recovery than people with severe lesions in the left anterior temporal lobe. The former group might have attention, planning, and organization problems precluding them from gaining the maximum benefit from the rehabilitation on offer, whereas the latter group, with language problems, could show considerable plasticity by transferring some of the language functions to the right hemisphere.

Nevertheless, Robertson and Murre (1999) make some interesting arguments and present a model of self-repair in neural networks based on a connectionist model of recovery of function. Plaut (1996) also uses a connectionist model to predict recovery. He argues that the degree of relearning and generalization varies considerably depending on the lesion location, and this in turn has implications for the nature and variability of recovery.

5 How much recovery takes place?

A few studies have looked at the natural history of 'recovery' of memory functioning over a period of years. Vargha-Khadem *et al.* (1997), for example, report on three children who sustained early bilateral hippocampal damage. These children were followed for several years and showed reasonable levels of language and general knowledge despite remaining severely amnesic. Thus they were able to learn information despite their impoverished memories. Broman *et al.* (1997) also describe a child who became amnesic following a cardiac arrest when he was 8 years old. He sustained bilateral hippocampal lesions and was followed for 19 years. At that time he was still severely amnesic showing no recovery. The most famous amnesic patient in the world is probably H.M., reported initially by Scoville and Milner (1957), who appears to have shown no recovery since his original operation to relieve epilepsy. Wilson *et al.* (1995) also describe a man with a dense amnesia following herpes simplex encephalitis at the age of 45 years. The follow-up covered a 10-year period with no change in his memory functioning.

It is possible that memory shows less natural recovery over time than other functions such as language (Kolb 1995; Wilson 1998). Nevertheless, there are hints that some people do show some recovery. Obviously, there is some recovery from posttraumatic amnesia, the period of confusion and disorientation following traumatic head injury and emergence from coma (Wilson *et al.* 1999*a*). Some recovery also occurs in the period following posttraumatic amnesia. A long-term follow-up study of 43 memory-impaired people (Wilson 1991) found that almost one-third of them showed evidence of

improved memory functioning when seen 5–10 years after discharge from a rehabilitation centre. Two-thirds had shown little change although almost all of the 43 were
compensating better. Victor *et al.* (1989) also found that about 21% of patients with
Korsakoff's syndrome showed almost complete recovery over a 3-year period, with a
further 53% showing some improvement.

Another factor appearing to influence recovery is the condition that caused the
memory problem. People with head injuries often do better than people with other
diagnoses. Newcombe (1996), for example, reported on a cohort of World War II veterans who survived missile wounds to the brain. This group has been followed since 1963
and is thus one of the most important follow-up studies of people with brain injury.
Newcombe found a striking preservation of ability in the group as a whole, despite the
fact that some members had selective impairments as a result of lesions in specific locations. In people with closed head injury (i.e. not from penetrating wounds), some have
found that age and coma duration predict recovery (Zwaagstra *et al.* 1996), despite contradictory findings on age mentioned earlier (Wilson *et al.* 1991). Fleming *et al.* (1997),
like others, found that psychosocial problems are more persistent than physical problems
1 year post-brain injury. People with encephalitis who remain with memory difficulties
several months post insult appear to show less recovery over time. McGrath *et al.* (1997)
found that 70% of encephalitis survivors showed memory impairment. The single-case
studies of Wilson *et al.* (1995) and Funnell and de Mornay Davies (1996) found little
change over time. A study looking at long-term outcome of 18 patients with hypoxic
brain damage (Wilson 1996) found that, several years postinsult, 11 had memory problems, usually together with other cognitive problems, and 4 were too severely intellectually impaired to be assessed on adult neuropsychological tests. Although recovery from
stroke has been studied (e.g. Robertson *et al.* 1997), most studies focus on recovery of
motor functions or attention. Robertson *et al.* found that ability to sustain attention was
associated with better functional recovery.

6 Can we improve on natural recovery?

Animal studies have shown that it is possible to regenerate cells in the dentate gyrus
through the provision of specific learning tasks (Gould *et al.* 1999) or through enriched
environments (van Praag *et al.* 1999; Young *et al.* 1999). Although until recently it was
believed that brain cells do not regenerate, an important recent paper shows that cells in
the hippocampal formation produce new neurons throughout adulthood, even in
humans (Eriksson *et al.* 1998). Thus it might be possible to enhance natural recovery
through enriched environments and focused rehabilitation strategies. Furthermore,
such programmes might indeed lead to neurogenesis in the human brain (see
McMillan *et al.* 1999 and Ogden 2000 for further discussion). Despite scepticism about
such recovery over the past decade or so (e.g. Glisky and Schacter 1986; Wilson 1995), we
now have the technology, through imaging procedures, to see whether it is possible
to improve memory functioning (rather than relying primarily on compensatory

approaches) and to see whether any observed behavioural change results in structural changes to the brain. Grady and Kapur (1999) suggest that imaging studies may enable us to measure specific changes occurring in the brain during recovery and therefore allow us to determine whether recovery is the result of:

+ reorganization within an existing framework; or

+ recruitment of new areas into the network; or

+ plasticity in regions surrounding the damaged area.

A few studies using imagery techniques to look at recovery from brain injury have appeared. One of the first papers in this area reported changes in regional cerebral blood flow (rCBF) after cognitive rehabilitation for people who had sustained toxic encephalopathy following exposure to toxins (Lindgren *et al.* 1997). Later the same year, positron emission tomography (PET) was used to identify the neural correlates of stimulation procedures employed in the rehabilitation of people with dysphasia (Carlomagno *et al.* 1997). Laatsch *et al.* (1997, 1999) used single-photon emission computerized tomography (SPECT) to evaluate rCBF during recovery from brain injury. The authors suggested that specific changes in rCBF appeared to be related to

+ the location of the injury;

+ strategies used in cognitive rehabilitation.

Continued improvements in the three patients in the 1997 study were documented in rCBF, functional abilities, and cognitive skills up to 45 months postinsult.

In 1998, Pizzamiglio *et al.* used functional imaging to monitor the effects of rehabilitation for unilateral neglect. The brain regions most active after recovery were almost identical to the areas active in control participants engaged in the same tasks. This would appear to support the view that some rehabilitation methods repair the lesioned network and do not simply work through compensation or behavioural change.

Is this true for memory rehabilitation? We do not yet know the answer to this question, but there is a growing interest in determining:

+ whether attempts to restore memory functioning and attempts to help people compensate result in structural changes to the brain;

+ whether any changes seen are different depending on the approach employed.

In reality, of course, the two approaches are not mutually exclusive and a combination of the two may prove to be the most practically useful.

7 Is treatment effective in helping people with memory and learning difficulties?

There would appear to be four major approaches to cognitive rehabilitation:

+ cognitive retraining through stimulation or exercises;

+ strategies derived from cognitive-neuropsychological theoretical models;

- techniques combining methodologies and theories from a number of different fields (particularly behavioural psychology, neuropsychology, and cognitive psychology);
- holistic approaches that address social and emotional problems alongside the cognitive ones.

The nature of these approaches together with their strengths and weaknesses are addressed in further detail by Wilson (1997a,b).

7.1 Compensatory approaches

There is increasing evidence to suggest that rehabilitation can improve cognitive functioning (e.g. Evans *et al.* 1998; Merzenich *et al.* 1996; Robertson 1999; Tallal *et al.* 1996; Wilson *et al.* 1994, 1997; Zihl 2000). In the field of memory disorders, the method of choice for reducing everyday problems (rather than improving memory functioning) is probably to teach compensatory approaches. Several publications show that people with memory impairments can function independently if they are able to use strategies to get round their difficulties. Wilson *et al.* (1997) describe J.C., a young man who became densely amnesic following a ruptured aneurysm on the left posterior cerebral artery. Over a 10-year period, J.C. developed a sophisticated system of memory aids enabling him to live alone, hold down a job, and be totally independent despite the fact that he remains severely amnesic. The paper describes the natural history of the development of J.C.'s compensatory system, which began by him writing on scraps of paper a few weeks after his stroke and over time developing his highly successful system.

Another encouraging study describes the rehabilitation of a young woman who became amnesic following status epilepticus (Kime *et al.* 1996). This woman was taught to use a personal organizer (datebook), refer to it regularly, and monitor a number of daily events. Over a period of several weeks, she was able to learn the different sections of a datebook and use this to manage her life. After leaving the rehabilitation centre, she worked in a voluntary capacity (still using her system) and eventually was taken on as a paid employee.

Even with those people who are unable to return to work, memory compensations can assist independent living. One instrument that has been helpful to a number of memory-impaired people is NeuroPage®, an alphanumeric pager attached to a belt worn by them that sends out daily reminders. In a pilot study (Wilson *et al.* 1997), 100% of 15 people with memory and/or planning problems showed a statistically significant improvement in achieving everyday target behaviours (e.g. taking medication, feeding the dog, collecting children from school) with the pager than they had achieved during a baseline period. Further work with the pager showed how effective this could be for individuals (Evans *et al.* 1998; Wilson *et al.* 1999b). Findings have since been replicated with a larger study of 143 people (Wilson *et al.* 2001).

7.2 'Errorless' learning

In addition to compensations in the form of external memory aids, techniques for improving learning in memory-impaired people are a major part of rehabilitation. It has been demonstrated that people with amnesia learn better if they are prevented from making mistakes during the learning process (Baddeley and Wilson 1994). Most of us benefit from trial-and-error learning if we can remember our previous mistakes. People with amnesia, of course, cannot do this because, once a mistake has been made, it may be strengthened or reinforced or be indistinguishable from the correct response. Consequently, it is better to prevent the incorrect response being made in the first place. Following the original Baddeley and Wilson (1994) paper, several studies have been carried out applying the 'errorless learning' principle to teaching real-life tasks (Clare *et al.* 1999, 2000; Squires *et al.* 1997; Wilson and Evans 1996; Wilson *et al.* 1994). Although a number of questions, both clinical and theoretical, remain to be answered about 'errorless learning', the principle would appear to be better than trial-and-error learning for teaching people with memory difficulties useful information for helping them cope in everyday life.

7.3 A holistic approach

Finally, a holistic programme for helping people with memory problems would address emotional problems such as anxiety and depression together with any cognitive deficits. In such a programme both group and individual therapy would be used to reduce both emotional and cognitive problems and would be embedded in a goal-planning approach. The goals would be negotiated between clients/patients, family members, and staff. Long-term goals are those that should be achieved by the time of discharge from the rehabilitation programme and short-term goals are the steps taken to reach the long-term goals. Thus, long-term aims might be to:

- 'develop a system for scheduling appointments';
- learn how to use a computer program for managing one's finances;
- learn the location of the nearest bank;
- reduce anxiety about meeting new people.

Short-term objectives for 'developing a system for scheduling appointments' might include:

- the occupational therapist accompanying the client in order to purchase an electronic organizer;
- the psychologist using an errorless learning procedure to teach the client how to enter an appointment;
- the client learning how to check a message when the alarm sounds;
- in the memory group the client will practise using the machine to schedule appointments and respond appropriately.

Each long-term aim would require a different set of short-term objectives.

Examples of this approach with individual clients can be found in Wilson *et al.* (in press) and Wilson *et al.* (2002). The important aspects of this approach are:

◆ addressing both emotional and cognitive difficulties;

◆ involving the client/patient and the family in the decision-making process;

◆ setting goals that are of practical everyday value as well as being realistic and achievable;

◆ monitoring and recording progress and, if unsuccessful, reasons for failure in achieving certain goals.

8 Summary and conclusions

People with memory problems typically show some resolution of deficits acquired as a result of an insult to the brain. Following traumatic brain injury the recovery process can continue for a number of years. In other conditions, such as encephalitis or hypoxic brain damage, the recovery process may not continue for such a long period. Age may have some bearing on the amount of recovery attainable, but other things, such as whether the lesion is focal or diffuse and the amount of time since the skill was originally learned, will also play a part.

The mechanisms of recovery are not well understood but several processes may be involved including regeneration of brain cells, diaschisis, and plasticity or reorganization of brain functions. Memory functions certainly show some recovery in the early days and weeks following an insult to the brain and, once again, the amount of recovery may depend on the cause of the brain damage (e.g. traumatic brain injury or encephalitis). It is not clear to what extent brain areas involved in memory can regenerate and whether such regeneration can be influenced by enriched environments, rehabilitation programmes, or other specific training strategies. Imaging techniques may enable us to answer some of these questions.

Rehabilitation can certainly reduce some of the everyday problems faced by people with memory deficits. Helping them to compensate for their poor memory skills is, at present, one of the most fruitful methods. Technology, including a new paging system, has significantly enhanced the ability to carry out everyday tasks in a recent randomized control cross-over design with 143 brain-injured people. Errorless learning techniques (i.e. avoiding trial-and-error learning) have proved beneficial in helping people to learn more efficiently. Holistic programmes addressing both emotional and cognitive problems are recommended in the rehabilitation of people with memory and learning difficulties, particularly when embedded in a goal-planning approach.

Selective references

Baddeley, A.D. and Wilson, B.A. (1994). When implicit learning fails: amnesia and the problem of error elimination. *Neuropsychologia* 32, 53–68.

Basso, A. and Farabola, M. (1997). Comparison of improvement of aphasia in three patients with lesions in anterior, posterior, and antero-posterior language areas. *Neuropsychol. Rehabil.* 7, 215–30.

Broman, M., Rose, A. L., Hotson, G., and Casey, C.M. (1997). Severe anterograde amnesia with onset in childhood as a result of anoxic encephalopathy. *Brain* 120, 417–33.

Carlomagno, S., VanEeckhout, P., Blasi, V., Belin, P., Samson, Y., and Deloche, G. (1997). The impact of functional neuroimaging methods on the development of a theory for cognitive remediation. *Neuropsychol. Rehabil.* 7, 311–26.

Clare, L. and Woods, B. (eds.) (2001). *Neuropsychological rehabilitation: special issue on cognitive rehabilitation in dementia.* Psychology Press, Hove.

Clare, L., Wilson, B.A., Breen, E.K., and Hodges, J.R. (1999). Errorless learning of face-name associations in early Alzheimer's disease. *Neurocase* 5, 37–46.

Clare, L., Wilson, B.A., Carter, G., Breen, K., Gosses, A., and Hodges, J.R. (2000). Intervening with everyday memory problems in dementia of Alzheimer type: an errorless learning approach. *J. Clin. Exp. Neuropsychol.* 22, 132–46.

Eriksson, P.S., Perfilieva, E., Bjork-Eriksson, T., Alborn, A.M., Nordborg, C., Peterson, D.A., and Gage, F.H. (1998). Neurogenesis in the adult human hippocampus. *Nature Med.* 4, 1313–17.

Evans, J.J., Emslie, H., and Wilson, B.A. (1998). External cueing systems in the rehabilitation of executive impairments of action. *J. Int. Neuropsychol. Soc.* 4, 399–408.

Farmer, S.F., Harrison, L.M., Ingram, D.A., and Stephens, J.A. (1991). Plasticity of central motor pathways in children with hemiplegic cerebral-palsy. *Neurology* 41, 1505–10.

Finger, S. and Almli, C.R. (1988). Margaret Kennard and her 'Principle' in historical perspective. In *Brain injury and recovery: theoretical and controversial issues* (eds. S. Finger, T.E. LeVere, R. Almli, and D.G. Stein), pp. 117–32. Plenum Press, New York.

Finger, S. and Stein, D. (1982). *Brain damage and recovery.* Academic Press, New York.

Fleming, J.M., Strong, J., Ashton, R., and Hassell, M. (1997). A one-year longitudinal study of severe traumatic brain injury in Australia using the Sickness Impact Profile. *J. Head Trauma Rehabil.* 12, 27–40.

Funnell, E. and De Mornay Davies, P. (1996). JBR: a reassessment of concept familiarity and a category-specific disorder for living things. *Neurocase* 2, 461–74.

Glisky, E.L. and Schacter, D.L. (1986). Long-term retention of computer learning by patients with memory disorders. *Neuropsychologia* 26, 173–8.

Gould, E., Beylin, A., Tanapat, P., Reeves, A.J., and Shors, T.J. (1999). Learning enhances adult neurogenesis in the hippocampal formation. *Nature Neurosci.* 2, 260–5.

Grady, C.L. and Kapur, S. (1999). The use of imaging in neurorehabilitative research. In *Cognitive neurorehabilitation: a comprehensive approach* (ed. D.T. Stuss, G, Winocur, and I. Robertson), pp. 47–58. Cambridge University Press, New York.

Jennett, B. (1990). Scale and scope of the problems. In *Rehabilitation of the adult and child with traumatic brain injury* (ed. M. Rosenthal, E.R. Griffith, M.R. Bond, and J.D. Miller), pp. 3–7. F.A. Davis and Co, Philadelphia.

Jennett, B. and Bond, M. (1975). Assessment of outcome after severe brain damage. *Lancet* 1, 480–4.

Kapur, N. (1997). *Injured brains of medical minds: views from within.* Oxford University Press, Oxford.

Kennard, M.A. (1940). Relation of age to motor impairment in man and subhuman primates *Archives of Neurology and Psychiatry* 44, 377–97.

Kime, S. K., Lamb, D.G., and Wilson, B.A. (1996). Use of a comprehensive program of external cuing to enhance procedural memory in a patient with dense amnesia. *Brain Injury* 10, 17–25.

Kolb, B. (1995). *Brain plasticity and behaviour*. Lawrence Erlbaum, Hillsdale, New Jersey.

Laatsch, L., Jobe, T., Sychra, J., Lin, Q., and Blend, M. (1997). Impact of cognitive rehabilitation therapy on neuropsychological impairments as measured by brain perfusion SPECT: a longitudinal study. *Brain Injury* 11, 851–63.

Laatsch, L., Pavel, D., Jobe, T., Lin, Q., and Quintana, J.-C. (1999). Incorporation of SPECT imaging in a longitudinal cognitive rehabilitation therapy programme. *Brain Injury* 13, 555–70.

Lindgren, M., Osterberg, K., Orbaek, P., and Rosen, I. (1997). Solvent-induced toxic encephalopathy: electrophysiological data in relation to neuropsychological finding. *J. Clin. Exp. Neuropsychol.* 19, 772–83.

Luria, A.R. (1963). *Recovery of function after brain injury*. Macmillan, New York.

Marshall, J.F. (1985). Neural plasticity and recovery of function after brain injury. *Int. Rev. Neurobiol.* 26, 201–47.

Max, J.E., Lindgren, S.D., Smith, W.L., Sato, Y., Mattheis, P.J., Robin, D.A., Stierwalt, J.A.G., and Muhonen, M. (1997). Surprising neurobehavioral functioning and brief major depression following penetrating brain injury in an adolescent. *Neurocase* 3, 127–36.

McGrath, N., Anderson, N.E., Croxson, M.C., and Powell, K.F. (1997). Herpes simplex encephalitis treated with acyclovir: diagnosis and long-term outcome. *J. Neurol., Neurosurg., Psychiatry* 63, 321–6.

McMillan, T.M., Robertson, I.H., and Wilson, B.A. (1999). Neurogenesis after brain injury. *Neuropsychol. Rehabil.* 9, 129–33.

Merzenich, M.M., Jenkins, W.M., Johnston, P., Schreiner, C., Miller, S.L., and Tallal, P. (1996). Temporal processing deficits of language-learning impaired children ameliorated by training. *Science* 271, 77–81.

Miller, E. (1984). *Recovery and management of neuropsychological function*. Wiley, Chichester.

Newcombe, F. (1996). Very late outcome after focal wartime brain wounds. *J. Clin. Exp. Neuropsychol.* 18, 1–23.

Nirkko, A.C., Rösler, K.M., Ozdoba, C., Heid, O., Schroth, G., and Hess, C.W. (1997). Human cortical plasticity: functional recovery with mirror movements. *Neurology* 48, 1090–3.

Ogden, J.A. (2000). Neurorehabilitation in the Third Millenium: new roles for our environment, behaviors, and mind in brain damage and recovery. *Brain Cogn.* 42, 110–12.

Pizzamiglio, L., Perani, D., Cappa, S.F., Vallar, G., Paolucci, S., Grassi, F., Paulesu, E., and Fazio, F. (1998). Recovery of neglect after right hemispheric damage: H2(15)O positron emission tomographic activation study. *Arch. Neurol.* 55, 561–8.

Plaut, D. (1996). Relearning after damage in connectionist networks: towards a theory of rehabilitation. *Brain Language* 52, 25–82.

Ponsford, J. (1995). Mechanisms, recovery and sequelae of traumatic brain injury: a foundation for the REAL approach. In *Traumatic brain injury: rehabilitation for everyday adaptive living* (ed. J. Ponsford, S. Sloan, and P. Snow), pp. 1–31. Lawrence Erlbaum Associates, Hove, East Sussex.

Ramachandran, V.S., Stewart, M., and Rogers-Ramachandran, D.C. (1992). Perceptual correlates of massive cortical reorganisation. *NeuroReport* 3, 583–6.

Reeder, K.P., Rosenthal, M., Lichtenberg, P., and Wood, D. (1996). Impact of age on functional outcome following traumatic brain injury. *J. Head Trauma Rehabil.* 11, 22–31.

Robertson, I.H. (1999). Theory-driven neuropsychological rehabilitation: the role of attention and competition in recovery of function after brain damage. In *Attention and performance XVII: Cognitive regulation of performance: interaction of theory and application* (ed. D. Gopher and A. Koriat), pp. 677–96. MIT Press, Cambridge, Massachusetts.

Robertson, I.H. and Murre, J.M.J. (1999). Rehabilitation after brain damage: brain plasticity and principles of guided recovery. *Psychol. Bull.* 125, 544–75.

Robertson, I.H., Ridgeway, V., Greenfield, E., and Parr, A. (1997). Motor recovery after stroke depends on intact sustained attention: a two-year follow-up study. *Neuropsychology* 11, 290–5.

Scoville, W.B. and Milner, B. (1957). Loss of recent memory after bilateral hippocampal lesions. *J. Neurol., Neurosurg., Psychiatry* 20, 11–21.

Squires, E.J., Hunkin, N.M., and Parkin, A.J. (1997). Errorless learning of novel associations in amnesia. *Neuropsychologia* 35, 1103–11.

Stern, R.A. (2000). *What is cognitive reserve?* Workshop presented to The International Neuropsychological Society meeting, Denver, Colorado, February 2000.

Stern, R.A., Silva, S.G., Chaisson, N., and Evans, D.L. (1996). Influence of cognitive reserve on neuropsychological functioning in asymptomatic human immunodeficiency virus-1 infection. *Arch. Neurol.* 53, 148–53.

Stern, Y., Tang, M.X., Denaro, J., and Mayeaux, R. (1995). Increased risk of mortality in Alzheimer's disease patients with more advanced educational and occupational attainment. *Ann. Neurol.* 37, 590–5.

Symonds, G.P. (1937). Mental disorder following head injury. *Proc. R. Soc. Med.* 30, 1081–94.

Tallal, P., Miller, S.L., Bedi, G., Byma, G., Wang, X., Nagarajan, S.S., Schreiner, C., Jenkins, W.M., and Merzenich, M.M. (1996). Language comprehension in language-learning impaired children improved with acoustically modified speech. *Science* 271, 81–4.

Thomsen, I.V. (1984). Late outcome of very severe blunt head trauma: a 10–15 year second follow-up. *J. Neurol., Neurosurg., Psychiatry* 47, 260–8.

Van Praag, H., Kempermann, G., and Gage, F.H. (1999). Running increases cell proliferation and neurogenesis in the adult mouse dentate gyrus. *Nature Neurosci.* 2, 266–70.

Vargha-Khadem, F., Gadian, D. G., Watkins, K.E., Connelly, A., Van Paesschen, W., and Mishkin, M. (1997). Differential effects of early hippocampal pathology on episodic and semantic memory. *Science* 277, 376–80.

Victor, M., Adams, R.D., and Collins, G.H. (1989). *The Wernicke-korsakoff syndrome and related neurologic disorders due to alcoholism and malnutrition*, 2nd edn. Philadelphia, PA: Davis.

von Monakow, C. (1914). *Die Lokalisation im Grosshirn und der Abbau der Funktion durch kortikale Herde.* J. F. Bergmann, Wiesbaden.

Whyte, J. (1990). Mechanisms of recovery of function following CNS damage. In *Rehabilitation of the adult and child with TBI*, 2nd edn (ed. M. Rosenthal, E.R. Griffith, M.R. Bond, and J.D. Miller), pp. 79–87. F.A. Davis and Co, Philadelphia.

Wilson, B.A. (1991). Long term prognosis of patients with severe memory disorders. *Neuropsychol. Rehabil.* 1, 117–34.

Wilson, B.A. (1995). Life after brain injury: long-term outcome of 101 people seen for rehabilitation 5–12 years earlier. In *Treatment issues and long-term outcomes: Proceedings of the 18th Annual Brain Impairment Conference* (Hobart, Australia, 1994) (ed. J. Fourez and N. Page), pp. 1–6. Australian Academic Press, Bowen Hills, Queensland.

Wilson, B.A. (1996). Cognitive functioning of adult survivors of cerebral hypoxia. *Brain Injury* 10, 863–74.

Wilson, B.A. (1997). Cognitive rehabilitation: how it is and how it might be. *J. Int. Neuropsychol. Soc.* 3, 487–96.

Wilson, B.A. (1998). Recovery of cognitive functions following non-progressive brain injury. *Curr. Opin. Neurobiol.* 8, 281–7.

Wilson, B.A., Emslie, H.C., Quirk, K., and Evans, J.J. (2001). Reducing everyday memory and planning problems by means of a paging systtem: a randomised control cross over study. *Journal of Neurology, Neurosurgery and Psychiatry*, 477–82.

Wilson, B.A. and Evans, J.J. (1996). Error free learning in the rehabilitation of individuals with memory impairments. *J. Head Trauma Rehabil.* **11**, 54–64.

Wilson, B.A., Vizor, A., and Bryant, T. (1991). Predicting severity of cognitive impairment after severe head injury. *Brain Injury* **5**, 189–97.

Wilson, B.A., Baddeley, A.D., Evans, J.J., and Shiel, A. (1994). Errorless learning in the rehabilitation of memory impaired people. *Neuropsychol. Rehabil.* **4**, 307–26.

Wilson, B.A., Baddeley, A.D., and Kapur, N. (1995). Dense amnesia in a professional musician following herpes simplex virus encephalitis. *J. Clin. Exp. Psychol.* **17**, 668–81.

Wilson, B.A., Evans, J.J., and Keohane, C. (2002) Cognitive rehabilitation: a goal planning approach. *Journal of Head Trauma Rehabilitation,* **17**, 542–55.

Wilson, B.A., Evans, J.J., Emslie, H., and Malinek, V. (1997). Evaluation of NeuroPage: a new memory aid. *J. Neurol., Neurosurg., Psychiatry,* **63**, 113–15.

Wilson, B.A., Evans, J.J., Emslie, H., Balleny, H., Watson, P.C., and Baddeley, A.D. (1999*a*). Measuring recovery from post traumatic amnesia. *Brain Injury* **13**, 505–20.

Wilson, B.A., Emslie, H., Quirk, K., and Evans, J. (1999*b*). George: learning to live independently with NeuroPage®. *Rehabil. Psychol.* **44**, 284–96.

Wilson, B.A., Evans, J.J., and Williams, H. (in press). Memory problems. In *Rehabilitation after traumatic brain injury: a psychological approach* (ed. A. T. Tyerman). The British Psychological Society, Leicester.

Young, D., Lawlor, P.A., Leone, P., Dragunow, M., and During, M.J. (1999). Environmental enrichment inhibits spontaneous apoptosis, prevents seizures and is neuroprotective. *Nature Med.* **5**, 448–53.

Zihl, J. (2000). *Rehabilitation of visual disorders after brain injury.* Psychology Press, Hove, East Sussex.

Zwaagstra, R., Schmidt, I., and Vanier, M. (1996). Recovery of speed of information processing in closed-head-injury patients. *J. Clin. Exp. Neuropsychol.* **18**, 383–93.

Chapter 11

Assessment and treatment of disorders of visuospatial, imaginal, and constructional processes

Lilianne Manning

1 Introduction

The usual screening neuropsychological batteries have practically ignored the assessment of visuospatial, imaginal, and constructional deficits. The general tendencies underlying current approaches consist of:

- an early *assessment* of these functions;
- the introduction of everyday life parameters, particularly, in *rehabilitation*.

The first tendency can be achieved by adding simple measures in order to increase the sensitivity of routine tests and guide the clinician to detect, from the very beginning of the assessment, one or more nonverbal disorders of the type covered in this chapter. An example is the enhancement of the sensitivity of the Mini Mental Status Examination by adding a clock drawing.

The second current tendency, studying the relationships between a given disorder and some measures of activity in daily living, implies the construction of highly targeted programmes based on both the patient's description (whenever possible) of his/her most disabling symptom(s) and a comprehensive assessment of deficits *and* preserved cognitive functions. It is worthwhile noting that everyday function can improve with the appropriate treatment without there being any improvement in cognitive test scores. The current 'ecological' concern also consists of using assessment and rehabilitation based on virtual environment technology when working with the real environment is impossible or unsuitable (e.g. for elderly patients) and when the aim of the programme cannot be achieved by using traditional neuropsychological methods. It basically consists of dynamic three-dimensional stimulus environments, in which a wide range of nonverbal deficits can be recorded, particularly concerning visual, topographical, and constructional processes.

2 Defects in visuospatial processes

Visuospatial processing ability can be defined as the capacity to localize objects in relation to each other in space and to know the location of single objects with respect to oneself. The major clinically different forms of visuospatial disorders are:

- visual disorientation;
- defective complex visuospatial processing;
- unilateral visual neglect;
- Balint's syndrome.

Balint's syndrome is triggered predominantly by attentional defects as is visual neglect—however, the latter can also be of an intentional and representational nature. Balint's syndrome and visual neglect are both dealt with elsewhere in this volume (see Chapter 8). Several other less frequently observed visuospatial deficits, such as impaired performance on mazes, have not been included in this section. The two forms of visuospatial disorders covered here are visual disorientation and defective complex visual processing.

2.1 Visual disorientation

2.1.1 Clinical presentation

Patients are unable to localize single objects, and act as if they were blind.

- They have marked difficulty in directing voluntary eye movements towards an object. Patients asked to look at the examiner's face look at many different points and are unable to 'stop' voluntarily at the face in front of them.
- They also have problems in reaching for or pointing to an object. They will almost invariably position the hand at the wrong distance in one or more of the three spatial dimensions. This deficit, observed despite the object actually being seen, is called *optic ataxia*. Note that patients with optic ataxia have no difficulty in localizing their own body parts. If the patient succeeds (often with help) in picking up food with a fork, he/she will bring it with no hesitation whatever to his/her mouth.
- Attentional processes are also impaired (see Chapters 5 and 6).

2.1.2 Brain damage localization

The brain damage is usually observed in the dorsal, occipitoparietal projections, i.e. the 'where' pathway. Lesions are generally bilateral, though there are some reports of visual location deficit in the hemi-field contralateral to the lesion. Visual disorientation, after either bilateral or unilateral lesions, is rare and its most severe form is found in patients with Balint's syndrome.

2.1.3 Diagnosis

The diagnosis of visual disorientation, i.e. impaired single-object localization, applies to the patient who, besides normal visual acuity, is able to localize external sounds (e.g. correctly pointing to the source of a voice while blindfolded) and tactile stimulation on his/her own body. This is necessary to rule out motor deficits and demonstrate accurate body sensations and normal use of body parts.

2.1.4 Assessment

A neuropsychological examination should only be conducted in patients who have successfully completed an ophthalmological examination.

- Ask the patient to look at an object and to point at an object or a dot on a sheet of paper to test *simple localization.*

- Assess *depth discrimination* by asking him/her to estimate distance of objects in the natural environment and by showing the patient two objects either on the same horizontal plane or on different planes, one of the objects being clearly closer to him/her. Can the patient say whether or not they are at the same distance? Carry out the same task moving the patient's finger from one object to the other. This tactile test should be normal.

- To test *size discrimination* place different sized real objects at the same distance from the patient. Can he/she say which is larger? The number of trials and the comparative size of the objects presented will depend on the initial results.

- *Optic ataxia* needs two conditions of testing:

  —First, ask the patient to reach out and grasp an object that he/she is looking at.

  —Second, repeat the manoeuvre but with a screen (a file or similar) placed between the patient's head and his/her arm to prevent him/her from seeing the hand movement.

Optic ataxic patients succeed in the second condition only.

- Test the patient's *spatial scan* and single-point localization using a dot-counting task. Norms exist for different groups of brain-damaged patients and normal controls (Warrington and James 1991).

2.1.5 Recovery and rehabilitation

Spontaneous recovery has been observed after unilateral right hemisphere damage. 'Improvement' of visuospatial difficulties has been observed after non-specific training programmes on visual material reflecting a general increase in the level of attention and awareness. Rehabilitation programmes in patients presenting impaired visual fixation, difficulty in scanning dot arrays, and inability to reach objects on visual guidance have been carried out. New rehabilitation programmes can be developed to improve on existing programmes provided that the rationale behind the intervention, the articulation of stages, and the time required to obtain results are all compatible with the case at hand. See, for example, Zihl (2000, pp. 107–32). His rationale was to improve localization of objects by fixating and reaching. He designed a progressively complex training scheme, the last stage being reading treatment demanding a very high level of visual control of eye movement. The whole programme took nearly 100 sessions. The results are encouraging. The patient improved her vision in everyday life, and improved fixation and localization helped her to achieve better identification of objects.

2.1.6 Case report

Patient H.B., a 63-year-old woman, obtained a Verbal IQ of 100 (Wechsler Adult Intelligence Scale (WAIS-R). She was able to name objects from a description but unable to carry out the Performance IQ. This combination of preliminary results both oriented the interview and indicated a test of visual process. She showed poor visual acuity but relatively well preserved ability to perceive shapes. Colour and face perception were preserved. Preliminary *visual orientation* was tested by asking her to point to a finger and to 1 cm diameter coloured dots presented one by one in different positions on a sheet of white paper. Her performance was markedly impaired. It was observed that she retained the ability to localize points on her body and the source of the examiner's voice with eyes closed. These few results suggested that both diffuse neurodegenerative processes and shape disorders could be ruled out and pointed to a *differential diagnosis* of visual disorientation. It was decided to carry out several of the tests described above (see Section 2.1.4).

2.2 Complex visuospatial processing

Disorders in complex visuospatial processing are subdivided into two types:

◆ topographical disorientation;

◆ spatial analysis deficits.

2.2.1 Topographical disorientation

Clinical presentation   This deficit considerably hinders patients' everyday life. Characteristically, they have difficulty in finding their way from one location to another, despite intact basic visual processes. Moreover, they may present preserved topographical visual recognition and memory—they are able to recognize places while getting lost on familiar and/or simple routes or have difficulty in finding objects at home. The opposite pattern of performance, i.e. loss of topographical recognition and preserved spatial knowledge, results in an inability to recognize buildings and places while managing accurate accounts of journeys.

Brain localization   Predominantly right parietal damage.

Diagnosis   Diagnosis is based on interviews with the patient and a relative or carer about the extent and characteristics of topographical disorientation.

◆ Does the patient get lost in *familiar* surroundings?

◆ Is he/she unable to learn *new* simple routes?

◆ Was his/her way-finding good before the illness?

Take into account the fact that this disorder can be either a feature of dementia or a selective impairment with other functions well preserved (see 'Recovery and rehabilitation' in this section).

Assessment   Ask patient questions such as:

- How did you get here?
- Can you tell me how to get from X to Y? (X and Y being two places familiar to the patient).
- How do you go from this room to your ward?
- Can you describe your home/flat/room?

Maps or plans are often used for the patient to locate well known places in his/her country or city. It can also be useful to present a large square on a sheet of paper, to represent the patient's bedroom, and ask him/her to locate furniture, doors, and windows.

Recovery and rehabilitation

- Patients having difficulty in locating items in their familiar places benefit from written lists, e.g. of contents of cupboards.
- Patients getting lost on familiar routes can be helped by photographs of prominent environmental cues to be used as landmarks.
- Written instructions are also useful for some patients.
- To increase meaningful associations concerning well delimited locations of daily journeys between several places, teach the patient simple mnemonics combining names of streets and their location.
- A further real-life orientated treatment consists of walking with the patient in familiar surroundings, briefly or for a few minutes (depending on the patient's degree of deficit), then asking him/her to go back to the starting point. The length of time and the number of changes of direction are gradually increased. Finally, the patient can be asked to draw the route.

Rehabilitation programmes are more frequently constructed (and reported) when topographical disorientation is isolated rather than embedded in a diffuse clinical picture. However, it is important to bear in mind that the isolated presentation can be the result of combined effects of several impairments such as space perception and nonverbal memory. Treatment can focus on one of these. When deciding on the type of treatment it is helpful to have the patient's description of the most disabling symptom in his or her everyday life.

2.2.2 Spatial analysis deficits

- *Clinical presentation.* These deficits are often only revealed through testing. Patients suffering from spatial analysis deficits have difficulty in position discrimination and/or line orientation discrimination. Detection of discrimination impairments requires fairly elaborate tasks (see 'Assessment' in this section).
- *Brain localization.* Predominantly right parietal damage.
- *Diagnosis* of spatial analysis deficits is based on quantitative results in a series of specially constructed tests.

Assessment   The following tests assessing the patient's capacity to perceive the relative position of objects in two-dimensional space have been standardized (Warrington and James 1991).

♦ *Position Discrimination* consists of sets of two adjacent horizontal squares, one with a dot printed in the centre and one with a dot slightly off-centre. Ask the patient to point to the dot that is in the centre (cut-off, 17/20). Carry out the next task even if the patient's performance is normal.

♦ *Number Location* consists of sets of two non-adjacent squares placed one above the other. The bottom square contains one single dot corresponding to one of the randomly placed nine numbers of the top square. Ask the patient to say or point to the number that matches the position of the dot (cut-off, 7/10).

♦ *Cube Analysis.* The patient has to interpret three-dimensional space in two-dimensional representations (see Fig. 11.1). Ask the patient to count the number of solid bricks (cut-off, 6/10).

♦ Discrimination of *line orientation* is tested with a graded difficulty task consisting of two figures, one above the other, showing a 'sun ray' of lines of different orientation: the top figure shows two 'rays', the bottom figure shows 11 'rays' covering 180°. Ask the patient to match the two lines of the top figure to those that have the same slant in the 'sun ray' bottom figure. The task is fairly sensitive and provides norms for groups of brain-damaged patients and normal controls (Benton *et al.* 1983, pp. 56–62). (See Table 11.1 for a synopsis.)

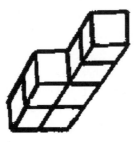

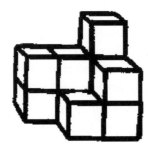

Fig.11.1 Example of stimuli from a spatial analysis test, the Cube Analysis task (Warrington and James 1991). (Reproduced by kind permission of the publisher, Thames Valley Test Company.)

Table 11.1 Visuospatial processes: synopsis of deficits and tests

Visuospatial disorientation	Complex visual processing	
	Topographical deficits	Spatial analysis deficits
Simple item localization	'How did you get here?'	Position Discrimination
Depth discrimination	'Go from X to Y'	Number Location
Size discrimination	'Show me . . . on this map'	Cube Analysis
Reaching out tests	'Draw your flat/room'	Line Orientation Test

Recovery and rehabilitation   Measurement of specific visuospatial abilities at time of admission may help the rehabilitation prognosis.

- Treatment could be attempted using the tactile versions of the cube analysis subtest or the line orientation test, with patients presenting deficits on spatial analysis in the visual modality only.

- A treatment using the tactile and the visual modalities consists of fitting different shapes into the correct holes in a board, as quickly as possible.

- Computer-generated virtual environments that can be explored in real time could be used to treat acquired visuospatial deficits.

- Finally, patients with some musical abilities could benefit from a rehabilitation programme combining increasing levels of difficulty, figures of cubes (of the type presented in Fig. 11.1), and musical isomers. It has been suggested that the latter facilitate visuospatial relations since the same holistic processes appear to be at work both in the perception of musical contour and in mental manipulations of two-dimensional figures.

> **Case report**   Patient C.S., a 73–year-old woman, obtained a verbal IQ of 99 and a performance IQ of 87 (WAIS-R). Naming on description was very good. Verbal recognition memory was adequate (it was orally presented). She was unable to recognize unusual views of common objects but recognized 20/20 when the canonical view was presented. This result led to her being asked to perform several visuoperceptual tasks (not commented on here) and visuospatial tasks. Concerning the latter, she failed the Position Discrimination test (8/20), and the Cube Analysis task (2/10). These preliminary results suggested that there was a deterioration affecting, in particular, perceptual and visuospatial skills, with verbal abilities remaining relatively intact. A further assessment session was decided with a view to obtaining a complete cognitive profile.

3 Deficits in imaginal processes

There are two forms of imaginal deficits: deficits in visual imagery and in spatial imagery. Visual or spatial imagery can be selectively impaired.

3.1 **Visual imagery**

Visual imagery is defined as the conscious reproduction of previously experienced events and objects, their shape, colour, size, and any other visual attributes that we know.

- *Clinical presentation.* Patients may not realize that the brain lesion has induced a loss of imaginal visual attributes. On the contrary, they may be surprised not to be able to perform some tests. Loss of visual imagery may be observed together with visual agnosia or in the context of preserved visual recognition. Patients frequently also have right homonymous hemianopsia. Right hemiplegia and/or language disturbances (particularly shortly after a stroke) can also be present.

- *Brain damage localization.* Left posterior lesions.

- *Diagnosis.* Loss of visual imagery can be diagnosed only if the capacity to copy models and describe their visual characteristics is preserved (see Manning 2000).

3.1.1 **Assessment**

- Ask the patient to draw from memory and then to copy from canonical models, objects such as a cube, a flower, etc. This very simple and informative task can be carried out even at bedside.

- Ask the patient questions rich in visual attributes (e.g. 'what's the name of the bird with a hooked beak, large, flat face, round head, large eyes, and soft plumage?') and questions concerning functions only (e.g. 'the bird that stays awake all night long, flies, and hoots?'). Results are fairly straightforward: patients with no aphasic symptoms and impaired visual imagery fail selectively the 'visual' questions.

- Present the patient with coloured line drawings of canonical views of animals. Ask the patient to indicate whether the tail of the animal is long or short relative to its body in each of the following three conditions:

  —the perceptual control condition, in which the patient has to respond while looking at the depicted animal; if failed, the test should be discontinued;

  —the test situation proper, in which the tail of the animal is masked;

  —the auditory condition, where only the name of the animal is given.

  This test allows comparisons to be drawn between the patient's ability to conjure up mental images from incomplete visual items and from auditory input. Patients with genuine loss of visual imagery will fail the test on the last two conditions.

- To test visual imagery of *colours*, administer the following tests:

- Control condition. Present the patient with 10 different coloured patches. Ask him/her to point to the same coloured patch as indicated by the examiner on a set of identical coloured patches distributed differently. If the patient fails this task, discontinue the colour examination.

- Present the patient with 10 or more uncoloured canonical line drawings and a good set of crayons. Ask him/her to fill in the line drawings with the appropriate colour.

– Auditory condition. Ask the patient the colour of different fruits (cherry, banana, tangerine), animals (tiger, elephant, parrot), and personal objects (his/her tooth-brush, front door, car).

3.1.2 Recovery and rehabilitation

A treatment using nonvisual information consists of a series of familiar (e.g. spoon, key, watch) and less familiar objects (e.g. stapler, funnel, pair of goggles) to be *tactilely* explored by the patient. Objects' surfaces, or part of them, are covered with fabrics of different textures, which are associated with colours. Instruct the patient to describe the shape, imagine the colour (from the texture), imagine the object on a table, in a bag, near the window, etc.

The issue of imaginal rehabilitation is crucial for patients with artistic activity. Copying sufficiently elaborated models may allow the patient to re-acquire at least some of his/her technical and artistic skills. Models to be copied, which should be very well known to the patient, could be presented with progressively fewer parts as training of visual imagery progresses.

3.2 Spatial imagery

Spatial imagery is the ability to conjure up images of the location and structure of objects in three dimensions. The capacity to manipulate images is crucial to mental spatial transformations.

♦ *Clinical presentation.* It is not unusual for patients with spatial imagery deficits to say that they have more difficulty in 'working things out' than they used to before the brain accident.

♦ *Brain damage localization.* Left posterior lesions.

♦ *Diagnosis.* Deficits in spatial imagery are diagnosed if the patient fails tests of mental transformations, regardless of his/her ability or inability to conjure up visual images.

3.2.1 Assessment

♦ Present the patient with a sheet of paper containing capital letters in random order, half of them upside-down. Ask the patient to indicate which letters are the right way up. This is probably the easiest task and it is useful to start with it in order to reduce anxiety in patients who feel ill at ease when asked to perform spatial tasks.

♦ Ask the patient to imagine a capital letter and to count the corners. This task is sensitive enough to indicate if extended testing on spatial imagery is necessary.

♦ Give orally a series of letters, with (Q, G, etc.) or without (L, E, etc.) curves. Ask the patient to imagine them in the upper-case form and to indicate whether or not they have curves.

♦ Present a series of drawings of a man holding a black disc sometimes in his right and sometimes in his left hand. The figure should be shown upright or upside-down and from the front or from behind. Ask the patient to indicate in which hand the 'manikin' is holding the black disc. This rotation task is particularly useful in cases of association of visual and spatial imagery, since the task elicits mental transformation but not generation of mental images.

3.2.2 Recovery and rehabilitation

A tactile training device utilizing a board with rotated, made fast letters can be used to treat spatial imagery.

4 Deficits in constructional processes

Constructional processes involve the ability to produce properly organized 'constructions' such as drawings and building tasks, i.e. to assemble patterns of simple arrangements made up of blocks, tokens, or sticks. They involve the ability of normal visual and motor systems to execute visuomotor tasks.

Clinicians use the term 'constructional apraxia' for convenience rather than as a term with a precise meaning. Different factors may provoke constructional difficulties. However, the symptoms are sufficiently distinctive to be defined independently of other classical apraxias and visuoperceptive deficits (see Andrewes 2001, pp. 35–81).

4.1 Clinical presentation

The patient is unable to grasp the way in which the component elements relate to the final model to be (re)-produced, and then to fit the components together in the correct spatial organization.

4.2 Brain localization

Either right or left parietal lesions. Incidence is higher after a right injury (right : left ratio of 3 : 1) and the deficit is more severe in right and bilaterally injured patients. Independently of the side, the predominantly posterior localization of lesions is confirmed by significant correlations between the damaged neural substrate of Brodmann's area 18 and constructional ability.

◆ *Left lesions* result in oversimplification of the model within the context of a relatively preserved spatial relation. The *cause* is failure in the organization of actions necessary for constructing tasks.

◆ *Right lesion* patients produce overelaborate, often irrelevant fragments showing spatial disorganization. The *cause* is failure in the organization of space.

4.3 Diagnosis

The patient's inability to perform drawing and construction tasks occurs in the context of the following preserved functions:

◆ visual form perception;

◆ spatial localization;

◆ ideomotor praxis.

Although 'pure' constructional apraxic patients are rarely encountered in everyday practice, at least a *relative* preservation of the above functions must be demonstrated before this can be diagnosed.

Note that relatively complex tasks make demands on sustained attention and therefore could be performed defectively without any clinical significance for constructional processes (e.g. the Complex Rey Figure Test). Should this be the case, base diagnosis on easier tasks (e.g. copy of a cube). Likewise, aphasic patients should have demonstrated their understanding of the verbal instructions before a constructional disability is diagnosed.

4.4 Assessment

♦ Ask the patient to carry out a spontaneous drawing. Note that it can be difficult to score drawings produced on verbal command (right lesion patients may produce marked lateral neglect drawings; left lesion patients may be unable to perform—see Section 4.2.).

♦ If this is the case, ask him/her to draw a bicycle (see Lezak 1995, pp. 74–81) and to comment on as many details as possible about the way in which the different parts relate to each other. (For example, a right parietal patient produced an elaborate defective bicycle with the pedals close to the saddle. Asked how she made it work, she told me, 'you have to bend your knees up'. Her verbal response was tailored to the defective relation of a component part to the whole, which she was unable to correct.)

♦ Ask the patient to copy a line drawing, an abstract design such as the Rey Complex Figure. Scoring procedures for this and some other copying tasks (e.g. the copying section of the Benton Visual Retention Test; Benton 1962) are reliable and norms exist for different groups of brain-damaged patients and normal individuals (but see Section 2.4). Time of completion can be important for the qualitative analysis.

♦ To assess greater demands on the spatial component of perception than those made by the drawing tests, present block construction tests. They test three-dimensional construction processes, which call upon a particular set of functions since they elicit deficits not shown on two-dimensional tests. The Benton Constructional Test, which has detailed norms, is frequently used together with two simple tasks from the Stanford–Binet battery, the Tower and the Bridge. The latter two tasks are useful for severely impaired patients.

♦ The Block Design test (WAIS subtest or similar) is one of the most frequently used clinical tools. The patient is normally instructed to reproduce the models within a time limit since this is an IQ subtest for which norms are reliable and can be found in many different countries. However, when the task is used to assess constructional processes, no time limit should be imposed.

♦ Constructing stick patterns and copying from stick patterns are both rapid and less demanding tasks, but norms are not readily available. Qualitatively, despite their simplicity, they have proved sensitive to constructional impairment.

The common and characteristic factor among these constructional tasks is that they all need to be carried out in extrapersonal space. On this basis, it is useful to bear in mind that right- and left-damaged patients fail constructional tests for different reasons: an inability to correctly organize the parts of an object and an inability to analyse those parts, respectively.

Note that visuoconstructional processes need to be assessed by at least two different tests, mainly due to only moderate intertest correlation coefficients and differing test sensitivity. Analysis of this latter point showed that clinicians relying on the WAIS Block Design alone could easily underestimate a high percentage of constructional apraxia patients whose impaired performance is apparent on the more sensitive Rey Complex Figure Test. A final point concerns constructional processes in neurodegenerative diseases. In demented patients of the Alzheimer type, impairments in constructional tests requiring access to semantic and lexical knowledge (e.g. drawing or constructing something meaningful) are present in the early phase of the disease, while impairments in constructional tests that do not require that access (e.g. copying the Rey Complex Figure) become evident in later phases. Digressions from this general pattern of deficits may prompt the clinician to envisage the administration of extended constructional batteries aiming at clarifying an early involvement of the posterior associative cortex in the onset of Alzheimer dementia in a given patient. In patients suffering from Parkinson's disease, performance on constructional tasks, particularly copying a cube, is associated with mobility in daily life and social cognition.

4.5 Recovery and rehabilitation

Spontaneous recovery has been observed in two-thirds of patients. The size of the lesion is not related to the rate of recovery from constructional disability. There is a difference in average recovery depending on the side of brain injury. Patients in the left-hemisphere group show better recovery a few months postonset than the right-hemisphere group. Rehabilitation programme reports are virtually non-existent in the literature. Compared to language or memory deficits, the inability to reproduce a line drawing or build a tower seems insignificant. 'Pure' cases are extremely rare and, whenever an intervention is reported, it is in the context of either motor or visuoperceptive impairments. Patients may never complain of being unable to reproduce patterns since this ability mostly involves non-ecological tasks.

Some empirical suggestions to be taken into account in a tailor-made rehabilitation programme follow.

◆ Analyse the patient's constructional errors concerning the whole, the parts, and the 'boundedness'. Observe the effects of time constraints. Some tasks (e.g. Block Design) are usually timed. It may be useful to obtain a score for standard time limit completion and a separate score for performance with no time constraints. However marginally patients may benefit from the extra time allowed them in terms of improved performance, comparisons of productions with and without a time limit might be helpful in determining whether different types of difficulty appear in each situation.

◆ Concerning daily life treatment, it is useful to bear in mind that

—there is a correlation between the WAIS-R Block Design subtest (see above) and meal preparation skills;

—some patients suffering from constructional apraxia may have difficulty in dressing (not the full-blown dressing apraxia picture), because a portion of the inability to dress is perceptual, not motor in origin. Constructional praxis treatment may produce some gains in the ability to dress.

Finally, computer-aided training programmes are available. The 'Visuoconstructive Abilities KONS' (Visuoconstructive Abilities Kons 1997) is intended for patients with mild or moderate constructional apraxia whose memory is preserved. The programme consists of 18 levels of difficulty. The authors state that the adaptive nature of the programme allows a great deal of variation in training. This has the advantage of ensuring maximum adjustment per patient, whose improvement is recorded. However, the programme makes no provision for quantitative data for groups of patients.

Table 11.2 'What to test and when': suggestions for everyday clinics for patients whose medical files and referral requests do not specify the symptoms (see text for more information)

Patient's characteristics	Suggested disorder to be tested
Defective pointing to and copying tasks; preserved shape recognition	Visual disorientation
Defective way and objects finding; preserved memory	Topographical disorientation
Defective or weak score on any subtest of the VOSP in routine examination	Visuospatial analysis disorder
Defective drawings from memory; preserved copies from models	Loss of visual imagery
Explicit complaint or loss of visual imagery	Loss of spatial imagery
Defective score on the Block Design task on routine assessment	Constructional apraxia

Table 11.3 Examples of treatments reported to have had positive effects on the patient's everyday life (see text for more information)

Disorder	Treatment	Everyday life
Visual disorientation	Fixating and reaching objects	Improved 'vision' in familiar surroundings
Topographical disorientation	Written lists and instructions Mnemonics to create associations Back to the starting point task	Find objects at home Find familiar routes Find familiar routes
Loss of visual imagery in artists	Copy and complete well-known pictures	Helps artistic production
Constructional apraxia	Training in constructional tasks	Meal preparation Ability to dress

5 Conclusion

◆ The deficits referred to in this chapter reflect a disturbance of the *processing* of sensory information, the sense organs usually remaining intact.

◆ Deciding 'What to test and when' considers both impaired and preserved functions, as shown in Table 11.2.

◆ To ensure that the patient receives appropriate treatment these syndromes must be diagnosed as early as possible. Table 11.3 lists the treatments that have been shown to have beneficial effects on everyday life.

Selective references

Andrewes, D. (2001). *Neuropsychology from theory to practice.* Psychology Press Ltd, Hove, East Sussex.

Benton, A. (1962) The visual retention test as a constructional praxis test. *Confina Neurologica* 22, 141–55.

Benton, A., Hamsher, K., Varney, N., and Spreen, O. (1983). *Contributions to neuropsychological assessment.* Oxford University Press, New York.

Lezak, M. (1995). *Neuropsychological assessment,* 3rd edn. Oxford University Press, New York.

Manning, L. (2000). Loss of visual imagery and defective recognition of parts of wholes in optic aphasia. *Neurocase* 6, 111–28.

Visuoconstructive Abilities KONS. (1997). *REHA COM.* Schuhfried, Moedling.

Warrington, E. and James, M. (1991) *The Visual Object and Space Perception Battery.* Thames Valley Test Company, Bury St Edmunds.

Zihl, J. (2000). *Rehabilitation of visual disorders after brain injury.* Psychology Press, Hove, East Sussex.

Chapter 12

Assessing disorders of awareness and representation of body parts

Carlo Semenza

1 Introduction

Disorders of awareness and representation of body parts traditionally encompass a number of very heterogeneous pathological conditions, whose links with one another share a common intuition that something about the representation of body has been damaged. This chapter acknowledges this tradition in the absence of a better way to cover the whole topic in a clinical handbook. Some provisos, however, must precede the description of single pathological entities.

For some time, the common factor grouping together these different behavioural pathologies was their effect on the so-called 'body schema'. This largely underspecified concept has enjoyed an immense, undeserved, and potentially damaging popularity. First, the concept has always been very vague. Second, a large variety of symptoms have been attributed to a 'disturbance of body schema' and then used to prove the validity of the concept. The circularity of this line of reasoning was first pointed out by Poeck and Orgass (1971), but it took several years for neuropsychologists to become aware of this problem and avoid the concept. Serious theorizing about disorders of bodily awareness and representation must thus be regarded, with the exception of a few studies, to be the result of a relatively recent enterprise that has taken place over the past 3 decades. This whole matter is dealt with, in detail, in several recent reviews (e.g. Denes 1989; Semenza 2001).

Quite apart from poor theorizing, the field has also suffered from inappropriate procedures and a failure to demonstrate body specificity for the effects emerging from clinical investigations. These all have seriously hampered traditional assessment and the theoretical conclusions derived from such methods. A good example is the request to draw one's own body as a method to test a subject's knowledge and sensory experience of their 'body schema'. Typically, such a procedure, suggested by authorities such as Schilder (1935), ignored the fact that drawing abilities were spared in all cases.

2 Overview: the variety of pathologies (representation and awareness)

One reason for the neglect of theory in the field is that the most significant patholog-ical conditions (Table 12.1) are, in general, rare and often difficult to spot, especially since most patients do not spontaneously complain about them.

◆ The cleareast example of body-specific representation disorder is *autotopoagnosia*, a rare condition where the patient cannot locate body parts on verbal command. The neuropsychological instruments used to detect such a disorder are paradig-matic and were developed from principled criteria. Consequently, they will be mentioned first.

◆ Hemisomatoagnosia or personal neglect and related disorders such as allochiria and extinction of contralesional stimuli to bilateral tactile stimulation are tradi-tionally ascribed to malfunctioning of body awareness. Distal extinction on uni-lateral double stimulation is another interesting condition with a different clinical meaning. This group of quite commonly observed disturbances have been extensively investigated and clinicians can therefore profit from a large repertory of clinical tools.

◆ The alien hand syndrome, though sometimes overlapping conceptually with hemi-somatoagnosia, is an uncommon cluster of symptoms wherein involuntary limb movements are coupled with a sense of estrangement from or of personification of the limb.

◆ Somatosensory hallucinations and illusions mainly consist of the experience of a larger, a smaller, or even a duplicated body. Some patients also report being 'unable to recog-nize their body boundaries' or their posture. There is no established assessment for

Table 12.1 Disorders of body representation and awareness

Autotopagnosia
Somatosensory hallucinations and illusions

Hemisomatagnosia (personal neglect) and related disorders
    Allochiria
    Somatoparaphrenia
    Extinction of contralesional stimuli to bilateral stimulation

Distal extinction on unilateral double stimulation

Altered muscular proprioception
    Proprioceptive deafferentation
    Deafferentation after parietal lesions

Alien hand syndrome (including Anarchic Hand)
Phantom limb and related disorders
Body-specific cognitive biases in eating disorders

these disorders, most reports being anecdotal. They will, therefore, not be discussed here, except for the more common ones, i.e. those associated with personal neglect that concern the contralesional side of the body.

- The consequences of altered muscular proprioception, proprioceptive deafferentation, and deafferentation after parietal lesion will also be described here, although well reported cases are extremely rare.

- Consciousness of missing body parts, i.e. phantom limb and related phenomena, constitutes a less traditional domain for neuropsychological investigation, since no direct damage to the brain is involved (despite considerable reorganization of the cortical representation of missing body parts). A detailed assessment of these conditions, rather frequent in amputees, depends on careful observational and experimental studies.

- Finally, *body-specific cognitive biases in eating disorders* will be considered. The reason for including this is not that these problems are treated as 'body schema' or 'body image' disorders. However, it has been recently shown that such biases (basically consisting of misjudgements of size and weight) can be body-specific. These observations were derived from, among other things, neuropsychological data.

Theoretically motivated rehabilitation of all the above disorders has rarely been attempted, except in the case of personal neglect, and often only in severe cases, where the condition dramatically interfered with everyday life.

3 Autotopagnosia

Autotopagnosia is the inability to locate body parts in response to command. The nature of this disturbance is not well understood in terms of the mental representations and cognitive processes involved.

The main preoccupation for researchers has been to make sure that the observed phenomenon is related to experience of the body. This deficit has to be the primary deficit, i.e. it should not result from other cognitive disorders. In its assessment, as in any case of agnosia, other sources of error should be ruled out. It is therefore important to make sure that aphasia, attentional deficits (e.g. neglect), visual or tactile agnosia, apraxia, or reaching disturbances, as well as more peripheral motor and sensory disorders, cannot explain the observed inability. Other more subtle and less well known deficits must equally be ruled out, such as the inability to isolate parts from a whole—a rare disorder that, in the past, was thought to be the basis of what seemed, in all other respects, to be true cases of autotopagnosia (De Renzi and Scotti 1970).

The term 'autotopagnosia' itself is not without problems. As Gerstman (1942) observed, and as the prefix 'auto' implies, 'autotopagnosia should, in principle, refer to a difficulty in indicating one's own body parts and not the body parts of other persons, of mannequins or drawings of a body'. Gerstman proposed the term 'somatotopagnosia' to include difficulties with the body parts of others. Indeed, no reported case has

Table 12.2 Transcoding tasks used in the assessment of autotopagnosia

Stimulus	Example	Response
Pointing tasks		
Verbal command	'Show me the ear'	Pointing to self
		Pointing to other person
		Pointing to drawing (full size)
		Pointing to drawing (single parts)
Nonverbal command	Examiner touches self	Pointing to self
	Examiner touches the patient	Pointing to other person
	(who must keep the eyes closed)	Pointing to drawing (full size)
	Examiner shows a picture of isolated	Pointing to drawing (cut-out
	parts	single parts)
Verification tasks	'Am I touching the ear?'	Yes/no (verbal or nonverbal
		indication)
Construction tasks	From pieces of puppets, etc.	
Description tasks		
Structural description	'Is the nose above or below the mouth?'	
	'Is the wrist next to the forearm?'	
Functional description	'What is the nose for?'	
	'Is the nose for smelling?'	

been shown where the difficulty only concerns one's own body parts and not also those of other people. Thus, in a strict sense, pure autotopagnosia has never been described. The arguably more correct term 'somatotopagnosia', however, was never fully adopted, and 'autotopagnosia' remains the currently used name for the disorder.

A detailed theoretical treatment of autotopagnosia and the operational tasks used to reveal such a disturbance has never been attempted. Available empirical evidence, however, suggests that specific transcoding mechanisms support the localization of body parts. Various input (verbal, visual, tactile) and output (motor, verbal) modalities are involved, with or without the mediation of a body-specific representation in semantic memory. Both spatial and functional components have been identified as constituents of this representation (see later in this section), although it is still unclear as to what proportion these contribute and which tasks tap which component.

Assessment of the few known cases of autotopagnosia (Table 12.2) has been performed using four specific tasks (Semenza and Goodglass 1985; Semenza 2001; Semenza and Delazer, 2003) and several control tasks.

3.1 **Pointing tasks**

The request to point to body parts is the task that originally uncovered autotopagnosia as a clinical entity, when the subject showed an inability to carry it out. This task should be assessed in at least two conditions: a *verbal* and a *nonverbal* one. Failure in the verbal condition only may be attributed to aphasia (though not necessarily in an uninteresting way: if found to be specific for the names of body parts, for instance, a comprehension disorder would be a relatively rare category-specific aphasia).

Several transcoding subtests, varying in stimulus and response, are also required in order to:

♦ ascertain whether the symptom concerns parts of one's own and also those of other's bodies (though so far the two deficits have never been found to dissociate);

♦ be reasonably sure that the problem is not one of isolating one part within the whole (see later for further testing).

Of particular importance are tests in which the patient is touched while keeping his/her eyes closed and then requested to point to the stimulated part on someone else's body. The observed difficulty in this task allowed Semenza and Goodglass (1985) to conclude that authentic, body-specific, autotopagnosic errors could be detected after left-hemisphere brain damage.

Classification of the patient's errors is important and is indeed necessary to understand the nature of the mental representation whose disturbance is thought to result in the problem. Semenza and Goodglass (1985) divided autotopagnosic errors into three types of categories.

♦ *Contiguity (spatial) errors*, same limb as stimulus or face–head response for a face–head stimulus; this group includes errors that reflect misreaching.

♦ *Conceptual errors.* Different types of errors are included under this label: joint for joint, eye–ear–nose substitutions and *contiguity errors* where alternative response choices are presented as cut-out parts in a multiple choice display. This last type of error is not classified as spatial because it cannot possibly result from a spatially vague indication. It is indeed likely to derive from a disorder in the conceptual representation or in its output.

♦ *Random* errors include all the remaining.

A prevalence of conceptual or contiguity errors may indicate the type of autotopagnosia. It has been recently recognized that, in some of the reported cases (e.g. I.S. in Semenza 1988), a conceptual component is crucial to the defect, while in other cases (e.g. patients V.M. and D.A. in Denes *et al.* 2000) the spatial component appears to be overwhelming.

A sufficient number of body parts must appear in pointing tests (Semenza and Goodglass used 18), including parts of the head, of the limbs, and of the trunk. For special purposes, the investigator may want to include less prominent parts like wrists, nails, etc. No dissociation concerning these parts has, however, been described.

3.2 **Verification tasks**

Published cases of autotopagnosia have reported patients who perform this task flawlessly. Thus autotopagnosia does not affect recognition for body parts but rather affects transcoding tasks that include pointing to body parts as an output.

3.3 Construction tasks

These tasks require the subject to build up a two- or three-dimensional body (or just a head; Ogden 1985) from separate pieces. Typically, autotopagnosics cannot perform these tasks and tend to miss correct positions. Ogden's patient, for instance, put the ears where the eyes should go and vice versa or put the mouth at the top of the head.

Patients are invariably unhappy with their performance and appear puzzled on completion. They cannot, however, tell what exactly is wrong with their construction. While this behaviour underlines the importance of the spatial component, it also suggests that a functional component must be disturbed as well. Since simple recognition of single body parts (as shown in verification tasks) is unaffected, it appears that knowledge of their exact function, which would allow the patient, for instance, to spot a hand/foot confusion, is less than intact.

3.4 Description tasks

These tests are meant to tap knowledge of body parts as stored in the semantic system. Such tests require at least two different kinds of description: that of structural attributes and that of functional attributes. Either questions requiring a categorical response (yes/no) or more open questions involving different degrees of difficulty have been used. Questions implying structural descriptions include:

- Is the wrist next to the forearm?
- Is the mouth above or below the nose?
- Where is the elbow?

Examples of questions implying functional descriptions include:

- Is the mouth for eating?
- What is the mouth for?

Unfortunately, no published study of autotopagnosia has pursued a thorough investigation using these or similar tasks. Patients seem to be more disturbed on structural items than on functional ones. An isolated deficit for 'description' tasks has never been reported.

3.5 Control tasks

Body specificity should be the only defining feature of autotopagnosia. It is thus necessary to collect evidence of the patient's ability to locate parts of other complex objects. If the patient fails also in this task, he/she cannot be considered a 'genuine' autotopoagnosic. If the deficit cannot be attributed to more general problems, such as reaching inabilities, visual agnosia, etc., it must be attributed to the 'inability to locate parts within a whole', cases of which were described by De Renzi and Scotti (1970) and by De Renzi and Faglioni (1963) and never reported since.

A good control task was used in Semenza's (1988) study. The patient was asked to locate on verbal command parts of a bike, a shoe, and a pair of glasses. In a nonverbal condition, the same parts on the object were first pointed to by the examiner—the patient had then to point to the equivalent part on a different object of the same kind, but with a different shape. For instance the examiner pointed to the heel of a heavy boot and the patient had to point to the heel of a high-heeled elegant lady's shoe. Patient I.S. was flawless in both the verbal and the nonverbal condition.

Control tasks should also be devised for construction and description tasks. In the case of 'construction' tasks, a dissociation is unlikely to be found because constructional apraxia is likely to be a concurrent deficit. The diagnosis of autotopagnosia thus rests mainly on pointing tasks. Selective deficits or a selective sparing within semantic memory of bodily knowledge (functional and/or structural) have never been properly investigated.

4 Personal neglect and related disorders (see Chapter 6)

Unilateral spatial neglect and a number of less frequent but often associated disorders are a relatively common consequence of right hemisphere lesions (and, in particular, stroke). In addition to extrapersonal space and peripersonal space, unilateral neglect may affect one-half of the patient's body. This condition is called *personal neglect* or *hemisomatagnosia*. According to Bisiach and Vallar (2000), this phenomenon is less frequent than extrasomatic neglect. Somatic and extrasomatic neglect are usually found in association, but double dissociations have been observed. While, however, severe extrasomatic neglect may be found in many patients where somatic neglect is absent, severe somatic neglect unaccompanied by neglect of extrasomatic space is very infrequent (Bisiach *et al.* 1986; Bisiach and Vallar 2000).

Selective personal neglect mostly occurs after right-sided lesions. However, neglect of the right personal space may also be a consequence, in the early phases of the disease (Peru and Pinna 1997), of a left-sided lesion. Indeed, it often occurs in the form of paroxysmal symptomatology, most frequently in the course of epilepsy or migrane (De Renzi 1982). For further details concerning localization, including symptoms raising after left-sided lesions, the reader is referred to Bisiach and Vallar's (2000) review.

In the absence of relevant primary motor deficits, unilateral neglect may affect motor functions of contralateral limbs. In this condition automatic movements may, however, be relatively preserved.

4.1 Related disorders

4.1.1 Allochiria

Allochiria is a disorder, often associated with unilateral visual neglect, wherein tactile stimuli delivered to the contralesional side of somatic (or extrasomatic) space are referred to the symmetrical location on the ipsilateral side. Less frequently, analogous phenomena may be observed in the auditory or in the visual modality (but see Halligan *et al.* 1995).

4.1.2 Anton–Babinski's syndrome

A frequently associated disorder is *anosognosia* for deficits contralateral to the lesion, known as *Anton–Babinski's syndrome* (see Chapter 22). While Anton (1899) first noted this condition, Babinski (1914) recognized it as resulting from a focal cortical lesion. This disorder may or may not be accompanied by a generalized anosognosia for illness. This condition has been observed to double dissociate from somatosensory and motor neglect (Bisiach *et al.* 1986; Stone *et al.* 1993).

Patients who are anosognosic for deficits contralateral to their lesion may show all degrees of severity, from minimization to obstinate denial of illness or of possession of the affected limb, even in the face of demonstrations by the examiners. Furthermore, delusions and confabulation concerning the affected side may appear (*somatopara-phrenias*; Gerstman 1942), a typical instance of which is the attribution of a plegic limb to the examiner or to other people (Bottini *et al.* 2002). Other pathological attitudes include showing indifference (*anosodiaphoria*; Babinski 1914), an expression of dislike for the affected side (*misoplegia*), and *personification*, where affected limbs are spoken about in third person (he, she, etc.). These delusions may even include the belief that another person lies permanently on the affected side (Zingerle 1913; Nightingale 1982). This 'person' may elicit intense emotion and even erotic sensations. Concrete examples of delusions described in the literature are reported in Table 12.3.

Table 12.3 Examples of somatoparaphrenic delusions reported in the literature

- '[The left side of my body] belongs to a woman lying beside me' (Zingerle 1913)

- 'My old left hand began to shrink and a new hand has emerged, becoming fleshier and more voluminous' 'I have a nest of hands in my bed' (Ehrenwald 1930)

- '[This arm] is not mine: I found it in the bathroom, when I fell. It's not mine because it's too heavy; it should be yours. I can move and do everything; when I feel it too heavy, I put it on my stomach. It doesn't hurt me, it's kind.' (Rode *et al.* 1992)

- 'They took two fingers and joined them back together. The left hand, it's cut down the centre, but it still functions quite well. It's a nice hand.'

  'It's difficult . . . to live with a foot that isn't yours . . . . I came to the conclusion that it was a cow's foot . . . . But I adopted it.'

  My mother has a suitcase and there are at least three pairs of fingers in there, and they are all functional . . . we brought them through the customs. The customs men were all shocked when they saw these fingers in a box. It wasn't conducive to good relations.'

  I could never tell why the doctors were so interested in amputating my arms, or my fingers . . . or my legs.' 'I wake up with this arm lying in my bed with me . . . but I remember the hairs and this nick here, and I realize it's my arm. It was a bit strange and disconnected. It had come loose from its bindings and was covered in blood. Not a nice thing. Sometimes it goes away . . . It goes back to my mother's suitcase where it belongs . . . .'

  The same patient four years later:
  'A few years ago it was somebody else's leg, not mine. To start with, I didn't think that my left arm and leg were my own. I thought that the left foot I kept in a box under my bed . . . for safe keeping, for later . . . and that solved the problem . . . It's all very well to laugh at it now, but at the time it was pretty bloody terrifying, to say the least.' (Halligan *et al.* 1995)

4.1.3 Extinction of contralesional stimuli on bilateral stimulation (or double simultaneous stimulation)

This may be found in patients who can otherwise detect single contralesional stimuli (Oppenheim 1911; Bender *et al.* 1948; Head and Holmes 1911; Denny Brown *et al.* 1952). This phenomenon has been reported to occur in the tactile, auditory, visual, and olfactory modalities. While it equally affects all modalities, double dissociations have been reported (De Renzi *et al.* 1984; Vallar *et al.* 1994) among modalities and with personal and extrapersonal neglect.

Since Zingerle's (1913) early work, disorders related to spatial neglect, collectively labelled as *dyschiria*, have been viewed as a consequence of a disturbance of the conscious representation of one side of the body and (though with less emphasis, as Bisiach and Vallar 2000 have noted) of the extrapersonal environment. The appeal to the notion of the body schema as a cue to the understanding of the conditions (e.g. Brain 1941; Critchley 1953; Gerstman 1942) has been common in the past and, as Bisiach and Vallar (2000) have noted, may be considered the basis for Bisiach's own representational account (Bisiach and Luzzatti 1978; Bisiach 1995, 1999).

All these phenomena, however, have also been interpreted in terms of an attentional disorder. Whether attention is involved *per se* or as attention to an internal representation is still an open question (which, to a certain extent, reconciles attentional and representational interpretation of the phenomena). As Kinsbourne (1995) argued, if awareness of the body derived from selective attention to somatosensory input to various body parts, there would be no need for the *ad hoc* construct of a separate 'body schema'.

Whatever the interpretation, and despite the tradition of its inclusion in body schema disorders, personal neglect and related problems seem to say little about the content and the format of bodily representation—except to prove the independence of this representation from other representational contents and to be indicative of an analogous non-prepositional quality. This disturbance may be viewed as complementary to phantom limb sensation. Taken together the two disturbances may indeed be suggestive of a system, hardwired somewhere in the brain, imparting signals that 'this is my body, it is part of me'. One such system is considered by Melzack (1992) as a component of the 'neuromatrix' responsible for phantom sensations.

4.2 Clinical assessment

Patients with personal neglect may show the condition in various degrees of severity. Sometimes only a careful neuropsychological examination may detect the phenomenon. In other cases the presentation is more dramatic. The patient may be unable to dress properly, leaving one-half of the body unclothed, and showing signs of personal care only on one side, leaving the contralateral side very untidy. Proper assessment should contain at least a *checklist* of these behavioural anomalies related to body usage.

◆   When not so severe, the presence of personal neglect may be assessed by asking patients to touch contralesional body parts using the unaffected ipsilateral hand, or through tasks involving the patient's body, such as using a comb. Light touches or even pinprick stimulation of the afferent side may also be used. Patients may still deny pinprick stimulation while showing movements aimed at avoiding it.

- *Motor* neglect may be assessed (Bisiach and Vallar 2000) by requiring the patients *to extend their hands* or *to squeeze the examiner's fingers placed within the palms of their hands.* Motor neglect may vanish if the patient is invited to attend the neglected limb or is actively prevented from moving the non-neglected one.

- In order to systematically assess personal neglect, Cocchini *et al.* (2001) recently developed the *Fluff Test.* This test requires subjects to remove white cardboard circles (2 cm in diameter) attached by velcro, at regular intervals, located to the front of their clothes. These stickers are distributed, on both the right and the left side, along the central body areas, the legs, and the arm that is not performing the task. The subject sits blindfolded whilst the circles are attached. Still blindfolded they are asked to remove all the stickers. The percentage of targets detached from each side is then calculated. Normative data are available.

    Somewhat surprisingly, Cocchini *et al.* (2001) found no correlation and a double dissociation of the Fluff Test with the *Comb and Razor/Compact Test* (Beschin and Robertson 1997), a test requiring exploration of the face area. Their interpretation for this dissociation is still speculative. Further research is required to clarify this issue as well as the role of motor neglect in failing the test.

- *Self-evaluation tests* (Marcel and Tegner 1994; Berti *et al.* 1996) and *structured interviews* (e.g. Cutting 1978) that require the patient to carefully describe their problem may be useful in cases of anosognosia and somatoparaphrenia. Patients affected by these disorders may show dissociations in verbal reports on their abilities. They may consistently exhibit the belief that their affected limbs are perfectly functioning while showing, in contrast, a realistic self-evaluation. For example Berti *et al.*'s (1998) patient, C.C., assigned a score of 2/10 to her own ability to lift a glass with her left hand but, at the same time, claimed that she could perform the task perfectly.

As Halligan *et al.* (1995) pointed out, it is of the utmost importance to elicit full accounts of what such patients believe their condition to be. Such irrationalities may be important cues to the patients' mental contents. The evolution of symptoms over time may also be revealing. Halligan *et al.* (1995), reporting detailed abstracts of subsequent interviews with a somatoparaphrenic patient, showed how most symptoms could be interpreted as a delusional way of coping with new, unfamiliar sensations.

- *Extinction* is generally assessed by symmetrically presenting two identical stimuli at the same time. However (Critchley 1953), the phenomenon may appear even with different and asymmetrical stimulation (see, for instance, the 'face–hand test'; Fink and Bender 1952). Sometimes the contralesional stimulus is not entirely neglected, but just misperceived. Different types of material have been also used. Schwartz and co-workers (1979) used the Quality Extinction Test, which consisted of two sets of various common materials such as sandpaper, tin foil, velvet, etc. One set consisted of test items each of which was made entirely of the same material ('whole items') while the other consisted of items made up of two different materials side-by-side ('half and half items'). In the test, each item is brushed against the subject's fingers so that both hands are stimulated simultaneously. Stimulation with the 'half-and-half' is arranged so that a different material stimulates each hand at the same time. An 'extinction' trial is recorded if the subject names only one when in fact two have been presented. The total score is derived by subtracting the number of omissions made by the other hand and converting the difference into a percentage. Errors in naming are not scored.

4.3 Rehabilitation (see Chapter 6)

Patients with severe and persisting unilateral neglect are seriously handicapped in everyday life and rehabilitation should therefore be attempted as soon as possible. Neglect is not only handicapping, but it has been demonstrated (Denes *et al.* 1982) to interfere in general rehabilitation. A major obstacle to rehabilitation efforts is the frequent co-occurrence of anosognosia.

Rehabilitation of unilateral neglect has been attempted with different techniques and different success (see Zoccolotti 1999 and Robertson and Halligan 1999 for comprehensive reviews). They mostly consist of repeated lateralized stimulation to the affected side and, in general, employ a series of sensory suggestions orientating or anchoring the patient's attention to the side of the target stimuli.

Visual stimuli have been most frequently used but somatosensory-proprioceptile and vestibular stimulation has also been employed with some improvement. Vestibular stimulation, in particular (Rubens 1985; Cappa *et al.* 1987; Vallar *et al.* 1990; Bisiach *et al.* 1991; Rode *et al.* 1992), has been shown to temporarily reduce remission of unilateral neglect phenomena, including somatoparaphrenic delusions and even associated motor deficits.

Most current attempts are made on patients affected by both personal and extrapersonal neglect, without clear efforts to distinguish the two conditions. Positive results are (with some notable exceptions, e.g. Halligan *et al.* 1992) generally reported. The effects of treatment have been shown to surpass those of spontaneous recovery, to be specific for neglect, to be stable over time after dismissal, and to extend to tasks not involved in treatment, at least when rehabilitation is protracted enough (Antonucci *et al.* 1995; see Chapter 6, this volume).

4.4 Distal extinction to unilateral double tactile stimulation

Patients may show extinction of the distal stimulus on unilateral tactile double stimulation (Denny Brown *et al.* 1952; Bender *et al.* 1948). This phenomenon is relatively little known, although it has been considered an early sign of diffuse brain damage (e.g. dementia). Cohn (1951), however, described it as a common finding in 3–5-year-old normal children. Typically, subjects are stimulated on the face and on the hand, the face stimulus being invariably the one resistant to the extinction. Other locations (e.g. shoulder and hand) may be chosen and a rostral dominance is invariably shown in case of extinction. When hand and foot are simultaneously stimulated, the foot will be dominant (Bender *et al.* 1948).

5 **Alien hand syndrome** (See Chapter 19)

The alien hand syndrome is a loosely defined cluster of symptoms, characterized by involuntary movements of a limb in conjunction with an experience of estrangement from and personification of the limb itself (see Blakemore *et al.* (2002)). The limb is perceived as having a will of its own, though ownership is seldom denied. While the syndrome concerns upper limbs, it may affect the legs.

The underlying pathology involves lesions of two types.

- In the *anterior type*, the damage is either to the left frontal lobe and to the anterior corpus callosum or to the corpus callosum alone. In the first case the right, dominant limb is affected, while in the second case the symptomatology is found in the left limb.

- In the less frequent, *posterior type*, the damage consists of corticobasal degeneration or, in a few cases, of posterior vascular damage. The anatomical substrate is the parietal and posterofrontal cortex and the corresponding subcortical areas, bilaterally. Recently, however, Martì-Fabregas *et al.* (2000) have described a patient with a vascular lesion limited to the right parietal lobe. Generally, if not exclusively, posterior cases have been found to involve the nondominant limbs.

The clinical presentation includes several phenomena. The following is taken from Fisher (2000).

- Failure to identify an upper limb as one's own on palpating it behind the back or with the eyes closed. As Fisher (2000) observes, this was the original definition.

- Movement of a limb that the patient regards as foreign, unwilled, strange, uncooperative. The limb seems to act on its own, outside the patient's control. It may actively contradict the other limb (see Della Sala *et al.* (1991)).

- Stereotyped 'reflex' motor activity of the 'frontal' type: reaching out, groping and grasping with inability to release, utilization behaviour, tactile and visual oral reactions.

- Other: withdrawal of a limb; flinging movement of optico-sensory ataxia.

Alien hand symptoms following corticobasal lesions may be distinguished insofar as involuntary movements are typically non-purposeful and non-conflictual, and include such behaviours as arm levitation and finger-writhing (Bundick and Spinella 2000). The corticobasal, posterior variety, therefore, does not include 'frontal' symptoms.

Table 12.4 Examples of alien hand behaviour

◆ [On order to pick an object with the right hand] Picking the object, the right hand approaches it and pauses, the left hand comes over to approach the object, and then both hands pick the object (left hemisphere infarction; Liepmann 1900).

....

◆ Put on clothes with the right hand and pull them off with the left hand.

Open a drawer or a door with the right hand and simultaneously push it shut with the left hand. Dry the clean dishes and then put them back in the pan to be washed again.

When thirsty fill a glass with water and then pour it out (following callosotomy; Akelaitis 1945).

....

◆ Inability, on verbal command, to place the left hand behind the head or to use it to point to something.

Reaching across with the right hand to grab the left hand and place it in proper position (following callosotomy; Gazzaniga et al. 1962).

....

◆ Failure to recognize as one's own one of the hands, usually the left, when the hands were out of sight (callosal tumour; Brion and Jedynak 1972).

....

◆ Hands fighting each other: holding an envelope, each hand independently and simultaneously tries to hold and to release it, tugging at it, sometimes for as long as 10 minutes (anterior cerebral artery infarction; Watson and Heilman 1983).

....

◆ The right hand pays for an item in a store, the left hand withdraws the money; while purchasing something else the left hand picks up an orange (ruptured anterior cerebral artery; Papagno and Marsile 1995).

....

◆ While the left hand takes food to the mouth with the fork, the right hand brings the knife towards the eye with the risk of injury (corticobasal degeneration; Lhermitte et al. 1925).

....

◆ The left hand has a tendency to levitation and the fingers wander 'like the tentacles of an anemone' (corticobasal degeneration; Gibb et al. 1989).

Patients with alien hand are usually alert, cooperative, interested, and aware of the movements requested. Their reaction to their symptomatology varies from frustration and torment to amusement. Concrete examples of alien hand behaviour described in literature are provided in Table 12.4.

6 Altered muscular proprioception

The role of muscular proprioception and its contribution to bodily representation emerges from observations of patients suffering from proprioceptive deafferentation due to peripheral pathologies and deafferentation due to central lesions. These patients are extremely rare and no routine clinical assessment is available. However, existing detailed descriptions of the phenomenon suggest the framework for proper testing procedures (Cole and Paillard 1995; Paillard et al. 1983).

One type of patient has been observed with a very selective and complete loss of large sensory fibres, while motor and small sensory fibres are left intact. Muscular proprioception is lost but vestibular information as well as the senses of pain and temperature is retained.

These patients express the feeling of using their bodies as tools, relying heavily on visual feedback, concentration, and intellectual effort. Motor automatism is apparent to them. If their vision is precluded, their ability to preshape the grip posture to the size and shape of a target would be absent.

On clinical examination, these patients may be asked, when blindfolded, to point to a part of their skin where a thermal stimulus (which they perceive) had been delivered. They could not carry out such a task. In dramatic contrast, however, they would be able to verbally designate the point ('over my elbow') and later to show it precisely on the picture of a human body.

Patients with parietal lesions may suffer from deafferentation of a body area. For instance, in the case reported by Paillard *et al.* (1983), a parietal lesion provoked deafferentation of the forearm. The patient was unable, when blindfolded, to detect the presence of a tactile stimulus on the affected area, but was surprisingly able to indicate the place of stimulation with the other hand. Paillard *et al.* considered this phenomenon to be the equivalent of blindsight in the tactile modality.

7 Phantom limb and related phenomena

Most amputees experience the continued existence of the amputated limb or body part. Detailed descriptions of all aspects of this phenomenon, including the history of condition, may be found in Ramachandran and Hirstein (1998), Ramachandran and Rogers Ramachandran (2000), Semenza (2001) and Halligan (2002). This chapter is only concerned with clinical assessment and attempts at rehabilitation.

Phantoms involve not only limbs but also other body parts such as breasts, male genitalia, or facial parts like the jaw. Amputation is not essential for the occurrence of such phantoms. They have been reported in conditions such as brachial plexus avulsion, spinal cord damage, and even single spinal anaesthesia. Even patients with congenital absence of limbs experience phantoms.

Phantom sensations are spontaneous but may also be evoked with appropriate stimulation not only of the stump but also of distant body areas. For instance, the stimulation of the ipsilateral side of the face may evoke sensations in phantom hands (e.g. Halligan *et al.* (1993) and Halligan *et al.* 1999). Referred sensations are often topographically organized and may be modality-specific. Thus, for example, hot, cold, vibration, rubbing, metal, or massage are felt as hot, cold, vibration, rubbing, metal, or massage at precisely localized points of the phantom limb. Such sensations can occur even hours after amputation.

A thorough interview should be carried on to assess phantom limb phenomena, considering all the main factors characterizing phantoms. (see Fraser, Halligan, Robertson and Kirker 2001) Phantom sensations seem to vary considerably in their intensity and veridicality. The size and form of missing parts may change over time. The vividness of the phantom sensation is typically enhanced by imaginary tasks performed with the phantom limb. The phantom may change in form or disappear in consequence of particular movements, e.g. bringing the stump near to a wall. Absent limbs seem to coordinate with the rest of the body in movement.

Patients may be able to provide a correct evaluation of the size, length, and weight of the missing part; in other cases the missing part may be perceived as shortened or in a bizarre, anatomically impossible position. 'Islands' of phantom sensation may be all the patient feels, e.g. phantom hands may be felt as suspended in mid-air. A common distinctive phenomenon that occurs over time is 'telescoping'—a phantom may gradually retract in such a way that, in the end, peripheral parts seem to join to the stump.

Pain is the most typical feature of phantom sensation and occurs in approximately 70% of cases. When severe it is described as burning, cramping, or shooting. Complex sensations may also accompany phantoms—patients with lower cord injury may report the sensation of defecation; phantom penises experience ejaculation.

A less frequent and less known phenomenon is the felt presence of and hallucinatory belief in the real existence of supernumerary body parts. Such a condition may paradoxically coexist with denial of hemiplegia and feeling of nonbelonging of the contralesional limb (Halligan *et al.* 1993).

7.1 Rehabilitation attempts

Phantom limb phenomena appear dependent on neural reorganization after amputation or the equivalent (besides already indicated references, see, on this point, Karl *et al.* 2001).

On the basis of findings that phantom limb pain is closely associated with plastic changes in the primary somatosensory cortex and on animal data that show that behaviourally relevant training alters the cortical map, Flor *et al.* (2001), have recently devised a sensory discrimination training programme for patients with intractable phantom limb pain. The programme consists of 10 daily 90-minute sessions of feedback-guided sensory training, in which patients have to discriminate the frequency or the location of high-intensity nonpainful electric stimuli applied in a random fashion through electrodes attached to their stump. After this training, patients showed a significant improvement in discriminating both the location and the frequency of the stimuli as well as a significant reduction of pain.

Ramachandran and Rogers-Ramachandran (1996) required phantom limb patients to look at the reflection of their intact hand mirror-reflected on the felt location of their phantom hand. The patients were thus able, while moving the intact hand, to receive visual feedback that the phantom hand was obeying commands. A number of patients appeared to benefit from repeated use of such procedures, in that they were relieved of spasms and cramps, with elimination of associated pain.

8 Body-specific cognitive biases in eating disorders

Mental anorexia and bulimia have been considered to be disorders of body schema. Modern investigators, however, quite rightly believe (see a review by Hsu and Sobkiewic 1991) that this idea is unfounded. Nonetheless subjects affected by eating disorders have been shown to be unable to correctly judge the size of their bodies. This problem is nowadays attributed to a 'cognitive bias' that is thought to commonly accompany eating disorders (Thompson 1990).

Typically, patients with eating disorders have been found to misjudge hip-to-hip, armpit-to-armpit, and cheekbone-to-cheekbone distances or the size of the waist. Waist size and hip-to-hip distance seem the most likely to be grossly misjudged.

Despite the variety of detection techniques, surprisingly little has been done so far to ascertain with proper control conditions whether misjudgement of size is indeed body-specific as has been always assumed. A few investigations (e.g. Slade and Russell 1973; Franzen *et al.* 1988; Probst *et al.* 1998*a,b*) required estimation of the size of small tridimensional objects or of the length of short lines. While these control conditions seemed to indicate that, indeed, size misjudgements are body-specific, the choice of measures is far from being satisfactory, since in most investigations control distances are grossly different from body distances. No weight estimation has been properly controlled. No comparison has been made between misjudgements of one's own body and of other people's bodies, whether of females or males. No control has ever been made on the modality of response (e.g. whether verbal responses differ from nonverbal responses). Comparisons between different types of anorexia and bulimia have been rare (Probst *et al.* 1998*a,b*).

No routine clinical instruments are, therefore, available for evaluating cognitive biases in eating disorders. Ideally, however, their proper assessment should take into consideration the above observations.

Selective references

Akelaitis, A.J. (1945). Studies on the corpus callosum IV. Diagonist dyspraxia in epileptics following partial and complete section of the corpus callosum. *Am. J. Psychiatry* 101, 594–9.

Anton, G. (1899). Uber die Selbstwahrnehmung der Herderkrankungen des Gehirns durch den Kranken bei Rindenblindheit und Rindentaubheit. *Arch. Psychiatrie Nervenkrankh.* 32, 86–127.

Antonucci, G., Guariglia, C., Judica, A., Magnotti, L., Paolucci, S., Pizzamiglio, L., and Zoccolotti, P. (1995). Effectiveness of neglect rehabilitation in a randomised group study. *J. Clin. Exp. Neuropsychol.* 17, 386–9.

Babinski, J. (1914). Contribution a l'étude des troubles dans l'hémiplégie cérébrale. *Rev. Neurologique* 31, 365–7.

Bender, M.L., Wortis, S.B., and Cramer, J. (1948). Organic mental syndrome with phenomena of extinction and allesthesia. *Arch. Neurol. Psychiatry* 59 (3), 273–91.

Berti, A., Ladavas, E., and Della Corte, M. (1996). Anosognosia for hemiplegia, neglect dyslexia and drawing neglect. Clinical findings and theoretical considerations. *J. Int. Neuropsychol. Soc.* 2, 426–40.

Berti, A., Ladavas, E., Stracciari, A., Giannarelli, C., and Ossola, A. (1998). Anosognosia for motor impairment and dissociations with patients' evaluation of the disorder: theoretical considerations. *Cogn. Neuropsychiatry* 3 (1), 21–44.

Beschin, N. and Robertson, I.H. (1997). Personal versus extrapersonal neglect: a group study of their dissociation using a reliable clinical test. *Cortex* 33, 379–84.

Bisiach, E. (1995). Unawareness of unilateral neurological impairment and disordered representation of one side of the body. *Higher Brain Function Res.* 15, 113–40.

Bisiach, E. (1999). Unilateral neglect and related disorders. In *Handbook of clinical and experimental neuropsychology* (ed. G. Denes and L. Pizzamiglio), pp. 479–96. Psychology Press, Hove, East Sussex.

Bisiach, E. and Luzzatti, C. (1978). Unilateral neglect of representational space. *Cortex* 14, 129–33.

Bisiach, E. and Vallar, G. (2000). Unilateral neglect in humans. In *Handbook of neuropsychology* (ed. F. Boller, J. Grafman, and G. Rizzolatti), Vol. 1, pp. 459–502. Elsevier Publishers, Amsterdam.

Bisiach, E., Perani, D., Vallar, G., and Berti, A. (1986). Unilateral neglect: personal and extrapersonal. *Neuropsychologia* 24, 759–67.

Bisiach, E., Rusconi, M.L., and Vallar, G. (1991). Remission of somatoparaphrenic delusion through vestibular stimulation. *Neuropsychologia* 29, 1029–31.

Bottini, G., Bisiach, E., Sterzi, R. and Vallar, G. (2002). Feeling touches in someone else's hand. *Neuroreport* 13, 249–52.

Blakemore, S.J., Wolpert, D.M., and Frith, C.D. (2002). Abnormalities in the awareness of action. *Trends Cogn. Sci.* 6, 237–42.

Brain, W.R. (1941). Visual disorientation with special reference to lesions of the right hemisphere. *Brain* 84, 244–72.

Brion, S. and Jedynak, C.P. (1972). Troubles du transfert interhémispherique (callosal disconnection) a propos de 3 observations de tumeurs du corps calleux. Le signe de la main étrangère. *Rev. Neurologique* 4, 273–90.

Bundick, T. and Spinella, M. (2000). Subjective experience, involuntary movement, and posterior alien hand syndrome. *J. Neurol., Neurosurg., Psychiatry* 68, 83–5.

Cappa, S., Sterzi, R., Vallar, G., and Bisiach, E. (1987). Remission of hemineglect and anosognosia after vestibular stimulation. *Neuropsychologia* 25, 775–82.

Cocchini, G., Beschin, N., and Jehkonen, M. (2001). The Fluff Test: a simple task to assess body representation neglect. *Neuropsychol. Rehabil.* 11, 17–31.

Cohn, R. (1951). On certain aspects of the sensory organization of the human brain. *Neurology* 2, 119–22.

Cole, J. and Paillard, J. (1995). Living without touch and peripheral information about body position and movement: studies with deafferented subjects. In *The body and the self* (ed. J.L. Bermudez, A.J. Marcel, and N. Eilan), pp. 245–66. MIT Press, Cambridge, Massachusetts.

Critchley, M. (1953). *The parietal lobes*. Edward Arnold, London.

Cutting, J. (1978). Study of anosognosia. *J. Neurol., Neurosurg., Psychiatry* 41, 548–55.

Della Sala, S., Marchetti, C., and Spinnler, H. (1991). Right-sided anarchic (alien) hand: a longitudinal study. *Neuropsychologia*, 1113–27.

Denes, G. (1989). Disorders of body awareness and body knowledge. In *Handbook of neuropsychology* (ed. F. Boller and J. Grafman), Vol. 2, pp. 207–27. Elsevier Publishers, Amsterdam.

Denes, G., Semenza, C., Stoppa, E., and Lis, A. (1982). Unilateral spatial neglect and recovery from hemiplegia. A follow-up study. *Brain* 105, 543–52.

Denes, G., Cappelletti, J.Y., Zilli, T., Dalla Porta, F., and Galliana, F. (2000). A category-specific deficit of spatial representation: the case of autotopagnosia. *Neuropsychologia* 38 (4), 345–50.

Denny Brown, D., Meyer, J.S., and Horenstein, S. (1952). The significance of perceptual rivalry resulting from parietal lesions. *Brain* 75, 433–71.

De Renzi, E. (1982). *Disorders of space exploration and cognition*. Wiley and Sons, New York.

De Renzi, E. and Faglioni, P. (1963). Autotopoagnosia. *Arch. Psicol., Neurol. Psichiatria* 24, 1–34.

De Renzi, E. and Scotti, G. (1970). Autotopagnosia: fiction or reality? Report of a case. *Arch. Neurol.* 23, 221–7.

De Renzi, E., Gentilini, M., and Pattacini, F. (1984). Auditory extinction following hemisphere damage. *Neuropsychologia* 22, 733–44.

Eherenwald, H. (1930). Verandertes Erleben des Korperbildes mit konsekutiver Wahnbildung bei linkseitiger Hemiplegie. *Monatschr. Psychiatrie Neurologie* 75, 89–97.

Fink, M. and Bender, B. (1952). Perception of simultaneous tactile stimuli in normal children. *Neurology* 3, 27–34.

Fisher, C.M. (2000). Alien hand syndrome: a review with the addition of six personal cases. *Can. J. Neurol. Sci.* **27**, 192–203.

Flor, H., Denke, C., Schaefer, M., and Grusser, S. (2001). Effect of sensory discrimination training on cortical reorganisation and phantom limb pain. *Lancet* **357**, 1763–4.

Franzen, V., Florin, I., Schneider, S., and Meier, M. (1988). Distorted body image in bulimic women. *J. Psychosom. Res.* **32**, 445–50.

Fraser, C.M., Halligan, P.W., Robertson, I.H. and Kirker S.G. (2001). Characterizing phantom limb phenomena in upper limb amputees. *Prosthet Orthot Int* **25**, 235–42.

Gazzaniga, M.S., Bogen, J.E., and Sperry, R.W. (1962). Some functional effects of sectioning the cerebral commissures in man. *Proc. Natl Acad. Sci., USA* **48**, 1765–9.

Gerstman, J. (1942). Problems of imperception of disease and of impaired body territories with organic lesions. Relation to body scheme and its disorders. *Arch. Neurol. Psychiatry* **48**, 890–913.

Gibb, W.R.G., Luthert, P.J., and Marsden, C.D. (1989). Corticobasal degeneration. *Brain* **112**, 1171–92.

Halligan, P.W., Donegan, C.A., and Marshall, J.C. (1992). When a cue is not a cue? On the intractability of visuospatial neglect. *Neuropsychol. Rehabilitation* **2**, 283–93.

Halligan, P.W., Marshall, J.C., and Wade, D.Y. (1993) Three arms: a case study of supernumerary phantom limb after right hemisphere stroke. *J Neurol Neurosurg Psychiatry* **56** (2), 159–66.

Halligan, P.W., Marshall, J.C., and Wade, D.T. (1995). Unilateral somatoparaphrenia after right hemisphere stroke. A case description. *Cortex* **31**, 173–82.

Halligan, P.W., Marshall, J.C., Wade, D.T., Davey, J., and Morrison, D. (1993). Thumb in cheek? Sensory reorganization and perceptual plasticity after limb amptation. *Neuroreport* **4** (3), 233–6.

Halligan, P.W., Zeman, A., and Berger, A. (1999). Phantoms in the brain. *Br. Med. J.* **319**, 587–8.

Halligan, P.W. (2002). Phantom limbs: the body is mind. *Cog. Neuropsychiatry* **7**, 251–68.

Head, H. and Holmes, G. (1911). Sensory disturbances from cerebral lesions. *Brain* **34**, 102–254.

Hsu, L.K.G. and Sobkiewicz, T.A. (1991). Body image disturbance: time to abandon the concept for eating disorders? *Int. J. Eating Disorders* **10**, 15–30.

Karl, A., Birbaumer, N., Lutzenberger, W., Cohen, L.G., and Flor, H. (2001). Reorganization of motor and somatosensory cortex in upper extremity amputees with phantom limb pain. *J. Neurosci.* **21**, 3609–18.

Kinsbourne, M. (1995). Models of consciousness: serial or parallel in the brain? In *The cognitive neurosciences* (ed. M. Gazzaniga), pp. 1321–9. MIT Press, Cambridge, Massachusetts.

Lhermitte, J., Lévy, G., and Kyriako, N. (1925). Les perturbations de la représentation spatiale chez les apraxiques—a propos de deux cas cliniques d'apraxie. *Rev. Neurologique* **2**, 586–600.

Liepmann, H. (1900). Der Krankeit der Apraxie, motorischen Asymbolie. *Monatschr. Psychiatrie Neurologie* **11**, 15–44, 102–32, 182–97.

Marcel, A.J. and Tegner, R. (1994). Knowing one's plegia. Poster presented at the XII European Workshop on Cognitive Neuropsychology, Bressanone, Italy.

Martì-Fabregas, J., Kulisevsky, J., Barò, E., Mendoza, G., Valencia, C., and Martì-Villalta, J.L. (2000). Alien hand sign after a right parietal infarction. *Cerebrovasc. Dis.* **10**, 70–2.

Melzack, R. (1992). Phantom limbs. *Sci. Am.* **187**, 90–6.

Nightingale, S. (1982). Somatoparaphrenia: a case study. *Cortex* **18**, 463–7.

Ogden, J.A. (1985). Autotopagnosia. Occurrence in a patient without nominal aphasia and with an intact ability to point to parts of animals. *Brain* **108**, 1009–22.

Oppenheim, H. (1911). *Textbook of nervous diseases.* Foulis, Edinburgh.

Paillard, J., Michel, F., and Stelmach, G. (1983). Localization without content. A tactile analogue of blind-sight. *Arch. Neurol.* **40**, 548–51.

Papagno, C. and Marsile, C. (1995). Transient left-sided alien hand with callosal and unilateral fronto-mesial damage: a case study. *Neuropsychologia* **33**, 1703–9.

Peru, A. and Pinna, G. (1997). Right personal neglect following a left hemisphere stroke. A case report. *Cortex* 33, 585–90.

Poeck, K. and Orgass, B. (1971). The concept of the body schema: a critical review and some experimental results. *Cortex* 7, 254–77.

Probst, M., Vandereycken, W., Van Coppenolle, H., and Pieter, G. (1998*a*). Body size estimation in anorexia nervosa patients, the significance of overestimation. *J. Psychosom. Res.* 44, 451–6.

Probst, M., Vandereycken, W., Vanderlinden, J., and Van Coppenolle, H. (1998*b*). The significance of body size estimation in eating disorders: its relation with clinical and psychological variables. *Int. J. Eating Disorders* 24 (2), 167–74.

Ramachandran, V.S. and Hirstein, W. (1998). The perception of phantom limbs. The D.O. Hebb Lecture. *Brain* 121, 1603–30.

Ramachandran, V.S. and Rogers Ramachandran, D. (1996). Synesthesia on phantom limbs induced with mirrors. *Proc. R. Soc. London B* 273, 377–86.

Ramachandran, V.S. and Rogers Ramachandran, D. (2000). Phantom limbs and neural plasticity. *Arch. Neurol.* 57, 317–20.

Robertson, I.H. and Halligan, P.W. (1999). *Spatial neglect.* Psychology Press, Hove, East Sussex.

Rode, G., Charles, N., Perenin, M.T., Vighetto, A., Trillet, M., and Aimard, G. (1992). Partial remission of hemiplegia and somatoparaphrenia through vestibular stimulation in a case of unilateral neglect. *Cortex* 28, 203–8.

Rubens, A.B. (1985). Caloric stimulation and unilateral neglect. *Neurology* 35, 1019–24.

Schilder, P. (1935). *The image and the appearance of the human body.* International Universities Press, New York.

Schwartz, A.S., Marchok, P.L., Kreinick, C.J., and Flynn, R. (1979). The asymmetric lateralization of tactile extinction in patients with unilateral cerebral dysfunction. *Brain* 102, 669–84.

Semenza, C. (1988). Impairment in localization of body parts following brain damage. *Cortex* 24, 443–9.

Semenza, C. (2001). Disorders of body representation. In *Handbook of neuropsychology* (ed. R.S. Berndt), Vol. 3, pp. 285–303. Elsevier Publishers, Amsterdam.

Semenza, C. and Delazer, M. (2003). Pick's cases studies on bodily representation (1908, 1915, 1922). A retrospective assessment. In *Classic cases in neuropsychology*, Vol. 2 (ed. C. Code, C. Wallesch, Y. Joanette, and A.R. Lecours), pp. 233–40. Psychology Press, Hove, East Sussex.

Semenza, C. and Goodglass, H. (1985). Localization of body parts in brain injured subjects. *Neuropsychologia* 23, 161–75.

Slade, P. and Russell, G.F.M. (1973). Awareness of body dimensions in anorexia nervosa: cross-sectional and longitudinal studies. *Psychol. Med.* 3, 188–99.

Stone, S.P., Halligan, P.W., and Greenwood, R.J. (1993). The incidence of neglect phenomena and related disorders in patients with an acute right or left hemisphere stroke. *Age Ageing* 22, 46–52.

Thompson, J.K. (1990). *Body image disturbances: assessment and treatment.* Pergamon Press, New York.

Vallar, G., Rusconi, M.L., Bignamini, G., Geminani, G., and Perani, D. (1994). Anatomical correlates of visual and tactile extinction in humans: a clinical CT study. *J. Neurol., Neurosurg., Psychiatry* 57, 464–70.

Vallar, G., Sterzi, R., Bottini, G., Cappa, S., and Rusconi, M.L. (1990). Temporary remission of left hemianesthesia after vestibular stimulation. A sensory neglect phenomenon. *Cortex* 26, 123–31.

Watson, R.T. and Heilman, K.M. (1983). Callosal apraxia. *Brain* 106, 391–403.

Zingerle, H. (1913). Ueber Stoerungen der Wahrnehmung des eigenen Koerpers bei organischen Gehirnerkrankungen. *Monatsschr. Psychiatrie Neurol.* 34, 13–36.

Zoccolotti, P. (1999). Visual, visuospatial, and attentional disorders. In *Handbook of clinical and experimental neuropsychology* (ed. G. Denes and L. Pizzamiglio), pp. 875–86. Psychology Press, Hove, East Sussex.

Chapter 13

Assessment of acquired spoken language disorders

Claus-W. Wallesch, Helga Johannsen-Horbach, and Gerhard Blanken

1 Introduction

The acquired language and speech disorders comprise:

- aphasia;
- speech apraxia;
- dysarthria;
- neurological stuttering;
- the 'foreign accent syndrome';
- language impairments with dementia and confusional states.

Only the first three conditions will be considered in detail.

1.1 Definitions

1.1.1 Aphasia

The aphasias are disorders of language-processing resulting from acquired focal brain pathology. The underlying pathology affects the cerebral representations of linguistic rules and language-specific information. In most instances, aphasia is a supramodal deficit, i.e. both language production and perception and both spoken and written language are affected.

However, due to the existence of cognitive pathways that only subserve written, but not spoken language, written language disorders will be treated separately (see Chapter 16). Also, disorders of written language-processing may occur in the absence of aphasia (e.g. pure alexia, neglect dyslexia). In its strict use, the term 'aphasia' is reserved for patients, who suffer from circumscribed pathology and in whom language dysfunction constitutes a focus of cognitive impairment. Therefore, the frequent and characteristic language impairment with Alzheimer's disease would only be termed aphasia in the broader sense.

The aphasias affect the cerebral representation of a developed language system. Therefore, they are separated from disorders of language acquisition (*developmental dysphasia*). The term *childhood aphasia* is restricted to the effects of brain damage upon language functions that had been acquired previously.

1.1.2 Speech apraxia

The existence and definition of speech apraxia have been intensely debated. Today, a majority of researchers and clinicians accept its existence and Darley's definition: 'An articulatory disorder resulting from impairment, as a result of brain damage, of the capacity to program the positioning of speech musculature and the sequencing of muscle movements for the volitional production of phonemes. No significant weakness, slowness, or incoordination in reflex and automatic acts.' (Darley 1969, according to Rosenbek 1993). Speech apraxia, however, very rarely occurs in isolation. Usually it is combined with Broca's or global aphasia.

1.1.3 Dysarthria

The term *dysarthria* is used to describe the effects of a sensorimotor disorder resulting from neurological pathology on respiratory, phonatory, and articulatory functions involved in speech sound production. It has been argued that 'dysarthrophonia' or even 'dysarthrophonopneumia' may be terminologically more adequate, but these terms have not entered into clinical use. Dysarthria may co-occur with aphasia, especially acute nonfluent, Broca's and global aphasia.

2 Aphasia

2.1 Epidemiology

Aphasia is a common symptom of cerebral disease with an incidence of about 1/1000 (not including transient aphasia as a symptom of transient ischaemic attack (TIA)) and a prevalence of about 2/1000. Its most frequent cause is ischaemic infarction in the territory of supply of the left middle cerebral artery (about 75%). Other causes are haemorrhage, tumour, trauma, infarctions in other territories, cerebral infections (herpes encephalitis), and circumscribed atrophic pathology.

2.2 Symptoms of aphasia

Clinically and in aphasia test batteries, the analysis and description of an aphasic patient's language performance is based on two types of observations:

- the analysis of his/her linguistic and communicative performance in conversation;
- the comparison of linguistic proficiency across modalities, using tasks such as repetition, oral and written naming, writing to dictation, reading aloud, speech and script comprehension.

2.2.1 Spontaneous speech

In spontaneous speech, deficits and errors are analysed on the levels of phonology, lexicon/semantics, and syntax. Other important dimensions are the fluency of language production and the presence of repetitive speech (see the box below). Usually, the accuracy and speed of articulation and prosodic features are also described. For a glossary of neurolinguistic terminology, see Table 13.1.

How to describe an aphasic patient's spontaneous communication

- Can communication be established (if not, consider disorders of attention or consciousness)?
- Does the patient produce speech at all (if not, consider mutism, anarthria)?
- Is the patient's speech comprehensible (if not, is it because of phonemic or semantic errors, because of dysarthria or speech apraxia?)?
- Does the patient use propositional language (meaningful word combinations)?
- Is the patient's speech fluent or nonfluent?
- Are there agrammatic or paragrammatic errors?
- Are there phonemic and/or semantic errors?
- Are there pathological repetitive productions (automatism, echolalia, perseveration, stereotypy)?

Table 13.1 Glossary of aphasic symptoms

Speech automatism	The automatic and compulsive production of the same phrase, word, neologism, syllable, or sound contrary to intention
Agrammatism	Reduction of grammatical elements, such as inflections and function words (e.g. prepositions)
Echolalia	Repetition of utterances of the communication partner, frequently with adequate changes denoting the speaker ('How are you?' → 'How am I?').
Jargon, phonemic or neologistic	Phonemic paraphasia occurs to such an extent that speech is incomprehensible
Jargon, semantic	Semantic paraphasia occurs to such an extent that speech is incomprehensible
Neologism, phonemic	A word is incomprehensible because of phonemic paraphasia
Paraphasia, phonemic	Substitution, omission, addition, or perseveration of a phoneme or error of phoneme sequence
Paraphasia, verbal	Substitution of a presumably intended word by another
Paraphasia, semantic	Substitution of a presumably intended word by a meaning-related one
Perseveration	The recurrent production of a previous response out of context
Stereotypy	The repetitive and stereotyped use of a communicatively acceptable word or phrase without propositional meaning (e.g. 'yes', 'my God', 'I don't know', 'such is life') in the position of a pause

Phonological deficits and errors   The phonological structure of an utterance includes the appropriateness of phoneme selection and combination in order to form the sound structure of words. Impairment of phoneme production as such is not an aphasic symptom but would indicate the presence of dysarthria or speech apraxia (whether the interface between linguistic and sensorimotor processes can be defined so rigidly is being intensively debated).

The phonological structure of a word may be altered by omissions, substitutions, the addition of phonemes, errors of sequence, and perseverations. Some aphasics strenuously attempt to correct their phonological output, be it comprehensible or not. Both the production of phonemic paraphasias and disorders of output monitoring and correction may result in the characteristic behaviours of 'conduite d'approche' and 'conduite d'écart', i.e. approximations and digressions from the target, e.g. 'trurtle–tertle–turtle–trullet' (naming a turtle). Words that are phonemically so distorted that they are incomprehensible, are termed *phonemic neologisms*. The term *phonemic* or *neologistic jargon* is used, when the patient's speech is incomprehensible because of phonemic paraphasia.

Lexical/semantic deficits and errors   The analysis of lexical and semantic structure includes the processes of word access, word selection, and the differentiation of word meanings. *Impaired word-finding* is a symptom of all types of aphasia, but also of more diffuse pathology such as dementia and impaired consciousness. It may also occur in normal speakers, especially under stress, distraction, fatigue, and intoxication. Word-finding difficulties may manifest themselves as pauses, in the use of circumlocutions, or in the discontinuation of the phrase.

The term *verbal paraphasia* describes the incorrect use of a word. Verbal paraphasias can be related to the target by meaning similarity, form similarity, or both. Also (seemingly) unrelated verbal paraphasias can occur. Meaning-related errors (*semantic paraphasias*) form the most frequent type of word substitution. Semantic paraphasias typically stem from the target's semantic category (e.g. 'bus' for 'lorry'—close semantic paraphasia) or can be otherwise semantically associated (by situation, function, etc.). If productions are rendered incomprehensible by semantic paraphasia, the term *semantic jargon* is used.

Syntactic deficits and errors   Traditionally, syntactic errors in aphasia are classified as 'agrammatic' and 'paragrammatic'. Because pathological stereotypies may be grammatically appropriate, the analysis of the use of syntax is based only on newly created propositional utterances.

◆ An error is classified as *agrammatic*, when a necessary grammatical element, such as a bound inflectional morpheme, a function word, or an auxiliary verb in a complex verb phrase is missing. In severe cases of agrammatism, the patient almost exclusively uses nouns, verbs in the infinite form such as the present and past participles, adjectives, and adverbs. Function words, such as prepositions, and inflections are greatly reduced or lacking.

◆ In *paragrammatism*, grammatical rules are applied. Patients inflect nouns and verbs and use function words, but their speech deviates from the grammatical norm. Sentence structures are typically long and complex. Sentence boundaries may become obscured ('when I came home is my favourite place').

Fluency and nonfluency in aphasia   Kertesz (1979) denotes two prototypes of aphasic patients.

◆ The nonfluent aphasic struggles with every word and gives the impression of great effort required for speech production;

◆ The fluent aphasic exhibits little or no effort but usually produces many empty phrases or many paraphasic errors.

The fluency/nonfluency dimension is especially helpful for the description of acute aphasia.

Repetitive speech   There are various types of repetitive speech that may occur in aphasic language productions. The most common are speech automatism (recurring utterances), echolalia, perseveration, and stereotypy (for definitions, see Table 13.1). From a clinical point of view, it is important to note that speech automatisms almost exclusively occur in aphasia, whereas echolalia, perseveration, and stereotypy also occur with non-aphasic brain pathology and even in non-brain-damaged persons (for a review, see Wallesch 1990).

2.2.2 Performance in language modalities

Although it is a great simplification in view of neural networks, the Wernicke–Lichtheim model (Fig. 13.1) has had a great influence upon aphasiology (Wernicke 1874; Lichtheim 1885). In this model, (spoken) language is processed by three interconnected components:

◆ a sensory centre for auditory word forms;

◆ a centre for speech–motor word forms;

◆ a (semantic) concept centre.

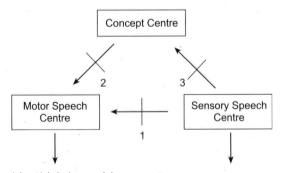

Fig. 13.1 The Wernicke–Lichtheim model.

Wernicke did not localize the concept centre in a circumscribed brain region, but assumed its representation in the interconnection of various association areas.

♦ The assumed connection between the sensory and the motor speech centres provided the ability to repeat without semantic analysis and also control and monitoring of speech output.

♦ The link between sensory and concept centres was necessary for comprehension.

♦ The link between concept and motor speech centres was necessary for naming.

With the exception of the concept centre, a parallel (or subordinate construction) was hypothesized for written language-processing. On the historical basis of the Wernicke–Lichtheim model, the vast majority of aphasia assessment batteries include the tasks of repetition, naming, and comprehension, in most instances both on the word and the sentence level (see box below).

Informal assessment of the aphasic patient

♦ Describe spontaneous communication (see previous box).

♦ Present single sounds ('a', 'm', 'p'), monosyllabic words ('house', 'car'), polysyllabics, and sentences for repetition. Watch for parapraxia (inadequate, mostly hesitant, and probing articulatory movements. If the patient does not repeat at all, ask him/her to imitate mouth movements with and without concomitant articulation (buccofacial apraxia?). If there is no response, ask him/her to imitate coughing (anarthria?, mutism?).

♦ Ask patient to name objects that are in easy reach (watch, cup, bottle). Try semantic ('you drink coffee from the . . .') and phonemic (. . . 'c . . .', 'cu . . .') cueing.

♦ Assess comprehension by simple commands ('point to the door', 'show me your thumb', 'open your mouth'. 'Close your eyes' is the easiest).

♦ If you want a quantification of severity of comprehension loss in aphasia, use the Token Test (see Section 2.4.1).

Errors in naming Table 13.2 summarizes error types in visual confrontation naming. For neurolinguistic analysis, naming has the advantage that the lexical target is known and errors can be more easily analysed linguistically than in spontaneous speech. Naming contains fewer degrees of freedom than spontaneous speech. Therefore, some aphasics may find naming comparatively easy. On the other hand, in most naming situations, only one response is appropriate. Aphasics with prominent disturbances of word access (e.g. with anomic aphasia) may be particularly impaired in naming (e.g. 'I cannot tell its name, but we have similar chairs at home').

Table 13.2 Error types in visual confrontation naming and their functional basis (based on Linebaugh 1990)

Error type	Functional basis
Delayed naming	Slowed activation or selection of lexical target
Self-correction	Recognition of error
Circumlocution	Failure to retrieve lexical target; alternative production of semantic information
Near semantic paraphasia	Retrieval of a lexical entry semantically related to the target
Unrelated word	Failure to access appropriate target
Visually related word	Error in visual object analysis
Perseveration	Failure to inhibit a previous response
Gesture	Compensation for failure to retrieve lexical target
No response	

Some patients have a specific impairment of visual object naming as compared to naming with other presentation modalities. This condition is called *optic aphasia* (Coslett and Saffran 1989). Its functional basis is a disconnection of the language region from the visual association cortex as it may occur with posterior watershed infarctions. These patients can easily be identified by their ability to produce names in response to questions (e.g. 'what do you open a lock with?').

Errors in repetition   In repetition, semantic and lexical search processes are usually not critically involved. Some patients, however, may have to rely on a semantic route in this task (Katz and Goodglass 1990). They cannot repeat 'nonwords' (phoneme sequences that do not constitute a meaningful word in the respective language). The assessment of repetition should include stimuli of varying length and lexical as well as nonlexical items.

A focal deficit of repetition may indicate a deficit of auditory-verbal short-term memory, an impairment of the memory for sequence, or of the transformation of a phonological representation into a phonetic string. The latter explanation is similar to the anatomical assumption of a disconnection between receptive and expressive speech areas to account for repetition deficits (Geschwind 1965).

Deficits in spoken language comprehension   Intactness or only mild impairment of spoken language comprehension is often wrongly assumed in aphasic patients, as the patient may make use of situational cues. In formal assessment, forced-choice decision tasks are often easier for the patient than those that demand production, both with respect to linguistic and neuropsychological processing demands (Wallesch and Kertesz 1993). To compensate for this effect, aphasia test batteries such as the Boston Diagnostic Aphasia Examination (Goodglass and Kaplan 1972), the Western Aphasia Battery (Kertesz 1979), or the Aachen Aphasia Test (Huber *et al.* 1983, 1984) use norms derived from aphasic patients to assign scaled scores or values.

2.3 **Syndromes of aphasia**

The term *syndrome* denotes the statistical co-occurrence of a cluster of symptoms. It is not imperative that all symptoms of a syndrome are present in a given patient. The statistical cluster is supposed to indicate an underlying cause of the various symptoms. Poeck (1983) pointed out that the underlying pathophysiological basis of the aphasia syndromes may be the vascular anatomy of the cerebral language representations rather than 'natural' linguistic structures. The importance of the syndromatic classification of a given patient has decreased in the last 20 years, since syndrome-specific treatments have been abandoned. Conversely, the description and interpretation of aphasic symptoms has increased in relevance.

Statistical cluster analysis reveals that most (about 70–80%) aphasic patients are grouped together and that these clusters relate to the clinical syndromes of acute or chronic aphasia (Kertesz 1979; Huber *et al.* 1983; Wallesch *et al.* 1992). Generally, patients with non-ischaemic aphasia syndromes correspond much less both to the clusters and clinical syndromes of chronic aphasia than patients who have suffered an ischaemic stroke.

To increase confusion even further, a number of classification systems are used. These can be grouped into three types.

- *Modality-oriented.* Syndromes are distinguished on the basis of assumed dissociations across modalities, resulting in categories such as 'motor'/'sensory' or 'expressive'/ 'receptive'. Recent examples are the classification systems of Goodglass and Kaplan (1972) and Kertesz (1979).

- *Anatomically-oriented* with syndromes such as 'anterior' versus 'posterior' (Benson 1967). Often, atypical aphasia syndromes are denoted by anatomical terms, e.g. 'subcortical' or 'thalamic' aphasia.

- According to the *linguistic deficit.* A very simple classification into 'fluent' and 'nonfluent' aphasia (Benson 1967) is based upon speed of production and phrase length.

The classification system described in more detail below is based on cluster analyses of the results of aphasia tests and therefore on the linguistic deficit.

The syndromes of acute and chronic aphasia will be treated separately. Obviously, there is no dichotomous distinction. However, acute aphasia, i.e. aphasia syndromes seen in the acute hospital and with progressive lesions such as tumours, differs in many ways from chronic aphasia, as seen in rehabilitation and afterwards (Table 13.3).

2.3.1 Syndromes of acute aphasia

Patients suffering from acute aphasia present symptoms of acute focal pathology in combination with the effects of diffuse cerebral dysfunction (Table 13.3), such as reduced consciousness, attentional impairment, and rapid fluctuations in performance. The deficits preclude detailed linguistic and neuropsychological assessment.

Table 13.3 Differences between acute and chronic vascular aphasia

	Acute	**Chronic**
Time postonset	Few weeks	Many months
Pathophysiology	Penumbra and diaschisis; enlarged functional lesion	Cerebral reorganization reduces functional deficit
Neuropsychology	Additional disorders of consciousness, attention, and awareness	Compensation, reorganization
Psychology	Distress	Coping
Social role	Illness	Handicap

Kertesz (1979) and Wallesch *et al.* (1992) analysed groups of patients 3 to 6 weeks after onset of aphasia by means of cluster analysis. The results of both studies converge with respect to syndromes of acute aphasia by finding clusters of:

1. mild aphasia with prominent word-finding difficulty;

2. mild aphasia with prominent comprehension deficit;

3. moderate aphasia with prominent repetition impairment ('acute conduction aphasia')

4. marked aphasia with (relatively) preserved repetition ('acute transcortical motor aphasia');

5. severe aphasia with (relatively) preserved comprehension;

6. severe aphasia with deficits in all modalities.

Clusters 1 and 2 are usually fluent; 4–6 nonfluent. Type 3 is fluent in stereotypies and mainly nonfluent in propositional utterances and repetition ('acute conduction aphasia'). A development towards chronic Wernicke's aphasia occurred in clusters 3 and 5, but not in 2 (Wallesch *et al.* 1992). A large number of patients from cluster 6 develop Broca's aphasia, and most patients from cluster 5 become anomic (Kertesz 1984). The frequency of a change of symptomatology ('Syndromwandel') speaks against the use of the terminology of chronic aphasia syndromes in the acute stage. Clusters 1 and 6 are the most frequent.

In the first hours and day after stroke or trauma, many patients are mute. Neurological mutism can result from aphasia, but also from severe apraxia, paresis, or akinesia. An analysis of nonverbal communication and comprehension may guide the initial differential diagnosis.

2.3.2 Syndromes of chronic aphasia

As has been pointed out, the classical aphasia syndromes describe best the symptomatology of stroke patients who have suffered a functional deficit due to a circumscribed lesion at one point in time and who have consequently developed adaptive and maladaptive compensatory strategies.

Global aphasia The term 'global' denotes that all language processes are severely affected. Propositional language is either almost absent, or reduced to single words or phrase fragments and is produced with great effort. A few stereotyped phrases may be preserved and used adequately in some situations. A subgroup of patients are able to produce highly overlearned sequences such as prayers, series such as the days of the week, or popular songs. With echolalia as an additional syndrome-unspecific symptom, repetition may be quite good. Speech automatisms (recurring utterances) can frequently (though not necessarily) be observed in global aphasia and seem to supersede intended more adequate utterances that in some cases can be realized by superior writing performance (see Blanken *et al.* 1990).

Global aphasia is the result of severe damage to the cerebral language representation in the area of supply of the left middle cerebral artery. Lesions of the deep periventricular white matter and/or the basal ganglia seem to be of special importance. Global aphasia is a syndrome of older patients. Subjects below the age of about 40 are likely to develop Broca's aphasia even with very large infarcts. Because stroke incidence is age-related, global aphasia is the most common chronic aphasia syndrome.

Broca's aphasia The syndrome of Broca's aphasia is different from the clinical status (global aphasia) and functional interpretation (similar to the modern concept of speech apraxia) of Broca's original patients. The principal feature of Broca's aphasia is a reduction of linguistic proficiency on the phonological (simplification of phonemic structure), lexical (word-finding difficulty), and syntactic (agrammatism) levels. Of these, the agrammatic deficits are quite specific for the syndrome and have been proposed to constitute an axial symptom. Severe agrammatism leads to the so-called 'telegraphic style' with a lack of function words and inflection forms ('skiing–bang–head–sick'). In mild cases, the patients' productions may be characterized only by a reduction in the use of subordinate clauses, multiple objects, or complex verb forms. In these cases, a premorbidly more elaborate use of language should be established. Case reports of patients with quite specific morphological or syntactic deficits, however, contradict a unitary view of agrammatism (Nadeau 1988).

Patients suffering from Broca's aphasia exhibit a deficit of lexical retrieval with time-consuming, laborious attempts at word finding. Phonological assembly and articulation are slowed down. A combination with speech apraxia is common. In a clinical situation, the comprehension deficit is mild. It has been shown that most patients have comprehension problems similar to their expressive symptomatology, namely, a prominent impairment of the understanding of grammatical constructions (Grodzinsky *et al.* 1999).

In the majority of cases, Broca's aphasia develops from a very severe deficit in all modalities, in most instances in a youngish (younger than 60 years) patient who suffers from a large infarct in the territory of the left middle cerebral artery. Their improvement indicates that reorganization (activation of lexical representations outside the damaged language region) and compensatory strategies (e.g. telegraphic style) contribute to the syndrome's phenomenology. Broca's aphasia is the second most common chronic aphasia syndrome.

Wernicke's aphasia This syndrome is characterized by its prominent 'para-symptomatology': phonemic and semantic paraphasia, neologisms, or jargon and paragrammatism. Speech production is usually fluent, with few attempts at error correction. With phonemic jargon, the syntactic structure cannot be analysed, although the presence of such structure can often be inferred, as undistorted function words frequently stand out and segment the utterance (Buckingham and Kertesz 1976) and inflectional morphemes may be used on neologisms. If the lexical content is sufficiently comprehensible, syntactic violations such as sentence blendings, choice of inadequate functors, and inappropriate inflections can be detected. Generally, language comprehension is more impaired in Wernicke's than in Broca's aphasia, although jargon may occur with little comprehension deficit.

Fluent paraphasic aphasia is frequent in the first 2 weeks postonset (20%; Willmes and Poeck 1984) but rare among chronic aphasics (3% in the same series). Most patients develop towards anomic or unspecific residual aphasia. This finding probably also indicates a process of reorganization by re-establishing monitoring and output control. The most common cause of chronic Wernicke's aphasia is posterior cerebral infarction in patients in whom reorganization is impaired, namely, those who are either elderly or have diffuse or multifocal brain pathology in addition. The average age of chronic Wernicke's aphasics is much higher than that of Broca's aphasics.

Anomic aphasia The core symptom of anomic aphasia is deficient lexical access and/or retrieval. Phonology and syntax are only mildly affected. The word-finding impairment results in pauses, circumlocutions, closely related semantic paraphasias, evasion of the target word by use of empty phrases or fillers without specific meaning ('thing'), circumscriptions by verbal or nonverbal means, or discontinuation of the ongoing phrase followed by variation of the statement. Most of these stragegies are communicatively acceptable. The deficit becomes striking, when only one lexical response is acceptable, such as in naming.

Anomic aphasia usually results from a lesion in the posterior border regions of the core language area. In most cases, the temporoparietal junction or the inferior parietal lobe is affected. Anomic aphasia is relatively frequent with non-ischaemic pathology, such as tumour or trauma.

Conduction aphasia Conduction aphasia was predicted by the Wernicke–Lichtheim model (Fig. 13.1) as a disconnection between the sensory and motor language centres. Wernicke predicted a deficit of output monitoring and control rather than a disorder of repetition (Köhler *et al.* 1998). Within the diagnositic category of conduction aphasia, two different types of patients have been distinguished (Shallice and Warrington 1977):

- those with a prominent repetition deficit due to an impairment of phonological short-term memory (Caramazza *et al.* 1981);

- those with an impairment of phonological output programming for single words, which together with relatively preserved monitoring results in frequent attempts at correction (conduites d'approche) that can be most prominent in repetition (Kohn 1984).

Only the latter patients form 'pure' cases of conduction aphasia. However, many conduction aphasics show deficits at both levels of performance. Conduction aphasia is frequent in the acute and rare in the chronic stage. When encountered with acute aphasia, its prognosis is good. Its association with a lesion of the arcuate fascicle, the anatomical connection between Wernicke's and Broca's areas, is disputed.

The transcortical aphasias   The syndromes of transcortical motor, transcortical sensory, and mixed transcortical aphasia are characterized by their preserved ability to repeat. They were predicted by the Wernicke–Lichtheim model as disorders in which the direct connections between sensory and motor speech areas were left intact.

Patients suffering from transcortical motor aphasia show greatly reduced language production, except for repetition, and rather preserved comprehension. This syndrome is usually encountered with lesions of the left frontal lobe outside Broca's area, especially in the vicinity of the supplementary motor area on the medial surface, and with lesions of the left basal ganglia. It has been related to a nonlinguistic mechanism involving initiative for speech. Repetition is least affected, because it involves the fewest degrees of freedom (Goldberg 1985).

Both transcortical sensory and mixed transcortical aphasia are rare. Patients are characterized by disinhibited echolalia. Most patients decribed in the literature have been demented. In transcortical sensory aphasia, language output is fluent with mainly semantic paraphasia. In mixed transcortical aphasia, language production is reduced to echolalia. Naming and comprehension are severely impaired in both syndromes. Mixed transcortical aphasia has been interpreted as an 'isolation of the speech area' (Geschwind *et al.* 1968), as these patients exhibit signs of linguistic processing in the absence of semantic analysis.

2.4 Diagnostic instruments

The experienced clinician does not require a formal test to detect the presence of aphasia and diagnose the syndrome. Tests subserve mainly three functions:

- establishing the severity of aphasia;
- analysing the neurospychological or neurolinguistic structure of the patient's deficits as a basis for treatment planning and evaluation by a test battery;
- analysing the effect of aphasia upon a patient's communication performance.

An overview of aphasia tests and their psychometric properties and problems is given by Willmes (1993).

2.4.1 Severity of aphasia

The Token Test (De Renzi and Vignolo 1962) is a simple and valid instrument to assess the severity of aphasia. It was originally designed as a test of language comprehension that would not include redundant information. The test consists of circles and squares of two different sizes and five different colours (Fig. 13.2), which the subject is required to point at or perform operations with at the request of the investigator. Contrary to the authors' intuition, the test scores correlate as highly with performance in expressive as in receptive language tasks. A linguistically more structured Revised Token Test has been devised by Mc Neil and Prescott (1978). This test is not very widely used, however, because it takes more time to administer.

2.4.2 Assessment of neurolinguistics structure

The most frequently used aphasia test is probably the Boston Diagnostic Aphasia Examination (Goodglass and Kaplan 1972). This battery includes 27 subtests that assess spoken and written language and associated functions. It provides norms from a collective of aphasics as Z-scores and assigns the patient's aphasia syndrome on the basis of test results. The Aachen Aphasia Test (Huber *et al.* 1983, 1984) assesses a more limited number of functions, but has psychometrical advantages, as it supports single-case statistics. Its English version has not been published yet. A brief, clinically oriented aphasia battery for nonspecialist use is the Frenchay Aphasia Screening Test (Enderby *et al.* 1987).

A very detailed instrument for the assessment of aphasic symptoms is the PALPA (Psycholinguistic Assessment of Language Processing in Aphasia; Kay *et al.* 1992). It provides an assessment of a wide variety of language processes intended for a mapping of a single case's deficits and dysfunctions upon a psycholinguistic model of normal language processing.

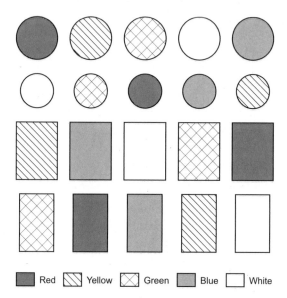

Fig. 13.2 The Token Test.   ▨ Red   ▨ Yellow   ▨ Green   ▨ Blue   ☐ White

2.4.3 Assessment of communication performance

The Amsterdam–Nijmegen Everyday Language Test (ANELT; Blomert *et al.* 1987) uses standardized everday situations in the form of role-play to assess aphasics' communicative use of verbal and nonverbal means of communications.

3 **Speech apraxia**

Speech apraxia describes the functional pathology of brain-damaged persons whose speech is more affected by articulatory symptoms such as distortions, substitutions, and dysprosody than is explained by sensorimotor, language, and cognitive deficits. The phenomenological boundaries of the apraxic dysfunction, e.g. towards dysarthria and conduction aphasia, remain unclear. The structure of the interface between linguistic and speech–motor processes is still unresolved. Speech apraxia has to be differentiated from oral (buccofacial) apraxia. Both conditions may co-occur but also occur separately.

Theoretically, speech apraxia denotes a deficit on the level of motor programming and execution that affects only speech-related movements.

◆ Sensorimotorically, speech is organized differently from other motor acts, in that sensorimotor feedback plays only a negligible role.

◆ On the phonetic level, speech apraxia is characterized by inconsistent errors variably related to the phonemic target, such as omission, substitution, distortion, addition, and errors of sequence. The errors are influenced by articulatory complexity. There are also effects of propositionality: stereotyped productions, such as expletives, are less affected. Usually, the beginning of a word is more impaired than sounds within a word. This finding can be explained on the level of motor processing, because the transition probabilities from one phoneme to the next are smaller within words than at word onset.

A very characteristic symptom of speech apraxia is the occurrence of *parapraxia*. Parapraxia is defined as errors on the level of movement elements, e.g. omission of a necessary element, addition, permutation, substitution, or perseveration. Without technical investigations, parapraxias can only be observed with the anterior articulators and inferred from the phonetic signal by an experienced examiner. Other typical symptoms are probe articulations in order to check auditorily and somatosensorily whether type and place of articulation are correct, and the use of the hands in order to place the articulators in the assumed correct position.

3.1 **Diagnostic instruments**

There is no generally accepted clinical instrument for the assessment of speech apraxia (see Collins 1989 and Rosenbek 1993 for discussions). The same technical investigations may be used as with dysarthria (see Section 4).

3.2 Other acquired disorders of motor–speech programming and execution

- *Neurological stuttering.* Occasionally, patients with subcortical lesions in either hemisphere, especially in the caudate nucleus, who did not suffer from developmental dysfluency, exhibit symptoms of (tonic, clonic, or tonic–clonic) stuttering (Ludlow *et al.* 1987).

- *Foreign accent syndrome.* Rarely, patients with left hemisphere subcortical lesions exhibit consistent alterations in linguistic, but not affective prosody that result in the impression of a foreign accent (Gurd *et al.* 1988).

4 Dysarthria

The dysarthrias are disorders of the sensorimotor performance of speech acts that are characterized by disturbances in speech musculature control due to paresis, slowness, incoordination, altered tone, or additional (dyskinetic) movements. They affect the respiration pattern required for speech, phonation, resonation, articulation, and prosody. As with the sensorimotor speed and quality of other (e.g. hand) movements, a number of neurological impairments can cause dysfunction:

- lesions of the first (spastic paresis) and second (flaccid paresis and atrophy) motor neuron;
- ataxia;
- akinesia;
- dys- and hyperkinesia;
- sensory impairment.

Accordingly, the dysarthrias are classified into a central and a peripheral paretic, a hypokinetic, an ataxic, and a dyskinetic variety. Clinically, some frequent neurological diseases result in mixed forms, as more than one sensorimotor mechanism is affected, e.g. amyotrophic lateral sclerosis (ALS) combines first and second motoneuron degeneration and multiple sclerosis frequently includes both spastic and ataxic symptoms.

4.1 Types of dysarthria

- Bilateral lesions of the first motor neuron of the corticobulbar tracts result in spastic (or, better, central paretic) dysarthria (because there is little spasticity in the involved muscles). It is characterized by impaired diadochokinetic motility of the articulatory musculature and a disinhibition of reflectory mass movements and synergisms (pathological laughter and crying, sucking, etc.). Speech is laboured, monotonous, and slow with imprecise consonants as the most prominent feature. It occurs in neurological diseases with prominent first motor neuron pathology, mainly diffuse or multifocal cerebrovascular disease ('pseudobulbar palsy').

- The symptomatology of lesions of the second (peripheral) motor neuron (or the neuromuscular junction (myasthenia gravis) or diseases of the relevant musculature, e.g. muscular atrophy and dystrophy, polymyositis) depends on the affected nerves or muscles. With diffuse disease, such as one form of ALS ('bulbar palsy'), bilateral affection of cranial nerves (e.g. Miller–Fisher syndrome), and myasthenia, speech is reduced in volume, monotonous, imprecise, and hypernasal.

- Hypokinetic dysarthria is phenomenologically similar to spastic dysarthria with imprecise articulation, slow speech, decreased prosody, and often decreased loudness. Speech in Parkinson's disease, the most frequent cause of hypokinetic dysarthria, is additionally characterized by variations in speech rate (tachyphasia) and rapid repetition of speech elements (palilalia).

- Ataxic dysarthria is characterized by variable articulatory errors and imprecisions with frequent omissions; rapid changes in speech rate, pitch, and loudness ('scanning speech'); and inadequate respiratory patterns.

- With dys- and hyperkinetic dysarthria, there is also a variable pattern of errors dictated by the involuntary movements. In view of the amount of dyskinesia, most patients articulate surprisingly well. A dissociation from respiration with phonation on inspiration, involuntary phonation, and diminished control of pitch and loudness are typical.

Table 13.4 describes characteristic features of the dysarthria types. For a detailed description of the dysarthrias, Darley *et al.* (1975) is still a most valuable source.

4.2 Diagnostic instruments

Clinically, the most frequently used assessment instrument is the Frenchay Dysarthria Assessment (Enderby 1983). It consists of a standardized investigation of speech and

Table 13.4 Characteristic features of the dysarthias

Type	Variability of errors	Symptoms	Pathognomonic features
Central paretic	None/little	Slow, monotonous, laboured speech	Disinhibited mass movements of facial muscles (e.g. crying)
Peripheral paretic	None/little	Depends on paretic muscles	Muscle atrophy when chronic
Hypokinetic	None/little	Monotonous, often laboured speech	With Parkinson's disease: acceleration, palilalia
Hyperkinetic	Pronounced	Hyperkinesia, surprisingly good intelligibility of speech	Visible hyperkinesia
Ataxic	Pronounced	Scanning speech (see text)	Rapid changes in rate, pitch, and loudness
Peripheral sensory	Yes	Numbness	Very recent visit to dentist; occasionally neurological disease

nonspeech motor acts of respiration and phonation, and speech and nonspeech movements of the articulators together with a rating of comprehensibility of the production of words, sentences, and spontaneous speech. Normative data for groups of patients are provided and aid differential diagnosis.

In addition, speech-related movements can be investigated by technical means, such as electroglottography, endoscopy, X-ray microbeam, and electromagnetic articulography, and phonetic signals by sound spectrography.

Selective references

Benson, D.F. (1967). Fluency in aphasia. *Cortex* 3, 373–94.

Blanken, G., Wallesch, C.W., and Papagno, C. (1990). Dissociations of language functions in patients with speech automatisms (recurring utterances). *Cortex* 26, 41–63.

Blanken, G., Dittmann, J., Grimm, H., Marshall, J.C., and Wallesch, C.W. (eds.) (1993). *Linguistic disorders and pathologies.* De Gruyter, Berlin.

Blomert, L., Koster, C., van Mier, H., and Kean, M.L. (1987). Verbal communication abilities of aphasic patients: The everyday language test. *Aphasiology* 1, 463–74.

Buckingham, H.W. and Kertesz, A. (1976). *Neologistic jargon aphasia.* Swets and Zeitlinger, Amsterdam.

Caplan, D. (1992). *Language. Structure, processing, and disorders.* MIT Press, Cambridge, Massachusetts.

Caramazza, A., Basili, A.G., Koller, J.J., and Berndt, R.S. (1981). An investigation of repetition and language processing in a case of conduction aphasia. *Brain Language* 40, 235–71.

Collins, M.J. (1989). Differential diagnosis of aphasic syndromes and apraxia of speech. In *Acquired apraxia of speech in aphasic adults* (ed. P. Square-Storer), pp. 87–114. Taylor and Francis, London.

Coslett, H.B. and Saffran, E.M. (1989). Preserved object recognition and reading comprehension in optic aphasia. *Brain* 112, 1091–110.

Darley, F.L., Aronson, A.E., and Brown, J.R. (1975). *Motor speech disorders.* Saunders, Philadelphia.

De Renzi, E. and Vignolo, L.A. (1962). The token test: a sensitive test to detect receptive disturbances in aphasia. *Brain* 85, 665–78.

Enderby, P.M. (1983). *Frenchay Dysarthria Assessment.* College Hill, San Diego.

Enderby, P.M., Wood, V.A., Wade, D.T., and Hewer, R.L. (1987). The Frenchay Aphasia Screening Test: a short, simple test for aphasia appropriate for nonspecialists. *Int. J. Rehabil. Med.* 8, 166–70.

Geschwind, N. (1965). Disconnection syndromes in animals and man. Part II. *Brain* 103, 337–50.

Geschwind, N., Quadfasel, F., and Segarra, J. (1968). Isolation of the speech area. *Neuropsychologia* 6, 327–40.

Goldberg, E. (1985). Supplementary motor area structure and function: review and hypothesis. *Behav. Brain Res.* 8, 567–616.

Goodglass, H. and Kaplan, E. (1972). *The assessment of aphasia and related disorders.* Lea and Febiger, Philadelphia.

Grodzinsky, Y., Pinango, M.M., Zurif, E., and Drai, D. (1999). The critical role of group studies in neuropsychology: comprehension regularities in Broca's aphasia. *Brain Language* 67, 134–47.

Gurd, J.M., Bessell, N.J., Bladon, R.A., and Bamford, J.M. (1988). A case of foreign accent syndrome, with follow-up clinical, neuropsychological and phonetic descriptions. *Neuropsychologia* 26, 237–51.

Huber, W., Poeck, K., Weniger, D., and Willmes, K. (1983). *Der Aachener Aphasie Test.* Hogrefe, Göttingen.

Huber, W., Poeck, K., and Willmes, K. (1984). The Aachen Aphasia test. In *Progress in aphasiology* (ed. F.C. Rose), pp. 291–303. Raven, New York.

Katz, R.B. and Goodglass, H. (1990). Deep dysphasia: analysis of a rare form of repetition disorder. *Brain Language* 39, 153–85.

Kay, J., Lesser, R., and Coltheart, M. (1992). *Psycholinguistic assessment of language processing in aphasia.* Lawrence Erlbaum, Hove, East Sussex.

Kertesz, A. (1979). *Aphasia and associated disorders.* Grune and Stratton, New York.

Kertesz, A. (1984). Recovery from aphasia. In *Progress in aphasiology* (ed. F.C. Rose), pp. 23–39. Raven, New York.

Köhler, K., Bartels, C., Herrmann, M., Dittmann, J., and Wallesch, C.W. (1998). Conduction aphasia—11 classic cases. *Aphasiology* 12, 865–84.

Kohn, S. (1984). The nature of phonological disorders in conduction aphasia. *Brain Language* 23, 97–115.

Lichtheim, L. (1885). Ueber Aphasie. *Deutsches Arch. Klin. Med.* 36, 204–68.

Linebaugh, C.W. (1990). Lexical retrieval problems: anomia. In *Aphasia and related neurogenic language disorders* (ed. L.L. LaPointe), pp. 96–112. Thieme, New York.

Ludlow, C.L., Rosenberg, J., Salazar, A., Grafman, J., and Smutok, M. (1987). Site of penetrating brain lesions causing chronic acquired stuttering. *Ann. Neurol.* 22, 60–6.

McNeil, M.R. and Prescott, T.E. (1978). *Revised Token Test.* Pro-Ed, Austin Texas.

Nadeau, S.E. (1988). Impaired grammar with normal fluency and phonology. Implications for Broca's aphasia. *Brain* 111, 1111–37.

Poeck, K. (1983). What do we mean by 'aphasic syndromes'? A neurologist's view. *Brain Language* 20, 79–89.

Rosenbek, J.C. (1993). Speech apraxia. In *Linguistic disorders and pathologies* (ed. G. Blanken, J. Dittmann, H. Grimm, J.C. Marshall, and C.W. Wallesch), pp. 443–52. De Gruyter, Berlin.

Shallice, T. and Warrington, E.K. (1977). Auditory verbal short-term memory impairment and conduction aphasia. *Brain Language* 4, 479–91.

Square-Storer, P. (ed.) (1989). *Acquired apraxia of speech in aphasic adults.* Taylor and Francis, London.

Wallesch, C.W. (1990). Repetitive verbal behaviour: neurological and functional considerations. *Aphasiology* 4, 133–54.

Wallesch, C.W. and Kertesz, A. (1993). Clinical symptoms and syndromes of aphasia. In *Linguistic disorders and pathologies* (ed. G. Blanken, J. Dittmann, H. Grimm, J.C. Marshall, and C.W. Wallesch), pp. 98–119. De Gruyter, Berlin.

Wallesch, C.W., Bak, T., and Schulte-Mönting, J. (1992). Acute aphasia—patterns and prognosis. *Aphasiology* 6, 273–85.

Wernicke, C. (1874). *Der aphasische Symptomencomplex. Eine psychologische Studie auf anatomischer Basis.* Cohn and Weigert, Breslau.

Willmes, K. (1993). Diagnostic methods in aphasiology. In *Linguistic disorders and pathologies* (ed. G. Blanken, J. Dittmann, H. Grimm, J.C. Marshall, and C.W. Wallesch), pp. 137–52. De Gruyter, Berlin.

Willmes, K. and Poeck, K. (1984). Ergebnisse einer multizentrischen Untersuchung über die Spontanprognose von Aphasien vaskulärer Ätiologie. *Nervenarzt* 55, 62–71.

Chapter 14

Treatment of spoken language disorders

Jane Marshall

1 Introduction

There are three broad types of speech disorder that can arise from brain damage:

+ dysarthria;

+ apraxia (or dyspraxia);

+ aphasia (or dysphasia).

The first two affect the muscular control or coordination of speech. In contrast, aphasia is a language disorder. Here the speech impairment is part of a complex of symptoms, typically involving several aspects of communication (see Chapter 13).

The different speech disorders can coexist, e.g. a person may have both aphasia and dysarthria, or aphasia and apraxia. Also, the speech problem may be just one aspect of a more global neurological condition that carries further implications for communication. For example, dysarthrias often co-occur with generalized motor difficulties that make it difficult for the person to write or use technological aids.

Numerous treatments for neurological speech problems have been attempted, a selection of which are summarized below. Although diverse, these are underpinned by some common principles.

+ Many therapies aim directly to recover lost skills or functions, e.g. through repeated and structured practice. If successful, these treatments may work by promoting a degree of neural reorganization.

+ Alternatively or additionally, treatments may aim to compensate for the difficulties. Such compensations may be made by the person with the speech problem, by drawing upon retained skills, or they may be employed by those in the person's environment.

+ The role of the environment in creating barriers for people with speech problems has been particularly emphasized in recent therapy literature (e.g. Pound *et al.* 2000). As a result, many treatments focus as much on that environment as on the individual with the disorder.

2 Therapy for people with dysarthria

Dysarthria ranges from a mild loss of intelligibility, e.g. due to damage to a single cranial nerve, to complete anarthria, due to a severe loss of the neuromuscular control of speech. Prognosis is equally varied. Some individuals, e.g. those with vascular aetiology, may expect a good recovery, while others are coping with progressive and terminal conditions. The social effects of dysarthria are wide-ranging, with implications for the person's working life, personal relationships, and ability to maintain family roles.

Given the diversity of the dysarthrias, we cannot look for a single 'dysarthria therapy'. Rather, clinicians employ a range of approaches, which vary across individuals, and within the treatment of the same individual over time.

2.1 Goals of therapy

Therapy aims to maximize the effectiveness, efficiency, and naturalness of communication (Duffy 1995). This entails a number of component aims.

- To restore or improve particular muscular functions, such as vocal cord closure. This is particularly relevant for those who can expect a degree of physiological recovery, e.g. stroke or trauma patients.

- To maintain neuromuscular function for as long as possible, e.g. in the case of some progressive disorders.

- To compensate for lost function, particularly when improvement of neuromuscular function is not achievable.

- To provide psychological support, e.g. to help the person deal with the profound life changes associated with dysarthria and, in some cases, plan for the progressive loss of speech. Support may consist of counselling, information and advice, and contact with relevant social and disability organizations.

2.2 Therapy regimes

Dysarthria calls for flexible therapy regimes. Some may be catered for in a single episode of intervention, while others require ongoing support, which changes in nature as the disease progresses. Therapy regimes should take account of the needs of family members, e.g. through relatives' support groups. Therapy settings should also be flexible. For example, therapy aiming to modify the person's environment is best conducted in that environment, while therapy employing instrumental feedback may have to be conducted in the clinic. It may be possible to administer group therapy, where individuals can benefit from working with others who share similar difficulties.

Individuals with complex neurological conditions typically receive input from a range of professionals. Coordination of multidisciplinary input is crucial to ensure compatible goals and to prevent patient confusion.

2.3 The role of assessment in planning therapy

Assessment has many roles.

- *To probe the individual's view about their problem,* e.g. about what impairs intelligibility, what helps, what situations are most difficult, what strategies they are already using, and the role of others in either easing or exacerbating the problem. Ideally, therapy is client-driven, e.g. by targeting the aspects of speech that most concern them, or by building upon strategies that they have already started.

- *To identify a target for intervention* by indicating which impairment to the speech mechanism most reduces intelligibility and where improvements are most likely to have effect.

- *To identify an approach,* e.g. focal or mild impairments may benefit from a speech-orientated approach, while degenerative conditions usually call for compensatory techniques.

- *To identify factors that may influence management decisions.* These include medical or personal factors that are likely to impact upon the individual's response to therapy, e.g. fatigue may preclude an intensive behavioural programme and low levels of literacy would argue against writing-based techniques.

- *To evaluate environmental factors.* Here client's insights can be supplemented with clinician observation, e.g. of the person's communication with significant others, and by structured questioning, e.g. about the layout of the home, social activities undertaken, and barriers confronted during those activities. This assessment is particularly crucial in planning communication-oriented approaches.

- *To provide a baseline against which to measure progress.* Baseline data may comprise quantitative or instrumental measures and/or intelligibility ratings. It should include measures of the dysarthric person's perspective, such as qualitative evaluations of their communication experiences.

2.4 Therapy approaches

2.4.1 Speech-orientated behavioural approaches (see examples in Table 14.1)

These involve exercises and drills aiming directly to improve neuromuscular function and hence speech. Tasks are hierarchically organized, progressing from readily attainable to more ambitious goals, and involve repeated and frequent practice. To achieve the latter, clinicians normally provide homework exercises. Ideally, the task is developed in consultation with the dysarthric person, since self-directed therapy achieves better retention and generalization than purely clinician-led approaches (e.g. Wertz *et al.* 1984). Feedback is important, with specific feedback, outlining the type and locus of errors, being more useful than general comments about intelligibility (Till and Toye 1988). In some settings, feedback may include instrumental techniques (see Section 2.4.6).

Table 14.1 Examples of speech-oriented approaches for dysarthria

Target parameter	Example exercises	Aim/rationale	Relevant dysarthria types
Respiration	Inspiratory checking (Netsell 1992); the person is instructed to 'take a deep breath' and 'now let the air out slowly'	To improve breath support for speech and prevent air wastage, e.g. where there is reduced vocal cord adduction; uses the inspiratory muscles to maintain relatively constant subglottal air pressure	Flaccid Ataxic Hypokinetic
Phonation	Pushing, pulling, and lifting exercises (e.g. Aronson 1990); effortful movements, such as pushing against the arms of a chair, are coordinated with phonation	To maximize vocal cord adduction and possibly improve vocal cord strength; appropriate for people with uni or bilateral vocal cord weakness	Flaccid dysarthria only
Articulation	Drill (Rosenbek and LaPointe 1985); an individual hierarchy of speech sounds is developed; targets are modelled by the clinician and cued, e.g. with illustrations of their production and hands on assistance in reaching articulatory placements; targets are practised and consolidated through drills	To improve accuracy and intelligibility in articulation; may promote compensatory strategies, e.g. by helping the person to attain acceptable articulatory substitutions for problem sounds	Flaccid Spastic Ataxic Hypokinetic Unilateral upper motor neuron

A typical therapy cycle involves:

- discussion and explanation, including the rationale for the exercise and how it relates to the person's problem;
- practice with hierarchically structured tasks;
- feedback and self-evaluation;
- repeated practice, possibly at a more demanding level;
- practice of the target skill in communicative/conversational tasks.

2.4.2 Compensatory behavioural approaches (see examples in Table 14.2)

These aim to develop strategies that improve intelligibility without necessarily changing neuromuscular function. A good example is therapy that compensates for poor articulation by reducing speech rate. Other compensatory approaches involve using prosthetic devices and alternative or augmentative communication.

Table 14.2 Examples of compensatory behavioural approaches for dysarthria

Target parameter	Approach	Aim/rationale	Relevant dysarthria types
Respiration	Optimal breath group (Linebaugh 1983); Assessment establishes the number of syllables that can be produced comfortably on one breath; the client practises segmenting utterances according to this figure; drills may aim gradually to increase the optimal breath group	Improve coordination between speech and respiration	Flaccid Spastic Ataxic Hypokinetic
Rate	Pause modification (Yorkston et al.1988); pause boundaries are identified, e.g. in a written sentence or passage; the client practises saying the target passage with the identified pauses; pauses are sustained for a given time	Rate reduction improves intelligibility by allowing more time for articulation; modifying pauses reduces rate but preserves natural speech rythms; pauses are easier to modify than speech duration	Flaccid Spastic Ataxic Hypokinetic Unilateral upper motor neuron
	Alphabet board supplementation (Beukelman and Yorkston 1977; Crow and Enderby 1989); the person points to the 1st letter of each word as they say it, using an alphabet board; the technique is practised with utterances of increasing length and in conversational contexts	The alphabet board helps the person controlspeech rate; aided speech is more intelligible than unaided speech, both because rate is reduced and additional information supplied by the letter cue	All

2.4.3 Communication-oriented approach (see examples in Table 14.3)

This approach may be offered in isolation, or as a supplement to behavioural therapy. It aims to develop strategies, which can be adopted by both the dysarthic person and their listener, to facilitate communication, despite continuing problems with intelligibility. Strategies should be developed in the light of environmental assessment findings. The client, and significant others, should play a major role in developing the ideas and should be provided with opportunities to practise and modify the strategies in therapy sessions.

2.4.4 Prosthetic devices used in dysarthria therapy

A number of prostheses play a role in dysarthria therapy, ranging from 'low tech' materials, such as alphabet boards, to more sophisticated devices, such as artificial larynxes.

Table 14.3 Examples of communication-oriented strategies

Strategies adopted by the dysarthric speaker
- Convey how communication is to take place, e.g. by showing a card explaing the dysarthria and outlining the person's preferred communication method

- Establish the topic of conversation, e.g. by pointing to an icon or spelling the topic on an alphabet board; signal changes in topic

- Modify content and length of utterances, e.g. by limiting production to key words or by *increasing* redundancy

- Monitor listener's comprehension and check whether utterances have been understood

Strategies adopted by the listener
- Reduce obstacles to comprehension in the environment, such as background noise and poor lighting

- Adopt active listening, e.g. feed back what has been understood so far; be prepared to initiate repair when comprehension fails

- Encourage the dysarthric person to employ alternative approaches to communication, e.g. 'can you spell that word out for me?'

Strategies adopted by both the speaker and listener
- Maintain good eye contact

- Agree upon methods of feedback, e.g. some diads may adopt a gesture to signal when comprehension has failed;

- Agree upon repair strategies, e.g. some dysarthric speakers may ask listeners to guess targets, while others may prefer that they remain silent and wait for clarification. Some speakers may value explicit feedback about where speech intelligibility broke down

Some prostheses are recommended when direct, behavioural therapy is unlikely to work. For example, hypernasality, due to velopharyngeal inadequacy, typically responds poorly to behavioural management (Duffy 1995; Theodorus and Thompson Ward 1998), but positively to palatal lifts (see Yorkston *et al.* 1988). These consist of a metal plate, fitting rather like a denture, with a posterior flap that aids elevation of the velum. Similarly, reduced volume, as occurs in hypokinetic dysarthria, may not be amenable to behavioural management, but might be assisted by a portable amplifier. Other devices can supplement behavioural approaches. A good example is a pacing board, which is a strip of wood marked with regular slots. This helps the client regulate speech rate by pointing to each slot as every word or syllable is produced.

2.4.5 Alternative and augmentative communication (AAC)

Where speech is severely affected it is practical to turn to alternative and augmentative methods of communication (AAC). AAC includes some of the strategies and protheses that have already been discussed. Other tools include:

- symbol charts;

- photographic communication books;

- icons;

- word and alphabet charts;
- word-processing software;
- e-mail;
- speech synthesizers;
- portable, commercially available aids, such as the Lightwriter.

Selection of AAC methods involves numerous factors such as client choice, attitudes to technology, cognitive and literacy skills, motor skills, and communicative need. The role of AAC for any individual may change over time. For example, people with progressive disorders may become increasingly dependent on AAC. In such cases, it is desirable to discuss and introduce possible methods before speech becomes unintelligible, so that the client is involved in the decision-making process.

2.4.6 Instrumental contributions to therapy

Dysarthric people have to regain control over a mechanism that, prior to the onset of their disabilities, was rapid and automatic. In effect, they are learning to speak again in a new, more conscious manner. Such learning benefits from feedback, one source of which is instrumentation. A selection of instrumentation used in dysarthria therapy is summarized in Table 14.4.

Therapies incorporating instrumentation can bring about significant gains. For example, Thompson and Murdoch (1995) used kinematic instrumentation to provide a patient with feedback about respiration patterns, and so improved phonation times. Electromyographic (EMG) feedback has been used positively in the treatment of impaired velar fuction, and Visispeech in the treatment of parkinsonian dysarthria

Table 14.4 Examples of instrumentation used in dysarthria therapy

U Tube manometer	Measures air pressures generated by exhalation; used in therapy aiming to improve breath support for speech (e.g. Rosenbeck and LaPointe 1991)
Kinematic instrumentation	Records movement of the chest wall; can help dysarthric people improve respiratory function (Theodoros and Thompson-Ward 1998)
Visipitch, Visispeech, Speech viewer	Provide visual feedback about various vocal parameters, such as fundamental frequency, intensity, and duration; used in therapy for phonatory and prosodic disorders (e.g. Johnson and Pring 1990; Le Dorze et al. 1992)
Nasopharyngoscopes	Positioned in the nasal cavity to provide a view of the velopharyngeal sphincter from above during speech, and so offer feedback about the elevation of the velum; used in therapy for velopharyngeal disorders
Nasometer	Measures nasal and oral accoustic energy and so provides the patient with feedback about the degree of nasal resonance during speech; used in therapy for velopharyngeal disorders
EMG feedback	Provides feedback about muscle activity, e.g. of tongue, lip, and other facial muscles; used in therapy for articulation disorders

Table 14.5 Examples of surgical procedures used in the treatment of dysarthria

Disorder	Treatment
Hyperadduction of vocal cords	Laryngeal nerve section (Dedo 1979). Paralyses one vocal cord and so prevents hyperadduction
	Injection of botulinum toxin into tyroarytenoid muscle (Aronson 1990) blocks release of acetylcholine from nerve endings, so denervating some of the thyroarytenoid muscle and preventing hyperadduction
Hypoadduction of vocal cords	Laryngoplasty (Koufman 1986). Implants cartilaginous material between the thyroid cartilage and inner thyroid perichondrium, so displacing the paralysed cord medially and facilitating cord approximation
	Teflon/collagen injection into submucosal tissue of paralysed vocal cord. Increases the bulk of cord and so facilitates approximation
Velopharyngeal incompetence	Pharyngeal flap surgery (Johns 1985)

(Johnson and Pring 1990 and see Theodoros and Thompson-Ward 1998 for review). Despite this, the application of instrumentation, at least in Britain, seems limited (Coventry et al. 1997).

2.4.7 Surgical and pharmacological approaches

In some settings treatments provided by speech and language therapists are supplemented by medical interventions, involving surgery or pharmacology.

Most surgical procedures are for disorders of phonation, and aim either to facilitate cord approximation, in the case of flaccid dysarthrias, or prevent hyperadduction, in the case of spastic dysarthrias (see summary in Table 14.5). Hypernasality, as a result of velopharyngeal incompetence, may be helped by phyaryngeal flap surgery, which, in effect, builds up the posterior pharyngeal wall and so facilitates closure with the velum (although the efficacy of this surgery is disputed; see Duffy 1995 for review).

Many neurological conditions are managed with drug treatments that have associated benefits for speech, such as mestinon for myasthenia gravis. The specific pharmacological management of dysarthric speech requires further investigation, but might involve antispasticity medications and interventions to combat tremor and choreiform movements (see Rosenfield 1991). Clinicians need to be aware of the medication taken by patients and any associated side-effects for speech.

3 Therapy for apraxia of speech

There is a huge debate about the nature of speech apraxia (see Ballard et al. 2000). However, most agree that it is an impairment of volitional speech production in the face of preserved linguistic and motor execution abilities. It differs from dysarthria in that there is no loss of strength or neuromuscular control. Rather the disorder is specific to the *planning* of speech movement.

Apraxia varies in severity. In mild cases, intelligibility may only be affected for long, phonologically complex words, or when rapid speech is attempted. In contrast, severe apraxia can cause complete loss of speech, with profound implications for the person's social and personal life.

Apraxia may occur in isolation, or with other communication problems, particularly aphasia. When other disorders are present the clinician has to decide which problem to treat. If the language problem is severe, this should be the focus of therapy. Conversely, apraxia should be treated if poor intelligibility is the main barrier to communication and if the person has sufficient language to benefit from improvements in speech.

Therapy for apraxia can aim to improve speech planning, and hence intelligibility, or to facilitate communication despite the speech problems. The former requires client-centred behavioural approaches. The latter takes more account of the communication environment and typically involves both the client and his or her key interactants. With many individuals, therapy tackles both aims, in sequence or parallel.

3.1 Therapies aiming to improve speech planning

Speech planning therapies typically involve repeated and structured practice of a hierarchy of speech sounds, normally progressing from single syllables/words, to phrases and more extended utterances. Therapy also seeks to extend skills from structured tasks to spontaneous production. A general hierarchy of difficulty is known to apply in apraxia (Darley *et al.* 1975). For example, within the consonants nasals are typically easiest, while affricates are more difficult, and clusters particularly so (although personal hierarchies may differ from the typical pattern). Therapy stimuli are designed in the light of this hierarchy. So, for example, drills may progress from /m/ + V words (May, more); to /m/ + V + /m/ words (maim, mime); to /m/ + V + C words (man, mine) and so on.

Some individuals with severe apraxia need help to phonate, before articulation drills can begin. Various techniques can be applied here, such as using a cough or sigh to elicit voice. Some may be able to use familiar songs or intoned speech, or automatic utterances such as counting or reciting the days of the week. One therapy for severe apraxia, the Voluntary Control of Involuntary Utterances, seeks to exploit islands of automatic speech, by bringing these under more conscious control.

A selection of programmes used in apraxia therapy is summarized in Table 14.6. Efficacy data for these programmes are variable. For example, Wambaugh and Doyle (1994) reviewed 28 treatment studies for apraxia of speech, and conclude that only eight achieved posttreatment retention of target skills, although since this review other studies have reported more positive outcomes (e.g. Freed *et al.* 1997; Wambaugh *et al.* 1998). A recent paper suggests that therapy should take more account of principles of motor learning, e.g. in the presentation of stimuli and feedback. When such principles are applied, better maintenance of effects may be achieved (Ballard *et al.* 2000).

Table 14.6 A selection of programmes used in treating apraxia of speech

Programme	Brief description	References
8 Step Continuum	A hierarchy of stimulus presentation ranging from imitation of the therapist to question/answer responses	Rosenbeck *et al.* 1973
Melodic Intonation Therapy (MIT)	Uses preserved singing skills to elicit speech, e.g. via 'intoned' utterances	Sparks *et al.* 1974
Prompts for Restructuring Oral Muscular Targets (PROMPT)	Uses physical prompts on the patient's face to facilitate articulation (e.g. tapping nose for nasal sounds)	Square *et al.* 1985; Freed *et al.* 1997
Minimal Pairs Treatment	Organized practice of minimal pair contrasts (e.g. 'sheet' versus, 'seat'; 'shame' versus, 'same', etc.)	Wambaugh *et al.* 1998

3.2 Communication-oriented approaches

These approaches aim to facilitate communication despite the impairment, and are rather similar to those used with dysarthric clients (see Table 14.3). Typical strategies are listed below:

◆ creating optimal environments for communication, e.g. with minimal background noise;

◆ providing information about topic before attempting to speak;

◆ modifying the rate, content, and length of utterances;

◆ developing strategies for dealing with communication breakdown;

◆ setting ground rules for communication, e.g. about the type of feedback provided by conversational partners;

◆ using communication aids, such as word charts and key board aids;

What are the clinical effects of apraxia therapy? As outlined above, some treatments may improve speech intelligibility, e.g. so that the person can clarify problem words or make better use of the phone. Compensatory approaches may enable apraxic people to participate more in conversation despite their problems, albeit in a new way. These approaches may also help the person recover from, or repair, communication breakdowns when they occur.

4 Remediation of spoken language impairments in aphasia

Aphasia causes diverse problems with spoken language. Some people cannot speak at all, or produce nothing but incomprehensible jargon. Those who can speak, may be frustrated by frequent word-finding blocks or problems in building sentences. Many aphasic people have reasonable comprehension, although not of abstract language or complex sentences; while others have virtually no understanding of speech. Aphasia also typically involves reading and writing problems, but these are covered elsewhere in the handbook (see Chapters 8 and 15).

Recent commentators have rightly argued that aphasia is more than a bundle of language impairments (e.g. Pound *et al.* 2000). The aphasic person is a social being, who interacts in numerous contexts, ranging from immediate family and friends to the wider community. Therapy based purely on an analysis of the language deficits is likely to fail the person. Rather, we need to pay attention to the social functions undertaken by the person and how to facilitate those functions.

Aphasia is typically a chronic condition, with initial severity being a strong predictor of outcome (Pedersen *et al.* 1995). A recent longitudinal study of 119 aphasic patients found that 43% still had significant aphasia at 18 months post onset; whereas only 24% had recovered (Laska *et al.* 2001). Clearly, therapy needs to respond to the long-term nature of the problem.

4.1 Setting goals in aphasia therapy

Goal-setting in aphasia therapy should start with the person.

- What communication are they attempting, and what difficulties do they encounter?
- What would they like to be able to do?
- What do they see as their main skills?

Care-givers' views are also crucial, e.g. about what most impairs communication, and what strategies are being adopted by the aphasic person or by family and friends.

Through such questions, the therapist and aphasic person start to pinpoint likely goals for intervention. Assessment is conducted in the light of these goals, i.e. it aims to identify obstructions to realizing the goals and useful skills. This may well involve investigations of the person's language, but also evaluation of their environment and those in contact with the person. At the end of the process we should arrive at goals that are specific, realistic, measurable, and of benefit to the person's daily communication (see box below for an example of goal setting).

Goal setting in aphasia therapy: a case example (Maneta *et al.* 2001)

Phillip was 84 and had jargon aphasia following a stroke 5 years ago. Previous therapy aimed to improve his speech, but with little progress. Phillip lived with his wife, Florrie, but had few other social contacts.

In the initial discussion Florrie said that telling Phillip anything was a 'nightmare'. She had to repeat information several times, and even then could not be sure that he had got it. Misunderstandings were common and could lead to conflict, e.g. when Phillip felt that Florrie was keeping things from him. It was agreed that therapy should aim to reduce communication breakdowns at home.

Goal setting in aphasia therapy: a case example (Maneta *et al.* 2001) *(continued)*

Assessment aimed to identify the nature of Phillip's input problem, e.g. using tests of word discrimination and comprehension, and to explore reading, to see whether this could compensate for the difficulties. An interactive assessment also looked at how Phillip and Florrie were dealing with communication. Florrie was given a number of written questions to convey to Phillip, using any method of communication that she liked. The transaction was videoed and analysed.

Here are the main assessment findings.

♦ Phillip's auditory input was severely impaired. Although he could discriminate environmental sounds, he could not discriminate, recognize, or understand spoken words.

♦ Phillip's reading was much better than his auditory input. For example, he could match written words to pictures, but failed when the same words were spoken.

♦ The interactive assessment confirmed that communication often broke down. Florrie tried to help Phillip, e.g. by repeating words and phrases, but often this did not work. She rarely wrote information down, despite Phillip's good reading.

The therapy goals were specified in the light of these findings.

♦ To improve Phillip's discrimination of speech sounds, at least in single words; If successful, this should enable him to recognize and comprehend spoken words more reliably, and so ease communication at home.

♦ To modify Florrie's communication with Phillip, e.g. so that she made more use of writing. This should reduce breakdowns and make exchanges between them more efficient and enjoyable.

4.2 Therapy for word comprehension problems

As suggested in the box, therapy may aim to alleviate the problems arising from a comprehension deficit. One approach aims directly to improve the person's input processing. The other aims to compensate for the problem, by changing the behaviours of those in the person's environment.

4.2.1 Direct therapy approaches

Therapy to improve word sound discrimination (Morris *et al.* 1996; Morris 1997)
Some comprehension problems arise from deficits in sound discrimination. This is signalled by difficulties with all auditory input tasks, including repetiton, and particularly by an inability to discriminate minimal pairs, such as 'cat' and 'bat'. People with this problem benefit from visual cues, such as lip reading (Shindo *et al.* 1991).

The therapy developed by Morris *et al.* (1996) aimed to improve discrimination, using carefully structured minimal pair tasks and lip reading cues (see the box for examples of tasks). After therapy, both participants demonstrated gains, e.g. in repeating words, but not in comprehension. A similar approach was attempted by Maneta *et al.* (2001, and see the box below), but again with disappointing results. To date, studies suggest that improving sound discrimination is difficult and, even if progress is made, this may not benefit comprehension.

Examples of therapy tasks to improve word sound discrimination

Same/different judgements

- Two CV syllables are spoken by the therapist, e.g. /ka/ /ta/. The aphasic person indicates whether they are the same or different.
- Two VC syllables are spoken, e.g. /ak/ and /at/. The aphasic person indicates whether they are the same or different.

Matching spoken to written words

- The aphasic person is given a written word (e.g. 'car'). The therapist says a word that is either the same as the written word or minimally different (e.g. 'tar'). The aphasic person indicates whether the spoken word matches the written word.
- The aphasic person is given several rhyming written words (e.g. car, tar, par, etc.). The therapist says one word that then has to be matched with its written target.

Matching sounds to letters

- The aphasic person is given several written letters, e.g. T, K, B, etc. The therapist says a sound (e.g. /t/) that then has to be matched to one of the letters.

All the above tasks are presented first with lip-reading information (where the aphasic person is encouraged to watch the therapist's face), then with 'free voice' (where the aphasic person looks away).

Therapy to improve semantic processing   Some comprehension problems appear to be due to a semantic disorder, as indicated by poor written and spoken comprehension, and comparable problems in production. In such cases, a semantic approach might be attempted, e.g. involving word to picture matching, picture and word categorization, and word association tasks. This approach was adopted by Grayson *et al.* (1997) with successful results. A subsequent stage of therapy successfully combined semantic and auditory therapy. For example, now the person had to match spoken words to pictures, but with rhyming foils (target: beer; distractors: deer and tear).

A recent treatment study involved a client who could not access semantic information from spoken words, even though his comprehension of written words was good (Francis *et al.* 2001). Two forms of therapy were attempted. One only involved written words, e.g. a written word is presented with a written definition and then has to be copied. The other involved comparable tasks, but now with spoken words. Both treatments were effective, in that treated words were understood better after therapy than untreated words. However, the spoken word tasks produced more durable effects.

4.2.2 An indirect approach to comprehension therapy

Indirect therapies aim to advise friends and relatives about the aphasic person's difficulties, and help them communicate in ways that tap into their strengths (e.g. Lesser and Algar 1995). A good example can be found in Maneta *et al.* (2001; see the first box, this chapter). Phillip had much better reading than auditory comprehension. Despite this, his wife Florrie rarely wrote things down for him and, when she did, she tended to produce long sentences that were hard for Phillip to understand. Therapy demonstrated how to simplify information, using strategies like chunking information and writing only key words. Florrie was given opportunities to practise these strategies with Phillip, while the therapist provided feedback. In post therapy assessment there were fewer communication breakdowns between Phillip and Florrie and those that did occur were resolved more rapidly.

4.2.3 Summary and conclusions

Comprehension problems are difficult to treat, not least because the impairment may obscure the person's understanding of therapy. There is some evidence that input skills can be enhanced through treatment, but often such direct work needs to be combined with indirect interventions with friends and relatives. Maneta *et al.* (2001) show that simply advising friends and relatives to change their communication is often not enough. Family members need time, guidance, and practice to develop new skills.

4.3 Therapy for production problems

An almost ubiquitious production problem is anomia, or a word-finding deficit. Research has shown that word-finding can fail for different reasons (e.g. Howard and Orchard Lisle 1984, Kay and Ellis 1987), which suggests that therapy should be tailored to the particular processing needs of the individual. Another important finding is that anomia usually reflects problems of *access* rather than loss of vocabulary. We know this because people may achieve a word on one occasion, but not another. Also, aphasic people often benefit from cues (e.g. Howard *et al.* 1985), which may consist of the first sound of the word (phonological cues) or information about its meaning (semantic cues). This suggests that practice may recover more permanent access to words. Finally, we know that production is affected by numerous variables, such as word frequency, imageability, and age of acquisition (see Nickels 1997), which has implications for the selection of vocabulary in therapy.

4.3.1 Word finding therapy

A typical programme of word finding therapy entails repeated practice with a target group of words. These are carefully selected for their personal relevance, e.g. they may be associated with a particular interest or life goal. A second control group of words may be tested but not treated. The content of therapy reflects a person's skills and weaknesses. For example, semantic approaches might be used if there are felt to be semantic difficulties or if semantic cueing seems to prime access to words. The programme should be intensive, e.g. at least two sessions a week. After this, retention of the vocabulary is tested, typically with a picture naming assessment. This may be administered again, after a pause, to see whether gains have been maintained. Approaches to naming therapy are summarized below.

Semantic approaches   Semantic tasks require the person to reflect upon the meaning of words, with the rationale that improved semantic processing may lead to better recovery of word forms (see examples in the box below). A number of studies demonstrate that repeated administration of such tasks can improve naming of the treated vocabulary, and with good maintenance of effects (e.g. Marshall *et al.* 1990; Nickels and Best 1996*a,b*). Best outcomes occur when semantic tasks are combined with exposure to target word forms (Le Dorze *et al.* 1994; Drew and Thompson 1999), i.e. the aphasic person should hear or see the target word, and think about its meaning.

Examples of semantic tasks to aid word finding

- *Word to picture matching* (e.g. Marshall *et al.* 1990). The person is given a picture, together with 5 written words comprising: the target, 2 words with similar meanings, and 2 words with similar forms. For example, the picture shows a television and the words are television, radio, computer, telescope, telephone. The person has to select the word that matches the picture and (optionally) read it aloud.
- *Semantic questions* (e.g. Barry and McHattie 1991). The person hears a question about each target word, which requires a yes/no answer. For example, 'is a microwave used for cooking food?'; 'does a microwave do the washing?'
- *Semantic associations* (Jones 1989). A target word is written in the centre of a piece of paper. Surrounding this are a number of other words that are either related or unrelated to the target. The person has to select the related words and explain their selection. For example, target word: car; words for selection: petrol, paraffin, garage, stable, wheels, rails, Ford, Microsoft.

Phonological therapy   Many aphasic people demonstrate good semantic knowledge about words that they cannot name; e.g. they can comprehend these words and may be able to convey information about them. Furthermore, semantic cues may be unhelpful, precisely because the person already knows the information provided by the cue. In such cases phonological therapy may be preferred.

Phonological therapies work on the premise that exposure to the phonological properties of a word will prime access. Tasks typically involve repeated naming with phonological cues, i.e. ones that provide the first sound of the word or its rhyme (see box for an example). Phonological therapies can improve access to words and with good maintenance of effects (e.g. Raymer *et al.* 1993; Robson *et al.* 1998*b*).

A phonological therapy programme (Robson *et al.* 1998a)

Gillian had jargon aphasia with incomprehensible speech and severe word-finding problems. Speech was her priority for therapy, a decision endorsed by her husband.

The speech problem seemed due to impaired phonological access, in that comprehension was good and naming benefited from phonological cues. Gillian suggested that some phonological recovery might be taking place, which was rapidly fading, e.g. she said of one word-finding block: 'I had it there and then it went'. Gillian had good phonological skills on input, e.g. could discriminate minimal pairs like 'bat' and 'hat' and could repeat words.

Therapy aimed to build up her phonological knowledge about words. If successful, naming should improve.

- *Stimuli.* 50 words were chosen for personal relevance. They all began with one of 8 phonemes and had one or two syllables. Fifty untreated words acted as controls.
- *Materials.* Pictures of therapy items, a chart providing the written form of the 8 initial phonemes.

Task 1. Syllable structure

- The therapist said the target word and Gillian had to indicate whether it had 1 or 2 syllables, by pointing to the numbers on a sheet of paper
- Gillian was given a target picture. She had to think of its name and indicate how many syllables were contained in the name, by pointing to the numbers on the paper.

Task 2. Initial phoneme

- The therapist said a target word and Gillian had to point to its first phoneme on the chart.
- Gillian was given a target picture. She had to think of its name and point to its first phoneme on the chart
- As in the previous step, but now Gillian was asked to say the name of the picture.

Outcome

Gillian's naming of both treated and control words improved and this was well maintained. Other language tasks that were unrelated to therapy were unchanged.

Relay therapy   Therapy may use intact skills to access words 'in a new way'. A good example is given by Nickels (1992). T.C. had severe problems both in naming and reading aloud, although his writing was better. Therapy helped him to develop letter to sound matching skills, i.e. he learned to associate the letter 't' with the sound /t/, 'k' with /k/, and so on. One effect of this was to improve his reading. Another was to give him a new route to naming, in that he could imagine the written name of an object, think of its first letter, convert that into a sound, and so give himself a phonological cue. Sure enough, after therapy, T.C.'s spoken naming became almost as good as his written naming (for a similar approach, see White-Thomson 1999).

4.3.2 Therapies aiming to compensate for speech production problems

Some individuals may be unable to improve their word finding at all and, even when therapy is effective, often only treated words improve. Therefore, therapy should also develop strategies to compensate for the word-finding problem.

Strategies typically engage alternative forms of output. One candidate is writing, which has been used successfully even with severely aphasic people (e.g. Robson *et al.* 1998*a*, in press; Beeson 1999). When writing is even more impaired than speech, non-verbal strategies, such as gesture and drawing, may be favoured (e.g. McIntosh and Dakin 1989; Sacchett *et al.* 1999).

A more comprehensive approach involves 'total communication' (Lawson and Fawcus 1999; Pound *et al.* 2000). Here the aphasic person is encouraged to communicate using any technique available to them, including speech, writing, drawing, communication books, facial expression, and gesture. Developing total communica-tion is complex. Typically, the person is first made aware of the various communication options. They may need help with particular skills, e.g. to produce recognizable drawings or gestures. Constrained tasks, e.g. ones in which the person has to communicate a hidden word or picture using total communication, can further develop the skills. Finally, therapy often needs to encourage the generalization of skills to settings beyond the clinic, e.g. by involving relatives or through communication assignments.

4.3.3 Summary and conclusions

Therapy can help aphasic people recover access to words and with good maintenance of effects. Furthermore, aphasic people can take considerable control of this aspect of their therapy, since self-administered tasks can be very effective (Marshall *et al.* 1990; Nickels and Best 1996*a*,*b*). The aphasic person should also select the vocabulary for therapy.

Other findings are less encouraging. For example, naming therapy often only benefits treated words, with no carry-over to controls. This result is still useful, particularly if the words are carefully chosen. However, it indicates that therapy should include compensatory strategies such as total communication, which provide aphasic people with a resource for what is likely to be a chronic problem.

Table 14.7 Examples of treatments for sentence processing disorders in aphasia

Approach	Rationale	Brief description of therapy content	References
Event Therapy	The aphasic person cannot determine the role structure of events, or who is doing what to whom	Making decisions about events shown on video, such as who instigated the action and who or what was changed by it	Marshall *et al.* (1993)
Mapping Therapy	The aphasic person has some syntactic skills, but cannot relate sentential word order to meaning	(i) Analysing written sentences, eg to find the verb, agent (instigator of action) and patient (person or object changed by an action)	Jones (1986) Schwartz *et al.* (1994)
		(ii) Matching reversible sentences to pictures, such as 'the woman chases the man'	Mitchum *et al.* (1995)
		(iii) Ordering sentence fragments to describe pictures	Byng (1988) Nickels *et al.* (1991)
		(iv) Interpreting and ordering 3 argument sentences, such as 'Bob lends £5 to John'	Marshall *et al.* (1997)
Verb Access Therapy	The sentence disorder is at least partly attributable to a impairment in verb retrieval	Naming verb pictures with cues; carrying out semantic tasks with verbs, such as odd one out tasks	Fink *et al.* (1992) Mitchum and Berndt (1994) Marshall *et al.* (1998) Marshall (1999)
Syntax Training	The aphasic person has a morpho-syntactic impairment, or cannot generate the surface forms of sentences	Hierarchical and cued production of target sentence structures	Doyle *et al.* (1987) Helm Estabrooks *et al.* (1981) Helm Estabrooks and Ramsberger (1986)
Linguistic Specific Treatment	The aphasic person cannot process complex structures, like questions and passives, where sentence elements have been moved from their deep structure positions	Practising the production of complex forms, such as questions and clefts; forming complex sentences from simple ones	Thompson *et al.* (1993) Thompson and Shapiro (1995) Thompson *et al.* (1997) Ballard and Thompson (1999)

4.4 Connected speech and conversation

Aphasia may leave single-word processing relatively unscathed, but severely impair sentences. This makes it difficult for the person to deal with language about events and relationships, the typical subject of most conversations.

Sentence processing can fail for different reasons, e.g. some people have problems with the meaning relationships of sentences, while others have problems in building surface forms (see Marshall *et al.* 1999). Such variations have stimulated a range of sentence therapies, a selection of which are summarized in Table 14.7.

There is evidence that therapy can improve sentence production and comprehension. However, the extent of change is variable. Some studies only improved treated structures, while others also benefited untreated forms, and, while some treatments changed spontaneous production, this was not always the case (see Marshall, 2002 for a review of sentence therapy outcomes).

The above limitations suggest that sentence therapy alone may not necessarily improve the aphasic person's ability to converse. An alternative, or additional approach is to create conversational environments that are accessible to aphasic people despite their impairments. Typically, this involves training conversational partners, who may be volunteers or friends and relatives of the aphasic person (e.g. Kagan and Gailey 1993; Pound *et al.* 2000). Such trained interactants can make it possible for even severely aphasic people to participate in conversations, and so regain access to one of the primary social functions of language.

4.5 Concluding comments

Aphasia therapy works. That is not to say that we can cure aphasia, but we can bring about numerous valuable changes, such as improved comprehension, word finding, and sentence building. We can also change the behaviours of those in the aphasic person's environment, and so reduce the effects of the impairment. Of course, not all these aims can be achieved with all people. So one of the key skills of aphasia therapy is to identify an approach that is relevant for the person and has some chance of succeess. Above all, we need flexible therapy regimes that enable the aphasic person to tackle different goals at different stages of their recovery.

Selective references

Aronson, A. (1990). *Clinical voice disorders.* Thieme, New York.

Ballard, K. and Thompson, C. (1999). Treatment and generalisation of complex sentence production in agrammatism. *J. Speech, Language, Hearing Res.* **42**, 690–707.

Ballard, K., Granier, J., and Robin, A. (2000). Understanding the nature of apraxia of speech: theory, analysis, and treatment. *Aphasiology* **14**, 969–95.

Barry, C. and McHattie, J. (1991). Depth of semantic processing in picture naming facilitation in aphasic patients. Paper presented to the British Aphasiology Society Conference, Sheffield, September 1991.

Beeson, P. (1999). Treating acquired writing impairment: strengthening graphemic representations. *Aphasiology* **13**, 767–85.

Beukelman, D. and Yorkston, K. (1977). A communication system for the severely dysarthric speaker with an intact language system; *J. Speech Hearing Dis.* **42**, 265.

Byng, S. (1988). Sentence processing deficits: theory and therapy. *Cogn. Neuropsychol.* **5**, 629–76.

Coventry, K., Clibbens, J., Cooper, M., and Rodd, B. (1997). Visual speech aids: a British survey of use and evaluation by speech and language therapists. *Eur. J. Dis. Commun.* **32**, 203–16.

Crow, E. and Enderby, P. (1989). The effects of an alphabet chart on the speaking rate and intelligibility of speakers with dysarthria. In *Recent advances in clinical dysarthria* (ed. K. Yorkston and D. Beukelman), pp. 99–107. Pro-Ed, Austin, Texas.

Darley, F., Aronson, A., and Brown, J. (1975). *Motor speech disorders.* Saunders, Philadelphia.

Dedo, H. (1979). Recurrent laryngeal nerve section for spastic dysphonia. *Annals of Otology, Rhinology and Laryngology* 85, 451–9.

Doyle, P., Goldstein, H., and Bourgeois, M. (1987). Experimental analysis of syntax training in Broca's aphasia: a generalisation and social validation study. *J. Speech Hearing Dis.* 52, 143–56.

Drew, R. and Thompson, C. (1999). Model-based semantic treatment for naming deficits in aphasia. *J. Speech, Language, Hearing Res.* 42, 972–89.

Duffy, J. (1995). *Motor speech disorders: substrates, differential diagnosis and management.* Mosby, St Louis.

Fink, R., Martin, N., Schwartz, M., Saffran, E., and Myers, J. (1992). Facilitation of verb retrieval skills in aphasia: a comparison of two approaches. *Clin. Aphasiol.* 21, 263–75.

Francis, D., Riddoch, J., and Humphreys, G. (2001). Cognitive rehabilitation of word meaning deafness. *Aphasiology* 15, 749–66.

Freed, D., Marshall, R., and Frazier, K. (1997). Long term effectiveness of PROMPT treatment in a severely aphasic speaker. *Aphasiology* 11, 365–72.

Grayson, E., Hilton, R., and Franklin, S. (1997). Early intervention in a case of jargon aphasia: efficacy of language comprehension therapy. *Eur. J. Dis. Commun.* 32, 257–76.

Helm-Estabrooks, N. and Ramsberger, G. (1986). Treatment of agrammatism in long-term Broca's aphasia. *Br. J. Dis. Commun.* 21, 39–45.

Helm-Estabrooks, N., Fitzpatrick, P., and Barrisi, B. (1981). Response of an agrammatic patient to a syntax stimulation program for aphasia. *J. Speech Hearing Dis.* 47, 385–9.

Howard, D. and Orchard Lisle, V. (1984). On the origin of semantic errors in naming: evidence from the case of a global dysphasic. *Cogn. Neuropsychol.* 1, 163–90.

Howard, D., Patterson, K., Franklin, S., Orchard Lisle, V., and Morton, J. (1985). The facilitation of picture naming in aphasia. *Cogn. Neuropsychol.* 2, 49–80.

Johns, D. (ed.) (1985). Surgical and prosthetic management of neurogenic velopharyngeal incompetency in dysarthria. In *Clinical management of neurogenic communication disorders.* Needham Heights MA, 153–78.

Johnson, J. and Pring, T. (1990). Speech therapy and Parkinson's disease: a review and further data. *Br. J. Dis. Commun.* 25, 183–94.

Jones, E. (1986). Building the foundations for sentence production in a non-fluent aphasic. *Br. J. Dis. Commun.* 21, 63–82.

Jones, E. (1989). A year in the life of EVJ and PC. Proceedings of the Summer Conference of the British Aphasiology Society Conference of the British Aphasiology Society, Cambridge.

Kagan, A. and Gailey, G. (1993). Functional is not enough: training conversational partners for aphasic adults. In *Aphasia treatment: world perspectives* (ed. A. Holland and M. Forbes). Singular, San Diego. 199–226.

Kay, J. and Ellis, A. (1987). A cognitive neuropsychological case study of anomia: implications for psychological models of word retrieval. *Brain* 110, 613–29.

Koufman, J. (1986). Laryngoplasty for vocal cord medialization: an alternative to teflon. *Laryngoscope* 96, 726–31.

Laska, A., Hellblom, A., Murray, V., Kahan, T., and Von Arbin, M. (2001). Aphasia in acute stroke and relation to outcome. *J. Intern. Med.* 249, 413–22.

Lawson, R. and Fawcus, M. (1999). Increasing effective communication using a total communication approach. In *The aphasia therapy file* (ed. S. Byng, K. Swinburn, and C. Pound), pp. 61–74. Psychology Press, Hove, East Sussex.

Le Dorze, G., Dionne, L., and Ryall, S. *et al.* (1992). The effects of speech and language therapy for a case of dysarthria associated with Parkinson's Disease. *European Journal of Disorders of Communication*, **27**, 313–24.

Le Dorze, G., Boulay, N., Gaudreau, J., and Brassard, C. (1994). The contrasting effects of a semantic versus a formal-semantic technique for the facilitation of naming in a case of anomia. *Aphasiology* **8**, 127–41.

Lesser, R. and Algar, L. (1995). Towards combining the cognitive neuropsychological and the pragmatic in aphasia therapy. *Neuropsychol. Rehabil.* **5**, 67–92.

Linebaugh, C. (1983). Treatment of flaccid dysarthria. In *Current therapy of communication disorders: dysarthria and apraxia* (ed. W. Perkins), pp. 59–67. Thieme, New York.

Maneta, A., Marshall, J., and Lindsay, J. (2001). Direct and indirect therapy for word sound deafness. *Int. J. Language Commun. Dis.* **1**, 91–106.

Marshall, J. (1999). Doing something about a verb impairment: two therapy approaches. In *The aphasia therapy file* (ed. S. Byng, K. Swinburn, and C. Pound). Psychology Press, Hove, East Sussex.

Marshall, J. (2002). The assessment and treatment of sentence processing disorders: a review of the literature. In *Handbook of adult language disorders* (ed. A. Hillis), pp. 351–72. Psychology Press: New York.

Marshall, J., Pound, C., White-Thompson, M., and Pring, T. (1990). The use of picture/word matching tasks to assist word retrieval in aphasic patients. *Aphasiology* **4**, 167–84.

Marshall, J., Pring, T., and Chiat, S. (1993). Sentence processing therapy: working at the level of the event. *Aphasiology* **7**, 177–99.

Marshall, J., Chiat, S., and Pring, T. (1997). An impairment in processing verbs' thematic roles: a therapy study. *Aphasiology* **11**, 855–76.

Marshall, J., Pring, T., and Chiat, S. (1998). Verb retrieval and sentence production in aphasia. *Brain Language* **63**, 159–88.

Marshall, J., Black, M., and Byng, S. (1999). *Working with sentences: a handbook for aphasia therapists*. Winslow Press, Telford.

McIntosh, J. and Dakin, G. (1989). Restoration of communication through Amer-Ind. Proceedings of the Summer Conference of the British Aphasiology Society, Cambridge.

Mitchum, C. and Berndt, R.S. (1994). Verb retrieval and sentence construction: effects of targeted intervention. In *Cognitive neuropsychology and cognitive rehabilitation* (ed. M. Riddoch and G. Humphreys), pp. 317–48. Lawrence Erlbaum Associates, Hove, East Sussex.

Mitchum C, Haendiges, A. and Berndt, R.S. (1995). Treatment of thematic mapping in sentence comprehension: implications for normal processing. *Cogn. Neuropsychol.* **12**, 503–547.

Morris, J. (1997). Remediating auditory processing deficits in adults with aphasia. In *Language disorders in children and adults* (ed. S. Chiat, J. Law, and J. Marshall), pp. 42–63. Whurr, London.

Morris, J., Franklin, S., Ellis, A., Turner, J., and Bailey, P. (1996). Remediating a speech perception deficit in an aphasic patient. *Aphasiology* **10**, 137–58.

Murdoch, B. (ed.) (1998). *Dysarthria: a physiological approach to assessment and treatment*. Stanley Thornes, Cheltenham.

Netsell, R. (1992). Inspiratory checking in therapy for individuals with speech breathing dysfunction. Presentation at American Speech-Language-Hearing Association Annual Convention.

Nickels, L. (1992). The autocue? Self-generated phonemic cues in the treatment of a disorder of reading and naming. *Cogn. Neuropsychol.* **9**, 155–82.

Nickels, L. (1997). *Spoken word production and its breakdown in aphasia.* Psychology Press, Hove, East Sussex.

Nickels, L. and Best, W. (1996*a*). Therapy for naming disorders (part 1).: principles, puzzles and progress. *Aphasiology* **10**, 21–47.

Nickels, L. and Best, W. (1996*b*). Therapy for naming disorders (part II).: specifics, surprises and suggestions. *Aphasiology* **10**, 109–36.

Nickels, L., Byng, S., and Black, M. (1991). Sentence processing deficits: a replication of therapy. *Br. J. Dis. Communication* **26**, 175–201.

Pedersen, P., Jorgensen, H., Nakayama, H., Raaschou, H., and Olsen, T. (1995). Aphasia in acute stroke—incidence, determinants and recovery. *Ann. Neurol.* **38**, 659–66.

Pound, C., Parr, S., Lindsay, J., and Woolf, C. (2000). *Beyond aphasia: therapies for living with communication disability.* Winslow Press, Telford.

Raymer, A., Thompson, C., Jacobs, B., and Le Grand, H. (1993). Phonological treatment of naming deficits in aphasia: model based generalisation. *Aphasiology* **7**, 27–53.

Robson, J., Pring, T., Marshall, J., Morrison, S., and Chiat, S. (1998*a*). Written communication in undifferentiated jargon aphasia: a therapy study. *Int. J. Language Commun. Dis.* **33**, 305–28.

Robson, J., Marshall, J., Pring, T., and Chiat, S. (1998*b*). Phonological therapy in jargon aphasia: positive but paradoxical effects. *J. Int. Neuropsychol. Soc.* **4**, 675–86.

Robson, J., Marshall, J., Pring, T., and Chiat, S. (2001). Enhancing communication in jargon aphasia: a small group strudy of writing therapy. *Int. J. Language Commun. Dis.* **36**, 471–88.

Rosenbeck, J. and La Pointe, L. (1985). The dysarthrias: description, diagnosis, and treatment. In *Clinical management of neurogenic communication disorders* (ed. D. Johns), pp. 97–152. Allyn and Bacon: Needham Heights MA.

Rosenbeck, J., Lemme, M., Ahern, M., Harris, E., and Wertz, R. (1973). A treatment for apraxia of speech in adults. *J. Speech Hearing Dis.* **38**, 462–72.

Rosenfield, D. (1991). Pharmacologic approaches to speech motor disorders. In *Treating disordered speech motor control* (ed. D. Vogel and M. Cannito), pp. 27–77. Pro-Ed, Austin, Texas.

Sacchett, C., Byng, S., Marshall, J., and Pound, C. (1999). Drawing together: evaluation of a therapy programme for severe aphasia. *Int. J. Language Commun. Dis.* **34**, 265–89.

Schwartz, M., Saffran, E., Fink, R., Myers, J., and Martin, N. (1994). Mapping therapy: a treatment programme for agrammatism. *Aphasiology* **8**, 19–54.

Shindo, M., Kaga, K., and Tanaka, Y. (1991). Speech discrimination and lip reading in patients with word deafness or auditory agnosia. *Brain Language* **40**, 153–61.

Sparks, R., Helm, N., and Albert, M. (1974). Aphasia rehabilitation resulting from melodic intonation therapy. *Cortex* **10**, 303–16.

Square, P., Chumpelik, D., and Adams, S. (1985). Efficacy of the PROMPT system of therapy for the treatment of acquired apraxia of speech. In *Clinical Aphasiology Conference Proceedings* (ed. R.H. Brookshire), pp. 319–20.

Theodoros, D. and Thompson-Ward, E. (1998). Treatment of dysarthria. In *Dysarthria: a physiological approach to assessment and treatment* (ed. B. Murdoch). Stanley Thornes, Cheltenham.

Thompson, C. and Shapiro, L. (1995). Training sentence production in agrammatism: implications for normal and disordered language. *Brain Language* **50**, 201–24.

Thompson, C., Shapiro, L., and Roberts, M. (1993). Treatment of sentence production deficits in aphasia, a linguistic specific approach to wh-interrogative training and generalization. *Aphasiology* **7**, 111–33.

Thompson, C., Shapiro, L., Ballard, K., Jacobs, B., Schneider, S., and Tait, M. (1997). Training and generalized production of wh- and NP-movement structures in agrammatic aphasia. *J. Speech, Language, Hearing Res.* **40**, 228–44.

Thompson, E.C. and Murdoch, B. (1995). Treatment of speech breathing disorders in dysarthria: a biofeedback approach. Paper presented at the Australian Association of Speech and Hearing Conference, Brisbane, Queensland. [Quoted in Theodoros Thompson-Ward (1998).]

Till, J. and Toye, A. (1988). Acoustic phonetic effects of two types of verbal feedback in dysarthric speakers. *J. Speech Hearing Dis.* **53**, 449.

Wambaugh, J. and Doyle, P. (1994). Treatment for acquired apraxia of speech: a review of efficacy reports. *Clin. Aphasiol.* **22**, 231–43.

Wambaugh, J., Kalinyak-Fliszar, M., West, J., and Doyle, P. (1998). Effects of treatment for sound errors in apraxia of speech and aphasia. *J. Speech Language Hearing Res.* **41**, 725–43.

Wertz, R., LaPointe, L., and Rosenbeck, J. (1984). *Apraxia of speech in adults: the disorders and its management.* Grune and Stratton, New York.

White-Thomson, M. (1999). Naming therapy for an aphasic person with fluent empty speech. In *The aphasia therapy file* (ed. S. Byng, K. Swinburn, and C. Pound). Psychology Press, Hove, East Sussex.

Yorkston, K., Beukelman, D., and Bell, K. (1988). *Clinical management of dysarthric speakers.* College Hill, San Diego.

Chapter 15

Neuropsychological assessment and treatment of disorders of reading

J. Richard Hanley and Janice Kay

1 Introduction

Brain injury can disrupt the reading abilities of individuals whose performance was previously quite normal in a variety of different ways. In the sections that follow, some of the most common and the most theoretically important types of reading impairment are discussed. The review starts with descriptions of the peripheral dyslexias (pure alexia, letter-by-letter reading, neglect dyslexia) in which reading appears to be affected prior to the point at which the word is recognized as a familiar visual form. Descriptions then follow of central dyslexic impairments (deep dyslexia, phonological dyslexia, surface dyslexia, and reading in dementia) in which reading processes generally appear to be intact up to the point at which the meaning or pronunciation of a word must be generated.

A summary of these different types of acquired dyslexia together with some of their most important associated attributes can be found in Table 15.1. However, it is appropriate to sound a note of caution. Grouping patients into categories such as these provides an economical way of summarizing a large body of literature, but the extent to which they represent groupings that are scientifically useful is highly controversial. For example, the nature of the reading problems suffered by two individual patients who both fit the criteria for surface dyslexia may differ in fundamental ways (see Section 7). Consequently, theorists such as Caramazza (1984) and Ellis (1987) have argued that the impairment that each individual patient has suffered should be explained by direct reference to a cognitive theory. They argue that there is no scientific value in first allocating a label such as 'surface dyslexic' to a patient. Similarly, we would encourage clinicians to discover the precise point(s) at which an individual's reading ability has broken down rather than to worry unduly about precisely which type of acquired dyslexic label best fits them. Of course, explaining patients' impairments case by case should not obscure the fact that a scientific theory should also be able to explain why, for example, so many different symptoms tend to co-occur in patients categorized as 'deep dyslexic' (see Section 5) or why there is an association between semantic memory loss and surface dyslexia (see Section 8).

Table 15.1 A summary of the impairments associated with different types of acquired dyslexia

Type of dyslexia	Impaired at reading	Characteristic responses to printed words	Ability relatively preserved	Common area(s) of brain injury
Pure alexia	All letters and words	No response or responds with unrelated words	Writing, recognition of orally spelled words	Left occipitotemporal, callosal lesions
Letter-by-letter reading	Long words; individual letters	Very slow responses; speed affected by number of letters	Writing; recognition of orally spelled words	Left occipitotemporal, callosal lesions
Neglect dyslexia	Words and/or text	Omissions or substitutions of letters on one side of word		Right parietal
Deep dyslexia	Nonwords; function words; words of low imageability	Semantic errors; visual errors; morphological errors	Reading of content words	Left frontotemporoparietal
Phonological dyslexia	Nonwords	Visual errors	Reading of familiar words	Left anterior perisylvian
Surface dyslexia	Irregular words	Regularization errors; visual errors	Reading regular words; high frequency words, and nonwords	Left temporal lobe
Dementia	Irregular words; unusual nonwords	Regularization errors	Reading regular words	Left temporal lobe

It must be acknowledged that, at the present time, there is considerable controversy as to which model is best to use when attempting to explain the reading impairments observed in acquired dyslexia. Coltheart (1985) advocated a three-route model that incorporated a *non-lexical* reading route and two separate *lexical* reading routes.

- The non-lexical route computes the pronunciation of a word on the basis of sub-lexical grapheme–phoneme correspondences (e.g. letter–sound associations). It is capable of reading accurately familiar and unfamiliar words whose pronunciation is consistent with those correspondences (often referred to as 'regular' words).

- The lexical reading routes can recognize a previously learned word by activating its representation in a store of familiar visual word forms ('orthographic lexicon').

  —The *lexical-semantic route* involves accessing the word's meaning, and would be heavily involved in silent reading of text. If required, the pronunciation of the word can then be accessed from its meaning.

  —The *direct-lexical route* is based on direct connections between a word's visual form and its representation in a phonological lexicon. It would be heavily involved in reading aloud.

  The lexical routes are equally capable of processing regular and irregular words so long as they have already been learned but are unable to deal with nonwords or unfamiliar words.

The status of the three-route model has been immeasurably strengthened by its successful implementation as a computational model capable of providing the pronunciation of written words (Coltheart *et al.* 1993, 2001) and simulating the effects of brain injury on word recognition. Nevertheless, the existence of the direct-lexical route is controversial; Hillis and Caramazza (1991) claim that the functions it provides can be performed by the interaction of the lexical-semantic and non-lexical routes.

A more radical alternative to the three-route model is provided by a computational model often referred to as the *triangle* model (Plaut *et al.* 1996; Seidenberg and McClelland 1989). Its advocates claim that it is not necessary to incorporate a separate non-lexical reading route. Plaut *et al.* argue that nonwords and regular words are generally read aloud via a direct orthography to phonology route (the triangle's first arm). Reading aloud of irregular words relies heavily on an orthography to semantics route (the triangle's second arm) and on the connections between semantics and phonology (the final arm of the triangle). Advocates of the triangle model (e.g. Patterson and Lambon Ralph 1999) also dispute the view that reading impairments reflect damage to mechanisms that are specific to reading. For example, Patterson and Lambon Ralph argue that:

- pure alexia reflects a primary visual impairment;
- surface dyslexia is caused by a semantic impairment;
- phonological dyslexia is the result of a phonological processing deficit.

The triangle model is clearly more parsimonious than Coltheart's model. To our mind, however, some of its explanations of acquired dyslexic performance are less plausible. For example, the triangle model has not provided an entirely convincing account as to why certain patients can read irregular words despite being ignorant of their meaning (see Section 8).

Many of the conditions discussed in this chapter are likely to affect profoundly the extent to which an individual can continue to derive any pleasure from reading books or newspapers. This is particularly likely to be true of the peripheral dyslexias and of central dyslexias caused by impairments that affect retrieval of a word's semantic representation. Where their reading problems reflect a primary phonological problem or a word-finding difficulty, however, individuals may continue to read books avidly (e.g. Hanley and McDonnell 1997). It is clear from cases such as these that comprehension of print can be entirely preserved even though an individual can no longer access the pronunciation of many familiar words.

In the sections that follow, we have included studies that attempt remediation of acquired reading problems. In determining whether to attempt to make use of any of these strategies, however, the clinician should bear in mind that they are likely to be time-consuming and must be tailored precisely to the needs and abilities of the individual concerned. In addition, it must be borne in mind that statistically significant gains in terms of increased reading speed or accuracy do not necessarily reflect clinically significant improvements that will increase a patient's quality of life. It is also the case that the reading impairments experienced by some patients will improve spontaneously in the months that follow their illness or injury, although those of others appear to remain stable across all the years that they have been studied.

Finally, it has unfortunately not been possible to include descriptions of some less extensively researched acquired reading problems. These include attentional dyslexia (Shallice and Warrington 1977), visual dyslexia (Hillis and Caramazza 1992; Lambon Ralph and Ellis 1997; Marshall and Newcombe 1973), semantic access dyslexia (Warrington and Shallice 1979), and word-meaning blindness (Lambon Ralph *et al.* 1996, 1998).

2 'Pure alexia' or 'alexia without agraphia'

2.1 Functional impairment

Detailed documented accounts of the functional impairments observed in pure alexia have been available since the end of the nineteenth century (Dejerine 1892; Hinshelwood 1895). Following a stroke, both of the patients described in these reports experienced sudden and complete loss of the ability to read any words despite intact speech production and comprehension, normal object recognition, and apparently unimpaired general intellectual functioning. Writing was entirely preserved in both patients (hence the term 'pure' alexia), although neither of them was subsequently able to read back what they had written. The reading problems did not appear to be the consequence of a basic visual problem since acuity, colour vision, and object naming were good when objects were presented in the preserved left visual field.

Dejerine's patient could see letters clearly because he could accurately copy and describe their visual form (e.g. he said that the letter Z looked like 'a serpent') but was completely unable to name them. Extremely poor naming of visually presented letters has consistently been observed in more recent reports of pure alexic patients who are unable to read words aloud (Caplan and Hedley-White 1974; Coslett and Saffran 1989, 1992; Miozzo and Caramazza 1998; Mycroft *et al.* 2002). However, all of these patients retained some ability to process letters. Caplan and Hedley-White's (1974) patient could correctly realign letter tiles that had been rotated away from their normal orientation. Coslett and Saffran's (1992) patient scored 10/10 at cross-case letter matching. Miozzo and Caramazza's (1998) patient was able to distinguish real letters from pseudoletters and could identify canonical letter orientations. Mycroft *et al.*'s (2002) patient could perform cross-case matching of visually presented letters despite a complete inability to name them. This did not occur because the patient was suffering from an anomia for letter names because she was able to name letters perfectly when asked to recite the alphabet or spell words orally. This suggests that some pure alexic patients can access the abstract identity of visually presented letters despite being unable to name them.

2.2 Anatomical issues

The classical account of the anatomical correlates of pure alexia derives from Dejerine (1892) and Geschwind (1965). A left hemisphere lesion produces a right-sided hemianopia, which means that visual information from the right visual field cannot be processed in the left hemisphere. Dejerine argued that the location of the left hemisphere lesion also made it impossible for visual information from the occipital lobe in the right hemisphere to access the angular gyrus in the left hemisphere (which, he believed, contained visual representations of words and letters). More recent accounts following Geschwind (1965) argue that a lesion of the corpus callosum prevents visual information from the left visual field crossing from the right to the left hemisphere.

This view has been developed in a most imaginative way by Coslett and Saffran (1989, 1992). They demonstrated that some patients are able to make lexical decisions (is this a word or a nonword?) and retrieve some basic semantic information (e.g. is this word the name of an animal?) about written words at above chance levels despite a complete inability to read words aloud. Coslett and Saffran claim that there is a rudimentary right hemisphere reading system and that, under appropriate circumstances, the right hemisphere can perform lexical decisions and retrieve some semantic information from visually presented words at above chance levels. An intact right hemisphere reading system would also explain why some pure alexic patients can access the abstract identity of written letters (see Section 2.1) despite being unable to name them. Coslett and Saffran claim that the right hemisphere is unable to provide the names of any words or letters. If words or letters are to be named, information about letter identity must be transferred across the corpus callosum to the left hemisphere (extremely difficult for pure alexics because of their callosal lesions).

2.3 **Remediation**

Dejerine's patient died just over 4 years after his initial cerebrovascular accident (CVA) having never recovered any ability to read words aloud. The only occasions on which he correctly named a letter were when he traced over their visual form with his finger. The speed at which he could name letters this way was unfortunately too slow to allow words to be recognized during reading. This strategy has been sometimes been reported in more recent accounts of pure alexia. For example, Case 3 (Benson *et al.* 1971) sometimes correctly identified a previously misnamed letter by tracing it with his finger. Maher *et al.* (1998) reported that a treatment for pure alexia based on finger spelling led to a 50% increase in reading speed with 100% accuracy.

An alternative remediation strategy is to attempt to teach pure alexic patients to name visually presented letters. If successful, this treatment should enable them to become letter-by-letter readers (see Section 3). Greenwald and Gonzalez-Rothi (1998) report a successful therapy programme of this kind. They suggest that this remediation strategy is likely to be beneficial so long as the patient's ability to recognize orally spelled words is preserved. It is worth adding a cautionary note, however. Hinshelwood (1900) reported that, after approximately 6 months, his alexic patient started to attempt to relearn the alphabet. He practised daily, and gradually came to read words 'slowly and laboriously, spelling out the words letter by letter' (Hinshelwood 1900, p. 13). Unfortunately, Hinshelwood (1917, p. 5) finally reported that this man did not persevere with reading in this way because it 'required such intense mental effort'.

Remediation strategies attempted with Mycroft *et al.*'s (2002) pure alexic patient included an attempt to teach her a small set of high-frequency words by sight, and an attempt to teach her to recognize groups of letters that co-occur frequently in English words. She had also been taught a strategy that encouraged her to recite the alphabet in an attempt to find the name of the letter that she was looking at. Unfortunately, none of these strategies proved at all effective, even though the patient felt highly motivated to try to learn to read again.

2.4 **Assessment**

Pure alexic patients will have great difficulty in reading aloud even simple lists of words (e.g. Psycholinguistic Assessment of Language Processing in Aphasia (PALPA) test 29, Kay *et al.* 1992) or letters (e.g. PALPA test 22). Writing of the same items should be preserved.

3 Letter-by-letter reading

3.1 Functional impairment

In letter-by-letter (LBL) reading, words are often read aloud accurately but reading is very slow and laborious. Reading times for single words increase in line with the number of letters in the word. For example, patient D.C. (Hanley and Kay 1996), who read relatively quickly for an LBL reader, took just over 2 seconds to read three-letter words aloud and approximately 5 seconds to read nine-letter words aloud. Patterson and Kay (1982) reported three patients who all took over 10 seconds on average to read a 3–4-letter word and over 30 seconds to read a 9–10-letter word. Nevertheless, the overwhelming majority of words were read correctly by these patients. The linear relationship between number of letters and reading times that is observed in LBL reading is not found in reading aloud by unimpaired individuals (Weekes 1997). It suggests that, unlike normal readers, LBL readers may be attempting to recognize a word by first naming its component letters. Consistent with this idea, some (though not all) LBL readers say the letter names aloud before the word is read.

There is now general agreement that LBL reading is associated with severe letter recognition deficits. In a major review of LBL reading, Behrmann *et al.* (1998) pointed out that 50/57 of the cases they surveyed showed clear evidence of slow and error-prone letter processing when *single* letters were presented in isolation to them. The other seven were not tested on speeded tasks. As Behrmann *et al.* (p. 23) put it, 'there is no single subject in whom letter recognition is definitively normal'. The widespread nature of the letter processing impairments has led several groups, including Behrmann *et al.* (1998), to conclude that it is the cause of the slow reading that LBL readers experience. Others have argued that the core impairment is a problem in recognizing letters *in parallel* (Kay and Hanley 1991; Patterson and Kay 1982). Consistent with this, there is evidence of serial left-to-right processing of the letters in a word by LBL readers, whereas normal individuals appear to read the letters in a word either in parallel or 'ends-in' (Kay and Hanley 1991). There is also considerable controversy over whether or not the letter-processing impairment is itself the consequence of a more basic visual processing impairment or whether it is specific to alphanumeric material (see Patterson and Lambon Ralph 1999 and Farah 2000 for interesting recent discussions of this issue).

It is widely assumed that the letter-processing deficit observed in LBL readers is qualitatively similar to that found in pure alexic patients who are unable to read words aloud (see Section 2). There is, however, surprisingly little evidence to substantiate this claim. In fact, whereas alexics who are unable to read words aloud appear to have particular problems in letter naming (see Section 2), it appears that letter-by-letter readers have difficulty in recognizing the *abstract identity* of visually presented letters (e.g. Arguin and Bub 1994; Reuter-Lorenz and Brunn 1990). Key evidence for this claim is the finding that all LBL readers so far tested are extremely inaccurate (Perri *et al.* 1996) or slow (Behrmann and Shallice 1995; Kay and Hanley 1991; Reuter-Lorenz and

Brunn 1990) at speeded cross-case matching of visually presented letters (e.g. does 'D' = 'b' or 'd'?). Further research on this issue is required.

It has been sometimes been claimed that the core impairment in LBL reading is a word-level deficit rather than a letter-level impairment, and that LBL reading reflects the use of the spelling system to read words aloud (Warrington and Shallice 1980). Indeed Warrington and her colleagues frequently refer to LBL reading as 'spelling dyslexia' (e.g. McCarthy and Warrington 1990). The discovery of word superiority effects in some LBL readers (e.g. Bub *et al.* 1989; Reuter-Lorenz and Brunn 1990) has cast doubt on this claim. Furthermore, spelling is severely impaired in some LBL readers, and it is sometimes impaired in a quite different way from reading (Hanley and Kay 1992; Rapcsak *et al.* 1990).

Nevertheless, some LBL readers appear to suffer from a word-level deficit in addition to their letter processing deficit. Whereas some patients (termed 'type 1' LBL readers by Patterson and Kay 1982) read words accurately given that they name the letters correctly, other patients (termed 'type 2' LBL readers by Patterson and Kay 1982) make errors even when letters are named correctly. This suggests that type 2 LBL readers have an additional impairment at the level of the orthographic lexicon or 'word form system' that is superimposed on top of their letter processing problem. An additional central impairment can explain why LBL reading is sometimes associated with visual errors (Hanley and Kay 1992), regularization errors (Friedman and Hadley 1992), semantic errors (Buxbaum and Coslett 1996), and imageability effects (Behrmann *et al.* 1998).

3.2 Anatomical issues

As is the case with pure alexic patients of the kind described in Section 2, LBL reading is frequently associated with lesions to the posterior part of the left hemisphere. Damage to the left occipitotemporal junction has been implicated as a probable cause of the difficulties experienced in recognizing words as wholes (Leff *et al.* 2001). Additional left hemisphere injuries, it is assumed, will produce a right-sided hemianopia. LBL reading is usually, though not invariably, also associated with lesions to the splenium of the corpus callosum (see Binder and Mohr 1992 for further anatomical evidence concerning alexics who do and do not read words letter-by-letter).

Leff *et al.* (2001) claimed that a right hemianopia that is caused by a lesion 'affecting either primary visual cortex on the left, or its geniculostriate afferents' can of itself produce a reading impairment in patients with no left occipitotemporal damage that can be confused with letter-by-letter reading. The impairment occurs because words can fall outside the patients' visual field and require one or more saccades before recognition is possible. In hemianopic alexia, they claim, reading times may show word-length effects but are quicker than for LBL readers (Leff *et al.* calculate a range of 51–162 milliseconds per letter), particularly with shorter words. They argue that it is important to diagnose hemianopic alexia accurately because there are remediation techniques available that can increase reading speed in these patients (Kerkhoff *et al.* 1992; Leff *et al.* 2000).

As in pure alexia, debate has centred on the precise role played by the left and right hemispheres in LBL readers. Shallice and Saffran (1986) showed that some LBL readers could make accurate lexical decisions and semantic classifications about visually presented words even when the words were presented so quickly that they could not be read by an LBL strategy. Saffran and Coslett (1998) argue that LBL readers who show these effects are using their right hemisphere reading system (see Section 2) to make these decisions. Similar abilities have been documented in some (but not all) LBL readers with whom these tasks have been attempted (Behrmann *et al.* 1998). Saffran and Coslett claim that LBL reading involves the use of the damaged primary left hemisphere reading system and that the left hemisphere inhibits the intact right hemisphere reading system. Behrmann *et al.* (1998), on the other hand, argue that an impairment to letter-level processors within a single reading system subserved by both left and right hemispheres could explain these effects so long as it is assumed that the system operates according to the principles of interactive-activation-and-competition computer models.

3.3 Remediation

A number of different remediation strategies have been attempted with LBL readers.

- Moyer (1979) and Moody (1988) employed multiple oral re-reading (MOR), in which the patient was encouraged to read the same passages of prose over and over again.
- Arguin and Bub (1994) employed a more theoretically driven technique by focusing on letter processing. They trained their patient to make cross-case matching decisions about pairs of letters in different-sized letter fonts.
- Behrmann and McLeod (1995) attempted to treat their patient by encouraging her to identify the letters at the end of a word before saying it aloud.

These techniques generally led to increased reading speeds that were statistically significant. Unfortunately, none of them produced clinically effective increases in the time it took to read words aloud—reading speeds remained disappointingly slow.

3.4 Assessment

Measure reading speed on a list of words that manipulates letter length (e.g. PALPA test 29, Kay *et al.* 1992).

4 Neglect dyslexia (see Chapter 6)

4.1 Functional impairment

In neglect dyslexia, portions of the left side of text are sometimes omitted when passages are being read. When individual words are being read, initial letters may be

- omitted (e.g. *cage* → 'age');
- substituted (e.g. *elate* → 'plate'); or
- added (e.g. *pan* → 'span').

Ellis *et al.*'s (1987) patient defined words consistent with her neglect error: (e.g. *rice* → 'price . . . how much for a paper or something in a shop').

It is often assumed that neglect dyslexia is just one of a number of features associated with a more general neglect of contralesional space. However, neglect dyslexia has been observed in a number of cases without other features of neglect (e.g. Baxter and Warrington 1983; Patterson and Wilson 1990). In discussing these studies, Riddoch (1990) has pointed out that reading may be a particularly demanding task and that evidence of generalized neglect might have emerged with more stringent testing of other visual stimuli. Whether or not neglect dyslexia always co-occurs with neglect of objects remains a controversial issue (Caramazza and Hills 1990; Haywood and Coltheart 2000).

There is clear evidence of fractionation of deficits within neglect dyslexia itself. Although word and text reading may both be affected in some patients (e.g. Ellis *et al.* 1987), reading of single words can be impaired selectively (e.g. Costello and Warrington 1987; Miceli and Capasso 2001), and reading of text can be impaired selectively (Kartsounis and Warrington 1989). Some patients make more neglect errors on non-words than words (Arguin and Bub 1997), but others show no lexicality effect (e.g. Ellis *et al.* 1987). When Ellis *et al.* (1987) rotated the page by 90 degrees, their patient no longer made any neglect errors. In contrast, patient N.G. (Caramazza and Hillis 1990) continued to make errors affecting the initial letters in a word regardless of whether it was presented in vertical orientation, mirror image, or inverted. Miceli and Capasso (2001) compared the performance of two neglect dyslexic patients using the same test materials and found that one of them (S.V.E.) made approximately the same number of errors regardless of whether words were presented horizontally or vertically, whereas the other (M.R.) made a much larger number of errors with horizontal presentation but no errors at all with vertical presentation.

Caramazza and Hillis (1990) suggested that any one of three distinct levels of representation (retina-centred, stimulus-centred, and word-centred) involved in the early stages of word recognition might be affected in neglect dyslexia.

◆ The *retina-centred* level represents the visual shape and location of visual forms (letters) within the viewer's visual field. Patients with retina-centred impairments will make errors only on words that are presented in the left hemifield so long as central fixation is maintained.

◆ *Stimulus-centred* representation maintains orientation but codes the location of letters relative to each other irrespective of their absolute location in visual space. Patients with left-sided neglect associated with stimulus-centred impairments will make errors regardless of whether or not a word is presented to the left or right of fixation but will not make errors on vertically presented words.

◆ The *word-centred* level represents the position and abstract identities of letters within a word irrespective of physical location (e.g. orientation). Patients such as S.V.E. (Miceli and Capasso 2001), who made neglect errors regardless of horizontal or vertical presentation and whether or not the word was presented to the left or right of a fixation point, are considered by Caramazza and Hillis to have a word-centred neglect.

Haywood and Coltheart (2000) reviewed the performance of 14 previously reported neglect dyslexic patients to whom suitable tests had been administered. They found that Caramazza and Hillis' theory provided a satisfactory account of all 14 of them.

4.2 **Anatomical issues**

Neglect dyslexia affecting the left side of text or words is generally associated with right occipitoparietal lesions. However, cases reported by Caramazza and Hillis (1990), Sieroff (1990), and Warrington (1991) all had left hemisphere lesions that correspondingly affected word endings and the right side of text.

4.3 **Assessment**

In neglect dyslexia, errors when reading words are visually related to the target word and consistently affect just one side of the word. In a patient with left-sided neglect, it is a good idea to use items that remain words when the first letter is omitted, and where the first letter can be substituted to make another word (e.g. cage, elate, peach, lever). Ellis *et al.* (1987) used a list of this kind.

5 **Deep dyslexia**

5.1 **Functional impairment**

The first cases were reported by Low (1931) and Goldstein (1948) (see Marshall and Newcombe 1980 for a historical review), although the term 'deep dyslexia' was first used by Marshall and Newcombe (1973). Marshall and Newcombe (1966, 1973) investigated the types of word that their patients found most difficult to read and examined systematically the nature of the errors that they made. They also attempted to explain their pattern of performance in terms of a model of reading derived from research in cognitive psychology. In so doing, Marshall and Newcombe provided a blueprint for subsequent cognitive neuropsychological investigations of acquired dyslexia.

Several decades of research into deep dyslexia have revealed a strikingly consistent pattern of reading impairment and associated language deficits (including agrammatism and phonological short-term memory problems). Deep dyslexics are almost completely unable to read nonwords and novel words aloud. They either respond with a visually similar real word or they make no response at all. The errors made by Marshall and Newcombe's patient (G.R.) included the following responses: *wux* → 'don't know'; *nol* → 'no idea'; *Zul* → 'Zulu'; *wep* → 'wet'; *dup* → 'damp'.

The probability that a familiar word can be read aloud correctly is closely related to its concreteness/imageability rating, with concrete words being much easier to read than abstract words. For example, L.W. (Newton and Barry 1997) read correctly 19/30 highly concrete words (e.g. house, snake) but only 1/30 medium concrete words (e.g. friend, joke), 2/30 medium abstract words (e.g. life, hint), and 4/30 highly abstract words (e.g. fate, hope). According to Paivio *et al.* (1968) imageability ratings are based on the capacity of a word to arouse *sensory experiences of objects, materials, or persons* whereas concreteness ratings are based on the extent to which a word *refers to objects, materials, or persons experienced in the physical world.* According to Paivio *et al.* concreteness and imageability are highly intercorrelated ($r = 0.83$) and, in deep dyslexia, they are almost certainly capturing the same dimension.

There is also a part of speech effect in deep dyslexia, whereby nouns are read better than adjectives and adjectives are read better than verbs. However, there is strong evidence that this effect only occurs when part of speech is confounded with imageability and/or frequency (Allport and Funnell 1981; Barry and Richardson 1988). Deep dyslexics also have particular problems with function words, often responding with a different function word (e.g. for → and; in → the; as → he). This problem occurs despite the fact that function words are amongst the most common words in English. Deep dyslexic patients appear to have lost knowledge about the syntactic role of function words (e.g. Morton and Patterson 1980). This might make it difficult for function words to be read accurately via the lexical-semantic route. Alternatively, the problem with function words might reflect their low concreteness/imageability.

- The errors made when reading content words include *semantic errors*, generally considered to be the hallmark of deep dyslexia. Examples include *uncle* read as 'cousin' (Marshall and Newcombe 1966), *hurt* read as 'injure' (Shallice and Warrington 1975) and *grass* read as 'lawn' (Saffran and Marin 1977). The majority of errors made by G.R. (Marshall and Newcombe 1966) were semantic.

- The most common errors made by several other deep dyslexics, however, are *visual errors* in which a word is read as a word that shares letters with the target word. Examples include *crowd* read as 'crown' (Marshall and Newcombe 1966), *fixed* read as 'mixed' (Shallice and Warrington 1975), and *proof* read as 'roof' (Saffran and Marin 1977). Visual errors are most common on words of low imageability, with the incorrect response typically being of higher imageability than the target word (Shallice and Warrington 1975).

- Sometimes errors are *both* visual and semantic. Examples include *earl* read as 'deaf' (Marshall and Newcombe 1966), and *stream* read as 'train' (Saffran and Marin 1977).

- Deep dyslexics also make *derivational errors* (Marshall and Newcombe 1966) in which the errors shares a root morpheme with the target word (e.g. heat → 'hot'). However, it must be borne in mind that morphological errors are also visually and semantically similar to the target word (for discussion of this issue, see Funnell 2000).

In terms of the three-route model of reading (Coltheart *et al.* 1993):

- Deep dyslexics would appear to have suffered severe damage to the non-lexical reading route (hence abolished nonword reading).

- There must also be severe damage to the direct-lexical route whereby familiar words are directly connected with their pronunciation in a phonological lexicon (hence poor reading of function words and words of low imageability).
- Deep dyslexics must therefore rely on the lexical-semantic reading route.

Newcombe and Marshall (1980) argued that semantic errors might be an automatic consequence of the output of the lexical-semantic route when it must operate in isolation. However, unimpaired individuals do not make semantic errors in picture naming (where the semantic route must also be operating without any phonological assistance) to anything like the same extent as made during reading by a deep dyslexic patient such as G.R. (Marshall and Newcombe 1966).

This raises the important question of where precisely the impairment to the lexical-semantic reading route in deep dyslexia lies. Even though some deep dyslexic patients perform poorly at visual lexical decision (Shallice and Coughlan 1980), an impairment at the level of the orthographic lexicon seems unlikely to be a primary cause of deep dyslexia. As Shallice (1988) pointed out, because it is considered to be pre-semantic, it is difficult to see how imageability/concreteness could exert such an effect on deep dyslexic reading if the impairment was to the orthographic lexicon. Shallice and Warrington (1980b) argued that at least three different types of deep dyslexia might exist.

- In *input deep dyslexia* there is a difficulty in *accessing* the semantic representations of low-imageability words. Consistent with this account, Shallice and Coughlan (1980) described a patient who was much better at auditory than written comprehension of low-imageability words.
- In *central deep dyslexia* there is said to be an impairment that affects the semantic representations themselves.

It is often assumed that deep dyslexics are suffering from a semantic-level impairment. Indeed, Plaut and Shallice's (1993) influential computational model of deep dyslexic reading hypothesizes that semantic features have been lost from semantic memory. They attempt to explain the imageability effect by assuming that abstract words contain fewer semantic features and are therefore less resistant to semantic feature loss. As Newton and Barry (1997) point out, however, the direct evidence for a semantic-level impairment in deep dyslexia is surprisingly sparse. There clearly are patients with central semantic deficits who make semantic errors in a variety of tasks (e.g. Hillis *et al.* 1990). However, Newton and Barry's review of the literature reveals that deep dyslexics typically perform well at written comprehension so long as they are tested appropriately.

- Newton and Barry's own deep dyslexic patient showed relatively normal written comprehension of low-imageability words that he could not read aloud, but widespread anomic word-finding problems. This corresponds to the third form of deep dyslexia (*output deep dyslexia*) suggested by Shallice and Warrington (1980b).

Newton and Barry's review revealed widespread evidence of speech production problems in deep dyslexia. Consequently, they suggested that the primary cause of deep dyslexia is a difficulty in lexicalization (the process whereby the lexical form of a word is accessed from its meaning) rather than with a semantic deficit *per se*. Lexicalization, they claim, is a particularly difficult process for words of low imageability/concreteness because these words tend to be more ambiguous than words of high imageability. A patient with a lexicalization problem is therefore likely to experience particular problems in producing low-imageability words.

5.2 Anatomical issues

Extensive left hemisphere damage is frequently observed in scans of deep dyslexic patients. Lambon Ralph and Graham (2000) reviewed 48 articles examining deep dyslexia and found evidence of damage to the left frontotemporoparietal region in 44 of them. The lesions were generally large 'encompassing at least the perisylvian area and often extending to include much of the left hemisphere'. Their review also revealed that, although there were a small number of cases of deep dyslexia following head injury, the majority occurred as a consequence of CVA. There were no cases of deep dyslexia associated with dementia.

A crucial issue is whether the extensive left hemisphere damage means that reading depends on a secondary right hemisphere reading system. Coltheart (2000) has recently been at pains to point out that the right hemisphere hypothesis does not require that orthographic processing, semantic processing, and phonological processing are all carried out by the right hemisphere: 'as long as any one of these three stages cannot be carried out by the left hemisphere, then some kind of right-hemisphere reading mechanism will be required if reading aloud is to be achieved.' In fact, Coltheart claims that the results of brain imaging studies of deep dyslexic patients (Price *et al.* 1998; Weekes *et al.* 1997) are consistent with the view that orthographic processing and semantic processing are carried out initially in the right hemisphere. There is then, he argues, transmission of information from semantic areas in the right hemisphere to semantic areas in the left hemisphere followed by phonological processing in the left hemisphere leading to spoken word production.

5.3 Remediation

De Partz (1986) attempted to improve the reading performance of a French deep dyslexic patient by trying to improve his non-lexical reading skills. She taught him to blend phonemes together to make words and nonwords and re-taught him grapheme–phoneme correspondences by associating letters with the phonemes at the start of familiar words. Phonemes that are represented by more than one grapheme were taught by an ingenious series of mnemonics that made use of the patient's preserved knowledge of whole word phonology. After 9 months of intensive therapy, the patient's reading accuracy for nonwords had improved from zero to 90%. Reading of all types of familiar words also improved dramatically, although irregular words were often regularized (see Section 7). Nickels (1992) used a similar technique with an English-speaking deep dyslexic. Unfortunately, this patient did not learn to blend phonemes together and so was unable to improve his ability to read nonwords and words of low imageability. The technique did, however, improve his ability to read words of high imageability, perhaps because knowledge of grapheme–phoneme associations enabled him to generate his own phonemic cues. These in turn may have enabled him to overcome lexicalization problems when trying to read high imageability words. Hillis and Caramazza (1994) present a series of theory-based studies that attempt to remediate lexical processing skills in patients who make semantic errors. The programmes used to improve phonological skills in phonological dyslexia (see Section 6) might also be appropriate for use with deep dyslexic patients.

5.4 Assessment

Investigate reading accuracy on words of low and high imageability (e.g. PALPA test 31, Kay *et al.* 1992). Examine responses for evidence of semantic errors in particular. Examine reading accuracy on functors (e.g. PALPA test 32) and nonwords (e.g. PALPA test 36).

6 Phonological dyslexia

6.1 Functional impairment

The defining characteristic of phonological dyslexia is a selective impairment of the ability to read nonwords relative to real words. Relative preservation of the ability to read familiar words is the probable reason why the first cases of phonological dyslexia were reported as recently as 1979 by Beauvois and Derouesne.

Although severely impaired, nonword reading ability can vary from one patient to another. For example, W.B. (Funnell 1983) virtually never read a nonword correctly, whereas J.D. (Farah *et al.* 1996) read 25–30% of nonwords correctly. In general, however, nonword reading is somewhat better preserved in phonological dyslexia than it is in deep dyslexia, with some patients making errors that are phonologically similar to the target item. Detailed investigations of the nature of the nonword reading problem in 11 phonological dyslexics (Berndt *et al.* 1996) revealed that all of them experienced problems in:

- graphemic parsing (how many phonemes does 'auk' contain?);
- poor grapheme–phoneme knowledge (providing the phonemes associated with single letters);
- blending auditorily presented phonemes.

A phoneme blending task does not involve any reading and, as a consequence of this type of impairment, some have argued that phonological dyslexia is primarily the consequence of a phonological processing deficit that affects reading rather than the consequence of an orthographic deficit *per se* (e.g. Patterson and Marcel 1992). In a similar vein, Friedman (1995) has argued that phonological dyslexics suffer from either a problem at the level of the phonological representations themselves or from a problem in accessing phonological representations directly from print.

Because nonwords have an unfamiliar phonological form relative to the phonological form of familiar words, they are more difficult for the phonological system to generate. Auditory repetition of nonwords is sometimes much more accurate than reading of nonwords (e.g. Patterson 1982), but repetition, Patterson and Marcel argue, places less onerous demands on the phonological system than reading. Whether or not there is a specifically orthographic deficit in phonological dyslexia is a crucial issue for future research to address (Coltheart 1996).

The ability to read real words aloud is never entirely normal in phonological dyslexia. W.B. (Funnell 1983) is often cited as a counterexample, but he read only 60/100 words correctly on the Schonell reading test, consistent with a reading age of 8.2 years. Some patients show imageabilty effects (Farah *et al.* 1996), and some patients such as A.M. (Patterson 1982) are worse at reading function words than content words. The errors made by A.M. on content words were visual/morphological and on function words were substitutions. Comprehension of familiar written words did appear to be entirely normal in A.M. (Patterson 1982), who was able to make visual lexical decisions and make semantic classifications about written words as accurately as control subjects despite poor nonword reading. W.B. (Funnell 1983), on the other hand, was above chance but severely impaired on written comprehension tasks using words she could read aloud. In terms of three-route models of reading (Coltheart *et al.* 1993), the obvious interpretation of these differences is that patients such as A.M. are reading via the lexical-semantic route whereas W.B. was reading via the direct-lexical route. However, advocates of two-route models such as Hillis and Caramazza (1991) have attempted to argue that W.B.'s reading of words might be explicable in terms of a partially functional semantic route and a partially functional non-lexical reading route. Coltheart *et al.* (1993) have argued that W.B.'s vastly superior ability to read words relative to nonwords plus his poor comprehension skills also pose problems for theoretical accounts that claim there is no need to postulate a separate non-lexical reading route (e.g. Seidenberg and McClelland 1989).

6.2 Anatomical issues

In a review of 37 papers on phonological dyslexia, Lambon Ralph and Graham (2000) found consistent evidence of 'damage focussed on the anterior perisylvian areas ranging from relatively circumscribed lesions typically of the left inferior, posterior frontal lobes to those patients with more extensive damage involving fronto-temporo-parietal areas'. A small number of patients had posterior left hemisphere lesions affecting the occipitotemporoparietal junction, and two had right hemisphere lesions. Apart from one case with head injury, one with Alzheimer's disease, one with Pick's disease, and one with hemispherectomy, all of the cases were associated with some form of CVA.

6.3 Remediation

Remediation is obviously a less pressing issue in a patient whose ability to read familiar words is relatively well preserved. Nevertheless, successful therapy programmes based on teaching of grapheme–phoneme correspondences (Kendall *et al.* 1998) and on teaching phonological awareness skills (Conway *et al.* 1998) have been reported. Gains were observed in both real word and nonword reading in these studies. It is interesting to note that patients who recover from deep dyslexia sometimes turn into phonological dyslexics. For example, Klein *et al.*'s (1994) deep dyslexic patient remained bad at reading nonwords (though nonword reading *did* improve), but the semantic errors and imageability effect disappeared with reading of words improving back to almost normal levels. Such observations suggest that deep and phonological dyslexia may reflect opposite ends of a continuum of severity from deep dyslexia (relatively severe) to phonological dyslexia (relatively mild). Friedman (1996) has suggested that the continuum represents the severity of a semantic impairment. Alternatively, Hanley and Kay (1997) argued that the continuum may represent the severity of the impairment to the non-lexical route and that, as Hillis and Caramazza (1991) argue, even a partially functioning non-lexical route is able to inhibit semantic errors in phonological dyslexia.

6.4 Assessment

Investigate reading accuracy on nonwords (e.g. PALPA test 36; Kay *et al.* 1992). Compare reading aloud accuracy on matched sets of words and nonwords (e.g. the items from PALPA 25).

7 Surface dyslexia

7.1 Functional impairment

Early accounts of surface dyslexic reading were provided by Marshall and Newcombe (1973) and it has been the focus of intensive investigation ever since. Because English does not employ a transparent alphabetic writing system, written English contains many irregular words whose pronunciation cannot be reliably generated on the basis of grapheme–phoneme rules. The two cardinal features of surface dyslexia are greater problems in reading irregular words than regular words (a 'regularity' effect) and regularized pronunciation of irregular words known as 'regularizations' (e.g. *island* → 'izland'; *trough* → 'truff'; *come* → 'comb'). For example, J.C. (Marshall and Newcombe 1973) correctly read 67/130 (52%) regular words (e.g. *bite*) but only 41/130 (32%) irregular words (e.g. *come*). M.K. (Howard and Franklin 1988) correctly read 90% of regular words (e.g. *shrug*) and 67% of irregular words (e.g. *shove*). M.P. (Behrmann and Bub 1992) correctly read 100% regular words (e.g. *summer*) and 80% irregular words (e.g. *island*). Most of the errors made by M.K. and J.C. were regularizations, but JC also made some visual errors (e.g. *reign* → 'region', *bargain* → 'barge', *bike* → 'bik'). It is therefore clear that the lexical reading route is impaired in surface dyslexia. According to the dual-route model, it is surface dyslexics' ability to use the non-lexical reading route that prevents their lexical impairment from causing semantic errors of the kind seen in deep dyslexia (Hillis and Caramazza 1991).

The nature of the impairment to the lexical route appears to differ from one patient to another (see Ellis *et al.* 2000 for detailed discussion). As Ellis *et al.* point out:

- Some patients such as N.W. (Weekes and Coltheart 1996), who was poor at distinguishing written words from nonwords, appeared to have difficulties in gaining access to the meaning of irregular written words.

- Others, such as M.P., who had difficulties in understanding both spoken words and written words, appeared to have a central deficit within the lexical-semantic reading route.

- Finally, there appear to be surface dyslexic patients such as E.S.T. (Kay and Patterson 1985), F.M. (Graham *et al.* 1994), and M.K. (Howard and Franklin 1988) whose problems reflect a lexicalization/word-finding problem rather than a central semantic deficit.

All surface dyslexics so far tested could read some irregular words correctly, however. In the case of M.P. (Behrmann and Bub 1992), the ability to do so appeared to be related to word frequency. M.P.'s ability to read regular words was unaffected by word frequency, but less common irregular words such as *anchor* and *echo* were read less accurately than more common irregular words such as *trouble* and *heart*.

It is sometimes claimed that nonword reading is normal in surface dyslexia, but this is true in only some of the published cases (e.g. Behrmann and Bub 1992; Shallice *et al.* 1983; Weekes and Coltheart 1996). M.P., for example, read 42/44 nonwords correctly, but M.K.(Howard and Franklin 1987) read only 25/30 nonwords correctly and J.C.'s nonword reading (Marshall and Newcombe 1973) was poorer still. There is, therefore, no guarantee that surface dyslexia will be associated with an unimpaired non-lexical reading route. Nevertheless, the finding that nonword reading can be unimpaired in a patient such as M.P. despite poor reading of irregular words is of considerable theoretical significance. This is because it represents a double dissociation with phonological dyslexics such as W.B. (Funnell 1983) and provides evidence consistent with the view that the reading system contains functionally distinct lexical and non-lexical reading routes. M.P. has posed a severe challenge to computational models of reading that dispense with a separate non-lexical phonological reading route (e.g. Plaut *et al.* 1996). It has not proved possible to reproduce the surface dyslexic symptoms observed in M.P. by lesioning a single phonological reading route. If a lesion to a single phonological route is severe enough to reduce performance on irregular words to the levels observed in M.P., it will also damage performance on regular words and nonwords.

Some surface dyslexics appear to comprehend words on the basis of the pronunciation that they assemble. For example, J.C. (Marshall and Newcombe 1973) read *begin* as 'beggin' and defined it as 'collecting money' and made comprehension errors on homophones (Newcombe and Marshall 1981). M.K. (Howard and Franklin 1988), on the other hand, whose surface dyslexia appeared to reflect a post-semantic impairment read only 52% of a set of irregular words correctly but defined 88% of them accurately. For example, he defined *steak* as 'good beef' but pronounced it as /stik/.

7.2 Anatomical issues

In a review paper, Vanier and Caplan (1985) found that surface dyslexia could occur following tumour, head trauma, and stroke. It is also associated with degenerative disease (see Section 8). Vanier and Caplan found that there was consistent evidence of damage to left temporal regions in published cases of surface dyslexia. Damaged areas frequently included the insula and the putamen.

7.3 Remediation

A successful technique for treating the symptoms of surface dyslexia is to repeatedly present words that the patient cannot read together with a picture that provides information about what the word means (Byng and Coltheart 1986; Coltheart and Byng 1989). This technique might help strengthen representations within the orthographic lexicon and\or strengthen connections between the orthographic lexicon and the semantic system. Such a technique is less likely to achieve improvement with a surface dyslexic patient whose reading difficulty is associated with lexicalization problems. Ellis *et al.* (2000) describe a technique in which the patient immediately hears a word's spoken form whenever the word is read incorrectly. The patient must then repeat the word whilst thinking about its meaning. Such a technique might prove successful in treating a number of different types of surface dyslexic patient.

7.4 Assessment

Compare reading accuracy on regular and irregular words (e.g. PALPA test 35; Kay *et al.* 1992). Examine responses for evidence of regularization errors.

8 Reading impairments in dementia

8.1 Functional impairment

The results from a number of studies show that there is an association between semantic memory loss and surface dyslexia (see Section 7). Patterson and Hodges (1992) investigated the reading performance of six patients with semantic dementia (progressive aphasia affecting semantic memory accompanying the temporal variant of frontotemporal dementia). All six turned out to be surface dyslexic. Graham *et al.* (1994) gave written word/picture matching tests to two further patients with semantic impairments who were also both surface dyslexic. They found that irregular words could be read aloud only if they could be matched with their appropriate picture. Irregular words that could not be matched with pictures were not read accurately. This suggests that the reading of an irregular word depends critically on access to the word's semantic representation and that, if the semantics for an item are missing or corrupted, it will not be read accurately. Such findings are evidence against the view that there is a separate lexical reading route that accesses pronunciation without going through meaning.

However, a small number of patients with semantic loss have been reported who are *not* surface dyslexic. This includes patients with Alzheimer's disease (Lambon-Ralph *et al.* 1995; Schwartz *et al.* 1980) and with semantic dementia (Cipolotti and Warrington 1995)

For example D.C. (Lambon Ralph *et al.* 1995) read correctly 40/42 of a list of irregular words. However, he defined only 24/42 of them correctly, even though a fairly lax criterion was used for accepting definitions. The existence of patients who can read irregular words aloud despite being unable to provide evidence that they know their meaning has been taken by many as core evidence in favour of the existence of a direct-lexical reading route (e.g. Coltheart *et al.* 1993). Advocates of two-route models argue that there may be enough semantic information still contained in semantic memory to permit accurate reading even though this information is insufficient to permit accurate performance in word–picture matching tasks (e.g. Hillis and Caramazza 1991).

8.2 Assessment

The National Adult Reading Test (NART; Nelson 1983) was designed to provide a measure of premorbid IQ based on the assumption that irregular word reading is relatively immune to the effects of dementia. However, it now appears that performance on the NART is correlated with dementia severity (Patterson *et al.* 1994) and there are a number of reports of a decline on this test as the disease develops (e.g. Fromm *et al.* 1991; Paque and Warrington 1995). Strain *et al.* (1998) suggest that decline on the NART can be observed as soon as the disease develops past the early stages, and Storandt *et al.* (1995) report a decline even in mild patients. Alzheimer patients have been shown to perform well at reading nonwords unless they are orthographically (Friedman *et al.* 1992) or phonologically unusual (Glosser *et al.* 1998).

Selective references

Allport, D.A. and Funnell, E. (1981). Components of the mental lexicon. *Phil. Trans. R. Soc. London B* 295, 397–410.

Arguin, M. and Bub, D. (1994). Pure alexia: attempted rehabilitation and its implications for interpretation of the deficit. *Brain Language* 47, 233–68.

Arguin, M. and Bub, D. (1997). Lexical constraints on reading accuracy in neglect dyslexia. *Cogn. Neuropsychol.* 14, 765–800.

Arguin, M., Bub, D., and Bowers, J. (1998). Extent and limits of covert lexical activation in letter by letter reading. *Cogn. Neuropsychol.* 15, 53–92.

Barry, C. and Richardson, J.T.E. (1988). Accounts of oral reading in deep dyslexia. In *Phonological processes and brain mechanisms* (ed. H. Whittaker), pp. 119–71. Springer Verlag, New York.

Baxter, D.M. and Warrington, E. (1983). Neglect dysgraphia. *J. Neurol., Neurosurg., Psychiatry* 46, 1073–8.

Beauvois, M-F. and Derouesne, J. (1979). Phonological alexia: three dissociations. *J. Neurol., Neurosurg., Psychiatry* 42, 1115–24.

Behrmann, M. and Bub, D. (1992). Surface dyslexia and dysgraphia. Dual routes, single lexicon. *Cogn. Neuropsychol.* 9, 209–51.

Behrmann, M. and McLeod, J. (1995). Rehabilitation for pure alexia. *Neuropsychol. Rehabil.* 5, 149–80.

Behrmann, M. and Shallice, T. (1995) Pure alexia. An orthographic not spatial disorder. *Cogn. Neuropsychol.* 12, 409–54.

Behrmann, M., Plaut, D.C., and Nelson, J. (1998). A literature review and new data supporting an interactive view of letter by letter reading. *Cogn. Neuropsychol.* 15, 7–51.

Benson, D.F., Brown, J., and Tomlinson, E.B. (1971). Varieties of alexia: word and letter blindness. *Neurology* 21, 951–7.

Berndt, R.S., Haendiges, A.N., Mitchum, C.C., and Wayland, S.C. (1996). An investigation of nonlexical reading impairments. *Cogn. Neuropsychol.* 13, 763–801.

Binder, J.R. and Mohr, J.P. (1992). The topography of callosal reading pathways. *Brain* 97, 1807–26.

Bub, D., Black, S. E., and Howell, J. (1989). Word recognition and orthographic context effects in a letter-by-letter reader. *Brain Language* 36, 357–76.

Buxbaum, L. and Coslett, H.B. (1996). Deep dyslexic phenomena in a letter-by-letter reader. *Brain Language* 54, 136–67.

Byng, S. and Coltheart, M. (1986). Aphasia therapy research. In *Communication and handicap* (ed. E. Helmquist and L.G. Nilsson), pp. 191–213. Elsevier, Amsterdam.

Caplan, L.R. and Hedley-White, T. (1974). Cueing and memory function in alexia without agraphia: a case report. *Brain* 115, 251–62.

Caramazza, A. (1984). The logic of neuropsychological research and the problem of patient classification in aphasia. *Brain Language* 21, 9–20.

Caramazza, A. (1997). *Access of phonological and orthographic forms:evidence from dissociations in reading and spelling.* Psychology Press, Hove, East Sussex.

Caramazza, A. and Hillis, A.E. (1990). Levels of representation, co-ordinate frames and unilateral neglect. *Cogn. Neuropsychol.* 7, 369–89.

Chialant, D. and Caramazza, A. (1998). Perceptual and lexical factors in a case of letter-by-letter reading. *Cogn. Neuropsychol.* 15, 203–38.

Cipolotti, L. and Warrington, E. (1995). Semantic memory and reading abilities: a case report. *J. Int. Neuropsychol. Soc.* 1, 104–10.

Coltheart, M. (1985). Cognitive neuropsychology and the study of reading. In *Attention and performance*, Vol. 11 (ed. M.I. Posner and O.S.M. Marin). Erlbaum, Hillsdale, New Jersey pp 3–37.

Coltheart, M. (1996). Phonological dyslexia: past and future issues. *Cogn. Neuropsychol.* 13, 749–62.

Coltheart, M. (1996). Phonological dyslexia: a special issue of *Cognitive Neuropsychology.* Psychology Press, Hove, East Sussex.

Coltheart, M. (2000). Deep dyslexia is right-hemisphere reading. *Brain Language* 71, 299–309.

Coltheart, M. and Byng, S. (1989). A treatment for surface dyslexia. In *Cognitive approaches to neuropsychological rehabilitation* (ed. X. Seron and G. Deloche), pp. 159–74. Erlbaum, Hillsdale, New Jersey.

Coltheart, M., Curtis, B., Atkins, P., and Haller, M. (1993). Models of reading aloud: dual-route *and* parallel-distributed processing approach. *Psychol. Rev.* **100**, 589–608.

Coltheart, M., Rastle, K., Perry, C., Langdon, R., and Ziegler, J. (2001). DRC: a dual route cascaded model of visual word recognition and reading aloud. *Psychol. Rev.* **108**, 204–56.

Conway, T.W., Heilman, P., Rothi, L.J., Alexander, A.W., Adair, J., Crosson, B.A., and Heilman, K.M. (1998). Treatment of a case of phonological alexia with agraphia using the auditory discrimination in depth (ADD) programme. *J. Int. Neuropsychol. Soc.* **4**, 608–20.

Coslett, H.B. and Saffran, E.M. (1989). Preserved object recognition and reading comprehension in optic aphasia. *Brain* **112**, 1091–110.

Coslett, H.B. and Saffran, E.M. (1992). Optic aphasia and the right hemisphere: a replication and extension. *Brain Language* **43**, 148–68.

Costello, A. and Warrington, E.K. (1987). Dissociation of visuo-spatial neglect and neglect dyslexia. *J. Neurol., Neurosurg., Psychiatry* **50**, 1110–16.

Dejerine, J. (1892). Contribution a l'étude anatomo-pathologique et clinique des differentes variétés de cécité verbale. *Mem. Soc. Biologique* **4**, 61–90.

De Partz, M.P. (1986). Re-education of a deep dyslexic patient: rationale of the method and results. *Cogn. Neuropsychol.* **3**, 149–78.

Ellis, A.W. (1987). Intimations of modularity, or the modelarity of mind. In *The cognitive neuropsychology of language* (ed. M. Coltheart, G. Job, and R.Sartori), pp. 397–408. Erlbaum, London.

Ellis, A.W., Flude, B., and Young, A.W. (1987). Neglect dyslexia and the early visual processing of letters in words and nonwords. *Cogn. Neuropsychol.* **4**, 439–64.

Ellis, A.W., Lambon Ralph, M.A., Morris, J., and Hunter, A. (2000). Surface dyslexia: description, treatment and interpretation. In *Neuropsychology of reading* (ed. E. Funnell), pp. 85–122. Psychology Press, Hove, East Sussex.

Farah, M.J. (2000). *The cognitive neuroscience of vision.* Blackwell, Malden, Massachusetts.

Farah, M.J., Stowe, R.M., and Levinson, K.L. (1996). Phonological alexia: loss of a reading specific component of the reading architecture? *Cogn. Neuropsychol.* **13**, 849–68.

Friedman, R.B. (1995). Two types of phonological alexia. *Cortex* **31**, 397–403.

Friedman, R.B. (1996). Recovery from deep alexia to phonological alexia. *Brain Language* **52**, 114–28.

Friedman, R.B. and Hadley, J.A. (1992). Letter-by-letter surface alexia. *Cogn. Neuropsychol.* **9**, 185–208.

Friedman, R., Ferguson, S., Robinson, S., and Sunderland, T. (1992). Dissociation of mechanisms of reading in Alzheimer's disease. *Brain Language* **43**, 400–13.

Fromm, D., Holland, A.L., Nebes, R.D., and Oakley, M.A. (1991). A longitudinal study of word reading ability in Alzheimers disease: evidence from the National Adult Reading Test. *Cortex* **27**, 367–76.

Funnell, E. (1983). Phonological access in reading: new evidence from acquired dyslexia. *Br. J. Psychol.* **74**, 159–80.

Funnell, E. (2000). Deep dyslexia. In *Neuropsychology of reading* (ed. E. Funnell), pp. 27–55. Psychology Press, Hove, East Sussex.

Geschwind, N. (1965). Disconnexion syndromes in animals and man. *Brain* **88**, 237–94, 585–644.

Glosser, G., Friedman, R.K., Kohn, S.E., Sands, L., and Grugan, P. (1998). Cognitive mechanisms for processing nonwords: evidence from Alzheimer's disease. *Brain Language* **63**, 32–49.

Graham, N., Hodges, J.R., and Patterson, K. (1994). The relationship between comprehension and oral reading in progressive fluent aphasia. *Neuropsychologia* **32**, 299–316.

Greenwald, M.L. and Gonzalez-Rothi, L.J. (1998). Lexical access via letter naming in a profoundly alexic and anomic patient: a treatment study. *J. Int. Neuropsychol. Soc.* **4**, 595–607.

Hanley, J.R. and Kay, J. (1992). Does letter-by-letter reading involve the spelling system? *Neuropsychologia* **30**, 237–56.

Hanley, J.R. and Kay, J. (1996). Reading speed in pure alexia. *Neuropsychologia* **34**, 1165–74.

Hanley, J.R. and Kay, J. (1997). An effect of imageability on the production of phonological errors in auditory repetition. *Cogn. Neuropsychol.* **14**, 1065–84.

Hanley, J.R. and McDonnell, V. (1997). Are reading and spelling phonologically mediated? Evidence from a patient with a speech production impairment. *Cogn. Neuropsychol.* **14**, 3–33.

Haywood, M. and Coltheart, M. (2000). Neglect dyslexia and the early stages of visual word recognition. *Neurocase* **6**, 33–43.

Hillis, A. and Caramazza, A. (1991). Mechanisms for accessing lexical representations for output: evidence from a category specific semantic deficit. *Brain Language* **40**, 106–44.

Hillis, A. and Caramazza, A. (1992). The reading process and its disorders. In *Cognitive neuropsychology in clinical practice* (ed. D.I. Margolin), pp. 229–62. Oxford University Press, New York.

Hillis, A. and Caramazza, A. (1994). Theories of lexical processing and rehabilitation of lexical deficits. In *Cognitive neuropsychology and cognitive rehabilitation* (ed. M. Riddoch and G. Humphreys), pp. 449–82. Erlbaum, Hove, East Sussex.

Hillis, A.E., Rapp, B.C., Romani, C., and Caramazza, A. (1990). Selective impairment of semantics in lexical processing. *Cogn. Neuropsychol.* **7**, 191–244.

Hinshelwood, J. (1895). Word blindness and visual memory. *Lancet* **2**, 1564–70.

Hinshelwood, J. (1900). *Letter, word, and mind-blindness.* Lewis and Co Ltd, London.

Hinshelwood, J. (1917). *Congenital word-blindness.* Lewis and Co Ltd, London.

Howard, D. and Franklin, S. (1988). *Missing the meaning.* MIT Press, Cambridge, Massachusetts.

Kartsounis, L.D. and Warrington, E.K. (1989). Unilateral neglect overcome by cues implicit in stimulus displays. *J. Neurol., Neurosurg., Psychiatry* **52**, 1253–9.

Kay, J. and Hanley, J.R. (1991). Simultaneous form perception and serial letter recognition in a case of letter-by-letter reading. *Cogn. Neuropsychol.* **8**, 249–73.

Kay, J. and Patterson, K. (1985). Routes to meaning in surface dyslexia In *Surface dyslexia: neuropsychological and cognitive studies of phonological reading* (ed. K. Patterson, J. Marshall, and M. Coltheart), pp. 79–104. Erlbaum, Hove, East Sussex.

Kay, J., Lesser, R., and Coltheart, M. (1992). *Psycholinguistic assessment of language processing in aphasia.* Erlbaum, London.

Kendall, D.L., McNeil, M.R., and Small, S.L. (1998). Rule-based treatment for acquired phonological dyslexia. *Aphasiology* **12**, 587–600.

Kerkoff, G., Munsinger, U., Eberle-Strauss, G., and Stogerer, E. (1992). Rehabilitation of hemianopic alexia in patients with postgeniculate visual fields disorders. *Neuropsychol. Rehabil.* **2**, 21–41.

Klein, D., Behrmann, M., and Doctor, E. (1994). The evolution of deep dyslexia. *Cogn. Neuropsychol.* **11**, 579–611

Lambon Ralph, M.A. and Ellis, A.W. (1997). 'Patterns of paralexia' revisited: report of a case of visual dyslexia. *Cogn. Neuropsychol.* **14**, 953–74.

Lambon Ralph, M.A. and Graham, N.L. (2000). Acquired phonological and deep dyslexia. *Neurocase* **6**, 141–3.

Lambon-Ralph, M.A., Ellis, A.W., and Franklin, S. (1995). Semantic loss without surface dyslexia. *Neurocase* **1**, 363–9.

Lambon Ralph, M.A. Sage, K., and Ellis, A.W. (1996).Word meaning blindness: a new form of acquired dyslexia. *Cogn. Neuropsychol.* 13, 617–39.

Lambon Ralph, M.A., Ellis, A.W., and Sage, K. (1998). Word meaning blindness revisited. *Cogn. Neuropsychol.* 15, 389–400.

Leff, A.P., Scott, S.K., Crewes, H., Hodgson, T., and Howard, D. (2000). Impaired reading in patients with right hemianopia. *Ann. Neurol.* 47, 171–8.

Leff, A.P., Crewes, H., Plant, G.T., Scott, S.K., Kennard, C., and Wise, R.J.S. (2001). The functional anatomy of single-word reading in patients with hemianopic and pure alexia. *Brain* 124, 510–521.

Maher, L.M., Clayton, M.C., Barrett, A.M., Schober-Peterson, D., and Rothi, L.J.G. (1998). Rehabilitation of a case of pure alexia: exploiting residual abilities. *J. Int. Neuropsychol. Soc.* 4, 636–47.

Marshall, J. and Newcombe, F. (1966). Syntactic and semantic errors in paralexia. *Neuropsychologia* 2, 169–76.

Marshall, J. and Newcombe, F. (1973). Patterns of paralexia: a psycholinguistic approach. *J. Psycholinguistic Res.* 4, 175–99.

Marshall, J. and Newcombe, F. (1980). The conceptual status of deep dyslexia: an historical perspective. In *Deep dyslexia* (ed. M. Coltheart, K. Patterson, and J Marshall), pp. 1–21. Routledge, London.

McCarthy, R. A. and Warrington, E.K. (1990). *Cognitive neuropsychology. A clinical introduction.* Academic Press, London.

Miceli, G. and Capasso, R. (2001). Word-centred neglect dyslexia: evidence from a new case. *Neurocase* 7, 221–37.

Miozzo, M. and Caramazza, A. (1998). Varieties of pure alexia: the case of failure to access graphemic representations. *Cogn. Neuropsychol.* 15, 203–38.

Moody, S. (1988). The Moyer reading technique re-evaluated. *Cortex* 24, 473–6.

Morton, J. and Patterson, K. (1980). Little words—no. In *Deep dyslexia* (ed. M. Coltheart, K. Patterson, and J. Marshall), pp. 270–85. Routledge, London.

Moyer, S.B. (1979). Rehabilitation of alexia: a case study. *Cortex* 15, 139–44.

Mycroft, R., Hanley, J.R., and Kay, J. (2002). Preserved access to abstract letter identities despite abolished letter naming in a case of pure alexia. *J. Neurolinguistics* 15, 99–108.

Nelson, H. (1983) *National Adult Reading Test (NART).* NFER Publishing Co, Windsor.

Newcombe, F. and Marshall, J.C. (1980). Response monitoring and response blocking in deep dyslexia. In *Deep dyslexia* (ed. M. Coltheart, K. Patterson, and J. Marshall), pp. 160–75. Routledge, London.

Newcombe, F. and Marshall, J.C. (1981). On psycholinguistic classification of the acquired dyslexias. *Bull. Orton Soc.* 31, 29–46.

Newton, P. and Barry, C. (1997). Concreteness effects in word production but not word comprehension in deep dyslexia. *Cogn. Neuropsychol.* 14, 481–509.

Nickels, L. (1992). The autocue? Self generated phonemic cues in the treatment of a disorder of reading and naming. *Cogn. Neuropsychol.* 9, 155–82.

Paivio, A., Yuille, J.C., and Madigan, S.A. (1968). Concreteness, imagery and meaningfulness: Values for 925 nouns. *J. Exp. Psychol.* 76, 1–25.

Paque, L. and Warrington, E.K. (1995). A longitudinal study of reading ability in patients suffering from dementia. *J. Int. Neuropsychol. Soc.* 1, 517–24.

Patterson, K. (1979). What is right with deep dyslexic patients? *Brain Language* 8, 111–29.

Patterson, K. (1982). The relation between reading and phonological coding: further neuropsychological observations. In *Normality and pathology in cognitive function* (ed. A.W. Ellis), pp. 77–111. Academic Press, London.

Patterson, K., Graham, N., and Hodges, J.R. (1994). Reading in dementia of the Alzheimer's type; A preserved ability? *Neuropsychology* **8**, 395–407.

Patterson, K. and Hodges, J.R. (1992). Deterioration of word meaning: implications for meaning. *Neuropsychologia* **30**, 1025–40.

Patterson, K. and Kay, J. (1982). Letter-by-letter reading: psychological descriptions of a neurological syndrome. *Quart. J. Exp. Psychol.* **34A**, 411–41.

Patterson, K. and Lambon Ralph, M. (1999). Selective disorders of reading? *Curr. Opin. Neurobiol.* **9**, 235–9.

Patterson, K.E. and Marcel, A. (1992). Phonological ALEXIA or PHONOLOGICAL alexia. In *Analytic approaches to human cognition* (ed. J. Alegria, D. Holender, J. Junca de Morais, and M. Radeau), pp. 259–74. Elsevier Science Publishers, Amsterdam.

Patterson, K. and Wilson, B. (1990). A rose is a rose or a nose: a deficit in initial letter identification *Cogn. Neuropsychol.* **7**, 447–79.

Perri, R., Bartolomeo, P., and Silveri, M.C. (1996). Letter dyslexia in a letter-by-letter reader. *Brain Language* **53**, 390–407.

Plaut, D. and Shallice, T. (1993). Deep dyslexia, a case study of connectionist neuropsychology. *Cogn. Neuropsychol.* **10**, 377–500.

Plaut, D., McClelland, J., Seidenberg, M., and Patterson, K. (1996) Understanding normal and impaired word reading. *Psychol. Rev.* **103**, 56–115.

Price, C.J., Howard, D., Patterson, K., Warburton, E.A., Friston, K., and Frakowiak, R.S.J. (1998). A functional neuroimaging of two deep dyslexic patients. *J. Cogn. Neurosci.* **10**, 303–15.

Rapcsak, S.Z., Rubens, A.B., and Laguna, J.F. (1990). From letters to words: procedures for word recognition in letter-by-letter reading. *Brain Language* **38**, 504–14.

Reuter-Lorenz, P.A. and Brunn, J.L. (1990). A prelexical basis for letter-by-letter reading. *Cogn. Neuropsychol.* **7**, 1–20.

Riddoch, M.J. (1990). Neglect and the peripheral dyslexias. *Cogn. Neuropsychol.* **7**, 369–89.

Saffran, E.M. and Coslett, H.B. (1998). Implicit versus letter-by-letter reading in pure alexia, a tale of two systems. *Cogn. Neuropsychol.* **15**, 141–65.

Saffran, E.M. and Marin, O.S.M. (1977). Reading without phonology: evidence from aphasia. *Quart. J. Exp. Psychol.* **29**, 515–25.

Schwartz, M. Saffran, E.M., and Marin, O.S.M. (1980). Fractionating the reading process in dementia. In *Deep dyslexia* (ed. M. Coltheart, K. Patterson, and J Marshall), pp. 259–69. Routledge, London.

Seidenberg, M.S. and McClelland, J. (1989). A distributed, developmental model of word recognition and naming. *Psychol. Rev.* **15**, 169–79.

Shallice, T. (1988). *From neuropsychology to mental structure.* Cambridge University Press, Cambridge.

Shallice, T. and Coughlan, A.K. (1980). Word recognition in a phonemic dyslexic patient. *Quart. J. Exp. Psychol.* **43**, 866–72.

Shallice, T. and Saffran, E.M. (1986). Lexical processing in the absence of explicit word identification: evidence from a letter-by-letter reader. *Cogn. Neuropsychol.* **3**, 429–58.

Shallice, T. and Warrington, E.K. (1975). Word recognition in a phonemic dyslexic patient. *Quart. J. Exp Psychol.* **27**, 187–99.

Shallice, T. and Warrington, E.K. (1977). The possible role of selective attention in acquired dyslexia. *Neuropsychologia* **15**, 31–41.

Shallice, T. and Warrington, E.K. (1980*a*). Modality specific word comprehension deficits in deep dyslexia. *J. Neurol., Neurosurg., Psychiatry* **27**, 187–99.

Shallice, T. and Warrington, E.K. (1980*b*). Single and multiple component central dyslexic syndromes. In *Deep dyslexia* (ed. M. Coltheart, K. Patterson, and J Marshall), pp. 119–45. Routledge, London.

Shallice, T., Warrington, E.K., and McCarthy, R. (1983). Reading without semantics. *Quart. J. Exp. Psychol.* **35A**, 111–38.

Sieroff, E. (1990). Focusing on/in visual–verbal stimuli in patients with parietal lesions. *Cogn. Neuropsychol.* **7**, 519–54.

Storandt, M., Stone, K., and Labarge, E. (1995). Deficits in reading performance in very mild dementia of the Alzheimer type. *Neuropsychology*, **9**, 174–6.

Strain, E., Patterson, K., Graham, N., and Hodges, J.R. (1998). Word reading in Alzheimer's disease. *Neuropsychologia* **36**, 155–71.

Vanier, M. and Caplan, D. (1985). CT scan correlates of surface dyslexia. In *Surface dyslexia: neuropsychological and cognitive studies of phonological reading* (ed. K. Patterson, J. Marshall, and M. Coltheart), pp. 511–25. Erlbaum, Hove, East Sussex.

Warrington, E.K. (1991). Right neglect dyslexia: a single case study. *Cogn. Neuropsychol.* **8**, 193–212.

Warrington, E.K. and Shallice, T. (1979). Semantic access dyslexia. *Brain* **102**, 43–63.

Warrington, E.K. and Shallice, T. (1980). Word-form dyslexia. *Brain* **103**, 99–112.

Weekes, B. (1997). Differential effects of number of letters on word and nonword naming latency. *Quart. J. Exp. Psychol.* **50A**, 439–56.

Weekes, B. and Coltheart, M. (1996). Surface dyslexia and surface dysgraphia: treatment studies and their theoretical implications. *Cogn. Neuropsychol.* **13**, 277–315.

Weekes, B., Coltheart, M., and Gordon, E. (1997). Deep dyslexia and right hemisphere reading—a regional blood flow study. *Aphasiology* **11**, 1139–58.

Chapter 16

Neuropsychological assessment and rehabilitation of writing disorders

Pelagie M. Beeson and Steven Z. Rapcsak

1 Introduction

The act of expressing ideas in writing involves clarifying our thoughts, formulating sentences, and sequentially translating each word to its written form according to the spelling conventions for the language. Written communication may be impaired by damage to any of the cognitive, linguistic, or sensorimotor processes that support spelling and writing. The goal of neuropsychological assessment of writing is to discern the status of these component processes. Understanding of the nature and degree of impairment to specific processes, as well as the availability of residual abilities, provides guidance for rehabilitation that is appropriate for a specific patient.

2 A cognitive model of writing

The cognitive-linguistic and sensorimotor processes necessary for writing single words are specified in Fig. 16.1.

2.1 Central spelling processes

- *Semantic system*: knowledge of word meanings stored in long-term memory.
- *Orthographic output lexicon*: memory store of learned spellings.
- *Phoneme–grapheme conversion*: the process of spelling by converting units of sound to corresponding letters.
- *Graphemic buffer*: a working memory system that temporarily stores orthographic representations while they are being converted into output for handwriting (or typing or oral spelling).

2.2 Peripheral spelling processes

- *Allographic conversion*: the process by which abstract orthographic representations are converted into appropriate physical letter shapes.
- *Graphic motor programmes*: spatiotemporal codes for writing movements that contain information about the sequence, position, direction, and relative size of the strokes necessary to create different letters.

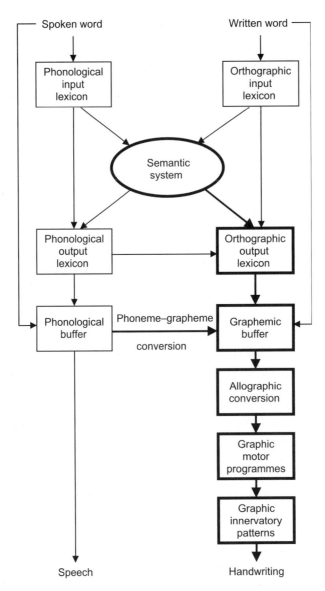

Fig. 16.1 A simplified model of information processing with writing processes in bold. Lexical–semantic spelling route: semantic system → orthographic output lexicon → graphemic buffer. Non-lexical spelling route: phonological buffer → phoneme–grapheme conversion → graphemic buffer. Peripheral writing processes: allographic conversion → graphic motor programmes → graphic innervatory patterns → handwriting.

- *Graphic innervatory patterns*: motor commands to specific muscle effector systems involved in the production of handwriting.

2.3 Other language-processing modules

- *Orthographic input lexicon*: memory store of familiar visual word forms critical for written word recognition.
- *Phonological input lexicon*: memory store of acoustic representations for familiar words used in auditory comprehension.
- *Phonological output lexicon*: memory store of sound patterns for familiar words used in speech production.
- *Phonological buffer*: a working memory system that temporarily stores phonological representations while articulatory planning for speech production is accomplished.

2.4 Lexical–semantic and non-lexical spelling routes

Written communication is most often motivated by the desire to convey conceptual information. To do so, the relevant semantic representations activate specific words in our orthographic output lexicon. Access to this lexicon via the semantic system is referred to as the lexical–semantic spelling route.

When the spelling of a word is unknown, one may rely on knowledge of sound-to-letter correspondences to assemble plausible spellings. This alternative means of spelling is depicted in Fig. 16.1 by the direct link from auditory input to the phonological buffer, and the subsequent phoneme–grapheme conversion process providing input to the graphemic buffer. Spelling in this manner is considered a non-lexical process, because spellings are not retrieved as whole words from the lexicon. Assembled spellings are likely to reflect regular spelling rules, so that irregularly spelled words might be regularized, for example, 'tough' might be spelled as *tuff*. This non-lexical route can provide an important compensatory spelling strategy when the lexical–semantic spelling route is impaired. This route is also used for spelling pronounceable nonwords (e.g. *chulf*) and unfamiliar words for which no representation exists in the orthographic lexicon.

Spellings generated by the lexical–semantic and non-lexical spelling routes are subsequently processed in the *graphemic buffer*. This buffer serves as an interface between central spelling processes and the peripheral procedures that support the production of handwriting. Peripheral writing procedures are accomplished through a series of hierarchically organized stages that include allographic conversion, motor programming, and the generation of graphic innervatory patterns.

3 Clinical assessment of spelling and writing

The initial goal of writing assessment is to determine whether an individual can meet their daily needs for written language production. Writing abilities should be considered relative to premorbid language skills. When agraphia is evident, careful

Table 16.1 Tasks used for the assessment of spelling. Check marks indicate those processes or representations that are necessary to accomplish the various tasks. (See discussion in text.)

Tasks	Lexical–semantic processes			Phonological processes (non-lexical): Phoneme–grapheme conversion	Central–peripheral interface: Graphemic buffer	Peripheral spelling processes		
	Syntax/grammer rules	Semantic representation	Orthographic output lexicon			Allographic conversion	Graphic motor programmes	Letter name selection
Conceptual								
Written narrative or picture description	✓	✓	✓		✓	✓	✓	
Written naming		✓	✓		✓	✓	✓	
Dictation								
Writing to dictation		✓	✓		✓	✓	✓	
Writing homophones		✓	✓		✓	✓	✓	
Typing or anagram spelling		✓	✓		✓			
Oral spelling		✓	✓		✓	✓		✓
Writing nonwords				✓	✓	✓	✓	
Copy								
Case conversion						✓	✓	
Direct copy							✓	

assessment should be performed to determine the functional integrity of the various processing components involved in writing. Comparing performance across various tasks allows for the relative isolation of the damaged components (Table 16.1).

3.1 Conceptually mediated writing

Conceptually medicated writing can be sampled by asking the patient to compose a written narrative on a specific topic or using picture description tasks from standardized tests (e.g. Kertesz 1982; Goodglass *et al.* 2001). Written narratives require grammatical and syntactic know-ledge, as well as higher level conceptual organization. Written naming can be assessed by using pictured stimuli from standardized tests (Kay *et al.* 1992; Kaplan *et al.* 2001).

3.2 Writing to dictation tasks

Writing to dictation tasks are selected to allow examination of various linguistic features known to affect spelling performance including word length, orthographic regularity, word frequency, concreteness, grammatical class, morphological complexity, and lexical status (word versus nonword) (Kay *et al.* 1992; Goodman and Caramazza 1984/2001). Certain lexical effects and characteristic error types are associated with damage to particular spelling processes and may result in specific agraphia syndromes (Table 16.2).

♦ *Semantic processing* is necessary for the composition of written narratives, written naming, and spelling words that sound the same but have different meanings (i.e. homophones, such as *bear, bare*). Although semantic activation typically occurs when words are spelled to dictation, these tasks may be accomplished by transcoding directly from sounds to letters, therefore bypassing semantics.

♦ *Activation of orthographic representations* is necessary to support spelling of familiar words.

♦ *Non-lexical spelling procedures* can be tested directly with the spelling of pronounceable nonwords (e.g. *merber*) that require conversion of phonemes to graphemes.

♦ *The graphemic buffer* holds orthographic information in short-term memory as sequential letters are written, typed, or spelled aloud.

3.3 Peripheral writing processes

Peripheral writing processes can be examined on all writing tasks shown in Table 16.1. Performance on these tasks may be compared to oral spelling, typing, and spelling by the arrangement of letters (i.e. anagrams) in order to identify potential dissociations between the various output modalities.

♦ *Allographic conversion* can be assessed by asking patients to write in a different case or style, or to transcribe from upper to lower case and vice versa.

Table 16.2 Summary of the primary features of various central agraphia syndromes

Central agraphia syndrome	Effect*						Characteristic errors
	Word length Short > Long	Spelling regularity Reg > Irreg	Word frequency HF > LF	Concrete Con > Abstr	Word class Cont > Func	Inability to read nonwords	
Lexical (or surface) agraphia		✓	✓				Phonologically plausible misspellings; homophone confusions
Phonological/deep dysgraphia			✓	✓	✓	✓	(Deep dysgraphia) semantic errors; functor substitutions; morphological errors
Graphemic buffer agraphia	✓						Letter omissions, substitutions, additions, transpositions

* ✓, Significant effect; Reg, regular spelling; Irreg, irregular spelling; HF, high frequency words; LF, low frequency words; Concrete, concreteness; Con, concrete; Abstr, abstract words; Cont, content words; Func, functors.

- *Graphic motor programs* and *graphic innervatory patterns* control the motor execution of handwriting movements. Poor control of movement speed, force, and amplitude may be readily apparent as the patient is observed in the act of writing. Peripheral writing processes may also be examined by asking the patient to copy words or single letters. Keep in mind that copying may be accomplished without activation of the orthographic output lexicon, letter shape selection, or graphic motor programmes if it is performed in a manner that is more like drawing a picture than writing.

3.4 **Comparison of writing abilities with related language and motor skills**

Writing abilities should be contrasted with performance on tasks that examine other input and output modalities, and relative to the performance of other skilled limb movements.

- Examine *single-word auditory comprehension* (point to picture in response to spoken word). Impairment will negatively affect performance on writing to dictation tasks.

- Examine *single-word reading comprehension* (match written word to picture) and the ability to recognize correctly spelled real words versus pseudowords, such as *flig* (visual lexical decision task). Poor word recognition abilities will impair the ability to detect spelling errors.

- Examine *reading aloud* to determine if written words provide access to appropriate entries in the phonological output lexicon. Good oral reading skills may provide strategies for self-detection of spelling errors.

- Examine *limb praxis* for tasks other than handwriting using an apraxia screening test or subtest (e.g. Kertesz 1982).

4 **Principles of agraphia classification and treatment**

The assessment of impaired and preserved writing processes should allow for the determination of whether a patient's performance fits the diagnostic criteria for a specific agraphia syndrome. Acquired disorders of writing can be subdivided into central and peripheral types.

- *Central agraphia syndromes* reflect damage to the lexical–semantic or non-lexical spelling routes, or the graphemic buffer, and result in similar impairments across different modalities of output (e.g. written spelling, oral spelling, typing). Central agraphia syndromes include lexical (or surface) agraphia, phonological agraphia, deep agraphia, and graphemic buffer agraphia (Table 16.2; Ellis 1988; Roeltgen 1993; Rapcsak and Beeson 2000).

- *Peripheral agraphia syndromes* reflect damage to writing processes that are distal to the graphemic buffer. Dysfunction primarily affects the selection or production of letters in handwriting. These syndromes include allographic disorders, apraxic

Table 16.3 Summary of the primary features of various peripheral agraphia syndromes

Peripheral agraphia syndrome	Distinctive features		Characteristic errors
	Impairment	Spared abilities	
Allographic disorders	Inability to generate or select correct letter shapes in handwriting	Oral spelling	Substitution of physically similar letter forms; case mixing errors. May be specific to case (upper versus lower) or style (print versus cursive)
Apraxic agraphia	Poor letter formation not attributable to allographic disorder or sensorimotor, cerebellar, or extrapyramidal dysfunction	Oral spelling, typing, spelling with anagram letters	Gross errors of letter morphology, spatial distortions, stroke insertions and deletions. Writing may be completely illegible
Nonapraxic disorders of motor function	Defective regulation of movement force, speed, and amplitude in handwriting	Oral spelling, spelling with anagram letters (typing may be impaired due to disordered motor function)	Micrographia (Parkinson's disease); disjointed and irregular writing movements (cerebellar disorders)

agraphia, and non-apraxic disorders of neuromuscular execution (Table 16.3; Rapcsak 1997; Rapcsak and Beeson 2000).

When an individual's agraphia profile does not conform to a recognized agraphia syndrome, it can be characterized by a description of the status of impaired and preserved processes.

4.1 Treatment principles and supporting evidence

Agraphia treatment may target central or peripheral components of the writing process. Treatments for central agraphias may be directed toward the lexical–semantic or non-lexical spelling routes, or the graphemic buffer. In contrast, treatments for peripheral agraphias are designed to improve the selection and implementation of graphic motor programmes for handwriting. In general, treatments are designed to strengthen damaged processing components and to take advantage of residual abilities.

A randomized controlled trial conducted with 94 individuals with aphasia (with alexia and agraphia) showed that patients who received treatment for spoken and written language made significantly greater improvement in writing than patients who did not receive treatment (Wertz *et al.* 1986). Writing treatment was characterized as individual 'stimulus–response treatment' provided by certified speech–language pathologists to a diverse population of individuals with acquired agraphia. These data serve to document the efficacy of writing treatment for agraphia. However, the underlying premise of a cognitive neuropsychological approach to treatment is that procedures are designed and adapted to suit the particular patient profile. Therefore, the treatments suggested in Sections 5–10 were selected from those shown to improve writing abilities in individuals with well-specified agraphia profiles using controlled, single-subject experimental designs. (For reviews see Beeson and Hillis 2001; Beeson and Rapcsak 2002; Behrmann and Byng 1992; Hillis and Caramazza 1994.) The procedures are likely to overlap with those used in the Wertz *et al.* (1986) study, but were selected with careful consideration of the specific nature of the writing impairment.

Individual agraphia syndromes and appropriate treatment approaches are detailed in Sections 5–10. The presumed neuroanatomical correlates of these syndromes are drawn from careful examination of lesions in patients with well-defined agraphia profiles. (For detailed reviews, see Rapcsak 1997; Rapcsak and Beeson 2002; Roeltgen 1993.)

5 Lexical agraphia (also called surface agraphia)

Lexical agraphia is a central agraphia syndrome that results from damage to the lexical–semantic spelling route. It is characterized by the loss or unavailability of word-specific spelling knowledge so that patients are forced to rely on spelling by a non-lexical strategy (i.e. phoneme-to-grapheme conversion). Patients tend to spell words as they sound.

5.1 Distinctive features

Spelling accuracy is strongly influenced by orthographic regularity in that regular words and nonwords are spelled correctly, but attempts to spell words with irregular sound-to-spelling relationships result in phonologically plausible errors (e.g. tomb → toom). Low-frequency irregular words are especially vulnerable to error. In addition, the loss of semantic influence on spelling creates difficulties in writing homophonic words that cannot be spelled correctly without reference to the word's meaning (e.g. dear → deer).

At a functional level, lexical agraphia often results in effortful, deliberate attempts to assemble spelling, rather than relatively automatic retrieval of spelling knowledge. Phonologically plausible spelling errors may be deciphered by the reader, but the loss of semantic influence on spelling can lead to homophone confusions.

5.2 Locus of neurological damage

Lexical agraphia is typically seen following damage to left extrasylvian temporoparietal regions. The syndrome has also been described in patients with Alzheimer's disease and in semantic dementia.

5.3 Treatment

Treatment for lexical agraphia may be directed toward improving the spelling of irregular words and homophones by strengthening word-specific links between the semantic system and the orthographic output lexicon. Treatments may also be directed toward restoring damaged orthographic representations. Positive treatment outcomes include improved spelling accuracy, reduction in time required for spelling, and improved ability to detect and self-correct errors.

5.3.1 Strengthening semantic–orthographic associations

- *Goal.* To re-learn spellings in an item-specific manner so that the link between corresponding semantic and orthographic representations is strengthened.

- *Task example(s).* Word-to-picture matching with corrective feedback, supplemented by repeated copying and writing to dictation of target words. Treatment may focus on homophone pairs that cause confusion, such as *red–read*, as well as irregularly spelled words that are difficult to spell in a non-lexical manner (e.g. choir). Homework may include looking up target words in the dictionary and copying the spelling and definitions, as a means to strengthen links between spelling and meaning.

- *Expectation.* Mastery of the spelling of targeted words is expected (Behrmann and Byng 1992; Behrmann 1987). Training of one word of a homophone pair may result in generalized improvement to the other homophone. Some generalized improvement in spelling irregular words may result if self-detection and correction of errors improves (Behrmann and Byng 1992).

5.3.2 **Restoring damaged orthographic representations**

◆ *Goal.* To strengthen specific orthographic representations for writing.

◆ *Task example(s).* Hierarchically ordered tasks with progressively increasing demands on spelling knowledge are appropriate. These include, for example, the arrangement of component letters (i.e. anagram task), direct copying of the target word, and delayed copying (after 10–15 second delays) of target words. A critical component of these treatment protocols is repeated, corrected spelling of the targeted words. The re-training of orthography should take place in the presence of pictured stimuli or in response to semantic information about the word, so that the link between semantics and restored orthographic representations is also strengthened. Another approach includes training to use an electronic spell checker so that phonologically plausible misspellings lead to retrieval of correct spellings (Beeson *et al.* 2000).

◆ *Expectation.* Improved spelling for targeted words with limited generalization to untrained words (Aliminosa *et al.* 1993; Hillis and Caramazza 1987; Carlomagno *et al.* 1994). Patients with lexical agraphia may be able to abandon non-lexical spelling strategies as representations in the orthographic output lexicon are restored. Other patients may combine partially spared (or recovered) orthographic knowledge with non-lexical (phonological) procedures to actively resolve spelling difficulties (Beeson *et al.* 2000).

6 **Phonological agraphia and deep agraphia**

Phonological agraphia and deep agraphia are central agraphia syndromes attributable to dysfunction of the non-lexical spelling route. In both syndromes, spelling is accomplished primarily via a lexical–semantic strategy and patients have difficulty spelling nonwords. In phonological agraphia, the spelling of familiar words (both regular and irregular) may be relatively spared. However, in deep agraphia, there is concomitant impairment to the lexical–semantic spelling route.

6.1 **Distinctive features**

In both phonological and deep agraphia, spelling accuracy is influenced by lexical–semantic variables (concreteness, word class, and frequency), consistent with reliance on a lexical–semantic strategy. Individuals with deep agraphia also produce semantic errors (e.g. boy → girl), indicating additional impairment of the lexical–semantic spelling route. Other spelling errors may include morphological errors (walked → walking), functor substitutions (while → into), and substitution of unrelated words (table → flower). As in any of the central agraphia syndromes, patients may recall only some of the letters of the target word.

Phonological and deep agraphia have been conceptualized as representing endpoints along a continuum of increasingly severe phonological and lexical–semantic spelling deficits. Consistent with this view, mild phonological agraphia may have limited clinical significance, whereas deep agraphia typically is associated with severe limitations in written communication.

6.2 **Locus of neurological damage**

Phonological and deep agraphia are associated with damage to the perisylvian language areas including Broca's area, Wernicke's area, and the supramarginal gyrus. Deep agraphia in patients with extensive left hemisphere lesions may reflect reliance on the right hemisphere for writing (Rapcsak *et al.* 1991).

6.3 **Treatment**

Treatment for phonological or deep agraphia may be directed toward improving the availability and use of non-lexical spelling procedures. In deep agraphia, additional treatment is required to restore the dysfunctional lexical–semantic spelling route in order to eliminate semantic errors.

6.3.1 Strengthening the non-lexical spelling route

- *Goal.* To re-establish phoneme–grapheme conversion skills so that patients can generate plausible spellings for words. Non-lexical spelling procedures may also help constrain the output of the unstable lexical–semantic spelling route, thus reducing the potential for semantic errors. Partial orthographic information derived by the application of sound-to-letter correspondences can also serve to cue the retrieval of word-specific spellings from the orthographic output lexicon.

- *Task example(s).* Establish a corpus of key words that can be used to derive orthography from phonology. For example, if the patient is able to say and spell the word *baby* then this will be the 'key word' used to derive 'b' when spelling other words. Retrieval of the first letter or two of a word may serve to cue retrieval of word-specific spellings and to block semantic errors in writing. Given that sound-to-letter correspondences for consonants are more predictable (i.e. less variable) than for vowels, it is best to begin with the establishment of key words for consonants (Beeson and Hillis 2001). Preserved spelling of proper or common nouns may be used to retrieve the spelling of consonants, vowels, consonant-vowel syllables, and whole words.

- *Expectation.* Using a lexical relay strategy, patients have been able to derive the spelling of untrained words, or to cue the recall of orthographic representations (Hatfield 1983; Hillis and Caramazza 1991; Cardell and Chenery 1999; Hillis Trupe 1986; Carlomagno and Parlato 1989). The establishment of key words to derive sound-to-letter correspondences may be a tedious process. However, daily homework may be implemented to accomplish the goal efficiently. Phonologically plausible spellings derived in this manner may also be typed into a portable computer that provides synthesized speech for communication (Hillis Trupe 1986) or into an electronic spell checker that offers possible correct spellings (Beeson *et al.* 2000).

6.3.2 Strengthening semantic processing

◆ *Goal.* To restore semantic representations for target words and to clarify the semantic distinctions between target words and semantically related errors.

◆ *Task example(s).* Written naming tasks followed by corrective feedback for semantic errors that highlights distinctive features of the target in contrast to other members of the semantic category. For example, if 'apple' is written for 'orange', the distinguishing features of colour would be highlighted for the two semantically related words. Thus, treatment tasks are directed toward semantic specification.

◆ *Expectation.* Treatment should result in a reduction of semantic errors in written naming and writing to dictation, and may also result in improved oral naming, and written and spoken comprehension of trained items (Hillis 1991). Generalization may also occur for untrained items in the same semantic category if treatment serves to enrich semantic representations and allow for more accurate distinctions among items in the treated categories.

6.3.3 Strengthening (and improving access to) the orthographic output lexicon

◆ *Goal.* To strengthen memory for specific orthographic representations, and to strengthen the link between semantic and orthographic representations in patients who make semantic errors as a result of faulty transmission of information between semantics and orthography.

◆ *Task example(s).* A cueing hierarchy for written naming of pictured stimuli may include tasks such as arrangement of component letters (i.e. anagram task), and direct and delayed copying of target words. The procedures should include corrective feedback to retrain or stabilize the association between concepts and written words, and to strengthen word-specific spellings. A relatively small set of words (about five) should be trained to mastery, with additional groups of words subsequently targeted for treatment.

◆ *Expectation.* Improved written naming of targeted items (Hillis 1989; Aliminosa *et al.* 1993; Beeson 1999). Generalization to untrained items in the same semantic category may also occur when semantic representations are strengthened (Hillis 1989). Such generalization is not likely in severely agraphic individuals for whom orthographic representations are degraded to the extent that they must be rebuilt one word at a time. However, item-specific response to treatment of single-word writing can provide a much-needed communication modality for individuals with severe impairments of spoken and written language (Beeson 1999).

7 Graphemic buffer agraphia

Graphemic buffer agraphia reflects impairment of the ability to retain orthographic representations in short-term memory as the appropriate graphic motor programmes are selected and implemented. Damage to the graphemic buffer leads to abnormally rapid decay of information relevant to the serial order and identity of stored graphemes.

7.1 Distinctive features

Spelling accuracy is notably affected by word length because each additional grapheme increases the demand on limited storage capacity. Spelling is not significantly influenced by lexical status (words versus nonwords), lexical–semantic features (concreteness, word class, frequency), or orthographic regularity (Table 16.2). Characteristic spelling errors include letter substitutions, additions, deletions, and transpositions (e.g. flower → florew). These errors are observed in all spelling tasks and across all modalities of output (handwriting, typing, oral spelling). Individuals with graphemic buffer agraphia may have relatively good spelling for words up to about four letters, but have increasing difficulty with longer words.

7.2 Locus of neurological damage

Lesion sites in patients with graphemic buffer agraphia have been variable, but left parietal and frontal cortical involvement is common.

7.3 Treatment

There is relatively little evidence to suggest that the graphemic buffer itself can be restored. However, several successful treatments have been documented that reduce spelling errors associated with graphemic buffer agraphia.

7.3.1 Strengthening the orthographic output lexicon

- ◆ *Goal.* To strengthen specific orthographic representations so that they are less subject to decay.
- ◆ *Task example(s).* Approaches for strengthening orthographic representations that were described for lexical and deep agraphia are also appropriate for treatment of graphemic buffer agraphia.
- ◆ *Expectation.* Improved spelling of words targeted for treatment, so that the word-length effect is diminished (Cardell and Chenery 1999; Hillis 1989).

7.3.2 Training segmentation of long words into shorter units

- ◆ *Goal.* To train segmentation of long words into shorter units that can be retained in the graphemic buffer.
- ◆ *Task example(s).* Long words that contain embedded words, such as *pen*cil or *base*-ment, are selected as target words in order to train the segmentation of words into smaller units. The lexical subsegments (i.e. embedded words) are underlined as the words are presented for study. Delayed copying of the target word is used to test

recall of spelling using the segmentation strategy. Homework involves studying and copying the segmented words.

◆ *Expectation.* de Partz (1995) documented improved spelling for trained words using the segmentation strategy in a patient with graphemic buffer impairment. Improvement was specific to trained words, and was greatest when long words had an embedded short word (i.e. a lexical subsegment).

7.3.3 Strengthening self-detection and correction of spelling errors

◆ *Goal.* To train self-detection and correction of spelling errors.

◆ *Task example(s).* A search strategy may be trained to detect errors, and to sound out each word as it is written in order to call attention to phonologically implausible misspellings.

◆ *Expectation.* If a patient is able to improve self-detection and correction of spelling errors, the spelling improvement should generalize to untrained words as well (Hillis and Caramazza 1987).

8 Allographic writing impairment

Allographic disorders are peripheral writing impairments that reflect the breakdown of procedures by which orthographic representations are mapped on to letter-specific graphic motor programmes.

8.1 Distinctive features

Allographic disorders are characterized by an inability to activate or select letter shapes appropriate for orthographic representations held in the graphemic buffer. Patients may have selective difficulty in writing upper- or lower-case letters, or they may produce case-mixing errors (e.g. tAblE). Other patients produce well-formed letter substitution errors that typically bear physical similarity to the target. Allographic disorders may occur in the presence of preserved oral spelling.

8.2 Locus of neurological damage

Allographic disorders are usually associated with damage to the left parieto-occipital region.

8.3 Treatment

◆ *Goal.* To improve letter selection and implementation of letter shape, or to develop compensatory strategies to overcome the allographic impairment.

◆ *Task example(s).* An alphabet card may be used to assist the patient when a model is needed for letter shapes, but treatment may be necessary to achieve effective use of this strategy. If oral spelling is preserved, self-dictation may provide a means to monitor letter selection and promote self-correction of errors. Repeated copying of target words followed by writing the word from memory, and case conversion tasks (e.g. transcoding words written in upper case into words written in lower case) may also be used to strengthen allographic conversion.

- *Expectation.* Use of the self-dictation strategy to prevent and self-correct errors has the potential to support generalized improvement in letter selection (Pound 1996). Repeated copying of target words may result in item-specific improvements, but has the potential for generalized improvement as allographic skills are strengthened (Ramage *et al.* 1998).

9 Apraxic agraphia

Apraxia agraphia is a peripheral writing impairment caused by damage to graphic motor programmes, or it may reflect an inability to translate information contained in these programmes into specific motor commands.

9.1 Distinctive features

Apraxic agraphia is characterized by poor letter formation that cannot be attributed to sensorimotor (i.e. weakness, deafferentation), basal ganglia (i.e. tremor, rigidity), or cerebellar (i.e. ataxia, dysmetria) dysfunction affecting the writing limb. Errors of letter shape include spatial distortions and stroke additions or deletions, frequently resulting in production of illegible handwriting. Oral spelling is typically preserved and, in some cases, typing remains intact.

9.2 Locus of neurological damage

In right-handers, apraxic agraphia is associated with damage to a left-hemisphere cortical network dedicated to the motor programming of handwriting movements. The major functional components of this neural network include posterior–superior parietal cortex (i.e. the region of the intraparietal sulcus), dorsolateral premotor cortex, and the supplementary motor area (SMA). Callosal lesions in right-handers may be accompanied by unilateral apraxic agraphia of the left hand.

9.3 Treatment

- *Goal.* To re-establish the ability to control hand movements necessary to write letters and words.
- *Task example(s).* Treatments for apraxic agraphia have not been well documented in the literature. When central spelling processes are intact, it may be possible to circumvent handwriting difficulties by using a keyboard for written communication. When copying skills are relatively preserved, treatment should include repeated

direct and delayed copying tasks to re-establish the ability to write letters and words. A task hierarchy should initially include deliberate and feedback-dependent writing to regain graphomotor control, with repeated productions to improve the automaticity of motor execution.

- *Expectation.* Limited evidence of improvement in apraxic agraphia is available. Several sessions of trial therapy should provide an indication of a patient's responsiveness to treatment.

10 Writing disorders due to impaired neuromuscular execution

Damage to motor systems involved in generating graphic innervatory patterns results in defective control of writing force, speed, and amplitude.

10.1 Distinctive features

Writing disorders due to impaired neuromuscular execution reflect the specific underlying disease or locus of damage. In the case of Parkinson's disease, micrographia results from reduced force and amplitude of movements of the hand. In patients with cerebellar dysfunction, movements of the pen may be disjointed and erratic. Patients with hemiparesis often have weakness and spasticity of the hand and limb that markedly impair their ability to write with the preferred hand.

10.2 Locus of neurological damage

Breakdown of graphomotor control in these neurological conditions suggests that the basal ganglia and the cerebellum, working in concert with dorsolateral premotor cortex and the SMA, are critically involved in the selection and implementation of kinematic parameters for writing movements.

10.3 Treatment

Although there are a variety of causes for impaired graphomotor control, there are relatively few rehabilitation reports. Successful rehabilitation strategies have been demonstrated for some patients with micrographia, and some with hemiparetic writing.

10.3.1 Treatment for micrographia

- *Goal.* To increase graphomotor control and thus improve legibility of handwriting.
- *Task example(s).* An increase in letter size may be accomplished by the provision of parallel lines or a template to facilitate the re-calibration of the range and force of movements for writing.

◆ *Expectation.* Improved letter formation is expected with provision of external cues (Oliveira *et al.* 1997). Maintenance of increased letter size is dependent upon establishing adequate self-monitoring abilities so that adjustments are made as legibility declines.

10.3.2 Hemiparetic writing

Writing with the nondominant hand can be mastered with practice. However, several investigators have reported on the use of various prosthetic devices to support the paralysed right hand during writing.

◆ *Goal.* To learn to write with the paretic dominant hand using a prosthesis.

◆ *Task example(s).* Using a custom-made splint with wheels that allows easy movement across the writing surface, the patient learns to move the affixed pen to form letters.

◆ *Expectation.* Some researchers have found that writing produced with the aided hemiparetic right hand proves to be linguistically superior to that written with the nondominant left hand (Brown *et al.* 1983; Leischner 1983; Lorch 1995).

11 Treatment schedule

11.1 Initiation of treatment

There are many reports of improved spelling and writing following agraphia treatment initiated long after onset of the neurological damage, suggesting that there is not a 'critical period' for the implementation of treatment.

11.2 Frequency of treatment

Reviews of the agraphia treatment literature reveal considerable variability in the frequency of treatment sessions that resulted in improved writing. Treatment schedules range from twice daily to once a week or even biweekly. However, daily practice is often incorporated in the treatment plan and appears to be important for bringing about enduring changes in writing. Therefore, regardless of the frequency of clinical treatment sessions, appropriate daily homework should accompany writing treatment protocols whenever possible.

11.3 Response to treatment

The likelihood that a patient will respond to a given treatment is based on several factors including the severity of the deficit, the status of the impaired and residual abilities, the nature of the neurological impairment, as well as the patient's motivation. In some cases, patients who appear to have similar functional deficits may respond differently to the same treatment. A patient's response to treatment may further clarify the nature of the writing impairment and subsequently prompt modification of procedures, provide guidance regarding the next stage of treatment or indicate that treatment should be terminated.

Acknowledgements

This work was supported in part by National Multipurpose Research and Training Center Grant DC-01409 from the National Institute on Deafness and Other Communication Disorders to The University of Arizona, and by the Cummings Foundation Endowment to the Department of Neurology at the University of Arizona.

Selective references

Aliminosa, D., McCloskey, M., Goodman-Schulman, R., and Sokol, S. (1993). Remediation of acquired dysgraphia as a technique for testing interpretations of deficits. *Aphasiology* 7, 55–69.

Beeson, P.M. (1999). Treating acquired writing impairment. *Aphasiology* 13, 367–86.

Beeson, P.M. and Hillis, A.E. (2001). Comprehension and production of written words. In *Language intervention strategies in adult aphasia*, 4th edn (ed. R. Chapey), pp. 572–604. Lippincott, Williams and Wilkins, Baltimore.

Beeson, P.M. and Rapcsak, S.Z. (2002). Clinical diagnosis and treatment of spelling disorders. In *Handbook on adult language disorders: integrating cognitive neuropsychology, neurology, and rehabilitation* (ed. A.E. Hillis), pp. 101–20. Psychology Press. Philadelphia.

Beeson, P.M., Rewega, M., Vail, S.M., and Rapcsak, S.Z. (2000). Problem-solving approach to agraphia treatment: interactive use of lexical and sublexical spelling routes. *Aphasiology* 14, 551–65.

Behrmann, M. (1987). The rites of righting writing: homophone mediation in acquired dysgraphia. *Cogn. Neuropsychol.* 4, 365–84.

Behrmann, M. and Byng, S. (1992). A cognitive approach to the neurorehabilitation of acquired language disorders. In *Cognitive neuropsychology in clinical practice* (ed. D.I. Margolin), pp. 327–50. Oxford University Press, New York.

Brown, J.W., Leader, B.J., and Blum, C.S. (1983). Hemiplegic writing in severe aphasia. *Brain Language* 19, 204–15.

Cardell, E.A. and Chenery, H.J. (1999). A cognitive neuropsychological approach to the assessment and remediation of acquired dysgraphia. *Language Testing* 16, 353–88.

Carlomagno, S. and Parlato, V. (1989). Writing rehabilitation in brain damaged adult patients: a cognitive approach. In *Cognitive approaches in neuropsychological rehabilitation* (ed. X. Seron and G. Deloche), pp. 175–209. Lawrence Erlbaum Associates, Hillsdale, New Jersey.

Carlomagno, S., Iavarone, A., and Colombo, A. (1994). Cognitive approaches to writing rehabilitation: From single case to group studies. In *Cognitive neuropsychology and cognitive rehabilitation* (ed. M.J. Riddoch and G.W. Humphreys), pp. 485–502. Lawrence Erlbaum Associates, Hillsdale New Jersey.

de Partz, M.-P. (1995). Deficit of the graphemic buffer: effects of a written lexical segmentation strategy. *Neuropsychol. Rehabil.* 5, 129–47.

Ellis, A.W. (1988). Normal writing processes and peripheral acquired dysgraphias. *Language Cogn. Processes* 3, 99–127.

Ellis, A.W. and Young, A.W. (1988). Spelling and writing. In *Human Cognitive Neuropsychology*, pp. 163–90. Psychology Press, Hove, East Sussex.

Goodglass, H., Kaplan, E., and Barresi, B. (2001). *Boston diagnostic examination for aphasia*, 3rd edn. Lippincott, Williams, and Wilkins, Philadelphia.

Goodman, R.A. and Caramazza, A. (1984). *The Johns Hopkins University dyslexia and dysgraphia batteries.* Published in Beeson, P.M. and Hillis, A.E. (2001). Comprehension and production of written words. In *Language intervention strategies in adult aphasia*, 4th edn (ed. R. Chapey), pp. 596–603. Lippincott, Williams and Wilkins, Baltimore.

Hatfield, F.M. (1983). Aspects of acquired dysgraphia and implication for re-education. *In Aphasia therapy* (ed. C. Code and D.J. Muller), pp. 157–69. Edward Arnold, London.

Hillis, A.E. (1989). Efficacy and generalization of treatment for aphasic naming errors. *Arch. Phys. Med. Rehabilitation* 70, 632–6.

Hillis, A.E. (1991). Effects of separate treatments for distinct impairments within the naming process. *Clin. Aphasiol.* 19, 255–65.

Hillis, A.E. and Caramazza, A. (1987). Model-driven treatment of dysgraphia. In *Clinical aphasiology* (ed. R.H. Brookshire), pp. 84–105. BRK Publishers, Minneapolis.

Hillis, A.E. and Caramazza, A. (1991). Mechanisms for accessing lexical representations for output: evidence from category-specific semantic deficit. *Brain Language* 40, 106–44.

Hillis, A.E. and Caramazza, A. (1994). Theories of lexical processing and rehabilitation of lexical deficits. In *Cognitive neuropsychology and cognitive rehabilitation* (ed. M.J. Riddoch and G.W. Humphreys), pp. 1–30. Lawrence Erlbaum Associates, Hillsdale, New Jersey.

Hillis Trupe, A.E. (1986). Effectiveness of retraining phoneme to grapheme conversion. In *Clinical aphasiology* (ed. R.H. Brookshire), pp. 163–71. BRK Publishers, Minneapolis.

Kaplan, E., Goodglass, H., and Weintraub, S. (2001). *Boston Naming Test*, 3rd edn. Lippincott, Williams, and Wilkins, Philadelphia.

Kay, J., Lesser, R., and Coltheart, M. (1992). *Psycholinguistic assessments of language processing in aphasia (PALPA).* Lawrence Erlbaum Associates, Hove, East Sussex.

Kertesz, A. (1982). *Western aphasia battery.* Grune and Stratton, New York.

Leischner, A. (1983). Side differences in writing to dictation of aphasics with agraphia: a graphic disconnection syndrome. *Brain Language* 18, 1–19.

Lorch, M.P. (1995). Laterality and rehabilitation: differences in left and right hand productions in aphasic agraphic hemiplegics. *Aphasiology* 9, 257–71.

Oliveira, R.M., Gurd, J.M., Nixon, P., Marshall, J.C., and Passingham, R.E. (1997). Micrographia in Parkinson's disease: the effect of providing external cues. *J. Neurol. Neurosurg. Psychiatry* 63, 429–33.

Pound, C. (1996). Writing remediation using preserved oral spelling: a case for separate output buffers. *Aphasiology* 10, 283–96.

Ramage, A., Beeson, P.M., and Rapcsak, S.Z. (1998). Dissociation between oral and written spelling: clinical characteristics and possible mechanisms, Presentation at the Clinical Aphasiology Conference, Ashville, North Carolina, June.

Rapcsak, S.Z. (1997). Disorders of writing. In *Apraxia: the neuropsychology of action* (ed. L.J.G. Rothi and K.M. Heilman), pp. 149–72. Psychology Press, Hove, East Sussex.

Rapcsak, S.Z. and Beeson, P.M. (2000). Agraphia. In *Aphasia and language: theory and practice* (ed. L.J.G. Rothi, B. Crosson, and S. Nadeau), pp. 184–220. Guilford Press, New York.

Rapcsak, S.Z. and Beeson, P.M. (2002). Neuroanatomical correlates of spelling and writing. In *Handbook on adult language disorders: integrating cognitive neuropsychology, neurology, and rehabilitation* (ed. A.E. Hillis), pp. 71–99. Psychology Press, Philadelphia.

Rapcsak, S.Z., Beeson, P.M., and Rubens, A.B. (1991). Writing with the right hemisphere. *Brain Language* 41, 510–30.

Roeltgen, D.P. (1993) Agraphia. In *Clinical neuropsychology*, 3rd edn (ed. K.M. Heilman and E. Valenstein), pp. 63–89. Oxford University Press, New York.

Wertz, R.T., Weiss, D.G., Aten, J.L., Brookshire, R.H., Garcia-Buñuel, L., Holland, A.L., Kurtzke, J.F., LaPointe, L.L., Milianti, F.J., Brannegan, R., Greenbaum, H., Marshall, R.C., Vogel, D., Carter, J., Barnes, N.S., and Goodman, R. (1986). Comparison of clinic, home, and deferred language treatment for aphasia. *Arch. Neurol.* **43**, 653–8.

Chapter 17

Assessment of executive function

Paul W. Burgess

1 Introduction

Executive function is probably the newest of the fields of neuropsychology. Although observations of patients showing symptoms of executive dysfunction have existed for over 150 years, and experimental investigation for at least half of that time, the area has only really become the focus of very widespread investigation in the last 20 years or so. And, since the translation of scientific findings into clinically useful techniques occurs relatively slowly, it is only recently that the experimental findings are being translated into procedures for clinical use. As a consequence, the practising clinician should take special care to follow the latest developments in this fast-moving field.

This chapter does not provide an exhaustive description of all the various tests of executive function available to the neuropsychologist since excellent summaries appear elsewhere (e.g. Lezak 1995; Spreen and Strauss 1998; Alderman and Burgess 2002). Instead, while we do briefly describe some of the most commonly used tests, the principal aim is to outline the philosophy of the assessment procedure, so that the reader can know what to look for, decide which tests to use, and understand the issues surrounding the possible choices of assessment procedure. This information is much harder to come by.

1.1 What are executive functions?

At the most basic level, executive functions are the abilities that enable a person to establish new behaviour patterns and ways of thinking, and to introspect upon them. This is required most in unfamiliar situations, where one doesn't know what to do, or in situations where established ways of behaving are no longer useful or appropriate. As such, the term 'executive function' refers to a whole range of adaptive abilities such as creative and abstract thought, introspection, and all the processes that enable a person to analyse what they want, how they might get it (i.e. form a plan, based often on recollections of past experience), and then carry that plan out. It is also widely accepted that executive functions play a critical part in complex social behaviour, such as understanding how others see us, being tactful, or deceitful. Therefore, there is probably no activity beyond the most routinized and practised ones that does not to some extent involve 'executive processing'. It is not clear, however, how much overlap there is between the processes underlying these various abilities. Identifying the processes and working out how they may relate to each other is the current focus of much exciting research, but we are just in the early stages.

These abilities are collectively referred to as 'executive functions' because it is believed that the region of the brain that supports them (the frontal lobes) operates in a 'supervisory' (Shallice 1988) or 'executive' (Pribram 1973) capacity over the rest of the brain. For many researchers, 'executive function' is synonymous with 'frontal lobe function'. However, the latter term is of little use to the practising clinician for two reasons.

- What is important clinically is the function that is impaired rather than the brain region that is damaged.

- Recent advances in cognitive neuroscience show that, whilst the frontal lobes play an important part in executive functions such as planning and organization of behaviour, the frontal lobe contribution is just one part of a wider network of brain involvement.

In the 1980s there was a move away from discussing 'frontal lobe function' towards use of the terms 'executive function' and 'dysexecutive symptoms' (to describe executive function impairments) in order to reflect this more function-oriented focus.

1.2 Symptoms of executive dysfunction

The 20 most commonly reported symptoms of executive dysfunction are shown in Table 17.1. This is by no means an exhaustive list, however, and there are also many other, generally less frequently encountered dysexecutive symptoms (e.g. utilization behaviour, alien hand sign).

Recent evidence suggests that at least some executive abilities may be impaired in neurological patients when others are not. The term 'dysexecutive syndrome', which is commonly used as shorthand to refer to executive function impairments, can therefore be misleading since it suggests that symptoms are invariably seen together. This is not the case. However, it is equally true to say that in normal clinical practice it is less common to see people with isolated problems than with clusters of them. There are probably two main reasons.

- Even apparently quite localized brain dysfunction is unlikely to affect only one brain system and, because of the highly interconnected nature of the brain, dysfunction in one region in any case can probably cause disruptions in others.

- Some researchers contend that there are some executive processes that are used in many situations (e.g. Duncan *et al.* 2000), e.g. those that govern attention and arousal, as well as others that are required in more specific situations, e.g. those requiring multitasking (Burgess *et al.* 2000).

1.3 The impact of executive dysfunction on everyday life

Even apparently quite mild deficits of executive function can have a devastating impact upon an individual's effectiveness in everyday life and their relationships with others.

Table 17.1 Frequency of 20 of the most common symptoms of executive dysfunction (adapted from Burgess and Robertson, 2002)

Symptom	Percentage reporting problem	
	Patients	Carers
Poor abstract thinking	17	21
Impulsivity	22	22
Confabulation	5	5
Planning	16	48
Euphoria	14	28
Poor temporal sequencing	18	25
Lack of insight	17	39
Apathy	20	27
Disinhibition (social)	15	23
Variable motivation	13	15
Shallow affect	14	23
Aggression	12	25
Lack of concern	9	26
Perseveration	17	26
Restlessness	25	28
Can't inhibit responses	11	21
Know–do dissociation	13	21
Distractibility	32	42
Poor decision-making	26	38
Unconcern for social rules	13	38

A key reason for this is the attributions that observers make about the causes of the behaviour they see. Many dysexecutive symptoms mimic exaggerated versions of behaviour that are sometimes seen in healthy people and therefore can easily be misunderstood. Take, for example, confabulation. All ordinary, healthy people at some time or another tell lies. This is a common event. So when a patient says something that is quite obviously untrue, it is easy for observers to assume that the patient is deliberately lying. Of course, this is not the case. Confabulation is caused by a problem with the cognitive control processes that govern recollection, leading to memories and thoughts becoming jumbled up with each other (see Burgess and Shallice 1996*b*). The patient can't help it. However, if one doesn't know this and has not seen confabulation before (as most spouses or relatives of neurological patients will not have), it is easy to make this mistake, and get irritated with the patient for 'lying' or 'making things up'. The same point can be made about many of the dysexecutive symptoms shown in

Table 17.1. Especially difficult to live with are the social changes such as lack of concern or increased aggressive reactions to troublesome situations. Relatives or partners might quite justifiably claim that these 'personality changes' mean that the patient 'is no longer the person she/he used to be'.

The non-social changes can also be a severe handicap, especially in the work situation. A good example is those patients who show relatively isolated multitasking deficits. These people may still be extremely intellectually gifted, with little or no (retrospective) memory, language, or other problems, and some are even very competent on most tests of executive function. However, for all reported cases in the literature, their return to work has been tragically unsuccessful, with employers complaining of tardiness and disorganization (see Burgess 2000 for review). Common complaints from the employers of these cases are that the patient starts many jobs but never completes any of them, and/or shows no awareness of the relative priorities of different jobs, treating the most trivial (e.g. the sticky tape needs replacing) as equally pressing as the most important (e.g. delivering an important letter to the company chairman). It is simply very difficult to work with someone who shows these sorts of symptoms—certainly more so in many contexts—than with a more predictable and obvious handicap (e.g. a language or visual impairment) for which compensatory methods exist and that can be readily understood by co-workers.

A further complication of executive dysfunction is that the associated problems are exactly the kinds of problems that interfere with learning new ways of behaving, or prevent patients from benefiting from therapy aimed at ameliorating other sorts of problems (e.g. physiotherapy). For this reason, combined with the typical lack of insight that accompanies these symptoms, dysexecutive problems present a real challenge for rehabilitation. (For further information see Burgess and Robertson, 2002.)

1.4 **Prognosis for executive deficits**

One of the reasons why the functions of the frontal lobes were described by a leading researcher over 30 years ago as a 'riddle' was that some apparently severe symptoms could resolve well in time, whereas other apparently milder problems could persist. This is just as true today: symptoms such as confabulation typically (but not always) resolve quite well on their own within a few weeks or months, but others (e.g. multitasking problems) when they persist beyond the initial stage of medical trauma are often best considered permanent handicaps requiring intervention before improvement will occur. We still do not understand why this should be the case, and this is an underresearched area. The wise clinician will freely admit this lack of knowledge to relatives, carers, or the patients themselves. There should be no embarassment in not knowing when there is nothing to know. Freely admitting that no one knows the answer has the advantage of removing the temptation to speculate whilst also avoiding seeming obscure or evasive.

2 Choosing the assessment approach

The ideal assessment would obviously attempt to assess all of the symptoms shown in Table 17.1, plus the less common signs of executive dysfunction (e.g. utilization behaviour, alien hand sign, subtle attentional changes). However, this is impractical in most clinical settings, and formal assessment measures do not yet exist for many of the symptoms. Moreover, relatively little is known about what many of the tests shown to be sensitive to frontal lobe lesions are actually measuring in these cases. (This is a theoretical problem that is far more complex than it seems at first.) One is left therefore with five choices of how to proceed:

- *Time.* Administer the greatest number of tests possible in the available time.
- *Psychometrics.* Base your choice of measures on test-based factors such as ease of use and cost, psychometric validity, how widely the tests are used, how often they have been used with a particular client group, etc.
- *Expectation.* Base assessment on what you expect to find, given knowledge of the medical history and/or previous assessments.
- *Observation.* Base assessment on symptoms already observed by carers or relatives.
- *Theory.* Adopt a particular theoretical stance and choose the tests that make most the sense according to it.

These methods are of different merit. Remarkably, perhaps, none is entirely meritless and, in practice, most experienced clinicians develop their own assessment procedure based on a personal weighting of these methods. In principle, this is appropriate. Too often, however, this choice has merely evolved haphazardly over time. Instead, the choice should be made deliberately and with good justification. If the same battery of tests is given to all clients, this choice should be reviewed regularly. The clinician should always be able to clearly articulate and defend the reasons behind his/her choice of procedures.

In practice, I have observed a further method of determining the assessment procedure: to just use whichever tests are most familiar and/or everyone else is using. This method might in some circumstances be most appropriate for students, but it would be dubious indeed for a qualified clinician, and this method will be considered no further.

Let us consider the legitimate approaches in turn.

2.1 Method 1. Time

This is not as unjustifiable as it might at first seem, for two reasons.

- As mentioned above, we know little about many of the traditional tests of executive function (e.g. Wisconsin Card Sorting Test, Stroop Test) or what they measure.
- The ecological validity of these tests (i.e. the extent to which they are indicators of real-world impairment) has not yet been clearly established. (It does, however, seem at present that the more modern tests designed to be more like real-life activities are often—but not always—better in this respect.)

Thus one solution to this problem is just to give as many tests as one can in the available time, in the hope of covering as many possible functions/situations as possible. The disadvantages of this approach are the following.

- As the number of tests administered rises, so does the likelihood of a false-positive result (unless the clinician statistically corrects for the number of tests administered, which is uncommon).

- Unless the clinician has at least some hypothesis about what he/she is measuring, it is difficult to know what might be usefully concluded from a task failure. Clinically, it is rarely sufficient to just baldly state 'this person failed this test', without further interpretation.

2.2 Method 2. Psychometrics

All people involved in the administration of psychometric tests should have at least some basic grounding in psychometric theory. This allows them to understand the relative merits of the measurement aspects of different tests, and to select accordingly. In particular, there may be times when some aspect of the psychometric dynamic of relative tests might strongly influence the clinician's choice, e.g. where parallel forms are required, where there is to be repeated testing using the same measure, or where various different people may make assessments on the same person.

In general, however, it is harder in the field of executive function to use psychometric values (e.g. test–retest and interrater reliability; interitem consistency, etc.) as a guide to test choice. This is because the tests are often measuring abilities such as response to novelty or strategy formation. These can subvert the theory behind traditional psychometrics, and render the values a poor guide to a test's actual clinical utility (see Burgess 1997 for more detail). In addition, there is another problem that is applicable to the use of most psychometric tests with pathological populations. This is that the construct validity of a task (i.e. the extent to which you are measuring what you intend to measure) alters with level of performance. Overall, these matters present a highly complex theoretical problem for someone trying to base their choice of assessment procedure upon psychometric values, especially when they are derived from the performance of a different population than the one you intend to test (e.g. healthy control subjects). In summary, *all other things being equal*, one should choose the test with the best psychometric validity. However, all other things are unlikely to often be equal.

2.3 Method 3. Expectation

If we knew more about what executive tests measure, this would probably be the most frequently appropriate single method. For success it does, however, rely upon at least four variables:

- The quality of the information, case history, or previous assessment that you have received.

- Your knowledge of the test's performance in different populations.
- How the test is affected by a variety of background variables (e.g. education, culture, age, etc.).
- The ecological validity of the task (i.e. how strongly you can make a prediction that your test measures the function that was observed to be impaired elsewhere).

This method therefore requires a high degree of knowledge and clinical judgement. This requirement should decrease as our knowledge of the performance of the tests and what they measure increases.

2.4 Method 4. Observation

Although the examinee should always be asked about the symptoms they notice since it is important to assess the patient's degree of insight and knowledge about their condition, it is unwise to base your assessment upon this report. Self-report of dysexecutive difficulties is notoriously inaccurate (e.g. Burgess and Robertson 2002). However, the reports of carers, relatives, or other people who know the examinee well can be very useful indeed, and should always be sought if possible.

The best witnesses are usually those who knew the person premorbidly, since *change* in behaviour is usually more instructive than comparisons of current behaviour with some population norm. This is important for executive function assessment since the behaviours under examination are often at the extreme of the range of behaviours that might be observed occasionally in the normal population. This is one of the important ways in which executive function assessment differs from assessment of other functions in neuropsychology. In, say, language assessment, or assessment of visuospatial skills, pathological symptoms (e.g. jargon aphasia, neglect) are rarely or never seen in the healthy normal population. However, many of the symptoms of executive dysfunction are seen occasionally in the healthy population, albeit perhaps under special circumstances, and in a milder form (e.g. confabulation (Burgess and Shallice 1996*b*), impulsivity, disinhibition). Since, therefore, it is often the extremity (i.e. severity, frequency) of the behavioural sign rather than its type that is at issue, it is important if possible to have an observer 'baseline' with which to compare current behaviour.

Once the clinician has collected the observations, however, he/she is faced with the challenge of interpreting them for the purposes of the examination procedure. There is no substitute for experience and knowledge in this respect. The job is made easier by some of the newer assessment procedures that are more like real-world situations, since one can ask the observer about situations in which the examinee experiences problems and then choose the closest test situations. However, for experienced examiners, more experimentally derived procedures also have their merits.

- Often the theory of how they work is more developed.
- They may be more specific in what they measure.
- The link with damage to certain brain regions may be more direct.

These factors can add up to a strong advantage if you have a clear idea what it is that you are looking for and have experience in interpreting the observations of others.

2.5 Method 5. Theory

All assessment and treatment has to start with some theory of what it is that is being studied, even if this is very basic. The assessment implications of all theories of executive function cannot be covered here. However a few of the leading ones will be selected as examples.

2.5.1 Single-process theories

These hold that damage to a single process or system is responsible for a number of different dysexecutive symptoms. An example is the theory of Cohen (e.g. Cohen *et al.* 1990). This holds that prefrontal cortex is used to represent 'context information', which is the 'information necessary to mediate an appropriate behavioural response' (Cohen *et al.* 1998, p. 196). Two functions of the prefrontal cortex may be effected by this system—active memory and behavioural inhibition—with both functions reflecting the operation of the context layer under different task conditions. Under the conditions of response competition the context module plays an inhibitory role by supporting the processing of task relevant information. But, when there is a delay until the execution of a response, the context module plays a role in memory by maintaining that information over time.

Following this theory, clinical assessment would include tests of response suppression (e.g. Hayling Test, Stroop) plus tests with a 'working memory' component (e.g. Wisconsin Card Sorting Test (WCST), Cambridge Neuropsychological Test Automated Battery (CANTAB) spatial working memory test).

2.5.2 Construct-led theories

Construct-led theories are those that propose a construct (i.e. a theoretical ability) such as 'working memory' or 'fluid intelligence' as a key function of the frontal lobe executive system.

Working memory theories   Two leading theorists in this area are Petrides and Goldman-Rakic.

- Petrides believes that the mid-dorsolateral prefrontal region (areas 9 and 46) supports a brain system 'in which information can be held on-line for monitoring and manipulation of stimuli' (Petrides 1998, p. 106). The mid-ventrolateral region, however, is used in explicit encoding and retrieval of information. Obvious suggested tests are therefore Petrides and Milner's (1982) Self-Ordered Pointing Test, and other memory tests that particularly stress explicit encoding and retrieval (e.g. recall of complex figures such as the Rey figure; recall of short stories or word lists).

- Goldman-Rakic's position is different in that she believes that the various different frontal lobe regions all perform a similar role in working memory, but that each processes a different type of information (Goldman-Rakic 1995). She suggests that dysfunction of this system can cause a variety of deficits on e.g. verbal fluency and Stroop tasks due to an inability to use working memory to initiate the correct response.

Duncan's theory of 'g' (e.g. Duncan et al. 1995, 2000)   Duncan suggests that the principal purpose of the frontal executive system is to support a single function that is used in many situations, called 'fluid intelligence' or Spearman's g. Of the commercially available tests, he believes Cattell's Culture-Fair Test and (by implication from his studies) the Six Element Test of the Behavioural Assessment of the Dysexecutive Syndrome (BADS) measure this function.

2.5.3 Multiple-process theories

These propose that the frontal lobe executive system consists of a number of components that typically work together in everyday actions.

Fuster's temporal integration framework (Fuster 1997)   This holds that the frontal lobe executive system performs three functions:

◆ working memory;

◆ set attainment;

◆ inhibition.

Suggested tasks are, therefore, WCST or CANTAB working memory tests, Brixton Test, Hayling Test, or Stroop.

Stuss's anterior attentional functions (e.g. Stuss et al. 1995; Stuss and Alexander 2000)   The focus of Stuss et al.'s theoretical approach is attention. They propose seven different attentional functions. The closest clinical test is probably the Test of Everyday Attention (TEA).

Shallice's supervisory attentional system (e.g. Norman and Shallice 1986; Shallice 1988; Shallice and Burgess 1991a,b, 1996; Burgess et al. 2000)   This is one of the longest established and best known theories. In this model, the frontal lobes support a cognitive system known as the supervisory attentional system (SAS). This plays a part in at least eight different processes, each of which may be impaired in isolation:

◆ working memory;

◆ monitoring;

◆ rejection of schema;

◆ spontaneous schema generation;

◆ adoption of processing mode;

◆ goal-setting;

◆ delayed intention marker realization;

◆ episodic memory retrieval.

On these grounds, and as the result of a study that examined the relationship between symptoms in everyday life and executive test performance, Burgess *et al.* (1998) recommend that *at the very least* an assessment of a dysexecutive patient should include the following.

◆ A general measure of inhibitory abilities (e.g. Hayling Test; however this function is probably also measured to varying degrees by many other tests, e.g. verbal fluency, Trail-Making).

◆ Measures of executive memory abilities both in the short-term (i.e. working memory tests) and long-term (i.e. accuracy of episodic recollection). Suggested tests would be WCST; Brixton Test; story, figure, and word list recall; and also observation of real-life ability to recollect events accurately.

◆ A measure of multitasking ability, e.g. Six Element Test from the BADS; Multiple Errands Test (Shallice and Burgess 1991*a*; Burgess *et al.* 1996*b*, 2000; Alderman *et al.* in press).

However, Burgess *et al.* (1998) make two further points.

◆ Neuropsychological tests of executive function do not measure well many of the emotional changes that can be part of the dysexecutive syndrome (e.g. euphoria, apathy). The formal tests need therefore to be supplemented by more general observation, preferably using a structured or semistructured interview, perhaps based around a symptom checklist or questionnaire such as the Dysexecutive Questionnaire (DEX; Burgess *et al.* 1996*a*) from the BADS test battery.

◆ Since many impairments can be seen in isolation, a true assessment will be as comprehensive as possible—the list above could be considered only as a basic screening assessment. For instance, one might also wish to supplement it routinely with measures of planning (e.g. Zoo-Map test of the BADS; abstract reasoning and judgement (e.g. proverb interpretation, cognitive estimates, or similar); initiation (e.g. Hayling Test section 1); problem-solving and strategy formation (e.g. Action Program and Key Search tests from the BADS); rule attainment and following (e.g. Brixton Test).

2.5.4 Single-symptom theories

These are theories of specific symptoms, such as confabulation (e.g. Burgess and Shallice 1996*b*; Burgess and McNeil 1999) or multitasking deficits (e.g. Burgess *et al.* 2000). In general, however, there are not tests specifically marketed to measure single symptoms. Clinicians therefore typically just make observations, or copy an experimental method.

3 Types of executive function test

The perfect test for most clinical applications would probably have the following characteristics (in addition to those that would be desirable in any psychometric test):

◆ perfect, and known correspondence to everyday life impairment;

◆ strong proven link to operation of one particular brain region or system;

◆ well understood psychometric dynamics;

◆ comprehensive theory as to what the test measures.

However as can be inferred from the discussions above, there is currently no test that could be said to have all these characteristics. Take for instance, probably the best-known executive test: the Wisconsin Card Sorting Task (WCST). This test was not originally designed for use with neurological patients (Berg 1948). Impairment of dorsolateral prefrontal lesioned patients was first demonstrated by Milner (1963), but there are few replications of this finding (see Stuss *et al.* 2000 for possible explanations). More positively, there is some early evidence about its relationship with everyday life impairments (Burgess *et al.* 1998), and there are various theories about what the test measures.

Similarly, the Stroop test, although widely used for the assessment of executive functions in neurological patients, was not designed with this purpose in mind. Moreover, in my opinion there is only one convincing demonstration of its sensitivity to frontal lesions (Perret 1974), and one convincing failure to replicate (Shallice 1982). There is disagreement about what the test measures (see MacLeod 1991), although there are some theories that have been made relevant to the assessment of executive functions, as outlined above. Moreover, there is little information that would allow one to predict from test impairment what deficits in real life might be expected.

Some of these shortcomings no doubt stem from the fact that the procedures were not designed with neuropsychological assessment in mind. In recognition of this situation, there have recently been tests invented for this specific purpose (e.g. BADS battery, Hayling and Brixton tests, CANTAB battery). Due to their newness, these tests have not, of course, yet been thoroughly put to the test of time (although there has been considerable work using the CANTAB in different populations), and it is possible that they will turn out not to fulfil the criteria above in any greater fashion than the older tests. However they do start with the advantage of being purpose-built.

3.1 Specificity and sensitivity

The *specificity* of a task refers to the degree to which a test measures the particular process or function of interest compared with other processes or functions that are not intended to be measured. The *sensitivity* of a task in this context refers to the degree to which any cognitive impairment can cause impairment on the task. There is some evidence that the different executive tasks differ greatly along these dimensions. For instance, the Cognitive Estimates Test does not seem to be particularly sensitive to any kind of neurological dysfunction *per se* (Burgess *et al.* 1998), but it does show consistent correlations with specific symptoms (e.g. fantastic confabulation), which suggests that it has good specificity. By contrast, the WCST appears to be more generally sensitive to cognitive decline, as well as to dysexecutive problems (e.g. Stuss *et al.* 2000). There is not room here for a discussion of the specificity and sensitivity of every test. However the clinician should consider matching the test to the clinical question under consideration. Using the current examples, for instance, the Cognitive Estimates test is probably not the best choice as a general screening measure for dysexecutive problems. However, its ecological validity is excellent and, if the clinical question instead concerns whether a patient has a specific executive problem rather than more general cognitive dysfunction, then the test is well suited to that application.

In many clinical settings the ideal test would have a combination of both characteristics, i.e.:

◆ sensitivity to a range of executive problems;

◆ relative insensitivity to non-executive cognitive impairments.

This compromise is generally closest in those tests that have been shown to be impaired in group studies of frontally lesioned patients compared with patients whose lesions were elsewhere in the brain (e.g. Hayling and Brixton Tests, Burgess and Shallice 1996*a,c*, 1997). Some tests appear to be both locally specific and more generally sensitive. For instance, impairment on the Six Element Test (a test of multitasking ability; see below) has been demonstrated in neurological patients with frontal lobe lesions who show no impairment on other executive function tests (e.g. Shallice and Burgess 1991*a*). However, this type of test is also more generally sensitive to executive (and to a lesser extent non-executive) impairments (Burgess *et al.* 2000). This combination of characteristics can make a test particularly useful in a wide range of settings. However, once a patient has failed a task, it generally requires that one should consider performances on other tasks in its interpretation (using this example, for instance, to find out whether the locus of the problem is a pure multitasking failure or, for instance, a more basic memory problem that prevents the examinee from learning the task rules).

3.2 Summary

Assessment of executive functions is probably the most technically and theoretically complex aspect of neuropsychological assessment. Executive test scores should always be administered in the context of a wider neuropsychological assessment since executive test performance can be affected by dysfunction in other cognitive systems (e.g. memory, etc.). The clinician's choice of tests and procedure should be made with careful consideration of the factors outlined above and, if not made on a case-by-case basis, they should be reviewed regularly.

Executive function as a subject area is one of the newest and fastest developing in neuropsychology, and there are still many gaps in our knowledge. However, since even relatively mild executive dysfunction has repeatedly been shown to greatly affect the long-term outcome of rehabilitation and recovery, any neuropsychological assessment is not complete without at least a basic evaluation of executive function abilities. New procedures and tests are appearing at a rapid rate. The assessment professional would therefore be wise to be circumspect when interpreting executive test scores, and make every attempt to benefit from the latest developments in the area as they appear.

4 Description of some key tests

There are many tests of executive function. A brief description of a few of the most commonly used is given in Sections 4.1–4.11. However, lack of inclusion in this list should not be seen as a failure of endorsement. There are a number of tests (e.g. the Test of Everyday Attention; Rey Complex Figure Recall) that could be seen as falling under the heading of 'executive function' but that have not been included since they also fall under other topic areas (e.g. attention, memory). There are also other methods that combine tests or aspects of them to increase specificity or sensitivity (e.g. the Frontal Lobe Score, see Ettlin *et al.* 2000; Wildgruber *et al.* 2000) and are worthy of consideration. Excellent summaries of the range of executive tests can be found in Lezak (1995) and Spreen and Strauss (1998) and, where publisher information etc. is not given below, it can be found in these texts. It should be borne in mind that dysexecutive problems demonstrate themselves as impairment on a wide range of neuropsychological tests, not just those specifically aimed at measuring 'executive function', so the *manner* of failure on a test can also be instructive.

4.1 Behavioural Assessment of the Dysexecutive Syndrome (BADS)

- *Original reference.* Wilson *et al.* (1998). Commercially available from various distributors worldwide. For details contact the Thames Valley Test Company, 7–9 The Green, Flempton, Suffolk, IP28 6EL UK. (tvtc@msn.com)

- *Test description.* The BADS is a test battery aimed at predicting everyday difficulties arising from the dysexecutive syndrome. It contains six tests (and a questionnaire (the DEX) that has two versions, one to be filled in by the patient and one by an independent rater, which can be used as the basis for a semistructured interview). The six different tests (Rule Shift, Action Program, Key Search, Temporal Judgement, Zoo-Map, and Six Elements Test) are designed to have high ecological validity, and scores from the tests can be combined to give an overall executive function measure that can be compared with measures of cognitive functioning.

4.2 Cambridge Neuropsychological Test Automated Battery (CANTAB)

- *Original reference.* Robbins *et al.* (1994).

- *Test description.* A computerized battery of 13 tests that evaluate more than executive functions alone. However, it contains two tests that are particularly oriented towards executive function assessment: ID/ED Shift and the Stockings of Cambridge test, which are developments of the WCST and Tower of London (Shallice 1982) tests, respectively.

4.3 Cognitive Estimates Test

♦ *Original reference.* Shallice and Evans (1978).

♦ *Test description.* Patients are asked 15 questions about everyday magnitudes where no rote knowledge or routine method seems available. Axelrod and Millis (1994) issued a shorter version (10 questions) adapted to the North-American population.

♦ *Scoring method.* Answers rated as normal, quite extreme, extreme, and very extreme according to how much they vary from the estimates of a control group.

4.4 Hayling and Brixton tests

♦ *Original references*

—Hayling: Burgess and Shallice (1996*c*).

—Brixton: Burgess and Shallice (1996*a*). Commercially available from various distributors worldwide; for details contact the Thames Valley Test Company, 7–9 The Green, Flempton, Suffolk, IP28 6EL UK. (tvtc@msn.com)

♦ *Test description.*

—Hayling: Patients have to complete 30 sentences from which the last word was omitted. In the first half (initiation condition), they complete the sentences with a word that makes sense. In the second half (inhibition condition) they have to supply a word that makes no sense in the context of the sentence (e.g. 'London is a very busy *banana*').

—Brixton: A nonverbal test of set attainment and rule detection. The patient is shown a 56-page stimulus book, one page at a time. All pages contain 10 circles in the same basic array (see Fig. 17.1(a)). Only one circle is filled on each page and the patient has to predict where the next filled position will be, based on what they have seen in the previous pages.

♦ *Scoring method.*

—Hayling: Sum of all response latencies for part 1; sum of all response latencies and error score for part 2.

—Brixton: Total number of errors (maximum is 54).

4.5 Multiple Errands Test (MET)

♦ *Original reference.* Shallice and Burgess (1991*a*).

♦ *Test description.* The test with probably the most obvious ecological validity in current use, this is a formalized version of a shopping task. It is conducted in a real shopping centre or mall, so a specific version has to be adapted to the local circumstances available to the clinician. There is also a version that can be carried out in most hospital environments (Knight *et al.* 2002). Appears to be highly sensitive both to brain damage in general, and to specific dysexecutive problems. Details of how to set up the test for your own local environment can be obtained from: Dr Nick Alderman, Consultant Clinical Neuropsychologist, Kemsley Brain Injury Rehabilitation Centre, St. Andrew's Hospital, Billing Road, Northampton, NN1 5DG, UK. (See also Alderman *et al.* 2003.)

◆ *Scoring method.* A number of different types of error are collected: rule-breaks; social rule-breaks; interpretation failures; inefficiencies; task failures.

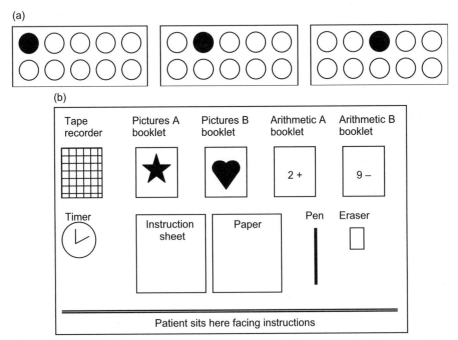

Fig. 17.1 (a) Sample sequence from the Brixton Test. Here one might reasonably expect the filled circle to be at number 4 on the next page (on the testing booklet, circles are numbered from 1 to 10 on each array to make it easier to refer to their position). (b) Materials used for the Six Elements Test.

4.6 **Proverbs Test**

◆ *Original reference.* Gorham (1956).

◆ *Test description.* Patients are asked to recognize and interpret a certain number of proverbs (e.g. 'Rome wasn't built in a day') in two different ways. In the first part, they must provide free verbal interpretations of each proverb. In the second part, they must choose one out of four possible answers provided for each proverb.

◆ *Scoring method.* Free verbal interpretations are scored on a 3-point scale according to their degree of 'concreteness'. In the multiple-choice test, there is only one correct response for each proverb (the other three are either wrong, partial, or concrete).

4.7 Six Elements Test (SET)

◆ *Original reference.* Shallice and Burgess (1991*a*).

◆ *Test description.* A modified version of this multitasking test for general clinical use (Burgess *et al.* 1996*b*) is commercially available as part of the BADS battery (see Section 4.1). Additionally, there are other versions of this test that have recently been developed by groups in Cambridge and Toronto, plus more extensive versions by the original authors (Burgess *et al.* 2000). Patients have 10 minutes to do three tasks (dictation, arithmetic, and picture naming; see Fig. 17.1(b)). Each task has two parts, called A and B. The two parts of each task cannot be carried out one after the other (for instance, dictation A immediately followed by dictation B, or vice versa). There are more items in the six tasks than can possibly be completed in the time allowed, so the aim is to do a bit of each part of each task within the 10 minutes and thus patients have to plan their time accordingly. The original, and some later versions also use weightings for certain items which gives them particular significance, but this is not used in the most widely used BADS subtest version of the SET.

◆ *Scoring method.* In the BADS version, a profile score is calculated from the number of tasks attempted minus the number of tasks where rule breaks were made. A further point is deducted if the maximum time on any one task is more than 271 seconds.

4.8 Stroop Test

◆ *Original reference.* Stroop (1935).

◆ *Test description.* In the Victoria version, patients are presented with three cards, each with a different stimulus: 24 coloured dots where one is asked to name their colour; 24 common words where one has to name the colour of the ink in which the words are printed; and 24 colour names, where the task is again to name the colour of the ink. There are other versions, for instance, using an additional card on which words are printed in black ink. Another version includes only two cards, both with colour names printed in different colour inks (first card, names are read; second card, the ink colour is named).

◆ *Scoring method.* For each card, the time to complete the task and the number of errors are recorded. The amount of time required for the interference card (name ink colour) is typically compared to the amount of time required in the other conditions(s).

4.9 Trail Making Test

◆ *Original reference.* Originally, the test was one of the Performance subtests of the US Army Individual Test Battery, published in 1944. Earliest use with neurological patients: Armitage (1946).

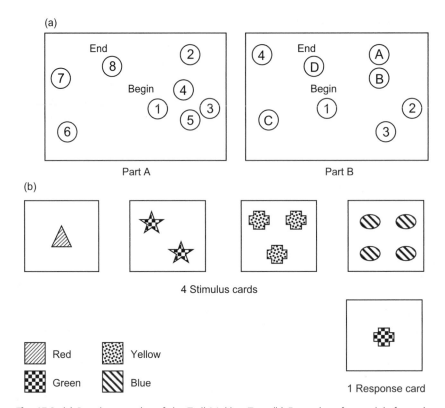

Fig. 17.2 (a) Practice samples of the Trail Making Test. (b) Examples of materials from the Wisconsin Card Sorting Test.

- *Test description.* In part A, examinees draw lines to connect consecutively numbered circles from 1 to 25 on a sheet of paper. Part B follows the same principle but this time the lines drawn must connect consecutively numbered and lettered circles (also 25 circles) by alternating between the two types of sequences (see Fig. 17.2(a)). There are various forms of this test.
- *Scoring method.* There is a separate score for Part A and Part B, which is the amount of seconds taken to complete each task.

4.9 Verbal Fluency Test

- *Original reference.* Thurstone (1938).
- *Test description.* Patients are asked to say as many words as they can, beginning with the letters F, A, and S (usually 1 minute per letter). They are asked not to give proper nouns or alternative forms of the same word (e.g. 'made' and 'making'). There are many alternate versions: written; semantic categories (e.g. animals); different letters.
- *Scoring method.* Total number of correct words; number of correct words for each letter.

4.11 **Wisconsin Card Sorting Test**

- *Original reference.* Milner (1963). (Originally invented by Berg 1948.)

- *Test description.* The patients sort 128 response cards under four stimulus cards according to colour, form, and number (see Fig. 17.2(b)). The aim is to work out the sorting category according to feedback from the examiner. Nelson (1976) introduced a shorter version with 48 cards, quicker shifts, and more feedback to the examinee.

- *Scoring method.* Number of categories achieved; total number of errors; nonperseverative errors; perseverative errors (definitions vary).

Acknowledgements

Paul Burgess is supported by Wellcome Trust grant ref: 049241/Z/96/Z/WRE/HA/JAT. I am grateful to Laure Coates, who gave valuable help with this manuscript.

Selective references

Alderman, N. and Burgess, P. W. (2002). Assessment and rehabilitation of the dysexecutive syndrome. In *Handbook of neurological rehabilitation*, 2nd edn (ed. R. Greenwood, T.M. McMillan, M.P. Barnes, and C.D. Ward). Psychology Press, Hove, East Sussex.

Alderman, N, Burgess, P.W., Knight, C., and Henman, C. (2003). Ecological validity of a simplified version of the multiple errands shopping test. *J. Int. Neuropsychol. Soc.* **9**, 31–44.

Armitage, S.G. (1946). An analysis of certain psychological tests used for the evaluation of brain injury. *Psychol. Monogr.* **60**, 91–6.

Axelrod, B.N. and Millis, S.R. (1994). Preliminary standardisation of the Cognitive Estimation Test. *Assessment* **1**, 269–74.

Berg, E.A. (1948). A simple objective technique for measuring flexibility in thinking. *J. Gen. Psychol.* **39**, 15–22.

Burgess, P.W. (1997). Theory and methodology in executive function research. In *Methodology of frontal and executive function* (ed. P. Rabbitt), pp. 81–116. Psychology Press, Hove, East Sussex.

Burgess, P.W. (2000). Strategy application disorder: the role of the frontal lobes in human multitasking. *Psychol. Res.* **63**, 279–88.

Burgess, P.W. and McNeil, J.E. (1999). Content-specific confabulation. *Cortex* **35**, 163–82.

Burgess, P.W. and Robertson, I.H. (2002). Principles of the rehabilitation of executive function. In *Principles of frontal lobe function* (ed. D.T. Stuss and R. Knight), pp. 557–72, Oxford University Press, Oxford.

Burgess, P.W. and Shallice, T. (1996a). Bizarre responses, rule detection and frontal lobe lesions. *Cortex* **32**, 241–60.

Burgess, P.W. and Shallice, T. (1996b). Confabulation and the control of recollection. *Memory* **4**, 359–411.

Burgess, P.W. and Shallice, T. (1996c). Response suppression, initiation and strategy use following frontal lobe lesion. *Neuropsychologia* **34**, 263–76.

Burgess, P.W. and Shallice, T. (1997). *The Hayling and Brixton Tests*. Thames Valley Test Company, Flempton.

Burgess, P.W., Alderman, N., Emslie, H., Evans, J.J., and Wilson, B.A. (1996a). The dysexecutive questionnaire. In *Behavioural assessment of the dysexecutive syndrome* (ed. B.A. Wilson, N. Alderman, P.W. Burgess, H. Emslie, and J.J. Evans). Thames Valley Test Company, Bury St. Edmunds.

Burgess, P.W., Alderman, N., Emslie, H., Evans, J.J., Wilson, B.A., and Shallice, T. (1996*b*). The simplified six element test. In *Behavioural assessment of the dysexecutive syndrome* (ed. B.A. Wilson, N. Alderman, P.W. Burgess, H. Emslie, and J.J. Evans). Thames Valley Test Company, Bury St. Edmunds.

Burgess, P.W., Alderman, N., Evans, J., Emslie, H., and Wilson, B.A. (1998). The ecological validity of tests of executive function. *J. Int. Neuropsychol. Soc.* **4**, 547–58.

Burgess, P.W., Veitch, E., Costello, A., and Shallice, T. (2000). The cognitive and neuroanatomical correlates of multitasking. *Neuropsychologia* **38**, 848–63.

Cohen, J.D., Dunbar, K., and McClelland, J.L. (1990). On the control of automatic processes: a parallel distributed processing account of the Stroop effect. *Psychol. Rev.* **97**, 332–61.

Cohen, L.D., Braver, T.S., and O'Reilly, R.C. (1998). A computational approach to prefrontal cortex, cognitive control, and schizophrenia: recent developments and current challenges. In *The prefrontal cortex: executive and cognitive functions* (ed. A.C. Roberts, T.W. Robbins, and L. Weiskrantz), pp. 195–200. Oxford University Press, Oxford.

Duncan, J., Burgess, P.W., and Emslie, H. (1995). Fluid intelligence after frontal lobe lesions. *Neuropsychologia* **33**, 261–8.

Duncan, J., Seitz, R. J., Kolodny, J., Bor, D., Herzog, H., Ahmed, A., Newell, F.N., and Emslie, H. (2000). A neural basis for intelligence. *Science* **289**, 457–60.

Ettlin, T.M., Kischka, U., Beckson, M., Gaggiotti, M., Rauchfleisch, U., and Benson, D.F. (2000). The frontal lobe score: part II: construction of a mental status of frontal systems. *Clin. Rehabil.* **14**, 260–71.

Fuster, J.M. (1997). *The prefrontal cortex: anatomy, physiology and neuropsychology of the frontal lobe*, 3rd edn. Lippincott-Raven, Philadelphia.

Goldman-Rakic, P.S. (1995). Architecture of the prefrontal cortex and the central executive. *Ann. NY Acad. Sci.* **769**, 212–20.

Gorham, D.R. (1956). A Proverbs Test for clinical and experimental use. *Psychol. Rep.* **1**, 1–12.

Knight, C., Alderman, N., and Burgess, P.W. (2002). Development of a simplified version of the multiple errands test for use in hospital settings. *Neuropsychological Rehabilitation* **12**, 231–55.

Lezak, M.D. (1995). *Neuropsychological assessment*, 3rd edn. Oxford: Oxford University Press, Oxford.

MacLeod, C.M. (1991). Half a century of research on the Stroop effect: an integrative review. *Psychol. Bull.* **109**, 163–203.

Milner, B. (1963). Effects of different brain lesions on card sorting. *Arch. Neurol.* **9**, 100–10.

Nelson, H.E. (1976). A modified card sorting test sensitive to frontal lobe defects. *Cortex* **12**, 313–24.

Norman, D.A. and Shallice, T. (1986). Attention to action: willed and automatic control of behaviour. In *Consciousness and Self-regulation*, Vol. 4 (ed. R.J. Davidson, G.E. Schwartz, and D. Shapiro). Plenum Press: New York.

Perret, E. (1974). The left frontal lobe in man and the suppression of habitual responses in verbal categorical behaviour. *Neuropsychologia* **12**, 323–30.

Petrides, M. (1994). Frontal lobes and working memory: evidence from investigations of the effects of cortical excisions in nonhuman primates. In *Handbook of neuropsychology*, Vol. 9 (ed. F. Boller and J. Grafman), pp. 59–82. Elsevier, Amsterdam.

Petrides, M. (1998). Specialized systems for the processing of mnemonic information within the primate frontal cortex. In *The prefrontal cortex: executive and cognitive functions* (ed. A.C. Roberts, T.W. Robbins, and L. Weiskrantz), pp. 103–16. Oxford University Press, Oxford.

Petrides, M. and Milner, B. (1982). Deficits on subject-ordered tasks after frontal- and temporal-lobe lesions in man. *Neuropsychologia* **20**, 249–62.

Pribram, K.H. (1973). The primate frontal cortex—executive of the brain. In *Psychophysiology of the frontal lobes* (ed. K.H. Pribram and A.R. Luria), pp. 293–314. Academic Press, New York.

Robbins, T.W., James, M., Owen, A.M., Lange, K.W., Lees, A.J., Leigh, P.N., Marsden, C.D., Quinn, N.P., and Summers, B.A. (1994). CANTAB: a factor analytic study of a large sample of normal elderly volunteers. *Dementia* 5, 266–81.

Shallice, T. (1982). Specific impairments of planning. *Phil. Trans. R. Soc. London B* 298, 199–209.

Shallice, T. (1988). *From neuropsychology to mental structure.* Cambridge University Press, New York.

Shallice, T. and Burgess, P.W. (1991*a*). Deficits in strategy application following frontal lobe damage in man. *Brain* 114, 727–41.

Shallice, T. and Burgess, P.W. (1991*b*). Higher-order cognitive impairments and frontal lobe lesions in man. In *Frontal lobe function and dysfunction* (ed. H.S. Levin, H.M. Eisenberg, and A.L. Benton), pp. 125–38. Oxford University Press, New York.

Shallice, T. and Burgess, P. W. (1996). The domain of supervisory processes and the temporal organisation of behaviour. *Phil. Trans. R. Soc. London B* 351, 1405–12.

Shallice, T. and Evans, M. (1978). The involvement of the frontal lobes in cognitive estimation. *Cortex* 14, 294–303.

Spreen, O. and Strauss, E. (1998). *A compendium of neuropsychological tests*, 2nd edn. Oxford University Press, Oxford.

Stroop, J.R. (1935). Studies of interference in serial verbal reaction. *J. Exp. Psychol.* 18, 643–62.

Stuss, D.T. and Alexander, M.P. (2000). Executive functions and the frontal lobes: a conceptual view. *Psychol. Res.* 63, 289–98.

Stuss, D.T., Shallice, T., Alexander, M.P., and Picton, T.W. (1995). A mulitidisciplinary approach to anterior attentional functions. *Ann. NY Acad. Sci.* 769, 191–211.

Stuss, D.T., Toth, J.P., Franchi, D., Alexander, M.P., Tipper, S., and Craik, F.I.M. (1999). Dissociation of attentional processes in patients with focal frontal and posterior lesions. *Neuropsychologia* 37, 1005–27.

Stuss, D.T., Levine, B., Alexander, M.P., Hong, J., Palumbo, C., Hamer, L., Murphy, K.J., and Izukawa, D. (2000). Wisconsin Card Sorting Test performance in patients with focal frontal and posterior brain damage: effects of lesion location and test structure on separable cognitive processes. *Neuropsychologia* 38, 388–402.

Thurstone, L.L. (1938). *Primary mental abilities.* Chicago University Press, Chicago.

Wildgruber, D., Kischka, U., Fassbender, K., and Ettlin, T.M. (2000). The frontal lobe score: part II: evaluation of its clinical utility. *Clin. Rehabil.* 14, 272–8.

Wilson, B.A., Alderman, N., Burgess, P.W., Emslie, H., and Evans, J.J. (1996). *Behavioural Assessment of the Dysexecutive Syndrome (BADS).* Thames Valley Test Company, Bury St. Edmunds.

Wilson, B.A., Evans, J.J., Emslie, H., Alderman, N., and Burgess, P. (1998). The development of an ecologically valid test for assessing patients with a dysexecutive syndrome. *Neuropsychol. Rehabil.* 8 (3), 213–28.

Chapter 18

The natural recovery and treatment of executive disorders

Andrew D. Worthington

1 Introduction

Consider a typical household at breakfast time, and it becomes easy to appreciate the organ-izational or executive skills that we normally take for granted. To prepare breakfast one needs to decide what to eat; to search for the relevant food items; recall how to boil an egg, make toast, or fry bacon; and carry out the steps in sequence so that everything is cooked safely and is ready to eat at the same time. During this activity other aspects of the environment are very probably being monitored too: keeping a check on the time; perhaps listening to the radio or television news, while simultaneously trying to stop the children squabbling and ensuring they are ready for school; mentally preparing for an important meeting at work; or trying to anticipate whether you will have time visit the bank in your lunch break. As if this were not complex enough, a barrage of irrelevant stimuli assault the senses—an irritating advertisement on the radio, a stray dog barking at the postman, a neighbour trying to start their car. All this information is processed, evaluated, and then discarded or accommodated within on-going behaviour. The ability to carry out such naturalistic activities successfully requires the coordinated and regulated implementation of many cognitive operations, especially those that have come to be associated with the term executive functioning. These include skills such as goal setting, planning, action initiation, self-monitoring, and behavioural inhibition. Disruption to any of these underlying processes as a result of brain injury produces characteristically impaired performance on many complex tasks that are fundamental to daily living. (see Chapter 17).

Consequently, treatment of executive functioning may be not only the most important part of an individual's rehabilitation, but also the most difficult, affecting the highest levels of cognitive ability, awareness, and self-regulation. If intervention is undertaken successfully, a person's life may be transformed in a manner more familiar to transplant surgeons than to psychologists. Effective treatment of severe executive disorder can enable a person to sustain a degree of employment, leisure activity, and family integrity previously inaccessible to them. In contrast, persistent dysexecutive problems may render an otherwise intelligent individual unable to undertake even the most rudimentary of everyday activities.

For practitioners, three facts make rehabilitation of executive skills particularly problematic.

- The manifestations of executive dysfunction are diverse, affecting cognition, mood, and behaviour.

- The problems are not readily encapsulated in the manner of traditional psychological assessment.

- There is no consensus regarding a conceptual or methodological approach to either investigation or treatment.

Effective rehabilitation depends on the therapist's skill in overcoming these fundamental difficulties. This chapter is intended to assist by providing an overview of the context and content of the management of executive dysfunction. Traditional approaches to this field tend to be structured in terms of various intervention types (Sohlberg *et al.* 1993; Evans 2001). In deliberate contrast, this chapter is organized around *a basic conceptual framework of normal executive functioning, and disorders that occur at each stage of the processing continuum are addressed in turn*. This is not a 'cookbook' approach to treatment, and its coverage is certainly not exhaustive, but the reader will find that this structure permits systematic discussion of practical intervention strategies for each of the most common executive dysfunctions. Repetition of interventions is limited to cross-references. The chapter has been organized pragmatically to help clinicians who are typically faced with problems and want to know what methods are available to manage the difficulties presented.

2 Natural recovery of executive disorders

Disorders of executive functioning are amongst the most persistent sequelae of brain injury. Paradoxically, they are often difficult to identify in hospital, due to the absence of appropriately skilled observers, the presence of ward routine, and the limited behavioural demands on patients. Furthermore, when they are apparent, executive disorders often exclude people from rehabilitation, leading to overly pessimistic prognoses (but beware the naïve optimism of the orthopaedic surgeon!). Finally, the manifestations of executive dysfunction are typically misunderstood in the community, with the result that many people fall by the wayside or come to the attention of psychiatric or forensic services. Many of the personality changes that follow serious brain damage are attributable to disorders of executive functioning. It is these changes, rather than physical or specific cognitive deficits, that cause long-term breakdown of relationships and status. The true severity of executive dysfunction may be apparent only after formal rehabilitation has ended and a person has returned home or back to work. However, significant improvements in everyday functioning can be made, even several years after the original injury, largely through compensatory interventions.

Recovery potential for executive disorders (see box, p. 324) is influenced by many factors. Important positive signs are:

- brain injury occurring in adulthood rather than childhood;

- single-incident brain injury without complications;

- circumscribed rather than diffuse cerebral involvement;
- motivation to participate in treatment (note that this is not the same as motivation to go home or return to work, which can be counterproductive);
- self-awareness of problems in thinking or personality;
- absence of severe behaviour disorders;
- no previous history of alcohol or substance abuse;
- no premorbid psychiatric history;
- supportive social and family circumstances.

Investigating rehabilitation potential for executive disorders

- Establish what organic basis there is for an executive disorder, before considering nonorganic factors.
- Certain neuropathology is especially likely to cause executive disorders: traumatic brain injury; herpes simplex encephalitis; aneurysms of the anterior communicating artery; certain tumours; dementia of frontotemporal type; subcortical infarcts involving the thalamus or internal capsule.
- Severe executive dysfunction in everyday life can occur in the absence of structural frontal lobe pathology on a magnetic resonance imaging (MRI) scan.
- Basal skull fractures/cerebellar lesions may be associated with significant executive deficits.
- Behaviour at home or work is a better index of executive problems than behaviour in hospital or formal assessment in a consulting room.
- Listen to what friends and family members say—give them permission to report changes in personality or behaviour.

3 A conceptual basis for the treatment of executive dysfunction

Clinicians can be forgiven for feeling that the burgeoning literature on executive functions and 'frontal lobology' is abstruse and bewildering. Even so, when faced with multiple executive problems, a simple framework is helpful in structuring treatment interventions, as diverse disorders of cognition and behaviour may be manifestations of the same underlying deficits. A rudimentary but robust framework for clinicians is shown in the box below. The role of action schemas is central to this model. An action schema is a representation of basic action, which, when arranged in hierarchical fashion with lower-level motor acts and higher-level organizational processes, forms part of the executive system for governing behaviour. For example, in the model shown in the box below, planning occurs at the level of assembly of action schemas relevant to a task.

A three-stage framework for prioritizing deficits for treatment

I Schema assembly

- Disorders of goal articulation and planning:
  —formulating intentions, clarifying goals, planning, and anticipation

II Schema activation

- Disorders of initiation and sequencing:
  —aspontaneity, action sequencing, prospective remembering

III Schema regulation

- Disorders of inhibition and control
  —utilization behaviour, impulsiveness, perseveration, disinhibition, aggression
- Disorders of monitoring and evaluation
  —attention and awareness, reasoning, judgement, decision-making, problem-solving, confabulation

A wide range of action and behaviour disorders can be encompassed within this simple scheme. In general, clinicians should begin intervention at the earliest stage at which there is a deficit. Therefore consider signs of impairment in the following stages:

- generation of an intent to act (goal articulation) and the formation of a plan;
- activating the plan and implementing the action to achieve the desired goal;
- monitoring progression towards the goal and regulating behaviour accordingly.

Most treatments can be considered to conform to one of three broad types (see box p. 326 for details), loosely based on putative mechanisms of effectiveness:

- environmental modification;
- cognitive remediation techniques;
- specific skills training.

We will now discuss interventions for particular disorders of executive control.

A broad taxonomy of intervention types

Environmental modification

Essentially a compensatory means of therapeutic intervention—changing the physical or social setting and modifying the contingencies of reward (e.g. changing layout of a room, using notebooks, diaries, pagers). Much underrated, often unfairly regarded as the therapist's last ditch option. Consider using for:

◆ deficits in initial goal setting, or in task execution;

◆ in situations of stimulus overload/competition;

◆ context-driven behavioural deficits, in the presence of other cognitive impairment.

Cognitive remediation techniques

Tasks aimed at restoring impaired cognitive processes—repetitive practice of a specific (sometimes rather contrived) task. Intervention delivered on structured exercises in set treatment sessions. Some promising results in the treatment of attentional deficits, but yet to demonstrate wider utility for executive problems (generalizability of treatment gains is poor). Be sceptical of interventions claiming to restore underlying cognitive processes (e.g. memory process training, organizational remediation).

Specific skills training

Variety of methods from cognitive and behavioural psychology intended to teach people how to perform very specific everyday activities. Often used in conjunction with environmental modifications to good effect. Includes training of metacognitive skills (e.g. monitoring, evaluation, feedback, and awareness). Not limited to classroom activities; can be employed in real-life settings. Most of the active interventions in this chapter conform to some kind of skills training approach.

4 Interventions for deficits in the creation of action plans

4.1 Impairments of planning and goal formulation

These can be defined as difficulty in formulating intentions or clear objectives before starting a task. The impairment is caused by inability to devise an appropriate action plan and commonly occurs with complex multistage tasks (Shallice 1982).

The clinician should *educate* (reiterate the importance of planning to eventual outcome) and *moderate* (consider changes in routine or the task environment).

◆ Some apparent planning impairments are really impulsive behaviours, and respond to self-instructional or verbal mediation interventions (e.g. Cicerone and Wood 1987).

- Poor planning may be improved by generating an appropriate action script by asking people to verbally rehearse what is required for a task (Zalla *et al.* 2001).

- Task-based checklists can also provide an explicit framework for developing plans (Burke *et al.* 1991).

- For complex deficits of strategic planning, consider training programmes with an early emphasis on goal articulation and planning (see *Goal Management Training*, stages 1–3; and *Problem Solving Therapy* in the box in Section 6.2.2).

- An alternative strategy is to focus upon time constraints, often neglected from planning. *Time Pressure Management* (TPM) training (Fasotti *et al.* 2000) offers a problem-solving framework that can be linked to self-instruction to help individuals plan more effectively. This kind of programme may be especially helpful where time constraints are critical.

4.2 Degradation of everyday action schema

This is characterized by problems in carrying out everyday routine activities. It is not really an executive deficit but manifests as one. It is caused by the breakdown of conceptual knowledge or 'schema assemblies' (Schwartz *et al.* 1991) for well-established actions and may manifest as part of an ideational or frontal apraxia. It may be associated with semantic impairments.

Treatment is as for *action disorganization* (Section 5.2). Ensure a good understanding of the task objectives and operations before commencing action. Follow this with online assistance (verbal prompts, physical cues) as necessary.

5 Interventions for deficits in the activation and implementation of action schema

Deficits in activating intentions or initiating behaviour cause poverty of action, an extremely debilitating condition. Manifestations may vary.

5.1 Aspontaneity

This is characterized by a marked reduction in spontaneous purposeful activity. This must be distinguished from the neurological conditions of abulia and akinesia and the neuropsychiatric syndromes of apathy and depression. Environmental cues and verbal prompts are often ineffective because the problem is not one of goal clarity but represents a difficulty in putting plans into action.

Solutions are as follows.

- Modify the environment to increase the salience of antecedent stimuli and reduce the significance of irrelevant stimuli (see *discrimination training*, Section 7.2).

- Self-prompting schedules can also be beneficial (Burke *et al.* 1991) but only if linked to clear rewards for the individual. Too often intervention fails because the person has no desire to engage in particular activities.

- Pharmacological agents may help (e.g. dopamine agonists).

5.2 **Action disorganization**

This involves problems with common everyday tasks (e.g. making a cup of tea). It is caused by disruption to the procedural knowledge base for over-learned actions (such as brushing one's teeth), rendering the activity dependent on inadequate executive control.

Intervention should ensure that conditions are optimal for action schema activation, and include procedures to improve behavioural regulatory functions in order to ensure efficient operation of the relevant action schema once activated. Treatment options include the following.

- ◆ Environmental simplification to minimize off-task errors.
- ◆ Provide a visual sequence of correct action stages to be followed.
- ◆ Use behavioural techniques. Where a desired response does not occur spontaneously such an action can be developed using the technique of shaping, which involves positively reinforcing successive approximations to the desired behaviour. Chaining techniques are recommended if the primary problem is in action sequencing.
- ◆ Use verbal self-regulation methods.

Clinicians usually select whatever seems likely to work, and then modify it accordingly (see Wilson 1999).

5.3 **Prospective remembering**

Deficits in prospective remembering involve the inability to carry out an intention to act at some future time. This is commonly associated with other executive deficits, but not necessarily with other memory problems. It needs to be distinguished from initiation disorder (see Section 5.1) and impairments of retrospective memory, as memory for the intent to act may be preserved.

Therapeutically, internal memory strategies have limited success. Likewise, the use of spaced retrieval methods (increasing the time lag between encoding and execution of intentions) has been disappointing (Sohlberg *et al.* 1992). Instead, external cueing systems should be considered (individualized checklists are a good example). Electronic aids can also be useful as long as the person can use the technology (Evans *et al.* 1998). If severe anterograde memory problems are also present, start with a very basic task and simple cues (e.g. prompt with telephone calls). Gradually, a self-cueing programme can be devised using a combination of checklists and external prompts to use the checklists, in order to develop a simple routine of action initiation. Many people develop their own idiosyncratic methods. These should be respected, but may be improved.

6 **Interventions for deficits in the regulation of behaviour**

For goal-oriented behaviour to be adaptive in the real world it has to be efficiently regulated. The majority of cognitive and behavioural disorders that characterize the dysexecutive syndrome arise from disturbance to regulatory control mechanisms. These comprise fundamental processes of attention and awareness, judgement, and inhibition.

6.1 Disorders of inhibition

Disorders of inhibition arise principally from a deficiency of executive control over lower-level action schemas, leading to unmodulated contention scheduling (see Chapter 17). The manifestations of impaired inhibitory control are varied. In some cases one observes a failure to exercise a socially acceptable degree of self-restraint in translating thoughts or feelings into action. In other instances, behaviour is clearly driven by external stimuli without any apparent cognitive mediation. Treatment of the most common manifestations is as follows.

6.1.1 Utilization behaviour

This is a non-planned and irrelevant response to an object that often interferes with an existing activity. It is caused by automatic activation of an action schema, usually triggered by a specific object, resulting in behaviour that may be socially unacceptable (drinking from someone's cup, answering their telephone). It is important to distinguish utilization behaviour from a simple frontal grasp reflex (objects do not have to be within immediate grasping range to elicit utilization behaviour) and 'alien hand'.

Verbal prompting does not usually help, as awareness may be preserved. Modifying the environmental triggers offers a partial solution, though the problem often resolves spontaneously.

6.1.2 Distractability

This involves responding to external stimuli (noise, people) at the expense of current activity. It is essentially a deficit in attentional control, allowing attention to be captured by task-irrelevant events. This can produce severe disability in everyday life, but it is amenable to treatment with cognitive and behavioural techniques. (See *Discrimination training* in Section 7.2 and also Chapter 6).

6.1.3 Impulsiveness

This is a tendency to act without pre-planning or thinking through the consequences. It is caused by inadequate executive control over behaviour—unconstrained contention scheduling and is commonly associated with other signs of dysregulation including mood.

The consequences of impulsive behaviour can be ameliorated to a degree by removing temptation, a simple but effective strategy at times. In treating impulsiveness itself, practical (and perhaps ethical) constraints prevent more widespread use of counterconditioning methods, massed practice, or paradoxical intention. Consequential learning methods can be used, where there is some incentive for demonstrating self-restraint. In practice this is better tied to a concurrent verbal task to capture attention, e.g. counting 1–5 and then carrying out the action. A personal favourite is the cue word 'WAIT!'—short, clear, and effective in interrupting action. It is also an acronym for 'what alternative is there?', which can be incorporated into a self-instructional programme.

6.1.4 Perseveration

This is a repetitive pattern of an action that is no longer relevant to the situation. Even if an action is triggered appropriately, there comes a time when it is redundant, due to changes in circumstances (e.g. a goal has been achieved). An inability to change action schema accordingly leads to inefficient, often highly inappropriate, behaviour.

The clinician should establish whether the behaviour is exclusively organically driven (*frontal perseveration*) or has been learned (*habitual behaviour*). Awareness may be preserved and the problem may improve within 6–12 months after brain injury.

- Training a person to use self-statements during perseverative acts can reduce the problem.
- There is some evidence that massed practice or 'cognitive over-learning' is effective in reducing verbal perseverative behaviour (Alderman and Ward 1991).
- Repetitive habitual behaviour needs a functional analysis, followed by appropriate cognitive–behavioural treatment to address the environmental contingencies helping to maintain the behaviour. In this way Matthey (1996) reduced perseverative behaviour, but effects did not generalize to the home environment, presumably because the external contingencies at home were different from the treatment environment. This problem could be minimized if the therapy specifically included the discharge environment as a legitimate treatment arena.

6.1.5 Disinhibition

This is acting or speaking in a manner that contravenes acceptable social conduct.

Disinhibited behaviour can take many forms, from mild overfamiliarity with strangers to acts of sexual indecency. Situations may vary and the first step in treatment is to conduct a comprehensive assessment of the context of the behaviour. Although organically derived, the behaviour is often exacerbated or sustained by reactions from others. Therefore, investigation should encompass social context, including antecedents and consequences, as the key to successful treatment. Amelioration has typically been based on principles of behaviour modification, including time-out from positive reinforcement (Wood 1990), though attention constraints associated with dysexecutive impairment may interfere with conditioning.

- Intervention should therefore be immediate, providing a *direct feedback* (usually a specific verbal response).
- For individuals with adequate memory, additional *delayed feedback* (up to 1 hour later) encourages reflection on behaviour and provides opportunity to rehearse alternative responses (thus developing a more acceptable action schema). Here *verbal mediation methods* (see box, p. 331) can help towards the development of a self-management approach (Wood and Worthington 2001).

Example of a verbal mediation dialogue

How are you this morning?
  Fed up, I missed my breakfast
What happened at breakfast?
  I had an argument with Jason, because he was staring at me.
Why do you think he did that?
  I don't know, maybe he was trying to annoy me. He was doing it on purpose.
How did that make you feel?
  I got angry; he was doing it on purpose to annoy me
What did you do then?
  I started shouting and calling him names
What happened next?
  He shouted back . . . we just kept shouting, until we got told to leave the dining room.
What else could you have done?
  I could have carried on eating my breakfast and ignored him.
How do you think Jason would have reacted then?
  He would have got fed up as I was ignoring him.
Would that have been better for you too?
  Yeah, because he's just a loser, but I would have had my breakfast.
So if you feel Jason is trying to wind you up at breakfast tomorrow, what will you do?
  I'll take no notice, and carry on.

6.1.6 Aggression

Aggression can be verbal or physical, towards objects or persons, including self-directed anger. It is often an attempt to intimidate rather than harm. Inability to articulate goals, solve problems, or communicate intentions can lead to frustrations and, if unchecked, to aggression. It is important to differentiate this from irritability and episodic dyscontrol. Remember also that aggression is a normal response to certain situations, but after frontal brain injury impaired behavioural control mechanisms mean that it becomes a default response in many situations. Once triggered, aggression may not be constrained by normal regulatory processes.

There are several approaches to treatment.

◆ Pharmacological intervention is usually necessary in severe cases, and can augment psychological methods. Medication alone is not a long-term solution.

◆ Modification of the environment can help reduce trigger events, but this is rarely adequate.

- The objective of treatment is usually to restore a degree of self-control. This can be done using behavioural methods alone, such as *cost–response techniques* that link the antisocial behaviour to a meaningful sanction (e.g. failure to earn privileges). Some understanding of response–consequence relationships is necessary for learning, so ensure learning intervals are brief where cognition is severely disturbed. Alderman and Burgess (1994) recommended cost–response techniques as especially useful in such cases.

- For higher-functioning individuals *cognitive–behavioural methods* can be used, either in a self-instructional programme or a problem-solving anger management intervention (Medd and Tate 2000).

In all cases the aim is to encourage the activation (consciously or otherwise) of an incompatible, more acceptable action schema in response to identifiable trigger stimuli.

- *Caveat.* Change on self-report measures of anger is not the same as spontaneous use of anger management strategies in everyday life, and generalization of treatment effects is problematic, especially after group interventions.

6.2 Disorders of evaluation and judgement

The inability to make sensible decisions or express sound judgements is a cardinal feature of executive dysfunction. In extreme cases, otherwise intelligent individuals mix with bad company, fritter away their savings on fruitless ventures, and generally go through life from one mishap to another, unless supervision is imposed. In such cases the matter of competency to manage one's affairs becomes important. In many other instances though, the deficiencies are subtle and may only be apparent some time after rehabilitation has ended.

6.2.1 Impairments of judgement and decision-making

First, establish whether impaired judgement is a specific or more general defect. For example, poor road safety judgement may be secondary to subtle perceptual deficits. Commonly, generalized impairments of judgement are accompanied by diminished self-awareness. The type of intervention depends on the likely underlying problem. Inability to select a single course of action from plausible options can produce impairments in both judgement and decision-making, or may even result in deficits of initiation. Therefore, distinguish between:

- a difficulty in making just about *any* kind of decision, which needs interventions aimed at clarifying the issues and generating solutions.

- a tendency to make poor decisions, which requires focus on the process of comparative evaluations and anticipated consequences.

Strategies used in training problem-solving (see Section 6.2.2) are valid in both cases.

6.2.2 Impairments of reasoning and problem-solving

Reasoning and problem-solving are two high-level skills that are often compromised as part of a dysexecutive presentation, but often the full magnitude of the deficits is only evident on real-life tasks (Shallice and Burgess 1991; Goel *et al.* 1997; Goel and Grafman 2000). Unfortunately, treatment for such deficits is still largely classroom-based (see Evans 2001).

◆ One comprehensive programme is *Problem Solving Training* (PST; von Cramon *et al.* 1991; von Cramon and Matthes-von Cramon 1992). The essence of the treatment (see box) is to train persons in key aspects of problem-solving. This kind of mental discipline training can improve performance on problem-solving exercises within a few weeks. However, the real difficulty is that patients with executive disorders can acquire knowledge and skills but may nevertheless fail to apply this spontaneously outside the treatment environment. Evidence to date suggests that effort would be better spent improving use of such skills in specific everyday environments (von Cramon and Matthes-von Cramon 1994).

◆ A related approach is employed in *Goal Management Training* (see box below; Robertson 1996). This is really another form of verbal mediation training intended to improve self-regulation, but with an abstract set of principles that can be applied across situations. This method can improve performance of everyday tasks (Levine *et al.* 2000) but, as with PST, it is not clear whether all the components are really necessary, and some stages may be more relevant than others for particular deficits.

Stages in problem-solving therapy

1. Problem formulation (defining the task objective);
2. Generation of solutions (brainstorming);
3. Deciding on a solution (weighing-up the options);
4. Verifying the outcome (recognizing errors, correcting mistakes).

Steps to goal management training

1. Problem orientation;
2. Problem definition (specifying the goal);
3. Listing (break down goals into relevant stages—subgoals);
4. Learning (encoding and retention of steps);
5. Monitoring (comparing outcome with intention).

6.2.3 Confabulation from memory

Confabulation is the production of false memories following brain injury, which the person confuses for, and cannot distinguish from, veridical recollection. It is generally associated with frontal—subcortical damage, and is considered to result from deficient executive control over memory retrieval—i.e. faulty verification procedures.

Improvement often occurs spontaneously, and there are few treatment studies. Given the purported nature of the deficit, self-monitoring techniques may prove useful in mild cases (see Section 6.3).

6.3 Impairments of self-monitoring

Another common form of impaired self-regulation is a defect in the normal feedback mechanism linking conscious intentions with the external world. Dysfunction of this system results in an inability to monitor one's behaviour, and its effect on others. This is why social disinhibition does not improve with experience alone. Excessively loud verbalizations are a common self-regulatory problem after brain injury. This is usually treated behaviourally, e.g. by first providing explicit feedback from another person and linking a reward to subsequent modification of speech volume (Burgess and Alderman 1990).

To promote generalization of gains clinicians should remember to include graded exposure to successively more challenging stimuli or situations. Self-instructional or self-management approaches (see box below for example) have been underused in brain injury. True, many cognitive skills packages (e.g. Goal Management Training) and behaviour modification techniques invoke an appeal to self-awareness and thereby to self-monitoring. But, few deal specifically with this crucial aspect of executive disorder.

A self-instruction programme

A self-instructional programme was employed to good effect with a 29-year-old woman 2 years after her severe head injury. She could take up to 3 hours to get washed and dressed in the morning as a result of severe distractability and obsessive behaviour. A programme was devised during which a support worker read out specific action prompts. These were repeated by the client as she performed the actions. These statements gradually came to act as internal prompts, improving her attention to task and increasing her speed to wash and dress to half an hour. Figure 18.1 shows the mean number of daily verbal prompts in a 2-week baseline period and for 4 weeks following withdrawal of the self-instructional programme.

A notable exception is the *Self-monitoring Training* (SMT) programme (see box, p. 335) reported by Alderman *et al.* (1995). This multistage programme is really a hybrid for improving self-awareness in combination with a procedure for reinforcing successively lower frequencies of target behaviour (DRL). Alderman and colleagues employed this method with a post-encephalitic patient to reduce frequency of inappropriate utterances.

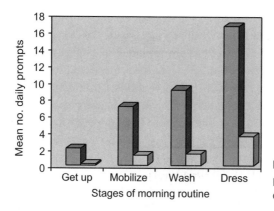

Fig. 18.1 Self-instructional programme for washing and dressing.

More recently it has also been used to reduce debilitating delusional confabulations (Dayus and van den Broek 2000). The technique is recommended for high-frequency problems and for its ease of use in community settings. For more able persons self-monitoring can be improved by completing a daily record or diary (Burke *et al.* 1991). However, personal experience suggests that increased self-awareness can be achieved within a few weeks, at most, but does not necessarily generalize to changes in behaviour. In many cases the problem is not one of self-evaluation, but an inability to divide attention between the task in hand and other pressures. In this case intervention could focus on the temporal aspect of the task (see *Time Pressure Management*, Section 4.1).

Components of Self-Monitoring Training (SMT)

1 Baseline assessment of frequency of target behaviour.
2 Spontaneous (i.e. unprompted) self-monitoring of target behaviour.
3 Prompted self-monitoring, with assistance of therapist.
4 Independent self-monitoring (with reward contingent on achieving a predetermined level of agreement in frequency ratings between therapist and client).
5 Independent self-monitoring and reduction of target behaviour (delivery of reward contingent upon graded reduction in frequency of target behaviour).

7 Issues in the treatment of executive disorder

7.1 Evaluating clinical efficacy

Well-designed rehabilitation studies for executive skills are a rare breed. The so-called dysexecutive syndrome encompasses a wide range of deficits, some presenting as behaviour problems, some manifesting as higher cognitive impairments. Treatment efficacy has to be evaluated for specific subtypes of executive disorder, indicating whether the behaviour or underlying cognitive processes are the focus of intervention. Evidence of effectiveness is limited to small group studies or single cases. While many of these seem to show good results (and clinical experience would support this), it is difficult to infer who benefits from which interventions. Comprehensive treatment packages may contain much redundant material and need to be examined in detail. In this light, studies comparing different interventions (e.g. Alderman and Burgess 1994) are particularly instructive.

7.2 The role of attention and self-awareness

Recruitment of attention is critical to improving many high-level executive skills, but attention is often impaired in conjunction with executive processes. Brain injury can also cause disorders of awareness and prevent use of attentional resources in regulating behaviour. This is why techniques based solely on positive reinforcement may be ineffective in modifying behaviour in the context of a dysexecutive syndrome. Rehabilitation can be focused on the attention deficit or the behavioural manifestation—the clinician must decide. In terms of self-regulatory disorders, attention *per se* is rarely the focus of intervention, but treatment does involve techniques for modifying attention to what is therapeutically important. This is the basis of *discriminative attention training*, which underpins much of the learning process in rehabilitation. Treatment methods, involving either environmental modification or manipulation of consequences of actions, focus on alternative or incompatible reactions to a situation. This allows selective reinforcement by therapists for certain actions and thereby increases the likelihood of the desired behaviours recurring. Such discriminative reinforcement techniques are reviewed by Wood (1990). Attentional re-directing is also integral to cognitive—behavioural approaches to improving social and functional skills, and is central to the development of self-monitoring programmes. Clinicians should establish first whether there is a significant attentional contribution to an executive disorder, as this is often the key to successful treatment. For a comprehensive review of attention disorders and remediation, the reader should refer to Chapters 5 and 6 on attentional disorders in this volume.

7.3 Designing effective interventions for executive disorders

The principles of sound clinical practice apply to rehabilitation of executive dysfunction. Thus budding therapists need to:

◆ carry out assessment of both spared and impaired abilities (i.e. a reliable baseline);

◆ decide on priorities for treatment;

◆ agree specific operational goals with family, client, and therapy team;

◆ devise a clear explicit intervention, based on a hypothesis of the nature of the executive dysfunction.

In addition, rehabilitation of executive deficits requires close attention to the following aspects of treatment design.

- Consider the conceptual basis for a deficit in order to rationalize choice of intervention strategy.
- Select practical tasks as targets for intervention.
- Avoid tasks reliant on regurgitation of old knowledge.
- Avoid highly constrained tasks where responsibility for correcting performance rests solely with therapist.
- Break down intervention into discrete stages.
- Consider most-to-least-prompts and spaced retrieval (using errorless learning principles).
- Deliver treatment in different settings to facilitate generalization.
- Start with a simple analogue but work towards increasing complexity of treatment environment.
- Assess similar non-treated tasks to investigate generalization of skills to related tasks.
- Assess non-treated domains of cognitive functioning to control for natural recovery.

The treatment of executive dysfunction is one of the least understood and most complex areas of brain injury rehabilitation. It is not sufficient to show improvements on a task with practice. To be effective an intervention must also address the problem of spontaneous application and self-evaluation of skills once acquired. The therapeutic techniques described are largely in their infancy. There is much we still have to learn about optimal methods for improving self-regulation (Muraven and Baumeister 2000). Nevertheless, if intervention is undertaken sensitively and rationally, executive functioning can be improved to the extent that real change can be effected in quality of life.

Selective references

Alderman, N. and Burgess, P. (1994). A comparison of treatment methods for behaviour disorder following herpes simplex encephalitis. *Neuropsychol. Rehabil.* 4, 31–48.

Alderman, N. and Burgess, P.W. (2001). Assessment and rehabilitation of the dysexecutive syndrome. In *Handbook of neurological rehabilitation*, 2nd edn (ed. R. Greenwod, T.M. McMillan, M.P. Barnes, and C.D. Ward). Psychology Press, Hove, East Sussex.

Alderman, N. and Ward, A. (1991). Behavioural treatment of the dysexecutive syndrome: reduction of repetitive speech using response cost and cognitive overlearning. *Neuropsychol. Rehabil.* 1, 65–80.

Alderman, N., Fry, R.K., and Youngson, H.A. (1995). Improvement of self-monitoring skills, reduction of behaviour disturbance and the dysexecutive syndrome: comparison of response cost and a new programme of Self-Management Training. *Neuropsychol. Rehabil.* 5, 193–221.

Ashley, M.J., Krych, D.K., Persel, C.S., and Persel, C.H. (1995). *Working with behaviour disorders. Strategies for traumatic brain injury rehabilitation.* Communication Skill Builders (Psychological Corporation), San Antonio, Texas.

Burgess, P.W. and Alderman, N. (1990). Rehabilitation of dyscontrol syndromes following frontal lobe damage: a cognitive neuropsychological approach. In *Cognitive rehabilitation in perspective* (ed. R.L.I. Wood and I. Fussey), pp.183–203. Taylor and Francis, London.

Burke, W.H., Zenicus, A.H., Wesolowski, M.D., and Doubleday, F. (1991). Improving executive function disorders in brain injured clients. *Brain Injury* 5, 241–52.

Cicerone, K.D. and Wood, J.C. (1987). Planning disorder after closed head injury: a case study. *Arch. Phys. Med. Rehabil.* 68, 111–15.

Dayus, B. and van den Broek, M.D. (2000). Treatment of stable delusional confabulations using self-monitoring training. *Neuropsychol. Rehabil.* 10, 415–27.

Evans, J.J. (2001). Rehabilitation of the dysexecutive syndrome. In *Neurobehavioural disability and social handicap following traumatic brain injury* (ed. R.L.I. Wood and T.M. McMillan), pp. 209–27. Psychology Press, Hove, East Sussex.

Evans, J.J., Emslie, H., and Wilson, B.A. (1998). External cueing systems in the rehabilitation of executive impairments of action. *J. Int. Neuropsychol. Soc.* 4, 399–408.

Fasotti, L., Kovacs, F., Eling, P.A.T.M., and Brouwer, W.H. (2000). Time pressure management as a compensatory strategy training after closed head injury. *Neuropsychol. Rehabil.* 10, 47–65.

Goel, V. and Grafman, J. (2000). Role of the right prefrontal cortex in ill-structured planning. *Cogn. Neuropsychol.* 17, 415–36.

Goel, V., Grafman, J., Tajik, J., Gana, S., and Danto, D. (1997). A study of the performance of patients with frontal lobe lesions in a financial planning task. *Brain* 120, 1805–22.

Jacobs, J.E. (1993). *Behaviour analysis guidelines and brain injury rehabilitation*. Aspen Publishers Inc, Maryland.

Levine, B., Robertson, I.H., Clare, L., Carter, G., Hong, J., Wilson, B., Duncan, J., and Stuss, D.T. (2000). Rehabilitation of executive functioning: an experimental–clinical validation of Goal Management Training. *J. Int. Neuropsychol. Soc.* 6, 299–312.

Matthey, S. (1996). Modification of perseverative behaviour in an adult with anoxic brain damage. *Brain Injury* 3, 219–27.

Medd, J. and Tate, R.L. (2000). Evaluation of an anger management therapy programme following acquired brain injury: a preliminary study. *Neuropsychol. Rehabil.* 10, 185–201.

Muraven, M. and Baumeister, R.F. (2000). Self-regulation and depletion of limited resources: does self-control resemble a muscle? *Psychol. Bull.* 126, 247–59.

Robertson, I.H. (1996). *Goal Management Training: A clinical manual*. Psyconsult, Cambridge, U.K.

Schwartz, M.F., Reed, E.S., Montgomery, M.W., Palmer, C., and Mayer, N.H. (1991). The quantitative description of action organisation after brain damage: a case study. *Cogn. Neuropsychol.* 8 381–414.

Shallice, T. (1982). Specific impairments of planning. *Phil. Trans. R. Soc. London B* 298, 199–209.

Shallice, T. and Burgess, P.W. (1991). Deficits in strategy application following frontal lobe lesions in man. *Brain* 114, 727–41.

Sohlberg, M.M., White, O., Evans, E., and Mateer, C. (1992). An investigation into the effects of prospective memory training. *Brain Injury* 6, 139–54.

Sohlberg, M.M., Mateer, C.A., and Stuss, D.T. (1993). Contemporary approaches to the management of executive control dysfunction. *J. Head Trauma Rehabil.* 8, 45–58.

von Cramon, D.Y. and Matthes-von Cramon, G. (1992). Reflections on the treatment of brain-injured patients suffering from problem solving disorders. *Neuropsychol. Rehabil.* 2, 207–29.

von Cramon, D.Y. and Matthes von Cramon, G. (1994). Back to work with a chronic dysexecutive syndrome? (a case study). *Neuropsychol. Rehabil.* 4, 399–417.

von Cramon, D.Y., Matthes-von Cramon, G., and Mai, N. (1991). Problem solving deficits in brain injured patients: a therapeutic approach. *Neuropsychol. Rehabil.* 1, 45–64.

Wilson, B.A. (1999). *Case studies in neuropsychological rehabilitation.* Oxford University Press, New York.

Wood, R.L.I. (1990). Conditioning procedures in brain injury rehabilitation. In *Neurobehavioural sequelae of traumatic brain injury* (ed. R.L.I. Wood), pp. 153–74. Taylor and Francis, London.

Wood, R.L.I. and Worthington, A.D. (2001). Neurobehavioral rehabilitation in practice. In *Neurobehavioural disability and social handicap following traumatic brain injury* (ed. R.L.I. Wood and T.M. McMillan), pp. 133–55. Psychology Press, Hove, East Sussex.

Zalla, T., Plassiart, C., Pillon, B., Grafman, J., and Sirigu, A. (2001). Action planning in a virtual context after prefrontal cortex damage. *Neuropsychologia* 39, 759–70.

Chapter 19

Neuropsychological assessment and treatment of disorders of voluntary movement

Georg Goldenberg

1 Introduction

Neuropsychology is concerned with 'higher-order' rather than 'elementary' disorders of movement. One class of such disorders is characterized by incorrect or awkward movements. They differ from 'elementary' motor disorders in that the same movements that give rise to errors in one condition can successfully be performed in other conditions and success or failure depend on nonmotor factors. Such factors may be the visual control of the movement, its communicative meaning, or its relationship to tools and objects. Another class of higher-order motor problems is constituted by well executed and apparently purposeful movements that do not conform to the subject's intentions. Table 19.1 gives an overview of disturbances fulfilling these criteria.

2 Incorrect and awkward movements

These can occur on one or both sides of the body. Kinaesthetic ataxia affects the hand and optic ataxia affects the visual field contralateral to the lesion. Face apraxia and limb apraxia are bilateral disorders resulting from unilateral, mainly left-sided, lesions. Callosal apraxia disturbs movements of the left-sided extremities.

Table 19.1 Higher-level motor disorders resulting from hemisphere damage*

Incorrect and awkward movements (parietal lesions†)		Movement outside voluntary control (frontal lesions)	
Contralesional	**Bilateral**	**Contralesional**	**Bilateral**
Kinaesthetic ataxia	Face apraxia	Grasping and groping	Motor perseverations
Optic ataxia	Limb apraxia	Anarchic hand	Utilization behaviour Imitation behaviour

* Callosal apraxia is not considered in this table.

† Persistent face apraxia may also result from frontal or deep lesions.

2.1 Kinaesthetic ataxia (parietal hand)

Patients need vision to compensate insufficient processing of kinaesthetic afferences. Shaping of the hand for grasp and manipulations is clumsy and needs visual attention. When out of visual control, the arm may unvoluntarily change its position but it does not unintentionally perform goal-directed action. Kinaesthetic ataxia is a very disabling condition. The need for visual control renders the hand unusable for swift and finely tuned manipulations.

♦ *Clinical diagnosis*
   —Note that patients spontaneously use visual control for all movements of the hand.
   —Observe palpation of objects given for stereognosis.
   —Ask blindfolded patient to replicate with the sound arm a passively induced position of the affected arm: they cannot do so because they lack kinaesthetic information.
   —Ask for history of involuntary displacement of the arm.
♦ *Lesion.* Anterior parietal lobe (Freund 1987).
♦ *Therapy.* Can be based on attempts to enhance kinaesthetic perception or on training of compensatory visual control.

2.2 Optic ataxia

Patients are unable to exploit visual information for exact guidance of goal-directed motor action of their hands. Inaccuracy and hesitancy of reaching to visually presented objects (e.g. the finger of the examiner) contrast with fast and accurate reaching to parts of the patient's own body (e.g. the tip of the nose or the finger of the other hand). Optic ataxia can be more severe in the periphery of the affected visual hemi-field than in foveal vision. If optic guidance of eye movements is preserved, patients can compensate optic ataxia by making a saccade to fixate a peripheral target and then reach it in the centre of the visual field. Optic ataxia affects reaching with either hand, but is sometimes more severe for the contralateral hand.

Bilateral lesions can cause optic ataxia of the whole visual field. Because of proximity of the responsible lesions bilateral optic ataxia can be associated with Balint's syndrome (see Chapter 8). Left-sided optic ataxia is frequently associated with hemineglect or visuospatial disturbances but should be clearly distinguished from these disturbances of the explicit representation of space. There are patients with optic ataxia who can perfectly analyse the location of targets they fail to reach, and most patients with hemineglect and visuospatial disturbances reach accurately to targets on the neglected side once they have noted them.

The ecological significance of optic ataxia depends on whether it is uni- or bilateral and whether reaching in central fixation is preserved. If only reaching in the periphery of one visual field is inaccurate, the impact on everyday functioning may be only moderate.

- ◆ *Clinical diagnosis*
    - —Sit opposite to the patient and ask the patient to fixate your eyes (as in confrontation perimetry). Raise a finger or a small object (e.g. a pencil) to different locations and ask patient to touch it with the index finger.
    - —To document preserved nonvisual pointing ask patient to touch their nose or fingers of the other hand.
- ◆ *Lesion.* Superior parietal and intraparietal sulcus. There is a possible role for subcortical extension of lesions interrupting fibres connecting visual areas with sensorimotor cortex (Perenin and Vighetto 1988).
- ◆ *Therapy.* If visual fixation is preserved, the strategy of self-cueing by visual fixation (see Section 2.1) can be trained.

2.3 Face apraxia

Patients have difficulties in performing facial or oral movements on command, although very similar movements are carried out spontaneously. For example, a patient may be unable to move the tongue into one cheek on command, but does the same movement when cleaning the mouth from remainders of a meal. Face apraxia may be associated with contralesional facial paralysis but can be demonstrated also on the ipsilesional side of face. Face apraxia is rarely noted by the patients themselves and has no impact on life outside the testing situation. It may, however, constitute an obstacle for speech therapy in patients with left brain damage and apraxia of speech.

- ◆ *Clinical diagnosis.* To avoid confusion with problems of language comprehension, movements are tested in imitation. Table 19.2 gives a list of items arranged by difficulty (Bizzozero *et al.* 2000).
- ◆ *Lesion.* Face apraxia can result from lesions of either hemisphere, but tends to be more persistent and more severe after left brain damage (LBD) than right brain damage (RBD). In contrast to limb apraxia (Section 2.4) there is no preponderance of parietal lesions. Persistent face apraxia may also result from frontal or deep lesions.

2.4 Limb apraxia (see box, p. 343)

Patients commit errors on performing some kinds of motor actions even when using the hand ipsilateral to the lesion, which shows completely normal skill on other kinds of actions. The affected domains of actions are imitation of gestures, performance of meaningful gestures, and use of tools and objects.

Table 19.2 Items for testing facial apraxia

A Lower face
B Easy
Open your mouth
Show your teeth
Blow
B Medium
Make a clip-clop noise with your tongue
Push the tip of your tongue against the inside of your left cheek
Move your jaw to right (and right to left) three times
B Difficult
Puff out your right cheek
Push out your lower teeth (prognathism)
Push your tongue against the inside of your lower lip
A Upper face
Wrinkle your forehead
Wrinkle your nose
Blink your right eye (tight)

Easy, medium, and difficult refer to the ease with which normals perform these gestures. All upper face items are medium to difficult. Performance should be considered pathological if patient produces random and amorphous movements, if response is preceded by additional, unsolicited movements, or if the required movement is incomplete or not performed at all. Items are from Bizzozero *et al.* (2000) where a complete list is given together with normative data.

Classification of apraxia

There is a traditional distinction between three forms of limb apraxia:

- ideational;
- ideomotor;
- limb-kinetic.

This classification goes back to a hierarchical model of motor control proposed by Liepmann about 100 years ago. He thought that patients with ideational apraxia cannot generate the idea or, respectively, mental image of the intended action, whereas ideomotor apraxia disrupts the transformation of this idea into appropriate motor commands. Limb kinetic apraxia should result from loss of 'motor engram' that each hemisphere possesses for directing overlearned routine actions of the opposite hand.

It is difficult to define clinical criteria that unequivocally distinguish between these forms. Consequently, they have received very different interpretations. The theoretical model underlying the classification does not accord well with current opinions on the neuropsychology of action planning and motor control. There are thus no convincing reasons for retaining the historical classification.

2.4.1 Imitation of gestures

Patients understand the request to imitate (if they do not, apraxia cannot be diagnosed) and try to attain a gesture resembling the demonstration, but the resulting posture is spatially wrong. The movement to the final position may be hesitant and searching, but there are patients who attain a wrong position by a fast and secure movement. The problem concerns the definition of the target posture rather than its motor execution, and patients commit errors also when asked to replicate the gestures on a manikin or to match photographs of the same gestures performed by different persons seen from different angles of view. Imitation of meaningful gestures may be preserved, as patients may be able to recognize the meaning of the gesture and reproduce it without actually copying the shape of the gesture.

Disturbed imitation of gestures is a very impressive and easily demonstrable symptom of high theoretical interest but, as imitation is rarely afforded outside the testing situation, it has little ecological significance. However, disturbed imitation may be an obstacle for efficient therapy of other motor impairments in physical and occupational therapy.

Clinical diagnosis: It is preferable to test meaningless gestures as they give an uncontaminated insight into the ability to imitate the shape of gestures. The examiner sits opposite the patient and demonstrates the gestures 'like a mirror' using the right hand for left hand imitation and vice versa. Patients should always use the hand ipsilateral to the lesion. The patient is allowed to start imitation only immediately after demonstration. Figure 19.1 shows 10 hand postures and 10 finger postures (Goldenberg 1996).

Lesion: LBD disturbs imitation of hand postures more than finger postures. RBD affects imitation of finger postures but spares hand postures. Within the left hemisphere, lesions of the inferior parietal lobe have the most severe effect on imitation. 'Strategically' placed left parietal lesions can cause 'visuo-imitative apraxia', i.e. defective imitation of meaningless gestures without other manifestations of apraxia and without accompanying aphasia.

Therapy: As it does not affect the patient's independence in daily living, disturbed imitation would not by itself justify therapeutical efforts. It may, however, be useful to train imitation of hand and finger postures as a prerequisite for acquiring the use of meaningful gestures to compensate aphasia.

2.4.2 Meaningful gestures

Patients are unable to demonstrate meaningful gestures on command. Such gestures may either have a conventionally agreed, more or less arbitrary, meaning like 'somebody is crazy', 'military salute', or 'okay', or they may indicate objects by miming their use. Outside the testing situation the deficit can be observed when aphasic patients try to express themselves in spite of severe language impairment. They either do not

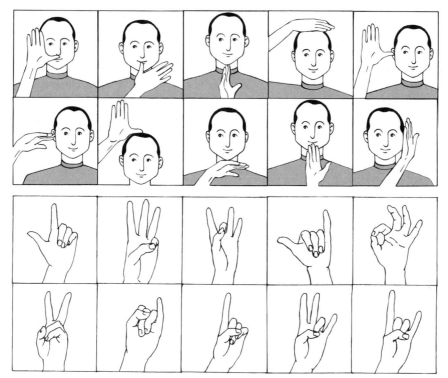

Fig. 19.1 Ten hand postures and 10 finger postures for testing imitation of meaningless gestures. When 2 points are credited for correct imitation on first trial, scores of 18 for hand postures and 16 for finger postures are borderline. Scores below these are pathological (Goldenberg 1996). (Taken with permission from Goldenberg *et al.* 2001*b*.)

employ gestures at all or produce amorphous, stereotypic, or incomprehensible gestures. Because it restricts the range of possible compensation for the language deficit, this manifestation of apraxia has ecological significance in patients with severe expressive language impairment.

Clinical diagnosis Usually, diagnosis concentrates on miming of object use, because aphasic patients may not understand the verbal label of gestures with conventional meaning, whereas comprehension of the object name can be facilitated by showing either the object (e.g. a hammer, a key, a screwdriver) or a picture of it. Even with this help, understanding of the instruction may be problematic. The demand to demonstrate the movements associated with object use without actually handling the object taxes not only speech comprehension but also 'abstract attitude' which is frequently compromised in patients with aphasia. A diagnosis of apraxia should be made only if patients respond to the presentation of the object with a movement of the hand that can be clearly distinguished from spontaneous 'baton' movements accompanying attempts of verbal expression. A further difficulty is posed by the great variability of gesture performance in normal subjects. For example, the replacement of the absent object by the hand ('body part as object', e.g. brushing teeth with the index rather than demonstrating the manipulation of a toothbrush) is a strategy frequently employed to indicate an absent object when the verbal label is lacking (e.g. when trying to buy a toothbrush in a country whose language you cannot speak). There are, however, errors that unequivocally indicate apraxia:

- perseveration of a more or less amorphic movement (e.g. a circling movement above the table or repeated hitting of the fist against one's chest);
- pointing to the location where the object should be applied (e.g. pointing to the mouth for a toothbrush or to the table for a pencil);
- searching movements of the hand and fingers that eventually result in a recognizable pantomime ('conduite d'approche').

Lesion: Apraxia for meaningful gestures is a symptom of LBD. It is virtually always associated with aphasia, but the severity of apraxia may differ from that of language impairment. Within the left hemisphere the preponderance of parietal lesions is less marked than it is for imitation.

Therapy: In patients with severe expressive language problems it may be worthwhile to train gesturing as an alternative channel for communication. To ensure use of trained gestures outside the laboratory it is advisable to involve the partners of the patients in the training and to concentrate on gestures that are important for everyday communication (e.g. I am hungry or tired, I need to go to the toilet, etc.).

2.4.3 Use of tools and objects

Use of tools and objects is awkward and faulty. For example, patients press the knife perpendicularly into the loaf rather than making a slicing movement or press the head of the hammer upon the nail and turn round rather than hitting the nail. Difficulties increase when patients perform chains of actions involving multiple tools and objects (e.g. preparing a meal), and when actions require comprehension of technical and mechanical constraints and mechanical problem-solving (e.g. household repairs or handling unfamiliar electronic equipment). The ecological significance of these difficulties is evident. However, some patients have less difficulty when performing activities at home with their familiar equipment and tools than in a testing situation.

Clinical diagnosis

- Present familiar, easy to use objects, such as a padlock with a key, a hammer and a nail, a comb, or a pair of binoculars, and ask patients to use them. For examining hemiplegic patients objects must be prepared for one-handed use (e.g. provide a wooden block with a hole in which the nail to be hammered can be fixed).
- More demanding probes are to provide a sheet of paper, a perforator, and a folder, and to ask the patient to punch the paper and insert it into the folder, or to ask the patient to put together a pocket lamp from its parts.

- Preparation of coffee or a meal and performance of technical tasks can be observed in occupational therapy.

Lesion: Misuse of familiar objects (e.g. hammer, knife, comb) is bound to LBD. Usually lesions are large. They involve the parietal lobe but are rarely restricted to it. Patients who commit errors with familiar objects are apraxic also for imitation and for performance of meaningful gestures. Errors and action slips in chains of actions with multiple tools and objects are less specific and can be observed also in LBD patients without other manifestations of apraxia as well as in patients with RBD, with frontal and with diffuse brain damage (Schwartz *et al.* 1999).

Therapy: Patients can relearn use of tools and objects and even performance of complex chains of actions by training. The most successful approach seems to be to guide the patients through the whole activity and gradually reduce support at the measure of increasing competency. Success of therapy remains restricted to the activity that has been trained and does not generalize to untrained activities. Therefore, it is advisable to train only activities that the patient needs and wants to master in everyday life (Goldenberg *et al.* 2001*a*). The therapeutic gains may even be specific to the individual tools and objects that have been used in therapy. Hence, the most effective approach is to train the patients within their permanent environment on tasks that they want to perform every day.

2.5 Callosal apraxia

Callosal disconnection deprives the right hemisphere of left hemisphere competence and renders the left hand apraxic. Like bilateral apraxia from LBD, left hand apraxia from callosal disconnection affects imitation, performance of meaningful gestures, and object use. Disturbed object use may be restricted to objects not normally used by the right hand (e.g. knife, but not fork). Because natural lesions destroying the corpus callosum frequently encroach on neighbouring mesial frontal regions, callosal apraxia can be associated with disorders of voluntary control of motor actions such as motor neglect, grasping and groping, or anarchic hand (see Section 3). On the other hand, destruction of callosal fibres is rarely absolute. Particularly when there is no additional mesial frontal lobe damage, imitation and object use by the left hand may recover due to enhanced employment of remaining callosal fibres or of ipsilateral motor pathways (Goldenberg *et al.* 2001*b*). Patients may, however, have lasting difficulties with tasks putting high demands on bimanual coordination.

Clinical diagnosis The hallmark of callosal apraxia is a discrepancy between apraxia of the left hand and normal praxis of the right hand. In addition, there are signs of sensory–motor, sensory–verbal, and verbal–motor disconnection.

- Blindfolded patients cannot indicate the location of touch on their left hand either verbally or by pointing with their right hand although they can point to the location with their left thumb.

- They cannot name objects put into their left hand although the left hand palpates them skilfully.
- They cannot move single fingers of their left hand on verbal command, although they can do so in imitation (note that imitation of finger postures depends less on left hemisphere than imitation of hand postures).

Lesion: Callosal apraxia is contingent upon destruction of the middle portion of the corpus callosum.

Therapy: We are not aware of therapeutic experiences.

3 Disturbed voluntary control of motor actions

The affected limbs either do not spontaneously participate in intended action (motor neglect) or do perform actions that are not intended (all other syndromes). Non-performance of intended actions and performance of non-intended actions are not mutually exclusive.

3.1 Motor neglect

Patients need an extra voluntary effort to make the affected limbs comply with their intentions. The limb is not used spontaneously, although force and coordination are preserved. In severe cases the affected limb may appear completely paralysed, but it is raised and moved readily on command. Motor neglect gets worse when attention is distracted. Thus, patients with mild paresis of a leg who can safely stand and walk may fall when attention is directed towards a simultaneous manual activity or external distractors. Simultaneous movement of the opposite limbs may also increase motor neglect, particularly if it is asymmetric.

If there has initially been paresis of the affected limbs, it may be difficult to distinguish motor neglect from 'learned non-use'—patients may have formed a habit of using preferentially the unaffected limbs even for tasks that could easily be accomplished by the affected limbs.

Motor neglect is a disabling condition as it prevents normal use of the affected limbs. Even very mild forms of motor neglect can be disastrous when combined with hemiparesis. Patients who have partly recovered from paresis and are able to stand and walk may neglect the affected limb when distracted and consequently fall and hurt themselves.

- *Clinical diagnosis.* Observe spontaneous motor behaviour and compare with explicit testing of motor function. Place an object (e.g. a glass) in different locations on a table before the patient and ask them to grasp it. They will use the non-affected hand even if the glass is placed on the affected side.
- *Lesion.* Extended lesions including the parietal lobes can cause motor neglect together with perceptual and representational neglect, but frontal or deep lesions can cause

pure motor neglect. Predominance of right-sided lesions is less conspicuous for motor than for sensory and representational neglect (Laplane and Degos 1983).

◆ *Therapy*

—Frequent reminders to use the contralesional limbs are integrated in physiotherapy and occupational therapy.

—Experimentally, technical devices have been tried that are fixed to a neglected leg and give acoustic feedback about its use (Robertson and Cashman 1991).

—It is questionable whether therapies aimed at alleviating visuospatial neglect (see Chapter 6) have an effect on accompanying motor neglect.

3.2 Grasping and groping

When getting in touch with an object, the affected hand grasps it. It may also grope for visually perceived objects located in its proximity and grasp them. Few patients are able to suppress the grasp reaction by an effort of will. The majority have to interfere using their sound hand to loosen the grasp. They may sit on their hand or permanently place an object into it to prevent it from clenching external objects. Groping and grasping are embarrassing and compromise use of the affected hand.

◆ *Clinical diagnosis*

—Move your finger or a comparable object (e.g. handle of reflex hammer) over palm exerting some pressure on skin. If patient grasps, advise them not to do so and repeat the manouevre.

—To elicit groping move an object (e.g. reflex hammer) close to patient's hand and withdraw it slowly if the hand moves towards it. If the hand follows the object, advise the patient not to do so and repeat.

◆ *Lesion.* Medial face of superior frontal lobe (cingulate gyrus and supplementary motor area). Unilateral lesions of either side can cause bilateral grasping (De Renzi and Barbieri 1992).

◆ *Therapy.* Spontaneous recovery is frequent, particularly when the lesion is unilateral. We are not aware of systematic attempts to institute therapy.

3.3 Anarchic hand (see Chapter 12)

One hand performs complex movements that are goal-directed and well executed but unintended. These unwanted movements cannot be voluntarily interrupted and may interfere with desired actions carried out by the other hand. Most of the unwanted actions are composed of seizing and pulling objects (e.g. pulling away a sheet on which the other hand is writing). Patients never deny that the hand is part of their own body but may accuse it of being disobedient and having a will of its own. Anarchic hand can be associated with forced grasping and with motor neglect. Anarchic hand is an impressive but rare phenomenon.

- *Clinical diagnosis.* Relies on complaints of patients and observation of spontaneous behaviour of the hand.

- *Lesion.* Mesial superior frontal lobe of opposite hemisphere. Lesions are large and frequently encroach on callosal fibres. Anarchic hand can be associated with callosal apraxia of the left hand (see Section 2.5), but there are cases of right-sided anarchic hand as well. The respective contributions of frontal lesion and callosal disconnection are a matter of debate (Marchetti and Della-Sala 1998).

- *Therapy.* We are not aware of therapeutic experiences.

3.4 Motor perseverations

Patients contuinue a motor action although its original purpose has been attained. For example, they may continue to peel all oranges in a basket after they have peeled one for eating, or they may be unable to stop toothbrushing or washing and spend hours in the bathroom. Patients may experience perseveration of actions as compulsive and against their own intentions, or they may justify them by ostensible motives (e.g. hygienic reasons for perseverative washing).

- *Clinical diagnosis.* Rests mainly on history taking and observation of patient. In examination motor perseveration can be provoked by asking patients to draw a series of figures each consisting of three consecutive loops. Patients will increase the number of loops.

- *Lesion.* Uni- or bilateral lesions of superior mesial frontal lobe, similar to the grasp reaction with which it may be associated. Persistent and severe motor perseverations are likely to afford large bilateral frontal lesions or additional diffuse brain damage.

- *Therapy.* If motor perseverations do not recover spontaneously and constitute an obstacle for activities of daily living, behavioural therapy and self-instruction can be tried.

3.5 Utilization behaviour

Patients use objects that happen to be within their grasp in a way that is appropriate to the object but not to the situation. For example, they may take glasses that the examiner has laid down and put them on their nose, or they may take a stamp and repeatedly press it on a sheet of paper. If occurring outside the test situation, utilization behaviour may be socially disturbing.

- *Clinical diagnosis.* Care must be taken to distinguish utilization behaviour from the enhanced suggestibility of brain-damaged patients. If, for example, the examiner interrupts testing and puts objects on the table without commenting on their purpose and waits for the patient's reaction (Lhermitte 1983), patients may understand this as a nonverbal invitation to use the objects. It is therefore preferable to have attractive objects (e.g. glasses, matchbox, cigarettes, a pack of cards, a filled bottle and a glass, etc.) already installed on the periphery of the table when the patient enters the room, to engage the patient in an unrelated conversation or test, and to observe their spontaneous behaviour (Shallice *et al.* 1989).

♦ *Lesion.* Large, bilateral mesial frontal lesions. It is possible that lesions must be associated with some diffuse brain damage to give rise to utilization behaviour.

♦ *Therapy.* Behavioural therapy may be worth a trial in patients who display utilization behaviour outside the testing situation.

3.6 Imitation behaviour

Although not requested to do so, patients imitate the gestures and actions of the examiner or other persons. For example, patients may take off their glasses when the examiner does so or repeat back questions rather than answering them. An explicit command not to imitate can stop imitation but introduction of a pause is sufficient for reappearance of imitation. When asked why they imitated patients are puzzled and say nothing or claim that they thought this was the implicit request made by the examiner (De Renzi *et al.* 1996). Like utilization behaviour, imitation behaviour will cause irritation when occurring outside the testing situation.

♦ *Clinical diagnosis.* Rests mainly on observation of spontaneous behaviour during conversation and testing. Avoidance of nonverbal requests to imitate can be very difficult when gestures are introduced explicitly for provoking imitation behaviour.

♦ *Lesions and therapy.* As in utilization behaviour (Section 3.5).

3.7 Voluntary motor control and social demands

The classification of utilization and imitation behaviour as disorders of voluntary control of movement can be called into doubt. The incriminated actions are wrong only with respect to the specific demands of the testing situation. The subtlety of their deviance from appropriate behaviour is highlighted by the fact that the very same actions—utilization of objects and imitation of gestures—are explicitly asked for when the examiner is interested in testing for apraxia (which may happen in the same session!). The observation that normal controls never utilize objects or imitate under the same conditions proves that they can easily understand such subtle distinctions whereas patients with frontal lobe damage cannot. It is, however, questionable whether this failure should be classified as a disorder of motor control or as a manifestation of the effects of frontal lobe damage on comprehension and observance of social demands.

Selective references

Bizzozero, I., Costato, D., Della Sala, S., Papagno, C., Spinnler, H., and Venneri, A. (2000). Upper and lower face apraxia: role of the right hemisphere. *Brain* 123, 2213–30.

De Renzi, E. and Barbieri, C. (1992). The incidence of the grasp reflex following hemispheric lesions and its relation to frontal damage. *Brain* 115, 293–313.

De Renzi, E., Cavalleri, F., and Facchini, S. (1996). Imitation and utilisation behaviour. *J. Neurol., Neurosurg., Psychiatry* 61, 396–400.

Freund, H.J. (1987). Abnormalities of motor behavior after cortical lesions in humans. In *Handbook of physiology*. Section 1: *The nervous system*. Volume 5: *Higher functions of the brain*, Part 2 (ed. V.B. Mountcastle, F. Plum, and S.R. Geiger), pp. 763–810. American Physiological Society, Bethesda, Maryland.

Goldenberg, G. (1996). Defective imitation of gestures in patients with damage in the left or right hemisphere. *J. Neurol., Neurosurg., Psychiatry* 61, 176–80.

Goldenberg, G., Daumüller, M., and Hagmann, S. (2001). Assessment and therapy of complex ADL in apraxia. *Neuropsychol. Rehabil.* 11, 147–69.

Goldenberg, G., Hermsdörfer, J., and Laimgruber, K. (2001*b*). Imitation of gestures by disconnected hemispheres. *Neuropsychologia* 39, 1431–42.

Laplane, D. and Degos, J.D. (1983). Motor neglect. *J. Neurol., Neurosurg., Psychiatry* 46, 152–8.

Lhermitte, F. (1983). 'Utilization behaviour' and its relation to lesions of the frontal lobes. *Brain* 106, 237–55.

Marchetti, C. and Della Sala, S. (1998). Disentangling the alien and anarchic hand. *Cogn. Neuropsychiatry* 3, 191–207.

Perenin, M.T. and Vighetto, A. (1988). Optic ataxia: a specific disruption in visuomotor mechanisms. I. Different aspects of the deficit in reaching for objects. *Brain* 111, 643–74.

Robertson, I. and Cashman, E. (1991). Auditory feedback for walking difficulties in a case of unilateral neglect: a pilot study. *Neuropsychol. Rehabil.* 1, 175–84.

Schwartz, M.F., Buxbaum, L.J., Montgomery, M.W., Fitzpatrick-DeSalme, E.J., Hart, T., Ferraro, M., Lee, S.S., and Coslett, H.B. (1999). Naturalistic action production following right hemisphere stroke. *Neuropsychologia* 37, 51–66.

Shallice, T., Burgess, P.W., Schon, F., and Baxter, D.M. (1989). The origins of utilization behaviour. *Brain* 112, 1587–98.

Chapter 20

Assessment and treatment of calculation disorders

N.J. van Harskamp and L. Cipolotti

1 Introduction

Acalculia is an acquired disorder of number processing and calculation skills following cerebral damage. Acalculia is not a unitary disorder and can take a variety of different forms. Table 20.1 provides an overview of the whole range of potential deficits that can be observed in acalculic patients. In this chapter, each of these disorders will be discussed individually. For recent reviews on acalculia see also Noël (2001), Cipolotti and van Harskamp (2001), and Miceli and Capasso (1999). In addition, two recent books (Butterworth 1999; Dehaene 1997) have been devoted to this topic.

1.1 Incidence

Acalculia is a not infrequent syndrome in patients with cerebral lesions. The incidence of acalculia in patients with left hemisphere lesions has been estimated as between 16%

Table 20.1 Overview of the potential deficits

Disorders of number processing		Disorders of calculation
Disorders of number production	Disorders of lexical processing	Disorders of arithmetical symbol processing
	Disorders of syntactical processing	
		Disorders of arithmetical fact retrieval
Disorders of number comprehension	Disorders of cardinal number meaning	
	Disorders of sequence number meaning	Disorders of calculation procedures
		Disorders of conceptual knowledge
		Subitizing

and 28%. Moreover, more than 90% of patients at the early stage of Alzheimer's disease present with acalculia (Carlomagno *et al.* 1999).

1.2 Secondary acalculia

Acalculia can be considered a secondary impairment, when poor performance on tasks that require the ability to process numbers and to calculate is underpinned by more generalized cognitive impairments. Thus, secondary acalculia may occur in the context of more general language impairment, dyslexia, dysgraphia, and visuoperceptual and visuospatial disorders.

2 Primary acalculia

Acalculia can be considered a primary impairment when the impairment in number processing and calculation is independent of other cognitive disturbances. For example, in 1991, Cipolotti *et al.* reported a patient C.G. who, following a cerebrovascular accident (CVA) in the region of the left middle cerebral artery, had largely preserved intellectual, language, memory, and visuospatial abilities. Moreover, the patient did not have:

◆ a more general semantic memory deficit;

◆ an impairment in dealing with quantities;

◆ an impairment in those reasoning skills thought to underlie the concept of numbers.

However, she presented with an unusually dense acalculia. The patient had lost the meaning of numbers above 4. For example, she was unable to say how many days there were in a week or whether 5 or 10 was the bigger number. Her deficit was so pervasive that it seriously limited her activities of daily living. For example, C.G. was unable to do her own shopping as she could no longer deal with money or check her change. She was no longer able to make phone calls, use a calendar, or read the time.

This finding indicates that acalculia can be the only deficit present following a cerebral lesion. It is now well established that numerical abilities can be largely independent from general intellectual skills (e.g. Remond-Besuchet *et al.* 1999) and other cognitive functions such as language (e.g. Rossor *et al.* 1995; Thioux *et al.* 1998) and short-term memory (e.g. Butterworth *et al.* 1995).

2.1 Clinical presentation

Patients may present with an impairment in either the processing of numbers, in calculation, or in both. It is of interest to note that patients may present with highly specific impairments in number processing and calculation. Several systematic single-case studies have shown that patients can present with severe impairments in calculation without any difficulty in number processing. For example, Sokol *et al.* (1991) reported a patient P.S. who, following a left CVA, showed very poor performance on single-digit multiplication problems. In contrast, she showed preserved performance on a series of number transcoding tasks (i.e. reading, writing to dictation, and repetition) as well as on number comprehension tasks. The reverse pattern, namely, a severe impairment in number processing without an impairment in calculation, is also on record (e.g. Cipolotti and Butterworth 1995). Moreover, cognitive neuropsychological studies have provided evidence for further dissociations within the number processing and calculation skills (see below).

3 Disorders of number processing

Several studies have demonstrated that patients with number processing impairments can have a selective deficit in either producing or in comprehending Arabic numerals (e.g. '5'), verbal numerals (e.g. 'five'), or both.

3.1 Disorders of number production

McCloskey and his colleagues have reported a series of patients with number reading disorders, not underpinned by comprehension deficits. For example, patient H.Y. was impaired in reading aloud Arabic numerals (McCloskey *et al.* 1986, 1990; Sokol and McCloskey 1988). When attempting to read aloud an Arabic numeral, he often made mistakes such as reading 5 as 'seven' and 29 as 'forty-nine'. Results from a series of number comprehension tasks showed that he was unimpaired in comprehending Arabic numerals. Thus, his impaired performance in reading aloud Arabic numerals reflected impairment in the number production system and not a deficit in comprehending the Arabic stimuli. As he owned and ran a construction company, he used numbers in many aspects of his work. Clearly, his reading deficit was extremely disruptive for his professional life.

Within the number production system two major cognitive mechanisms are thought to be involved—the syntactic and the lexical number production mechanisms.

- ◆ Syntactic processing involves the specification of the relationship among the elements of the number (e.g. *number class*, e.g. to read aloud 600, one needs to retrieve the correct number class (hundred)). Syntactic errors are errors where the wrong number class is selected (e.g. stimulus 5 → response 'fifty' or stimulus two thousand and thirty eight → response '2000308').

- ◆ Lexical processing involves the processing of individual elements in the number (e.g. to read aloud 600, once the correct class {hundred} has been retrieved, it is necessary to retrieve the correct element (6)). Lexical errors involve the incorrect production of one or more of the individual elements in a number (stimulus 29 → response 'forty-nine').

Patients making mainly lexical or syntactical errors have been reported. For example, patient H.Y.'s errors in reading aloud Arabic numerals were lexical errors. He appeared to be able to access the correct number lexical class (ones, teens, tens). However, he had difficulty in accessing the correct position within that class (e.g. stimulus 17 → response 'thirteen' or stimulus 902 → response 'nine hundred six'). The opposite pattern of errors was described in patient S.F. (Cipolotti 1995). This patient showed a selective impairment in reading aloud Arabic numerals. The majority of his errors were syntactic errors and could be best classified as 'quantity-shift' errors (e.g. 207 → 'two thousand and seven'; 80 → 'eight'). This deficit impacted seriously on the patient's everyday life activities. He used to work as a bank manager. As a result of his deficit he was no longer able to accurately read cheques or correctly verify bank statements and carry out payments. These difficulties forced him to take early retirement.

3.2 Disorders of number comprehension

A few studies have reported patients with a basic failure in number comprehension. For example, patient N.R. (Noël and Seron 1993) showed an impairment in understanding Arabic numerals. Thus, she could no longer point to the larger of two Arabic numerals (e.g. 345 and 785 or 265 and 2307). Moreover, she lost the ability to match spoken number names to the corresponding Arabic numeral. Delazer and Butterworth (1997) have provided further insight into different aspects of number meaning. The authors made the theoretical distinction between 'cardinal' number meaning and 'sequence' number meaning.

* *Cardinal number meanings* represent the numerosity of a set of entities and describe the manyness of the set.

* *Sequence number meanings* represent the position of a number word in the number sequence and do not refer to numerosities.

They reported a patient S.E. who showed a selective impairment in cardinal meanings, but preserved sequence meaning of numbers. Thus, S.E. was unable to add 1, an operation that according to the authors requires access to cardinal number knowledge. However, she was still able to give the next number in the sequence.

4 Disorders of calculation

It is widely accepted that in order to carry out calculation, specific independent calculation processes are required. These include the following.

* The processing of arithmetical symbols (e.g. $+$, $\times$, $-$).

* The retrieval of arithmetical facts. These are defined as a vocabulary of 'number combinations', such as $3 + 3 = 6$. These facts are directly retrieved from memory.

* The execution of calculation procedures. These procedures allow access to specific algorithms required to solve multidigit calculation. Specific examples are the carrying and borrowing procedures.

* The retrieval of conceptual knowledge. This allows understanding of the principles underlying arithmetical facts and procedures (e.g. the principle of commutativity, such as $a + b = b + a$).

Each of these different cognitive processes appears to be functionally independent and differentially susceptible to brain damage. Examples of selective calculation impairments are discussed in the following sections.

4.1 Disorders of arithmetical symbol processing

Very few patients with a selective impairment in the comprehension of written arithmetical symbols have been reported (e.g. Ferro and Botelho 1980). For example, Laiacona and Lunghi (1997) investigated a patient who misnamed and misidentified the arithmetical signs and performed written calculation according to their misidentification. Thus, for example the patient systematically plussed the times (see Fig. 20.1(a)). According to the authors, this deficit appeared to have little impact on the patient's everyday life. He continued to be completely autonomous. However, it is of interest to note that this deficit was not highly specific for arithmetical symbols, but part of a more general processing deficit for relational symbols. He also presented with an impairment in the use of punctuation marks.

4.2 Disorders of arithmetical fact retrieval

Several patients have been documented with a selective arithmetical fact retrieval impairment. Typically, these patients have severe problems on very simple single-digit addition, subtraction, multiplication, and division. They produce many errors (e.g. $5 + 7 = $ '13 roughly') and their response times are abnormally slow (e.g. >2 seconds.) However, their knowledge of arithmetical principles and procedures is intact. Typically, they are able to retrieve and apply the appropriate arithmetic steps to solve complex arithmetical problems. Moreover, they can define arithmetic operations adequately (e.g. Delazer and Benke 1997; Sokol *et al.* 1991; Warrington 1982). For this type of patient everyday activities such as checking their change or bank statement pose great difficulties.

Arithmetical fact impairment can also manifest itself in a highly selective manner. Selectively preserved and selectively impaired arithmetical facts according to the specific type of operation have been reported. For example, patients have been documented with selective impairments or selective preservations of multiplication (e.g. Dehaene and Cohen 1997; McCloskey *et al.* 1991*b*; Grafman *et al.* 1989; Delazer and Benke 1997) and subtraction facts (e.g. Dagenbach and McCloskey 1992; Pesenti *et al.* 1994; McNeil and Warrington 1994; Lampl *et al.* 1994; Dehaene and Cohen 1997). Selective impairments for addition and division are also on record. Cipolotti and de Lacy Costello (1995) reported a patient who could no longer solve $4 : 2$, while being able to solve 27×26. Recently, van Harskamp and Cipolotti (2001) described a patient with a selective addition impairment. The patient could no longer solve $2 + 3$, while still being able to solve $13 - 6$ and 8×9.

4.3 Disorders of calculation procedures

There have been only a few reports of patients with a selective impairment of calculation procedures. Girelli and Delazer (1996) described a patient M.T. who systematically subtracted the smaller number from the larger one, irrespective of whether the larger digit was at the top or on the bottom line (see Fig. 20.1(b)). His impairment in solving multidigit subtractions was attributed to a defective knowledge of calculation procedures. It is of interest to note that this deficit was selective for subtraction, as he was able to correctly carry out multidigit addition problems such as 78 + 26, involving the carry over procedure.

4.4 Disorders of conceptual knowledge

Delazer and Benke (1997) described a patient J.G. who completely lost conceptual knowledge, which is defined as '... an understanding of arithmetical operations and laws pertaining to these operations ...' (Hittmair-Delazer *et al.* 1994, p. 117). The study showed that the patient had a very good performance in the retrieval of multiplication tables (e.g. 9×9), despite severe problems in all tasks tapping conceptual knowledge. For example, the patient was encouraged to use any 'back-up strategies', such as counting with fingers for simple addition problems that she could no longer solve. This is a strategy normally spontaneously adopted by patients with arithmetical fact retrieval impairments. However, J.G. never succeeded in representing problems with her fingers and stated that '... they were of no use in this task ...' (Delazer and Benke 1997, p. 705). She did not even apply very basic principles such as commutativity in multiplication ($4 \times 12 = 12 \times 4$). Moreover, she was unable to recognize that multiplication can be transformed into repeated addition ($4 \times 12 = 12 + 12 + 12 + 12$).

The opposite side of the dissociation (intact conceptual knowledge and impaired fact retrieval) was reported in two single-case studies (Hittmair-Delazer *et al.* 1994, 1995). These authors described two patients who, despite a severe acalculia, demonstrated excellent conceptual knowledge. For example, the author reported a patient B.E. who showed a profound impairment in single multiplication and division problems. However, the patient showed a preserved knowledge only of the $N \times 2$, $N \times 10$, and $N : 2$ facts. This preserved fact knowledge coupled with very sophisticated preservation of conceptual knowledge allowed him to solve the $M \times N$ problems. For example, when confronted

(a)	48		59	(b)	923		171
	× 67		× 29		− 644		− 48
	115		88		321		127

(c) $8 \times 10 = 80; 80 \div 2 = 40; 40 + 8 = 48$

Fig. 20.1 (a) Example of patient E.B. with a selective impairment in arithmetical symbol processing (Laiacona and Lunghi 1997). The patient systematically interpreted the times symbol as a plus symbol. (b) Examples of patient M.T. with a calculation procedure impairment. He showed 'smaller from larger' subtraction errors (Girelli and Delazer 1996). (c) Example of patient B.E. with impaired arithmetical fact retrieval, but preserved conceptual knowledge. When confronted with a problem such as 8×6, he adopted the strategy shown (Hittmair-Delazer *et al.*, 1994).

with a problem such as 8×6, he adopted the following strategy $8 \times 10 = 80$; $80 : 2 = 40$; $40 + 8 = 48$ (see Fig. 20.1(c)).

Another example of well preserved conceptual knowledge despite severe acalulia is that of a second patient, who was no longer able to solve simple elementary arithmetical facts such as $2 + 3$. However, despite this severe impairment, he showed an excellent understanding and use of abstract equations such as $(b \times a) : (a \times b) = 1$ and $(cd + ed) : d = c + e$. These observations have been interpreted as demonstrating that conceptual knowledge is a functionally independent component of calculation.

5 Subitizing

When people are presented with small sets of four or fewer items such as dots for a limited amount of time they can rapidly and accurately determine their number. This ability has been called *subitizing*. However, for over four items, visual object enumeration is slow, more error-prone, and is thought to require counting. Several theories have been proposed to account for this dichotomy. The most popular view assumes that the processing underlying subitizing and counting is different in nature, both functionally and anatomically (e.g. Trick and Pylyshyn 1993; Sathian *et al.* 1999). For example, Trick and Pylyshyn (1993) proposed that subitizing of small sets depends on a limited-capacity preattentive visual process. Counting of more numerous objects requires serial shifts in spatial attention. However, an alternative view has also been put forward. Some investigators have proposed that subitizing and counting simply reflect two different levels along a continuum of difficulty and do not have separate dedicated neural systems (e.g. Balakrishnan and Ashby 1992; Piazza *et al.* 2002).

In neuropsychological data, evidence for a dissociation between subitizing and counting is sparse. Dehaene and Cohen (1994) reported simultanagnosic patients who showed intact subitizing despite severely impaired counting. However, the subitizing range was rather limited (sets of 1, 2, and, rarely, 3 items). The above discussed patient C.G. was still able to count to four, while unable to subitize a range of 1 or 2 items (Cipolotti *et al.* 1991). To date, the question as to whether subitizing and counting require functionally and possible anatomically distinct processes remains unanswered.

6 Localization of lesions

Brain lesions causing acalculia have been well documented. A recent overview of both group studies and single-case studies has suggested that numerical skills have a discrete and independent brain substrate (Cipolotti and van Harskamp 2001). The majority of patients with number production and/or number comprehension impairments had left posterior lesions, almost always involving the parietal lobe. Similarly, the majority of patients with arithmetical fact retrieval impairments had lesions mainly implicating the left parietal lobe. It is of interest to note that this is even the case for the majority of patients with arithmetical fact retrieval impairment selective for specific types of operations. In particular, patients with impairments for multiplication or subtraction mostly presented lesions encroaching upon the left parietal lobule. Very few patients with a deficit in arithmetical procedures have been reported. Although the evidence available is sparse, a more anterior localization site has emerged.

Recent neuroimaging studies investigated the neuronal correlates underpinning number processing and calculation. They often report large neuronal networks including bilateral inferior parietal activations and other regions such as the prefrontal cortex (e.g. Pesenti *et al.* 2000; Dehaene *et al.* 1999).

7 Diagnosis and assessment tools

The diagnosis of acalculia relies on establishing with appropriate tools the presence of a number processing and/or calculation impairment in a subject who premorbidly had acquired normal calculation skills. The diagnosis of primary acalculia can only be made when the investigator can exclude that the deficit in numeracy skills is not a secondary consequence of other cognitive deficits. In other words, one needs to exclude that a generalized impairment in language, attention, or visuospatial functions is underpinning the failure of number processing and calculation.

A formal assessment of the patient's numeracy skills requires a detailed evaluation of number processing and calculation skills. In order to assess individual number processing skills both number production and number comprehension need to be evaluated.

- *Number production skills* can be assessed by number reading, writing to dictation, and repetition tasks. The stimuli can be presented as either Arabic numerals (e.g. '8') or written (*eight*) or spoken number names ('eight'). The patient can be simply asked to read, write, or repeat the given numeral.

- *Number comprehension skills* are usually assessed by a variety of tasks.

    —One of the most used tests is the Magnitude comparison task. In this test the subject is asked to indicate the larger of two numbers (i.e. 6 or 9, which is the bigger?).

    —Another test of number comprehension is the Poker chips test. In this test the subject is asked to select poker chips (poker chips ranging in value from 1 to 500) corresponding to the value of the presented Arabic numeral or spoken number name.

Calculation skills are assessed by tests tapping arithmetical signs processing skills, arithmetical facts, and arithmetical procedures.

- To evaluate the ability to process the *arithmetical signs* (e.g. $+$, $-$, $\times$) the subject is usually required to read, point at, and write the arithmetical signs.

- To evaluate simple *arithmetical fact retrieval*, the subject is given single-digit problems with operands between 0 to 9 across the four basic operations such as $4 + 2$, 3×4, or $5 - 2$.

♦ The access to *arithmetical procedures* is usually assessed by performing multidigit calculations, such as 294 + 12 = 306, either in the written or in the oral modality.

Such a detailed functional assessment of the patient's number processing and calculation skills is needed to establish which specific components within the number processing or calculation system are impaired. There are a series of research batteries that evaluate in detail numerical skills along this line (e.g. McCloskey *et al.* 1991*a*).

However, only a few standardized tests have been developed. One of these is the EC301 composite battery, which allows the detailed evaluation of both calculation and number processing abilities in brain-damaged adults (Deloche *et al.* 1994). However, this battery is rather lengthy and requires approximately 1 hour to administer. A revised and shorter form (EC301R) is also available (Deloche *et al.* 1995, 1996). In this version there are fewer tasks, which makes it possible to assess mathematical abilities in less time (about 30 minutes). Another advantage of this battery is represented by the fact that it also evaluates some aspects of mathematical knowledge necessary for everyday life (e.g. numerical knowledge such as the number of days in the week).

A standardized test that evaluates mental calculation is the graded difficulty arithmetic (GDA) test (Jackson and Warrington 1986). This test comprised 12 multidigit additions and subtractions, graded in difficulty, including relatively easy problems such as '15 + 13 = ?' and rather difficult problems such as '244 + 129 = ?'. This is a timed test that requires the subject to give an answer within 10 seconds.

Error analyses, although usually not included in standardized tests, are very useful additions to the assessment, insofar as they can provide information about the locus of damage. Thus, when patients have problems in reading and writing of numerals, a common analysis of errors is the distinction between lexical or syntactical errors (as discussed in Section 3.1). When patients have problems in the retrieval of arithmetical facts, a common analysis is the error classification proposed by McCloskey *et al.* (1991*c*). Hence, errors can be classed as:

♦ *operand errors*, if the incorrect answer is the correct answer to a problem that shares one of the operands (e.g. 6 × 5 = 25);

♦ *operation errors*, if the incorrect answer is the correct answer to another problem involving the same operands, but a different operation (e.g. 3 + 4 = 12);

♦ *table errors*, if the incorrect answer is an answer that is a product of two other single-digit numbers (e.g. 4 × 4 = 25);

♦ *non-table errors*, if the incorrect answer is not an operand, table, or operation error (e.g. 9 × 8 = 52).

8 Natural recovery of acalculia

Although acalculia is a frequent disorder in left-brain-damaged patients, relatively little is known about its prognosis. Only one study has investigated the natural evolution of acalculia in patients with left hemisphere vascular lesions (Caporali *et al.* 2000). This study indicates that some patients completely recovered from acalculia in the first months post-stroke even without a specific rehabilitation. Apparently, this improvement was also present in severely acalculic patients. This suggests that the initial severity of acalculia may not significantly influence recovery. The authors suggested that the recovery might be due to the resolution of the diachises in the first months after stroke (up until the 3–6 months period). However, besides this more general and 'passive' recovery, the authors suggested that a more specialized functional reorganization might have played a role several months post-onset (>7 months). This suggestion was made to account for the fact that a few patients continued to improve even several months after the stroke. For example, one patient, first seen 5 months post-onset, improved significantly on an acalculia test in the following 7 months. However, it is not clear whether the recovery was specific for acalculia. In fact, most patients improved in other cognitive domains, such as language.

9 Rehabilitation of number-processing and calculation skills

The high-frequency and disabling consequences of acalculia underline the importance of developing remediation techniques and intervention for arithmetical disorders. A complete and detailed assessment of the patient's numerical processing and calculation skills is essential to understand the nature of the numeracy impairment (Girelli and Seron 2001). According to the specific type of acalculia, different kinds of rehabilitative intervention may be required.

Thus, a detailed assessment of a patient's number processing and calculation skills will constitute the basis for designing a suitable rehabilitation programme. For example, a patient may show a highly selective impairment in the retrieval of simple multiplication facts. However, he/she may still be able to perform simple addition and subtraction. The re-acquisition of multiplication facts may then be facilitated by the use of back-up strategies based on addition (e.g. counting-on procedure: $3 \times 6 = 6 + 6 + 6$).

A recent review by Girelli and Seron (2001) has showed that very few studies have been devoted to the rehabilitation of numerical skills. These few studies concentrated on the rehabilitation of number transcoding deficits (e.g. Deloche et al. 1989; Sullivan et al. 1996) and the rehabilitation of arithmetical facts retrieval (e.g. Hittmair-Delazer et al. 1994; Girelli et al. 1996; Whetstone 1998).

9.1 Rehabilitation of transcoding skills

The rehabilitation of transcoding skills has concentrated on the ability to translate numerical stimuli into different codes (e.g. 'four' → 4). As an example we will discuss an interesting rehabilitation programme implemented by Deloche et al. (1989). They treated a patient with selective difficulties in the production of written verbal numerals from Arabic numerals (i.e. 7001 → seven thousand zero one). This deficit was very pronounced. Indeed, he showed a 45% error rate. His errors were mostly syntactic (e.g. 114 → one hundred ten four). Deloche *et al.*'s rehabilitation programme consisted in reteaching, step by step, a set of explicit transcoding rules. They used highly specific exercises that targeted a single transcoding rule. There were several facilitation procedures (e.g. colour cues, vocabulary panels) to help the patient with his learning process. For example, they rehabilitated the patient's ability to transcode a 2-digit Arabic numeral such as *73* into the corresponding written verbal numeral *seventy-three*, by explicitly stating the rule 'transcode the left digit by a ten name and the right digit by a unit name'. During the training the vocabulary panel in two coloured columns was placed in front of him. The red part of the vocabulary panel contained TENS names (ten, twenty, thirty, etc. up to ninety) and the blue part of the vocabulary panel contained UNIT names (one, two, etc. up to nine). After 25 training sessions of 30 to 60 minutes each, the patient's performance was close to ceiling. Interestingly, the long-term effects of the treatment were reassessed 7 months post-training. Only a very small increase in error rate relative to post-training evaluation was reported (6%). Overall, the patient continued to perform better than before training (45% error rate retraining).

9.2 Rehabilitation of arithmetical facts

The rehabilitative intervention for arithmetical fact retrieval impairments primarily consists of attempts to re-teach 'lost' knowledge via extensive practice. The underlying assumption is that practice may 're-create' and 're-strengthen' the lost associations between problem and answer. Thus, for example, two patients, T.L. and Z.A., with a specific multiplication fact retrieval impairment underwent twice-weekly training sessions over a period of 8 weeks (Girelli *et al.* 1996). During the training session the arithmetical problems were presented in written form and simultaneously read aloud by the examiner. The patients were asked to answer, either verbally whilst pointing to the number on a table or by writing the Arabic numeral. Errors were always corrected immediately. Patient T.L. relearned the answers as 'labels' by reciting one operand's table (e.g. $4 \times 3 = 4, 8, 12$). Patient Z.A. relearned the answers as serial addition (e.g. $4 \times 3 = 3 + 3 + 3 = 12$). At the end of the session, both patients improved considerably and showed a stable recovery at 1-month follow-up. Strikingly, after treatment, their overall error rate dropped to 10% from pretreatment error rates of 91% (T.L.) and 81% (Z.A.). Interestingly, not only did the error rate decrease dramatically over the course of the remediation programme for both patients, but the nature of the errors also changed. This change in error patterns was interpreted as due to the different strategies used by the patients to relearn their facts. As described above, patient T.L. relied on the recitation of $N \times 1$ forward until she could access the solution to the problem. Patient Z.A. relied on the strategy of repeated addition of the second operand. Thus, back-up strategies may certainly play a facilitating role in the re-acquisition of simple arithmetic. A similar training programme for the rehabilitation of arithmetical fact impairment was adopted by, e.g. Hittmair-Delazer *et al.* (1994) and Whetstone (1998).

In their review, Girelli and Seron (2001) also stressed the importance of minimizing the opportunity to make mistakes, since repeated errors may strengthen the wrong associations between problems and answers. Moreover, the use of back-up strategies based on the principles underlying arithmetical facts such as the order-irrelevant principle e.g. $8 \times 6 = 6 \times 8 = 48$, decomposition strategies like $4 \times 8 = 2 \times 8 + 2 \times 8 = 32$, or repeated addition of the second operand ($3 \times 5 = 5 + 5 + 5 = 15$) seems important in rehabilitation of arithmetical facts. Overall, the findings indicated that the patients benefited significantly from the training undertaken. Importantly, the improvement was retained over time and, in some cases, the training effects spontaneously generalized.

9.3 Conclusion

It is apparent from this short review that there are several important aspects of numerical skills for which no specific interventions have been developed. For example, currently there are no specific programmes available for the rehabilitation of calculation procedures impairment nor for the rehabilitation of conceptual knowledge or number comprehension impairments. Therefore, it seems necessary in the near future to develop studies aimed at providing guidelines on the treatment of the different calculation impairments. Moreover, it seems important to develop studies looking specifically at the efficacy of the methods in calculation rehabilitative interventions. Importantly, rehabilitation programmes including more ecological tasks such as handling real money need to be developed. It still remains an open question whether the facilitation effects of the training session generalize to real-life situations—the purpose of any rehabilitation programme.

Selective references

Balakrishnan, J.D. and Ashby, F.G. (1992). Subitizing: magical numbers or mere superstition? *Psychol. Rev.* **54**, 80–90.

Butterworth, B. (1999). *The mathematical brain*. Macmillan, London.

Butterworth, B., Cipolotti, L., and Warrington, E.K. (1995). Short-term memory impairments and arithmetical ability. *Quart. J. Exp. Psychol.* **49A**, 251–62.

Caporali, A., Burgio, F., and Basso, A. (2000). The natural course of acalculia in left-brain-damaged patients. *Neurol. Sci.* **21**, 143–9.

Carlomagno, S., Iaverone, A., Nolfe, G., Bourene, G., Martin, C., and Deloche, G. (1999). Dyscalculia in the early stages of Alzheimer's disease. *Acta Neuropsychol. Scand.* **3**, 166–74.

Cipolotti, L. (1995). Multiple routes for reading words, why not numbers? Evidence from a case of Arabic numeral dyslexia. *Cogn. Neuropsychol.* **12**, 313–42.

Cipolotti, L. and Butterworth, B. (1995). Toward a multiroute model of number processing: impaired number transcoding with preserved calculation skills. *J. Exp. Psychol. Gen.* **124** (4), 375–90.

Cipolotti, L. and De Lacy Costello, A. (1995). Selective impairment for simple division. *Cortex* **31**, 433–49.

Cipolotti, L. and van Harskamp, N.J. (2001). Disturbances of number processing and calculation. In *Handbook of neuropsychology* (ed. F. Boller and J. Grafman), pp. 305–31. Elsevier, Amsterdam.

Cipolotti, L., Butterworth, B., and Denes, G. (1991). A specific deficit for numbers in case of dense acalculia. *Brain* **114**, 2619–37.

Dagenbach, D. and McCloskey, M. (1992). The organisation of arithmetical facts in memory: evidence from a brain-damaged patient. *Brain Cognition* **20**, 345–66.

Dehaene S. (1997). *The number sense: how the mind creates mathematics.* University Press, New York.

Dehaene, S. and Cohen, L. (1994). Dissociable mechanisms of subitizing and counting: neuropsychological evidence from simultanagnosic patients. *J. Exp. Psychol.: Hum. Percept. Perform.* **29** (5), 958–75.

Dehaene, S. and Cohen, L. (1997). Cerebral pathways for calculation: double dissociation between rote verbal and quantitative knowledge of arithmetic. *Cortex* **33**, 219–50.

Dehaene, S., Spelke, E., Pinel, P., Stanescu, R., and Tsivkin, S. (1999). Sources of mathematical thinking: behavioral and brain-imaging evidence. *Science* **284**, 970–4.

Delazer, M. and Benke, T. (1997). Arithmetic facts without meaning. *Cortex* **33**, 697–710.

Delazer, M. and Butterworth, B. (1997). A dissociation of number meanings. *Cogn. Neuropsychol.* **14**, 613–36.

Deloche, G., Seron, X., and Ferrand, I. (1989). Re-education of number transcoding mechanisms: a procedural approach. In *Cognitive approaches in neuropsychological rehabilitation* (ed. X. Seron and S. Deloche), pp. 249–87. Lawrence Erlbaum, Hillsdale, New Jersey.

Deloche, G., Seron, X., Larroque, C., Magnien, C., Metz-Lutz, M.N., Noel, M.N., Riva, I., Dordain, M., Schils, J.P., Ferrand, I., Baeta, E., Basso, A., Cipolotti L., Claros-Salinas, D., Gaillard, F., Goldenberg, G., Howard, D., Mazzuchi, A., Stachowiack F., Tzavaras, A., Vendrell, J., Bergego, C., and Pradat-Diehl, P. (1994). Calculation and number processing: Assessment battery; role of demographic factors. *J. Clin. Exp. Neuropsychol.* **16**, 195–208.

Deloche, G., Hannequin, D., Carlomagno, S., Agniel, A., Dordain, M., Pasquir, F., Pellat, J., Dennis, P., Desi, M., Beauchamp, D., Metz-Lutz, M.N., Cesaro, P., and Seron, X. (1995). Calculation and number processing in mild Alzheimer's disease. *J. Clin. Exp. Neuropsychol.* **17**, 634–9.

Deloche, G., Dellatolas, G., Vendrell, J., and Bergego, C. (1996). Calculation and number processing: neuropsychological assessment and daily life difficulties. *J. Int. Neuropsychol. Soc.* **2**, 177–80.

Ferro, J.M. and Botelho, M.A.S. (1980). Alexia for arithmetical signs: a cause of disturbed calculation. *Cortex* **16**, 175–80.

Girelli, L. and Delazer, M. (1996). Subtraction bugs in an acalculic patient. *Cortex* **32**, 547–55.

Girelli, L. and Seron, X. (2001). Rehabilitation of number processing and calculation skills. *Aphasiology* **15** (7), 695–712.

Girelli, L., Delazer, M., Semenza, C., and Denes, G. (1996). The representation of arithmetical facts: evidence from two rehabilitation studies. *Cortex* **32**, 49–66.

Grafman, J., Kampen, D., Rosenberg, J., Salazar, A., and Boller, F. (1989). Calculation abilities in a patient with a virtual left hemispherectomy. *Behav. Neurol.* **2**, 183–94.

Hittmair-Delazer, M., Semenza, C., and Denes, G. (1994). Concepts and facts in calculation. *Brain* **117**, 715–28.

Hittmair-Delazer, M., Sailer, U., and Benke, T. (1995). Impaired arithmetic facts but intact conceptual knowledge—a single case study of dyscalculia. *Cortex* **31**, 139–48.

Jackson, M. and Warrington, E.K (1986). Arithmetic skills in patients with unilateral cerebral lesions. *Cortex* **22**, 611–20.

Laiacona, M. and Lunghi, A. (1997). A case of concomitant impairment of operational signs and punctuation marks. *Neuropsychologia* **35**, 325–32.

Lampl, Y., Eshel, Y., Gilad, R., and Sarova-Pinhas, I. (1994). Selective acalculia with sparing of the subtraction process in a patient with left parieto-temporal haemorrhage. *Neurology* **44**, 1759–61.

McCloskey, M., Sokol, S.M., and Goodman, R.A. (1986). Cognitive processes in verbal–number production: inferences from the performance of brain-damaged subjects. *J. Exp. Psychol. Gen.* **115** (4), 307–30.

McCloskey, M., Sokol, S.M., Goodman-Schulman, R.A., and Caramazza, A. (1990). Cognitive representations and processes in number production: evidence from cases of acquired dyscalculia. In *Advances in cognitive neuropsychology and neurolinguistics* (ed. A. Caramazza), pp. 1–32. Lawrence Erlbaum Associates, Hillsdale, New Jersey.

McCloskey, M., Aliminosa, D., and Macaruso, P. (1991*a*). Theory-based assessment of acquired dyscalculia. *Brain Cognition* **17**, 285–308.

McCloskey, M., Aliminosa, D., and Sokol, S.M. (1991*b*). Facts, rules and procedures in normal calculation: evidence from multiple single-patient studies of impaired arithmetic fact retrieval. *Brain Cognition* **17**, 154–203.

McCloskey, M., Harley, W., and Sokol, S.M. (1991*c*). Models of arithmetic fact retrieval: an evaluation in light of findings from normal and brain-damaged subjects. *J. Exp. Psychol.: Learning, Memory, Cognition* **17**, 377–97.

McNeil, J. and Warrington, E.K. (1994). A dissociation between addition and subtraction with written calculation. *Neuropsychologia* **32**, 717–28.

Miceli, G. and Capasso, R. (1999). Calculation and number processing. In *Handbook of clinical and experimental neuropsychology* (ed. G. Denes and L. Pizzamiglio), pp. 583–612. Psychology Press, Hove, East Sussex.

Noël, M.P. (2001). Numerical cognition. In *The handbook of cognitive neuropsychology: what deficits reveal about the human mind* (ed. B. Rapp), pp. 495–518. Taylor and Francis, Psychology Press, Hove, East Sussex.

Noël, M.P. and Seron, X (1993). Arabic number reading deficit: a single case study. *Cogn. Neuropsychol.* **10**, 317–39.

Pesenti, M., Seron, X., and Van Der Linden, M. (1994). Selective impairment as evidence for mental organisation of arithmetical facts: BB, a case of preserved subtraction? *Cortex* **30**, 661–71.

Pesenti, M., Thioux, M., Seron, X., and De Volder, A. (2000). Neuroanatomical substrates of Arabic number processing, numerical comparison, and simple addition: a PET study. *J. Cogn. Neurosci.* **12** (3), 461–79.

Piazza, M., Mechelli, A., Butterworth, B., and Price, C.J. (2002). Are subitizing and counting implemented as separate or functionally overlapping processing? *NeuroImage* **15** (2), 435–46.

Remond-Besuchet, C., Noël, M.P., Seron, X., Thioux, M., Brun, M., and Aspe, X. (1999). Selective preservation of exceptional arithmetical knowledge in a demented patient. *Math. Cognition* **5** (1), 41–63.

Rossor, M.N., Warrington, E.K., and Cipolotti, L. (1995). The isolation of calculation skills. *J. Neurol.* **242**, 78–81.

Sathian, K., Simon, T. J., Peterson S, Patel, G.A., Hoffman, J.M., and Grafton, S.T. (1999). Neural evidence linking visual object enumeration and attention. *J. Cogn. Neurosci.* **11** (1), 36–51.

Sokol, S.M. and McCloskey, M. (1988). Levels of representation in verbal number production. *Appl. Psycholinguistics* **9**, 267–81.

Sokol, S.M., McCloskey, M., Cohen, N.J., and Aliminosa, D. (1991). Cognitive representations and processes in arithmetic: inferences from the performance of brain-damaged subjects. *J. Exp. Psychol. Learning, Memory, Cognition* **17** (3), 355–76.

Sullivan, K.S., Macaruso, P., and Sokol, S.M. (1996). Remediation of Arabic numerals in numeral processing in a case of developmental dyscalculia. *Neuropsychol. Rehabil.* **6**, 27–53.

Thioux, M., Pillon, A., Samson, D., de Partz, M.P., Noël, M.P., and Seron, X. (1998). The isolation of numerals at the semantic level. *Neurocase* **4**, 371–89.

Trick, L.M. and Pylyshyn, Z.W. (1993). What enumeration studies can show us about spatial attention: evidence for limited capacity preattentive processes. *J. Exp. Psychol.: Hum. Percept. Perform.* **19** (2), 331–51.

Van Harskamp, N.J. and Cipolotti, L. (2001). Selective impairments in addition, subtraction and multiplication: Implications for the organisation of arithmetical facts. *Cortex* **37**, 363–88.

Warrington, E.K. (1982). The fractionation of arithmetical skills: a single study. *Quart. J. Exp. Psychol.* **34**, 31–51.

Whetstone, T. (1998). The representation of arithmetic facts in memory: results from retraining a brain-damaged patient. *Brain Cognition* **36**, 290–309.

Chapter 21

Assessment and treatment of emotional disorders

Guido Gainotti

1 Introduction

The juxtaposition, in this and in most other books of neuropsychology, of emotional disorders and disorders of language, memory, attention, visuospatial exploration, etc. could implicitly suggest that a basic similarity exists among all these 'neuropsychological' disorders. This suggestion, however, is misleading from both the conceptual and the pathophysiological points of view. Conceptually, emotions cannot be placed under the same general heading as the above-mentioned cognitive functions. Pathophysiologically, the relationship between brain damage and clinical symptomatology is different in the cases of cognitive and of emotional disorders.

1.1 Emotion as a general 'adaptive system'

From the 'conceptual' point of view, language, memory, attention, etc. must be viewed as 'functional systems' that can be considered to be components of a general, phylogenetically advanced, adaptive system (the 'cognitive system'). Emotion, on the other hand, should be considered as a second (more primitive) general adaptive system, also composed of different functional subsystems. The adaptive nature of both the emotional and the cognitive system has been stressed by Oatley and Johnson-Laird (1987), who claimed that, in order to face a partially unpredictable environment and to select the most appropriate response pattern, the organism makes use of two operative (the emotional and the cognitive) systems.

- The *emotional system* is considered to be an automatic emergency system, based on processes involved in the quick appraisal of external events and the immediate activation of a small number of innate operative patterns. These action patterns correspond to a few basic emotions (e.g. fear, rage, joy, sadness, surprise, and disgust) that reflect, at the level of interpersonal communication and of proneness toward action, the most important interactive schemata for the human species.

- The *cognitive system* can be considered, in contrast, to be a powerful propositional adaptive system, based on the exhaustive computation of sensory data and on the selection of complex strategic plans, but one that requires much more time to carry out its adaptive function (see Gainotti 2000 for a more detailed discussion of this issue).

If we turn now to the different pathophysiology responsible for cognitive and emotional disorders resulting from brain injury, we can say that the relationship between brain damage and clinical symptomatology is immediate (and the functional defect closely related to the anatomical locus of lesion) in various kinds of cognitive disorders. This relation, however, is at least in part indirect (and the behavioural pattern only in part related to the anatomical locus of damage) in the case of emotional disorders. In fact, cognitive disorders observed in patients with focal brain damage typically result from the disruption of brain structures subserving specific components of the cognitive system, but this general principle does not account for emotional disorders. Many of these disorders result from a more general process, namely, from the emotional appraisal that the patient makes of his actual situation.

1.2 Emotional reactions to the consequences of brain damage

According to most theorists of emotions (e.g. Lazarus 1982), the process of emotional appraisal (or emotional evaluation) is a fundamental step of every kind of emotional reaction and consists of the subjective evaluation:

♦ of the personal significance of a situation or event;

♦ of the capacity to cope adequately with this event.

Now, since a stroke, brain injury, or other cause of brain damage is an event that can have tremendous personal meaning for the patient, a significant emotional reaction to the brain damage is to be expected, irrespective of the extent and of the anatomical location of the brain lesion. Furthermore, an appraisal process similar to the one required in response to the unexpected event causing the brain damage will be provoked by the long-term behavioural consequences of the brain lesion, since disorders of communication, loss of independence in daily living activities, and loss of social role and of social relations constitute further challenging situations for the emotional equilibrium of the patient. We can, therefore, conclude that, if language, memory, and visuospatial disorders are the net consequence of the underlying brain damage, emotional disorders observed in the same patients can result not only from neurological factors, similar to those subserving cognitive disorders, but also from psychological/psychodynamic reactions and psychosocial factors.

2 Taxonomies of emotions and their underlying theoretical models

The theoretical debate between biologically and cognitively oriented authors about the nature of emotions has been dominated in recent years by a controversy about the relationships between emotion and cognition. On the one hand, authors such as Zajonc (1980), Panksepp (1982), and LeDoux (1996) have stressed the biological foundations of emotions, maintaining that emotion and cognition must be considered as independent systems. On the other hand, cognitively oriented authors, such as Lazarus (1982), Frijda (1986), and Scherer (2000), have argued that there are not two independent adaptive systems, but that cognition plays an integral part in emotion. This controversy was reflected in Section 1, where I first stressed the independence between emotional and cognitive systems, but then claimed that the emotional reaction of brain-damaged patients derives from a cognitive process of emotional appraisal. This conflict (and the apparent inconsistency that I have just mentioned) stems from the facts that human emotions are very complex, hierarchically organized phenomena (Gainotti 2001) and that the levels of emotions taken into account by biologically oriented and by cognitively oriented authors, respectively, can be very different.

- The biologically oriented authors, being interested in brain–behaviour relationships and drawing on Darwin's (1872/1965) seminal work on the survival value of the social aspects of emotions, focus their attention on the simplest aspects of emotion, as they appear in animals and in the early stages of human development. Their taxonomies of emotions are, therefore, based on a small number of basic emotions that are deemed to be at least in part innate and devised to solve in a stereotyped manner some basic problems of the human species.

- The cognitively oriented authors, attracted by the complexity of emotional phenomena, focus their attention on the subtleties of human interactions, consider the biological approach as inappropriate and reductionistic, and base their taxonomies of human emotions on various types of situational antecedents and of appraisal criteria (Scherer 2000).

Biologically oriented authors are therefore right in considering that, from the phylogenetic and from functional points of view, emotion and cognition constitute two partly independent adaptive systems and are subserved by different brain structures. However, cognitively oriented theorists are also right in stressing the interaction that exists between the two systems and the integral role that cognition plays in functions of emotional appraisal.

Trying to construct a bridge between these two different but not necessarily alternative positions, Leventhal (1974) has proposed an ontogenetic model of emotions that implicitly acknowledges both the earlier autonomy and the later dependency of the emotional on the cognitive system. The distinction between biologically grounded basic levels of emotions and psychologically oriented emotional reactions can allow us to understand why emotional disorders can result in some cases from neurological factors and in other instances from psychological or psychosocial factors.

3 Neurological, psychological, and psychosocial factors causing emotional disorders in brain-damaged patients

3.1 Neurological factors

Emotional disorders are due to neurological factors when they result from the encroachment of the lesion upon 'limbic' structures (such as the fronto-orbital cortex, the cingulate gyrus, the amygdala, or the ventral striatum) specifically involved in various

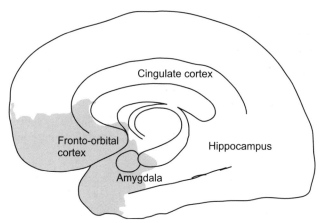

Fig. 21.1 A schematic representation of the fronto-orbital cortex, the cingulate gyrus, and the amygdala mapped on to a medial view of a cerebral hemisphere. The hatched parts of the figure indicate the brain structures usually damaged in patients with a severe closed head injury.

aspects of emotions (see Gainotti 2001 for a survey of this subject). A schematic representation of these structures, mapped on to a medial view of a cerebral hemisphere, is shown in (Fig. 21.1).

3.1.1 Emotional disorders as long-term sequelae of closed head injury

Of the various categories of diseases that can provoke brain damage, closed head injury is probably the one that shows the most direct link between structural brain lesions and emotional disorders. This is due to the fact that, in patients who report a typical road accident of the acceleration–deceleration type, the injury mostly involves the axial brain structures and the mesiobasal parts of the frontal and temporal lobes (Adams *et al.* 1980). Particularly damaged, therefore, are structures such as the fronto-orbital cortex, the anterior part of the cingulate gyrus, and the amygdala (Fig. 21.1), which are critically involved in various aspects of emotional and motivational processes. The clinical counterpart of the preferential encroachment of the lesion upon these limbic structures is a prevalence of emotional and of behavioural disorders (rather than of motor, sensory, or aphasic disturbances) as the long-term sequelae of severe head injury. These emotional disorders usually consist of:

♦ a severe apathetic syndrome, with a lack of emotional reaction to pleasant or unpleasant events and of goal-directed behaviour;

♦ a marked inability to keep under control socially unacceptable emotional reactions, such as aggressive outbursts when experiencing frustrating situations;

♦ less specific anxious or depressive reactions.

These mental changes, which usually affect young or very young persons and are associated with significant memory disorders and poor awareness of cognitive and behavioural disturbances, are extremely important from the clinical point of view. They hamper resumption of gainful employment and also place a heavy burden upon family members, who must cope with the patient's childishness, impaired initiative, low tolerance of frustration, and impulsive or aggressive reactions. Several pharmacological, behavioural, and psychological treatment methods for these disruptive emotional disturbances have, therefore, been proposed and will be discussed in Section 6. It must, however, be acknowledged that the prognosis of this condition is often very poor, that return to a productive lifestyle is sometimes impossible, and that the attainment of a relative independence and the re-establishment of more satisfactory interpersonal relationships often are the only realistic endpoints of the rehabilitation process.

3.2 **Psychological factors**

Emotional disorders due to psychological or psychodynamic (rather than to neurological) factors result from the process of appraisal:

- evaluating the personal significance that the consequences of the brain damage will have for the subject;
- evaluating his/her capacity to cope with these consequences.

A factor that critically contributes to the outcome of this (implicit or explicit) appraisal process is the awareness of the brain damage and of its consequences. When this awareness is full and painful, as in many patients with a Broca's aphasia and a right-sided hemiplegia, the emotional response often consists of 'catastrophic reactions' following frustrating attempts at verbal expression and also of a more stable anxious–depressive disorder. When, on the contrary, this awareness is poor (as in patients with a frontal lobe lesion resulting from a traumatic brain injury, or in stroke patients with a right hemisphere lesion and a syndrome of neglect for the left half of the body and of extrapersonal space), a lack of concern or apathetic behaviour is usually observed.

It must be acknowledged, however, that an (apparent) unawareness of the functional defect and of the resulting disability ('anosognosia') can sometimes be considered to be a primitive form of coping mechanism, rather than as a factor influencing the appraisal process. In this case it seems preferable to use the term 'denial of illness', rather than the term 'unawareness of the disability', to mean that the patient is somehow aware of his/her disabilities but, being unable to accept them, is forced to verbally deny their existence.

3.2.1 Anosognosia of left-sided hemiplegia (see Chapter 12)

The more impressive form of 'denial of illness' is often observed in patients who have sustained a massive stroke in the territory of the right middle cerebral artery but who verbally deny their left-sided hemiplegia or behave as if this side of their body is perfectly normal (see Chapter 22). The reactive nature of this pattern of behaviour is suggested by a qualitative analysis of the first manifestations and of the temporal evolution of the patient's anosognosia. In the first days after the stroke the patient shows a 'real obstinacy not to admit his hemiplegia and a resistance to its recognition that is truly striking and a little disconcerting' (Barré *et al.* 1923). In the days that follow, he/she begins to admit that there is something wrong in the paralysed limbs, but alleges trivial reasons (such as rheumatism or the pain provoked by injections) to excuse their poor performance. Only at a later stage does the patient really acknowledge his left-sided hemiplegia, but at this point he/she appears frustrated and depressed.

The existence of a 'denial syndrome' due to general psychodynamic mechanisms and not directly resulting from brain damage is suggested by several lines of evidence. One of these is that a denial syndrome is often observed in life-threatening conditions, e.g. cancer or myocardial infarction, independently of brain damage. Another line of evidence stems from Weinstein and Kahn's (1955) observation that premorbid personality factors, such as a strong need for prestige and independence or an almost exclusive reliance upon personal skills and capabilities (leading the patient to consider illness and dependency a source of intolerable anxiety), can play an important role in the development of 'denial of illness'.

Difficulty in determining whether an emotional behaviour is a consequence of a process of emotional appraisal or is, instead, due to a biologically determined factor that influences the outcome of this process is frequently experienced in brain-damaged patients. This problem may concern not only the awareness of the disease, but also other important aspects of emotional behaviour, such as a depressive mood or an apathetic state.

3.2.2 Poststroke depression

The syndrome of major 'poststroke depression' (PSD), which is observed in a high proportion (20–25%) of stroke patients, is considered by Robinson *et al.* (1984; Robinson 2001) to be a biological consequence of stroke, resulting from disruption of monoaminergic pathways running from the brainstem to the cerebral cortex. These conclusions, however, have been criticized on methodological grounds by Gainotti *et al.* (1997), who have reanalysed the question using a new instrument (the Post-Stroke Depression Rating Scale) specifically constructed with a view to the symptoms and problems of stroke patients. These authors showed that major PSD is phenomenologically different from the 'endogenous' forms of major depression and concluded that PSD must be considered to be a motivated form of depression, provoked by the serious obstacles that the consequences of brain damage put in the way of the patients' attainment of their personal goals. The emphasis on the personal nature of the emotional problems caused by brain damage to each patient underlines the weakness of the main objection of supporters of the 'neurological' model to the psychological interpretation of PSD, namely that, since in some studies no significant association has been found between degree of disability and severity of PSD, no relationship should exist between psychological factors and PSD. The weakness of this argument consists in its assumption that a linear and objective relationship must exist between disability and emotional reaction. This assumption does not take into account the subjective nature of the process of emotional appraisal. This subjective component implies that a motivated form of depression does not result from the objective consequences of brain damage, but from the personal significance that the subject attributes to these consequences, in terms of social roles and of personal goals. Thus, a mild language disorder can have devastating effects for the professional achievements of a lawyer, but only a minor importance for the work adjustment of a violinist, whereas a loss of fine motor control in the left hand will have just the opposite effect, in terms of achievement of social roles and of personal goals.

3.3 Psychosocial factors

Emotional disorders can be due to psychosocial factors rather than to the appraisal of the immediate consequences of brain damage, when they result from the long-term consequences of this event on the full range of activities, social roles, and social relationships of the patient. The most important of these social consequences is perhaps represented by the process of social isolation, which increases over time, extending from the patient to his or her family.

This process implies two major modifications in the patient's social network:

- a reduction in its size, as the number of people interacting with the patient progressively decreases;
- an increase in its intensity, since the only persons remaining in contact with the patients are those who are committed to a lasting relationship with them, i.e. family members, closely related to each other.

From the emotional point of view, the first modification leads patients to become apathetic, lonely, and depressed, whereas the second modification usually leads to an increasing strain among the members of this isolated group, with development of feelings of resentment and hostility.

3.3.1 Circular interactions between patients and their families

It is important to note in this context that the circular interactions that can develop between patients and their families can, not surprisingly, have either a positive or a negative influence on the patient's own emotional attitude and, consequently, on the rehabilitation process and outcome. Thus, if close relatives are unable to tolerate the emotional problems of these patients and the associated role changes that the patients' disabilities introduce in the family system, then their negative attitude will further decrease the self-esteem of the patients and their motivation toward rehabilitation. If, on the contrary, family members warmly support their relative and assume a realistically positive attitude toward his or her condition, then this positive attitude will be taken on board by the patient, restoring his or her self-esteem and increasing motivation toward rehabilitation.

4 The major types of emotional disorder following brain damage

As I mentioned previously, depression, anxiety, apathy, and lack of control over disruptive emotional outbursts are among the most prevalent and clinically relevant forms of emotional disorders observed in brain-damaged patients. The prevalence of these disorders and their clinical characteristics are different, however, following different categories of brain damage and during different stages in the evolution of the same disease. The anatomical locus of the lesion and the time elapsed from onset are very important determinants of this heterogeneity in the patterns of emotional behaviour shown by different clinical categories of brain-damaged patients.

In particular, the anatomical locus of the lesion, which is the more powerful source of variance from this point of view, probably acts through two main mechanisms:

♦ the encroachment of the lesion upon limbic structures (or neurochemical circuits) crucially involved in emotional functions;

♦ the level of awareness of physical and cognitive disorders provoked by lesions of different functional systems.

Since the first mechanism has already been covered when discussing the 'neurological factors' subserving emotional disorders of patients with severe head injury and the neurochemical interpretation of major PSD put forward by Robinson *et al.* (1984; Robinson 2001), this section will not dwell further on this issue. This section will, however, analyse in some detail the emotional disorders corresponding to some important clusters of physical and cognitive disorders that are usually provoked by the encroachment of the lesion upon well defined cortical areas. The aim of this description is twofold:

♦ to illustrate how some of the most frequent emotional phenomena present clinically;

♦ to show that these different kinds of emotional reactions are mainly due to a different level of awareness of physical and cognitive disorders.

The emotional disorders that will be discussed here correspond to the early stages following infarcts affecting the territories of:

♦ the anterior branches of the left sylvian artery;

♦ the posterior branches of the same artery;

♦ the right middle cerebral artery.

4.1 The 'catastrophic reaction' of patients with Broca's aphasia

Lesions involve the inferior part of the left frontal lobe and the patient clinically presents with a severe sensorimotor defect on the right side of the body, affecting hand and face. From the (cognitive) linguistic point of view, the most striking defect is severe Broca's aphasia, characterized by difficulty in engaging in any form of propositional speech, very low speech rate, effortful speech production, and inability to produce fluent and well formed verbal utterances, but relatively spared comprehension of oral and written language. The emotional counterpart of this cluster of motor and speech disorders is a marked tendency to 'catastrophic reactions' (i.e. to show increasing signs of anxiety and/or to suddenly burst into tears) because of the frustrating and repeated attempts at verbal expression. These catastrophic reactions often emerge from a background of discouragement, depressed mood, and a tendency to avoid situations of potential emotional danger for the patients.

4.2 The anosognosic 'excitement' of patients with severe Wernicke's aphasia

Here the vascular lesion encroaches upon the temporoparietal areas of the left hemisphere, involving Wernicke's area, and produces a quite different pattern of sensorimotor, linguistic, and emotional disturbances. Sensorimotor disorders are absent or very mild, and usually only a partial visual defect for the right half space can be detected. The verbal production of these patients appears fluent, harmonious, and well formed, but its meaning cannot be understood, since the most informative parts of speech (i.e. names and other content words) are substituted by phonemic or semantic transformations, producing a quite incomprehensible jargon. Equally important (and, if possible, even more striking) are disorders of language comprehension that hamper these patients' understanding not only of the content of verbal messages addressed to them, but also of the pathological nature of their own verbal production. The emotional behaviour of these subjects sharply contrasts with the catastrophic attitude of patients affected by a Broca's aphasia, since these patients usually appear unaware of their language disorders and appear overtalkative, excited, and often even aggressive against people who appear not to understand their verbal communications.

4.3 The 'indifference reaction' of right-brain-damaged patients

This cluster of physical, cognitive, and emotional disorders results from a focal brain lesion that affects the territory of the right sylvian artery, involving in particular the right parietal lobe. From the physical point of view, these patients usually present a severe left-sided hemiplegia and a marked deviation toward the right side of space of all the components of their body-orienting apparatus, i.e. trunk, head, and eyes. From the cognitive point of view, the most striking defect consists of a strong tendency to neglect the left half of the body and of extrapersonal space with an automatic capture of attention by stimuli rising on the right half space. From the emotional point of view, these patients show a composite pattern of emotional disorders that can be grouped into three sets of emotional abnormalities.

- The first and most important set, 'emotional indifference', includes an apparent lack of appropriate concern for the disability and an attitude of indifference toward other kinds of emotionally laden events.

- The second set, labelled 'verbal disinhibition', consists of a tendency to joke in a fatuous ironic or sarcastic manner.

- The third set includes verbal denial of left-sided hemiplegia (considered in Section 3.2.1) and other related phenomena that all suggest an implicit attitude of denial of illness. These last features often suggest feelings of rejection of the paralysed limbs that are felt not to belong to the patient ('somatoparaphrenia') or described with expressions of hatred, couched in a grotesque or exaggerated language ('misoplegia'; see Chapter 22).

4.4 **Factors underlying the awareness of the disorder (see also Chapter 22)**

From the clinical point of view, the 'catastrophic reactions' of patients with Broca's aphasia, the anosognosic excitement of patients with severe Wernicke's aphasia, and the abnormal cluster of indifference, anosognosia, and misoplegia shown by right-brain-damaged patients represent the most striking and frequent emotional abnormalities of stroke patients.

From the pathophysiological viewpoint, one of the most important factors that can explain these different patterns of emotional behaviour is the different extent of awareness of the defect following disruption of the functional systems subserved by these different anatomical regions. This awareness could in turn be related both to neurological and to psychological factors. From the psychological point of view, the level of awareness of a defect could result from the amount of attention and of effort requested to the patients to overcome their functional defect. This could explain why patients with Broca's aphasia, being obliged to make a sustained conscious effort to mobilize their articulatory apparatus and to overcome their difficulties of speech production, are acutely aware of their communication difficulties, whereas patients with Wernicke's aphasia, having a fluent speech and a severe comprehension disorder that do not allow them to monitor their meaningless utterances, are unaware of their language disorders. Analogously, right-brain-damaged patients with a left sided hemiplegia and an ipsilateral neglect may be unable to automatically orient their attention toward the paralysed limbs and this fact could explain the most important aspects of their emotional disturbances.

4.5 **The stigma of language expression disorders**

A final mechanism that may explain the different emotional behaviours of patients with lesions located in different parts of the brain consists in the different meaning and psychosocial impact that different kinds of cognitive and communication disorders can have for the patient. In particular, the high level of depression and of discouragement often shown by left-brain-damaged patients with expressive aphasia may be due to the feelings of inadequacy, embarrassment, and self-depreciation that communicative disorders understandably provoke in these subjects. Several authors (e.g. Hurwitz and Adams 1972) have, indeed, observed that aphasic patients feel particularly stigmatized and report lowered self-esteem and feelings of shame as a consequence of their communication disorders.

Obviously, the different kinds of emotional disorders observed in patients with different clusters of physical and cognitive defects only represent common or typical patterns of emotional behaviour shown by brain-damaged patients. It is not possible to consider here the complex problem of the many other facets that emotional disorders can have following various categories of brain damage and during the various stages of

Table 21.1 Pathophysiology and prevalence of the most important kinds of emotional disorders in various categories of brain damage

Categories of brain damage	Stroke	Brain injury	Alzheimer's disease
Pathophysiology			
Anxiety and depression			
Psychological factors. 'Painful' awareness of the adverse effects of handicaps and disabilities on the patient's social role and personal goals	Very common (40–50%) in hospitalized patients and less common (20–30%) in community settings	Rather uncommon in the earliest posttraumatic periods; tend to develop with the increased awareness of handicaps and disabilities	Rather common (40%) in the first stages of the disease; tend to disappear in later stages with the progression of dementia
Neurological factors? (major PSD). Disruption of monoaminergic pathways relaying the brainstem to the cerebral cortex	According to some authors more common after left than right hemisphere damage		
Apathy			
Neurological factors. Lesions encroaching upon the mesial parts of the frontal lobes, the anterior cingulate gyrus and the mesolimbic dopaminergic system	More common after right (20–25%) than left (10–15%) hemisphere stroke	Very frequent and due to neurological factors in the earliest stages and to psychosocial factors in late periods	Very frequent (30–80%). Its frequency and severity increase with the progression of dementia
Psychological factors. Can result from the tendency to avoid the frustrations resulting from handicaps, disabilities, and communication disorders			
Lack of control over disruptive emotional outbursts			
Neurological factors. Lesions encroaching upon the orbitofrontal cortex and the fibres connecting these structures to the amygdala	Very uncommon	Very frequent after the earliest posttraumatic periods	Rather common in the most advanced stages of the disease progression

evolution of the disease. For simplicity's sake, Table 21.1 summarizes the most important points concerning the pathophysiology and prevalence of three broad categories of emotional disorders (anxiety and depression, apathy, and poor control of disruptive emotional outbursts) following three important kinds of brain damage, namely, stroke, closed head injury, and Alzheimer's disease (see also Starkstein and Manes 2001 for a recent review of this subject).

The data reported in Table 21.1 are relevant from both the epidemiological and the pathophysiological point of view. On the one hand, they show that all these kinds of emotional disorders are widely, although unevenly distributed in different clinical forms of brain damage or in different stages of evolution of the same disease. On the other hand, they confirm that anxiety and depression are mostly due to psychological factors, whereas apathy and disruptive emotional outbursts usually result from neurological factors. The relationship between anxiety/depression and a painful realization of the consequences of the disease is, in fact, present not only in stroke patients but also in closed head injury or in dementia of the Alzheimer's type (DAT). However, in the last two categories of brain damage, these emotional disorders are only observed in the stage of evolution of the disease characterized by the highest level of awareness, namely, in the earliest stages of DAT and in the late stages of brain injury. Very different is the context in which disruptive emotional outbursts and apathetic disorders are usually observed.

- Disruptive emotional outbursts are mainly observed in patients with a severe traumatic injury of the fronto-orbital cortex (and in the most advanced stages of DAT).

- Apathetic disorders are particularly severe in patients with lesions encroaching upon the anteromesial parts of the frontal lobes, but are also observed in patients with an extensive infarct impinging upon the the right parietal region and in the advanced stages of DAT.

5 Assessment of emotional disorders following brain damage

In recent years, the behavioural and emotional disorders of brain-damaged patients have attracted more and more attention in the field of neurorehabilitation for two main reasons.

- These disorders constitute an important obstacle not only to the resumption of productive activities, but also to the rehabilitation process. They are indeed responsible for the lack of collaboration of the patient, which impedes the improvement of potentially treatable physical and cognitive defects.

- The fact that emotional and personality disorders are the consequence of brain damage is likely to be difficult to accept for most family members. These disorders are, therefore, the factors that most frequently trigger the negative circular interactions between patients and their families briefly described in Section 3.3.1.

A careful assessment of emotional and behavioural disorders is, therefore, critical to the process of evaluation of the specific needs of each brain-damaged individual and is crucial when establishing comprehensive (holistic) rehabilitation programmes. Furthermore, the recent development of evidence-based rehabilitation medicine stresses the need for using a large array of standard psychometric instruments that could be appropriate to the assessment of emotional disorders of brain-damaged patients and that could, in turn, be used as outcome measures for various kinds and stages of neuropsychological rehabilitation (see Fleminger and Powell 1999 for a survey of the state of the art in this area). Obviously, the in-depth assessment required to understand individual problems and to establish personalized rehabilitation programmes overlaps only in part with the standard psychometeric assessment required by evidence-based rehabilitation medicine. Consequently, this chapter will only deal with two forms of evaluative processes:

◆ the personalized assessment;

◆ the psychometric instruments currently used for a standard assessment of emotional disorders.

5.1 Personalized assessment of the significance of emotional disorders

The subjective, personalized assessment of the significance of emotional disorders consists of two main steps:

◆ distinguishing the neurological from the motivated (psychological or psychosocial) components of these disorders;

◆ delineating the main problems and psychosocial resources of the patient.

The former can be identified by trying to understand the process of emotional appraisal of the patient; the latter by evaluating strength and weakness of his/her most significant personal relationships.

5.2 The standard psychometric assessment of emotional disturbances

The standard psychometric assessment is much less relevant for the evaluation of individual problems and difficulties, but has the virtue of being more objective and quantitative. It is, therefore, much more reliable as a method of assessment for the negative effects that emotional disturbances can exert on the rehabilitation process. Important methodological objections have been raised against the use of these psychometric measures of emotional and affective disorders. These will be considered briefly and then, in Table 21.2, some information about a few instruments commonly used for the assessment of anxiety or depression, apathy, or some disruptive behavioural disorders will be given.

5.2.1 Methodological objections

◆ One general problem for all of these instruments, and in particular for those assessing anxious-depressive disorders, consists of the fact that they have usually

Table 21.2 Main instruments used for the standard neuropsychological assessment of the most important kinds of emotional disorders

Emotional disorder	Instrument	Reference	Comments
Anxiety	Hamilton Anxiety Scale	Hamilton (1959)	Designed for psychiatric settings
	Hospital Anxiety and Depression Scale	Zigmond and Snaith (1983)	Self-report instrument for detecting anxiety and depression in hospitalized medical and neurological patients
Depression	Hamilton Depression Rating Scale	Hamilton (1960)	Designed for psychiatric settings
	Poststroke Depression Rating Scale	Gainotti et al. (1997)	Clinician-rated scale specifically constructed for stroke patients
	Wimbledon Self-report Scale	Coughlan and Storey (1988)	Self-report scale devised to assess mood in brain-damaged patients
Apathy	Apathy Evaluation Scale	Marin et al. (1991)	Self-informant and clinician-rated versions of this scale exist
Disruptive behavioural disorders	Overt Aggression Scale	Yudowsky et al. (1986)	Designed to be rated by nursing staff in psychiatric setting; is also used in brain injury patients
General neurobehavioural disorders	Neurobehavioral Rating Scale	Levin et al. (1987)	Sensitive to behavioural disorders related to frontal lobe injury
Rating scales	Neuropsychiatric Inventory	Cummings et al. (1994)	Clinician-rated instrument developed as an assessment tool for patients with dementia

been developed for psychiatric patients and that their transfer into the field of organic brain damage may produce misleading results. In particular, false-positive errors may result from attributing to a major depression symptoms, such as weight loss, fatigue, or lack of concentration, that in these patients may be a consequence of the brain damage *per se*. It is for this reason that some authors have developed instruments specifically constructed for well defined groups of brain-damaged patients, such as the already mentioned 'Post-Stroke Depression Rating Scale', designed by Gainotti *et al.* (1997) to clarify the meaning of major depressive disorders frequently observed in stroke patients.

◆ A different, but equally important, problem can be raised for the use of self-report instruments, such as the 'Beck Depression Inventory'(1961), the Zung Self-Rating Inventory' (Zung *et al.* 1965), the 'Hospital Anxiety and Depression Scale' (Zigmond and Snait 1983), or the 'Wimbledon Self-Report Scale' (Coughlan and Storey 1988). Since patients with dementia or with severe brain injury may well be unaware not only of their physical problems, but also of their cognitive or emotional difficulties, the assessment based on the use of self-report scales must be considered quite unreliable.

6 Treatment of emotional and behavioural disorders in brain-damaged patients

The treatment of emotional disorders in brain-damaged patients is based on a large array of methods and techniques ranging from pharmacological treatment in the most severe emotional disorders, through the behaviour management techniques, used to modify inertia or disruptive patterns of social behaviour in patients with severe brain injury, to various kinds of group treatments and individual psychotherapies. The latter aim to support the difficult process of adaptation to a new condition (and sometimes to a new identity) required of a patient with a severe brain injury. The following paragraphs will be limited to a brief discussion of some aspects of the behavioural management techniques and of the group treatment of emotional and behavioural disorders of patients with severe brain injury. Then the pharmacological treatment of depression, apathy, and disruptive behavioural disorders in various groups of brain-damaged patients will be discussed. Finally, the role of rehabilitation in restoring the emotional equilibrium of these patients will be briefly considered.

6.1 Group treatment of emotional and behavioural disorders

Group treatment of the emotional and behavioural disorders of patients with severe brain injury has several advantages.

◆ It increases the level of awareness of the patients' defects and capabilities, allowing them to check the adequacy of their current behaviour.

◆ It promotes interactions that, on one hand, increase the level of initiative and of personal involvement of the patients and, on the other hand, improve their control over irritability, overt aggression, or other disinhibited patterns of behaviour.

♦ It improves the level of participation in shared activities, favouring some degree of competition and, consequently, a more independent attitude.

In particular, the 'role-playing' procedures, which clearly define the role of each participant and the general rules adopted by the group, are very useful for improving the social/behavioural disorders of these patients, making a firm distinction between acceptable and unacceptable patterns of behaviour and explicitly declaring the positive and negative consequences of the patient's behaviour.

6.2 Behavioural management techniques

Behavioural management techniques tend to induce an implicit learning of the suggested behavioural modifications by means of (classical or operant) conditioning methods. These techiques make use of positive and negative reinforcements to increase favourable changes (e.g. the development of intentional action schemata in patients with inertia or severe apathy) and to inhibit socially unacceptable emotional outbursts. Wood (1987) has suggested, for example, the systematic use of the 'time-out' procedures (which consist in the complete suspension of every kind of reaction to the onset of undesirable behavioural patterns), since the patient implicitly learns from this unexpected lack of response that his or her provocative behavioural patterns are unable to produce any effect on the external milieu.

6.3 Pharmacological treatment of emotional disorders

As for the pharmacological treatment in those cases of severe emotional disorders, the data in Table 21.3 clearly show that several drugs are able to ameliorate the depressive disorders, apathy, and disruptive behavioural outbursts of brain-damaged patients.

This does not mean, however, that purely biological methods are sufficient to treat in the long term the emotional problems and disorders of brain-damaged patients. Pharmacological treatments are necessary to improve the most severe emotional disorders of these patients and to re-establish a physiological process of emotional appraisal, but the emotional problems of these patients will lose their dramatic nature only when the outcome of this process becomes more acceptable to them. From this point of view, it is probably correct to say that the rehabilitation process is the most powerful instrument that we can use to improve the long-term emotional equilibrium of these patients.

6.4 The role of rehabilitation in improving the long-term emotional equilibrium of the patient

Rehabilitation, by decreasing the level of impairments, handicaps, and disabilities, allows patients to draw a less dramatic representation of the consequences of brain damage. In addition, the active role played by the patients in the rehabilitation process allows them to understand that the results obtained are the consequence of their own personal effort. They, therefore become more aware of being able to cope with the

Table 21.3 Drugs used for the treatment of poststroke depression, apathy, and behavioural disorders of brain-damaged patients

Therapeutic approach	Reference
Poststroke depression	
Selective serotonin re-uptake inhibitors (SSRI)	
Fluoxetine	Gainotti *et al.* (2001)
Citalopram	Andersen *et al.* (1994)
Others	
Trazodone	Reding *et al.* (1986)
Nortriptyline	Robinson *et al.* (2000)
Apathy	
Dopamine agonists	
Bromocriptine	Campbell and Duffy (1997)
Pergolide	
Stimulant drugs	
Methylphenidate	Marin *et al.* (1995)
Aggression and other behavioural disorders	
Atypical antipsychotic medications	
Risperidone	Lavretsky and Sultzer (1998)
Clozapine	Carlyle *et al.* (1993)

difficult consequences of the brain injury. Furthermore, the positive results obtained help restore the self-esteem of these patients. This is of paramount importance in the difficult transition from their disrupted (pre-brain damage) identity to the new self-image that they are now forced to develop.

Selective references

Adams, J.H., Scott, G.P., Parker, L., Graham, D.I., and Doyle, D. (1980). Contusion index: a quantitative approach to cerebral contusions in head injury. *Neuropathol. Appl. Neurobiol.* 6, 319–24.

Andersen, G., Vestergaard, K., and Lauritzen, L. (1994). Effective treatment of poststroke depression with the selective serotonin reuptake inhibitor citalopram. *Stroke* 25, 1099–104.

Barré, J.A., Morin, L., and Kaiser, D. (1923). Etude clinique d'un nouveau cas d'anosognosie de Babinski. *Rev. Neurologique* 29, 500–4.

Beck, A.T. (1961). An inventory for measuring depression. *Arch. Gen. Psychiatry* 4, 561–71.

Campbell, J.J. and Duffy, J.D. (1997). Treatment strategies in amotivated patients. *Psychiatric Ann.* 27, 44–9.

Carlyle, W., Ancill, R.J., and Sheldon, L. (1993). Aggression in demented patients: a double-blind study of Clozapine vs Haloperidol. *Int. Clin. Psychopharmacol.* 8, 103–8.

Coughlan, A.K. and Storey, P. (1988). The Wimbledon Self-Report Scale: emotional and mood appraisal. *Clin. Rehabil.* 2, 207–13.

Cummings, J.L., Mega, M., Gray, K., Rosenberg-Thompson, S., Carusi, D.A., and Gornbein, J. (1994). The Neuropsychiatric Inventory: comprehensive assessment of psychopathology in dementia. *Neurology* 44, 2308–14.

Darwin, C. (1872). *The expression of the emotions in man and animals.* Murray, London [Reprinted Chicago University Press, Chicago, 1965].

Fleminger, S. and Powell, J. (eds.) (1999). *Evaluation of outcomes in brain injury rehabilitation.* Psychology Press, Hove, East Sussex.

Frijda, N.H. (1986). *The emotions.* Cambridge University Press, New York.

Gainotti, G. (1999). Neuropsychology of emotions. In *Handbook of clinical and experimental neuropsychology* (ed. G.F. Denes and L. Pizzamiglio), pp. 613–63. Psychology Press, Hove, East Sussex.

Gainotti, G. (2000). Neuropsychological theories of emotion. In *The neuropsychology of emotion* (ed. C. Borod), pp. 214–36. Oxford University Press, New York.

Gainotti, G. (2001). Emotions as a biologically adaptive system: an introduction. In *Emotional behaviour and its disorders* (ed. G. Gainotti), pp. 1–15. Vol. 5, *Handbook of neuropsychology* (ed. F. Boller and J. Grafman). Elsevier, Amsterdam.

Gainotti, G., Azzoni, A., Razzano, C., Lanzillotta, M., Marra, C., and Gasparini, F. (1997). The Post-Stroke Depression Rating Scale: a test specifically devised to investigate affective disorders of stroke patients. *J. Clin. Exp. Neuropsychol.* **19**, 340–56.

Gainotti, G., Antonucci, G., Marra, C., and Paolucci, S. (2001). Relation between depression after stroke, antidepressant therapy, and functional recovery. *J. Neurol., Neurosurg., Psychiatry* **71**, 258–61.

Hamilton, H. (1960). A rating scale for depression. *J. Neurol., Neurosurg., Psychiatry* **23**, 56–62.

Hamilton, M.A. (1959). The assessment of anxiety states by rating. *Br. J. Med. Psychol.* **32**, 50–5.

Hurwitz, L.J. and Adams, G.F. (1972). Rehabilitation of hemiplegia: indices of assessment and prognosis. *Br. Med. J.* **1**, 94–8.

Lavretsky, H. and Sultzer, D. (1998). A structured trial of risperidone for the treatment of agitation in dementia. *Am. J. Geriatr. Psychiatry* **6**, 127–135.

Lazarus, R.S. (1982). Thoughts on relations between emotion and cognition. *Am. Psychol.* **37**, 1019–24.

LeDoux, J. (1996). *The emotional brain.* Simon and Schuster, New York.

Leventhal, H. (1974). *Emotions: a basic problem for social psychology: classic and contemporary integrations.* McNally, Chicago.

Levin, H.S., High, W.M., Goethe, K.E., *et al.* (1987). The neurobehavioural rating scale: assessment of the behavioural sequelae of head injury by the clinician. *J. Neurol., Neurosurg., Psychiatry* **50**, 183–93.

Marin, R.S., Biedrzycki, R.C., and Firinciogullori, S. (1991). Reliability and validity of the Apathy Evaluation Scale. *Psychiatry Res.* **38**, 143–62.

Marin, R.S., Fogel, B.S., Hawkins, J., *et al.* (1995). Apathy: a treatable syndrome. *J. Neuropsychiatry Clin. Neurosci.* **7**, 23–30.

Oatley, K. and Johnson-Laird, P. (1987). Toward a cognitive theory of emotions. *Cognition Emotion* **1**, 29–50.

Panksepp, J. (1982). Toward a general psychobiological theory of emotions. *Behav. Brain Sci.* **5**, 407–67.

Reding, M.J., Orto, L.A., Winter, S.W., Fortuna, I.M., Di Ponte, F., and Mc Dowell, F.H. (1986). Antidepressant therapy after stroke: a double blind trial. *Arch. Neurol.* **43**, 763–5.

Robinson, R.G. (2001). The neuropsychiatry of stroke. In *Contemporary neuropsychiatry* (ed. K. Miyoshi, C.M. Shapiro, M. Gaviria, and Y. Morita), pp. 116–27. Springer-Verlag, Tokyo.

Robinson, R.G., Kubos, K.L., Starr, L.B., Rao, K., and Price, T.R. (1984). Mood disorders in stroke patients: importance of lesion location. *Brain* **107**, 81–93.

Robinson, R.G., Schultz, S.K., Castillo, C., *et al.* (2000). Nortriptyline versus fluoxetine in the treatment of depression and in short-term recovery after stroke: a placebo-controlled, double-blind study. *Am. J. Psychiatry* 157, 351–9.

Scherer, K.R. (2000). Psychological models of emotion. In *The neuropsychology of emotion* (ed. C. Borod), pp. 137–62. Oxford University Press, New York.

Starkstein, S.E. and Manes, F. (2001). Neural mechanisms of anxiety, depression and disinhibition. In *Emotional behaviour and its disorders* (ed. G. Gainotti), pp. 263–84. Vol. 5, *Handbook of neuropsychology*, 2nd edn (ed. F. Boller and J. Grafman). Elsevier, Amsterdam.

Weinstein, E.A. and Kahn, R.L. (1955). *Denial of illness: symbolic and physiological aspects.* Charles C. Thomas, Springfield, Illinois.

Wood, R.L. (1987). *Brain injury rehabilitation: a neurobehavioural approach.* Croom Helm, London.

Wood, R. and McMillan, T. (2000). *Neurobehavioural disability and social handicap after traumatic brain injury.* Psychology Press, Hove, East Sussex.

Yudowsky, S.C., Silver, J.M., Jackson, W., Edicott, J., and Williams, D.W. (1986). The Overt Aggression Scale for the objective rating of verbal and physical aggression. *Am. J. Psychiatry* 143, 35–9.

Zajonc, R.B. (1980). Feeling and thinking: preferences need no inferences. *Am. Psychol.* 2, 151–76.

Zigmond, A.S. and Snait, R.P. (1983). The Hospital Anxiety and Depression Scale. *Acta Psychiatrica Scand.* 67, 361–70.

Zung, W.W.K., Richards, C.B., and Short, M.F. (1965). Self-rating depression in an outpatient clinic: further validation of the SDS. *Arch. Gen. Psychiatry* 13, 508–15.

Chapter 22

Assessment and rehabilitation of anosognosia and syndromes of impaired awareness

George P. Prigatano

1 Clinical presentation

'Anosognosia refers to the clinical phenomena in which a brain dysfunctional patient does not appear to be aware of impaired neurological and/or neuropsychological functioning which is obvious to the clinician and other reasonably attentive individuals. The lack of awareness appears specific to individual deficits and cannot be accounted for by hypoarousal or widespread cognitive impairments' (Prigatano 1996*a*, pp. 80–81). One may witness frank anosognosia for hemiplegia, aphasia, visual field losses (i.e. for hemianopia or quadrantanopsia), complete cortical blindness, apraxia, and even amnesias. In the case of anosognosia for hemiplegia, patients may exhibit hemiplegia but report no disturbance whatsoever with motor function. Careful examination of patients often reveals other associated disturbances such as disorientation for time and/or place, hemispatial neglect, disturbances in the perception of facial affect, and failure to show normal concern about their illness or impairments (Starkstein *et al.* 1992; Cutting 1978).

An important feature of this class of disturbances is that they often change with time and may develop into different syndromes (similarly to aphasic syndromes). The disassociation of anosognosia for one neurological disturbance (e.g. hemiplegia) and a concomitant apparent awareness of another disturbance (e.g. aphasia) have been reported (Breier *et al.* 1995) and has important theoretical implications. Monitoring these changes and patterns of partial or complete recovery may provide clues about the underlying disturbed neural structures and neural networks responsible for the various syndromes of impaired awareness.

Thus, disorders of awareness, of which anosognosia represents the most dramatic form, may vary because they appear to reflect a disturbance in the 'highest level of organization' of a given function (Bisiach *et al.* 1986). Therefore, various types of neuropathological disturbances to different regions of the cerebral hemispheres (and possibly brainstem (Evyapan and Kumral 1999) and cerebellum) may produce different types of altered consciousness and associated disturbances in self-awareness.

Progressively, there has been an appreciation that disturbances of self-awareness may be associated with neuropsychological impairments, even when frank anosognosia subsequently 'disappears' (Prigatano 1999). However, correlations between measures of impaired awareness and standard neuropsychological test scores are seldom found. This lack of correlation does not mean that impaired awareness is unrelated to neuropsychological deficits—only that standard tests fail to capture the most salient features (Prigatano 1999). For example, patients with severe traumatic brain injury (TBI) may exhibit socially inappropriate behaviour months or years after brain injury. When their behaviour is brought to their attention, they may honestly be perplexed by the feedback and appear not to experience the inappropriateness of their comments or actions. Their phenomenological experience appears to be disturbed. Assessing this class of disturbances is delicate. Clinicians must constantly keep in mind the differential diagnosis of 'organically mediated' impaired self-awareness versus some form of psychiatric defence mechanism in which denial, projection, or both may be prominent features.

The hallmark of a disorder of (self)awareness, however, is the presence of clear neurological or neuropsychological impairments that are obvious to clinical observers. Patients confronted with such impairments or deficits explicitly state that the deficits either do not exist or are substantially less severe than what may be painfully obvious to those around them. A key issue addressed below is how this class of disturbance is assessed, through both a brief clinical examination and a more extensive neuropsychological investigation.

2 Incidence

The incidence of anosognosia and related disorders of awareness varies depending on (see Prigatano 1999):

◆ when the patient is examined;

◆ how the patient is examined;

◆ the nature of the brain disorder involved;

◆ possibly on a patient's premorbid cognitive and personality characteristics.

After an acute cerebrovascular accident (CVA), the incidence of frank anosognosia for hemiplegia is typically between 20% (Pedersen *et al.* 1996) and 30% (Starkstein *et al.* 1992). The incidence of anosognosia for hemiplegia associated with a right cerebral hemisphere CVA is higher. Cutting (1978) estimated 50–60%. Pedersen *et al.* (1996) suggested the figure could be as high as 81%. Stone *et al.* (1993) reported an incidence figure of 28% after right hemisphere CVA and 5% after left hemisphere CVA. Like other investigators, they note that language deficits associated with left hemisphere CVA make it difficult to assess anosognosia and related disorders in this patient group.

The incidence of impaired awareness of visual field deficits associated with stroke may be even higher (Bisiach *et al.* 1986), but no clear estimates exist. One small study estimated the incidence at 62.5% (Celesia *et al.* 1997). Patients with quadrantanopsia or hemianopsia often fail to report a visual field difficulty spontaneously, particularly a problem with the left visual field. Many are completely unaware of their visual field loss. Some form of natural compensation seems to exist. Conversely, the brain may simply lack the appropriate template or comparison system to register such a disturbance and therefore the impairment remains outside conscious awareness (Bisiach and Geminiani 1991).

By definition, all patients with a severe TBI (admitting Glasgow Coma Scale (GCS) scores of 3 to 8) have a disorder of consciousness. On emerging from coma, these patients often show continued signs of impaired awareness and associated memory disturbances (posttraumatic amnesia, PTA). Postacutely (6–12 months or longer after injury), however, how many of these patients show a residual disturbance of impaired awareness? No firm statistics are available. One behavioural study suggested that several months after TBI more than 30% of such patients do not fully experience or at least underestimate their neuropsychological impairments compared to reports from their relatives (Prigatano and Altman 1990).

Other investigators have reported that diseases such as parkinsonism may begin without the patient being aware of a motor disturbance. In contrast, in other disease states such as Alzheimer's disease, patients may be aware of their problem before others. As time progresses, however, anosognosia may worsen (Starkstein *et al.* 1997). Anosognosia has also been assessed after intracarotid amobarbital injections. Meador *et al.* (2000) reported that 88% of 62 patients were unaware of their hemiparesis after the injection.

3 Neural correlates of anosognosia

Clinicians studying computerized tomography (CT) and magnetic resonance imaging (MRI) findings of patients with anosognosia for hemiplegia have repeatedly found it difficult to identify specific lesion locations to account for the symptom picture. Nevertheless, some important observations have been made.

Starkstein *et al.* (1992) noted that patients who demonstrated anosognosia generally had larger frontal horn, lateral ventricle, and third ventricle ratios. That is, there were greater signs of cerebral atrophy involving both cortical and subcortical structures. They also note in their series that right temporal parietal as well thalamic lesions were common in anosognostic patients. Starkstein *et al.* (1993), studying a smaller group of individuals, specifically noted the potential role of frontal lobe dysfunction in anosognosia.

Small and Ellis (1996) reported that lesions in the deep white matter are frequently associated with anosognosia for hemiplegia. They also noted that involvement of the corona radiata and the caudate nucleus is commonly observed. An earlier case report by House and Hodges (1988) emphasized the important role of subcortical damage when persistent anosognosia for hemiplegia exists. They reported on a patient who showed persistent anosognosia following a right internal capsule lesion affecting also the globus pallidus and corona radiata.

These findings become even more interesting in light of a recent single-photon emission computerized tomography (SPECT) study that implicates the role of hypometabolic activity in the basal ganglia, particularly the head of the caudate nucleus in patients who show conversion hysteria affecting the movement of the arm and leg (Vuilleumier *et al.* 2001).

4 **Anosognosia and prognosis**

Pedersen *et al.* (1996) note that the presence of anosognosia predicted the level of functioning at discharge following stroke rehabilitation. More interestingly, they noted that the likelihood of death during hospitalization increased dramatically in patients who were anosognostic. Jehkonen *et al.* (2000) also noted that impaired awareness was related to poor functional outcome after cerebral infarction. Patients who were acutely anosognostic for hemiplegia had a poorer functional outcome 1 year postonset than that of patients who were aware of their hemiparesis. This finding matches other clinical experiences. Prigatano (1999) notes that anosognosia is often associated with poor psychosocial outcome after TBI. This point has also been made by Sherer *et al.* (1998*a*).

5 **Methods of assessment**

By definition, disturbances of (self)awareness involve a disturbance of consciousness. There are no direct measures of consciousness, only measures of unconsciousness (i.e. failure to respond to the environment as measured by such instruments as the GCS). Disturbances of awareness can only be measured indirectly. As yet, science has not progressed enough to permit the direct measurement of patients' subjective experience.

There are two common methods of assessing impaired awareness. The first is clinicians' ratings based on observing and talking to patients. The second involves comparing patients' verbal responses (or ratings) with the judgements of someone who has known them well before injury and who interacts with them daily after injury (e.g. relatives). The work of Starkstein *et al.* (1992) is an example of the first type of measurement. These workers acutely assessed anosognostic patients using an Anosognostic Questionnaire (Table 22.1). On the basis of patients' responses to an examiner's questions, they were classified as showing no anosognosia, mild anosognosia, moderate anosognosia, or severe anosognosia.

Azouvi *et al.* (1996) asked patients 10 questions related to hemineglect. The patients' responses were then compared to their actual performance on 10 items that reflect neglect in everyday life. The disparity between the two scores is another useful index of mild, moderate, or severe anosognosia for neglect. In this instance, patients' actual behaviour is compared to what they report verbally as it relates to daily activities.

Prigatano *et al.* (1986) developed the Patient's Competency Ratings Scale to assess awareness in postacute TBI patients. Patients with moderate to severe TBI were predicted

Table 22.1 Anosognosia questionnaire

Anosognosia questionnaire
1. Why are you here?
2. What is the matter with you?
3. Is there anything wrong with your arm or leg?
4. Is there anything wrong with your eyesight?
5. Is your limb weak, paralysed, or numb?
6. How does your limb feel?

If denial is elicited ask the following:
(a) (arm picked up) What is this?
(b) Can you lift it?
(c) You clearly have some problem with this?
(d) (asked to lift both arms) Can't you see that the two arms are not at the same level?
(e) (asked to identify finger movements in and out of the abnormal visual field) Can't you see that you have a problem with your eyesight?

Scoring
0: The disorder is spontaneously reported or mentioned following a general question about the patient's complaints
1: The disorder is reported only following a specific question about the strength of the patient's limb or about visual problems
2: The disorder is acknowledged only after its demonstration through routine techniques of neurological examination
3: No acknowledgment of the disorder

* Taken with permission from Starkstein *et al.* (1992).

to be able to evaluate their abilities to perform self-care activities objectively, but to exhibit notable problems in being aware of difficulties in controlling their emotional responses and in behaving in a socially appropriate manner. The questionnaire was constructed with these clinical observations in mind. The initial hypothesis was supported (Prigatano *et al.* 1990) and later replicated (Prigatano 1996*b*). During postacute stages of injury, patients can be asked more extensive questions to help quantify the degree to which they exhibit impaired awareness of neuropsychological disturbances. Acutely, measures of impaired awareness often focus on the assessment of frank neurological impairments; postacutely, awareness measures are used to assess neuropsychological deficits. Sherer *et al.* (1998*b*) have also reported the usefulness of clinicians' ratings and a questionnaire for assessing disturbances of awareness after TBI. They used the measures to predict return to work.

From these two approaches, a hybrid approach has emerged. Prigatano and Klonoff (1997) developed a clinician's rating scale to differentiate impaired self-awareness from denial of disability after head injury. Patients' responses to questions and their failure to report difficulties spontaneously were used to help decide whether individuals exhibited impaired awareness. Clinicians can also rate how individuals respond to feedback and their responses during neuropsychological testing.

All of these approaches have merit in different clinical and research settings. The measurement of impaired awareness, however, continues to be limited by the lack of a theoretical model for classifying these disturbances. Relatively straightforward but reliable techniques for assessment are lacking. Prigatano (1999) has presented a model that helps explain the heterogeneity of disorders of self-awareness. This model is discussed briefly, and its implications for assessment and rehabilitation are considered.

6 Complete and partial syndromes of impaired awareness after brain damage: a theoretical perspective

As in other neuropsychological disturbances, different degrees or levels of impaired awareness can be observed. Early after brain injury, a complete syndrome of impaired awareness is common. In this case, there is no subjective experience of an impairment or deficit. This condition reflects frank anosognosia.

With time, however, individuals may experience some disturbance but their knowledge of the disturbance remains partial. This clinical reality led to the differentiation between complete and partial syndromes of impaired awareness (Prigatano 1999). It is beyond the scope of this article to discuss this model in detail. Theoretically, however, complete syndromes of impaired awareness are often present when there is evidence of bilateral cerebral dysfunction. Partial syndromes tend to emerge with primarily unilateral cerebral dysfunction. Again, perhaps, the best example is anosognosia for hemiplegia.

Although a stroke may be on one side of the brain, behavioural and positron emission tomography (PET) studies suggest that, soon after injury, cerebral hypometabolism is often bilateral (Perani *et al.* 1993; Prigatano and Wong 1997). As the hypometabolism decreases in the affected and the so-called unaffected hemisphere, individuals seem to exhibit partial awareness of their deficits. Failure to show a return to normal metabolic activity in the so-called unaffected cerebral hemisphere may result in a persistent and severe form of anosognosia.

What complicates this simple dichotomy, however, is that regional areas of cerebral dysfunction may produce different syndromes of unawareness. This helps explain why patients may be aware of, for example, hemiplegia but not hemianopsia or aphasia. Postacutely, patients who are aware of a language disturbance may not necessarily be aware of socially inappropriate behaviours. Presumably, such individuals would have relatively intact temporal lobe-mediated functions, but poor frontal lobe-mediated functions. Four basic syndromes of impaired awareness after brain injury are often seen clinically. Broadly, these syndromes have been referred to as

- the frontal heteromodal syndrome;
- the parietal heteromodal syndrome;
- the temporal heteromodal syndrome;
- the occipital heteromodal syndrome.

An evaluation of impaired awareness should therefore assess whether a patient exhibits a complete or parietal syndrome associated with one of these four hetero-modal regions. Specific behavioural steps can be followed to assess the presence or absence of a complete or partial syndrome (Table 22.2). In this way, an algorithm can be followed to assess disorders of impaired awareness. If an individual exhibits partial awareness, the clinician must further evaluate whether the patient exhibits evidence of a defensive or nondefensive method of coping. This approach avoids making the common error of dichotomizing the patient as showing impaired awareness, which is neuro-logically based, or denial of disability, which appears to be psychiatrically based.

Given this model, the clinician would repeatedly assess a patient's neurological and neuropsychological function. Consequently, the diagnostic impression of the nature of the patient's level of awareness may change as the patient's clinical condition changes. Residuals of disturbances of awareness are probably more common than recognized and should be assessed as a part of any neuropsychological examination.

7 Methods of rehabilitation

Anosognosia clearly relates to rehabilitation outcome (Pedersen *et al.* 1996; Jehkonen *et al.* 2000). Yet, rehabilitation of patients with disorders of awareness remains chal-lenging. The administration of 10 mm of ice-cold water to the left ear of patients with dense hemineglect and anosognosia for hemiplegia has produced a short-term recog-nition of their impairments, but the effects are short-lived (Bisiach *et al.* 1991; also see Ramachandran, 1994). During the acute phase following the onset of a true anosognosia, little can presently be done except to make patients comfortable and to help them avoid dangerous situations or decisions. Patients who are anosognostic for hemiplegia are frequently compliant and show little distress about their condition.

In contrast, some patients have significant awareness deficits for neuropsychological functioning and are anything but cooperative. The classic examples are patients with a severe TBI who insist that they need no treatment and who wish to leave the hospital or rehabilitation setting prematurely. Trying to 'reason' with these patients is often ineffective—they simply do not experience what others around them observe.

In the acute and postacute phases of rehabilitation of such individuals, the establish-ment of a trusting, therapeutic relationship is critical to their rehabilitative care. During this time, patients truly may not recognize their disturbances, but they may fol-low the guidance of their clinician simply because they know the clinician wants to work on their behalf. Even nonpsychodynamically oriented therapists have come to recognize the importance of establishing a trusting, nonconfrontational therapeutic alliance with such patients (Bieman-Copland and Dywan 2000).

7.1 Rehabilitation of partial syndromes of impaired awareness

The more interesting and challenging question is whether patients who show partial syndromes of impaired awareness can be helped by rehabilitative interventions. At this

Table 22.2 Assessment strategy for evaluating disorders of self-awareness

---

Step 1. Is there evidence of a complete syndrome present (i.e. a true anosognosia)?

If yes	If no
(1) Document anosognosia for specific neurological disturbances (using such scales as the Anosognostic Questionnaire (Starkstein *et al.* 1992))	(1) Is there evidence of a partial syndrome present? If yes: Go to step 2 If no: Stop
(2) Monitor changes in the syndrome over time	
(3) Document associated neurological or neuropsychological disturbances	

Step 2. Determine if a partial syndrome is present.

If yes:	If no:
(1) Document and describe what areas of neuropsychological disturbances apparently are not experienced by the patient (using a variety of measures such as the PCRS*, Sherer *et al.*'s (1998*b*) Awareness Questionnaire, etc.)	(1) Is there evidence of psychiatric disorder? If yes: obtain a psychiatric consultation If no: stop
(2) Determine if the unawareness of deficits/ impairments cluster (i.e. combine so as to suggest certain regions of brain dysfunction or systems dysfunction)	

If yes:	If no:
(a) Can dysfunction be described as reflecting frontal, parietal, temporal, or occipital heteromodal disturbances?	(1) List areas of reduced awareness
	(2) Monitor changes over time
	(3) Go to step 3

If yes:
(a) Document and relate to neuroimaging and neuropsychological findings
(3) Monitor changes and symptoms/syndromes over time
(4) Go to step 3

Step 3. If there is a partial syndrome of impaired awareness, does the patient appear to use nondefensive methods of coping with partial knowledge?

If yes:	If no:
(1) Document method of coping	Is the patient using a defensive method of coping?
(2) Document patient's response to feedback	If yes: Go to step 4 If no: Stop
(3) Document patient's response to rehabilitation	

Step 4. If there is a partial syndrome of impaired awareness, does the patient appear to be using defensive methods of coping?

If yes:	If no: Stop
(1) Document the method of coping	
(2) Document how the presumed defence is being clinically approached	
(3) Document reaction of the patient to the methods of intervention/rehabilitation	
(4) Document the patient's course over time	
(5) Has the partial or complete syndrome of impaired awareness resolved?	
If yes, document and stop treating this disturbance.	If no, document and try to manage the patient in light of the reality that some permanent deficit in awareness exists.

---

* PCRS, Patient Competency Rating Scale.

point, the work that has been done is still within the realm of clinical impressions. No clear protocol has been established for working with patients who have frontal, parietal, temporal, or occipital syndromes of partial impaired awareness. Moreover, no clear methods have been established for working with patients who exhibit nondefensive compared to defensive methods of coping. Some clinical examples of how such work has been attempted in individual patients are outlined below.

A patient with a right parietal syndrome of impaired awareness insisted that he could return to teaching as a college professor even though he showed obvious problems with organization, visuospatial planning, and the logic of his thought processes. He was, however, nondefensive about how he dealt with his partial awareness. He knew that some aspects of his teaching capacity might have been affected but was unconvinced that it would substantially affect his performance as a teacher. The patient agreed to let an experienced occupational therapist attend his lectures to observe how well he organized his presentation to his students. It was agreed that, if he neglected to present important information, presented information in a fragmented or unclear manner, or performed in any way that reflected a lack of his being able to grasp the complexity of the information that he was presenting to his students, he would stop teaching and work with the occupational therapist before proceeding. Based on the feedback of an experienced occupational therapist, the professor slowly began to appreciate that he was unable to meet the demands of his profession, at least during the first 6 months after his right CVA.

Patients with a partial temporal lobe syndrome of impaired awareness may show memory impairments as well as disorders of language. One method that has been suggested for working with patients who show language impairments but who fail to recognize their impairment is to record their speech via tape recorder and later play it back to them. Patients often recognize their voices and realize that they are making more language errors than they had thought. This technique has not been tested systematically. In a few clinical cases, however, it seems to have been helpful.

More challenging is helping patients who are partially aware of their memory impairment but who use a defensive method of coping. Sometimes therapists want to force patients to recognize that their memory impairment is worse than it actually is. As described elsewhere (Prigatano 1999), therapists may purposely let patients forget things and experience anxiety about their memory failure to convince them that they have a severe memory problem. Such approaches, however, only erode patients' trust in their therapist. Only by determining why patients deny the extent of a memory problem can therapeutic progress be made (Prigatano 1999).

In daily clinical practice, it is perhaps patients with frontal temporal lobe pathology and associated disturbances of self-awareness who often prove most problematic. Such individuals may be impulsive, socially inappropriate, and use poor judgement in planning. Therefore, they make decisions that place them at high risk for dangerous consequences or severely negative social feedback. The more extensive their problems with awareness, the more they fail to interpret feedback correctly. In fact, later some develop delusions (Prigatano 1999). Many of these patients need a day-treatment programme that helps them to receive feedback from individual therapists and group interactions in gradual steps. The combination of such feedbacks can help patients to recognize their deficit in awareness. This technique is the hallmark of any form of rehabilitation dealing with anosognosia and its various manifestations.

Selective references

Azouvi, P., Marchal, F., Samuel, C., Morin, L., Renard, C., Louis-Dreyfus, A., Jokic, C., Wiart, L., Pradat-Diehl, P., Deloche, G., and Bergego, C. (1996). Functional consequences and awareness of unilateral neglect: study of an evaluation scale. *Neuropsychol. Rehabil.* **6** (2), 133–50.

Bieman-Copland, S. and Dywan, J. (2000). Achieving rehabilitative gains in anosognosia after TBI. *Brain Cognition* **44**, 1–18.

Bisiach, E. and Geminiani, G. (1991). Anosognosia related to hemiplegia and hemianopia. In *Awareness of deficit after brain injury. Clinical and theoretical issues* (ed. G.P. Prigatano and R.L. Schacter), pp 17–39. Oxford University Press, New York.

Bisiach, E., Vallar, G., Perani, D., Papagno, C., and Berti, A. (1986). Unawareness of disease following lesions of the right hemisphere: anosognosia for hemiplegia and anosognosia for hemianopia. *Neuropsychologia* **24** (4), 471–82.

Bisiach, E., Rusconi, M.L., and Vallar, G. (1991). Remission of somatophrenic delusion through vestibular stimulation. *Neuropsychologia* **29**, 1029–31.

Breier, J.I., Adair, J.C., Gold, M., Fennell, E.B., *et al.* (1995). Dissociation of anosognosia for hemiplegia and aphasia during left-hemispheric anesthesia. *Neurology* **45**, 65–7.

Celesia, G.G., Brigell, M.G., and Vaphiades, M.S. (1997). Hemianopic anosognosia. *Neurology* **49**, 88–97.

Cutting, J. (1978). Study of anosognosia. *J. Neurol., Neurosurg., Psychiatry* **41**, 548–55.

Evyapan, D. and Kumral, E. (1999). Pontine anosognosia for hemiplegia. *Neurology* **53** (3), 647–9.

House, A. and Hodges, J. (1988). Persistent denial of handicap after infarction of the right basal ganglia: a case study. *J. Neurol., Neurosurg., Psychiatry* **51**, 112–15.

Jehkonen, M., Ahonen, J-P., Dastidar, P., Laippala, P., and Vilkki, J. (2000). Unawareness of deficits after right hemisphere stroke: double-dissociations of anosognosias. *Acta Neurol. Scand.* **102**, 378–84.

Meador, K.J., Loring, D.W., Feinberg, T.E., Lee, G.P., and Nichols, M.E. (2000). Anosognosia and asomatognosia during intracarotid amobarbital inactivation. *Neurology* **55** (6), 816–20.

Pedersen, P.M., Jorgensen, H.S., Nakayama, H., Raaschou, H.O., *et al.* (1996). Frequency, determinants, and consequences of anosognosia in acute stroke. *J. Neurol. Rehabil.* **10** (4), 243–50.

Perani, D., Vallar, G., Paulesu, E., Alberoni, M., and Fazio, F. (1993). Left and right hemisphere contribution to recovery from neglect after right hemisphere damage—an [18F] FDG PET study of two cases. *Neuropsychologia* **31**, 115–25.

Prigatano, G.P. (1996a). Anosognosia. In *The Blackwell dictionary of neuropsychology* (ed. J.G. Beaumont, P.M. Kenealy, and M.J.C. Rogers). Blackwell, Cambridge, Massachusetts, 80–4.

Prigatano, G.P. (1996b). Behavioral limitations TBI patients tend to underestimate: a replication and extension to patients with lateralized cerebral dysfunction. *Clin. Neuropsychologist* **10**, 191–201.

Prigatano, G.P. (1999). *Principles of neuropsychological rehabilitation*. Oxford University Press, New York.

Prigatano, G.P. and Altman, I.M. (1990). Impaired awareness of behavioral limitations after traumatic brain injury. *Arch. Phys. Med. Rehabil.* **71**, 1058–64.

Prigatano, G.P. and Klonoff, P.S. (1997). A clinician's rating scale for evaluation of impaired self-awareness and denial of disability after brain injury. *Clin. Neuropsychologist* **11** (1), 1–12.

Prigatano, G.P. and Wong, J.L. (1997). Speed of finger tapping and goal attainment after unilateral cerebral vascular accident. *Arch. Phys. Med. Rehabil.* **78**, 847–52.

Prigatano, G.P., Fordyce, D., Zeiner, H.K., Roueche, J.R., Pepping, M., and Wood, B.C. (1986). *Neuropsychological rehabilitation after brain injury.* Johns Hopkins University Press, Baltimore.

Prigatano, G.P., Altman, I.M., and O'Brien, K.P. (1990). Behavioral limitations that traumatic-brain-injured patients tend to underestimate. *Clin. Neuropsychologist* **4**, 163–76.

Ramachandran, V.S. (1994). Phantom limbs, neglect syndromes, repressed memories, and Freudian psychology. *Int. Rev. Neurobiol.* **37**, 291–372.

Sherer, M., Bergloff, P., Levin, E., High, W.M. Jr, Oden, K.E., and Nick, T.G. (1998*a*). Impaired awareness and employment outcome after traumatic brain injury. *J. Head Trauma Rehabil.* **13** (5), 52–61.

Sherer, M., Bergloff, P., Boake, C., High, W. Jr., and Levin, E. (1998*b*). The Awareness Questionnaire: factor structure and internal consistency. *Brain Injury* **12** (1), 63–8.

Small, M. and Ellis, S. (1996). Denial of hemiplegia: an investigation into the theories of causation. *Eur. Neurol.* **36**, 353–63.

Starkstein, S.E., Fedoroff, J.P., Price, T.R., Leiguarda, R., and Robinson, R.G. (1992). Anosognosia in patients with cerebrovascular lesions. A study of causative factors. *Stroke* **23**, 1446–53.

Starkstein, S.E., Fedoroff, J.P., Price, T.R., Leiguarda, R., and Robinson, R.G. (1993). Neuropsychological deficits in patients with anosognosia. *Neuropsychiatry, Neuropsychol. Behav. Neurol.* **6**, 43–8.

Starkstein, S.E., Chemerinski, E., Sabe, L., Kuzis, G., Petracca, G., Teson, A., and Leignarda, R. (1997). Prospective longitudinal study of depression and anosognosia in Alzheimer's disease. *Br. J. Psychiatry* **171**, 47–52.

Stone, S.P., Halligan, P.W., and Greenwood, R.J. (1993). The incidence of neglect phenomena and related disorders in patients with an acute right or left hemisphere stroke. *Age Ageing* **22**, 46–52.

Vuilleumier, P., Chicherio, C., Assal, F., Schwartz, S., Slosman, D., and Landis, T. (2001). Functional neuroanatomical correlates of hysterical sensorimotor loss. *Brain* **124**, 1077–90.

Part 4

Developmental and paediatric neuropsychology

Chapter 23

Neuropsychological assessment of developmental disorders

Christine M. Temple

1 Background issues

1.1 Objectives of assessment

The neuropsychological assessment of children is motivated by different objectives. Regardless of aetiology, there may be a query about whether or not a child has a problem in a particular area. It is the task of the neuropsychologist to determine whether the level of performance exhibited constitutes a problem and also to identify the specificity of the difficulty, with intact skills being of interest as well as those that are impaired. A child may also have a specific syndrome known to be linked to a particular disability, but the degree or precise form of the disability in the child may be unknown. In research, there may also be interest in contrasting performance across tasks thought to address different components of cognitive systems.

1.2 Comparison to normal function

In formulating judgements about the existence of a disorder, the performance of the child is compared to that of other children. For many assessments, the comparison children are the population whose norms are reported with the published psychometric test. Where there is no appropriate psychometric test or there is not one with relevant norms for children, new or modified tasks may be derived from adult tasks or the research literature. For such tasks, supplementary norms or control data are often published. In making judgements about the specificity of a disorder, cross-task comparisons are also made of performance by the same child on different measures.

1.3 Slowed development versus qualitatively abnormal development

If the issue is whether a child is impaired in comparison to peers then a chronological age comparison group is appropriate. However, if there is an issue of whether impaired performance reflects slowed development or qualitatively abnormal development, it may be more relevant to compare the child to younger children matched for overall ability in the area of question to determine whether the pattern of performance differs from that of this group. The match, for example, might be made on mental age or language age or reading age, depending on the question being asked. In each case, the issue would be whether the child being assessed differs from the ability-matched group, in which case development would be abnormal rather than slowed.

1.4 Decisions about impairment

In making judgements about differences in performance between or within children, there will be an issue about the relevant cut-off for the difference to be reliable or significant. Dependent on the question being asked, the method of deciding this may vary. For many psychometric tests, tables of norms indicate what constitutes abnormality in the view of the test producers. For tasks in which normative data is more limited, the cut-off may be:

* performance outside the control range;

* the performance level that fewer than 1 in 20 normal children attain, which would be the equivalent of a 5% cut-off for normative data;

* performance where z is statistically significant with z derived from the mean and standard deviation (SD) of the control/normative sample. As an alternative to z, where the normative sample is small, it may be more appropriate to use a modified t-test. Rather than assuming that the parameters of the control group apply directly to the population from which it has been sampled, the modified t-test treats the control group as a group to compare with a group represented by the assessed child. See Crawford and Howell (1998) for discussion and website link for a straightforward program to compute results.

Deficits, not apparent on initial testing may appear after a delay post-injury or late in development, perhaps because tasks for older children become more complex or place more specific demands upon the child. Follow-up into middle childhood is of importance where initial assessment takes place at an early age.

1.5 Issues affecting assessment quality

Assessment should be rigorous, systematic, and objective but not rigid. The nature of the child in question and the issues in the case should moderate the tasks selected, the data used for control comparison, the cut-off decision in deciding about impairment, and the interpretation of the results. Preconceptions about the development of skills in children will also affect both task selection and the interpretation of results. Different neuropsychologists may interpret the same results in different ways, particularly when the tasks employed tap several functions. For example, abnormal digit span may be interpreted as a short-term memory problem, or as a sequencing problem, or as a difficulty with numbers. The correct interpretation may depend upon performance on other comparison tasks.

The most critical thing to determine before starting any assessment is what it is that you wish to measure. Administration of tasks because they happen to be available but without a clear idea of what one is trying to measure will render the interpretation of results limited. Large batteries are often not particularly helpful. If subtests are employed because the test producers have generated them, rather than because they measure something that has already been identified as needing to be measured, then assessment time is simply wasted. The tasks discussed below are inevitably selective but represent some of those best suited to address the assessment of specific identified functions.

2 **Testing status**

- Prior to assessment a detailed history of development is usually taken to determine the background against which the assessment occurs. This may include family history, medical history, developmental progress, and parental concerns. Whilst lacking specialist knowledge, the perceptiveness of many parents in highlighting the key areas of their children's difficulties should not be underestimated.

- Ideally, there should be recent confirmation that visual acuity or corrected visual acuity with glasses/lenses is normal.

- The shape detection subtest of the Visual Object and Space Perception (VOSP) Battery (Warrington and James 1991) can be used as a rough screener for those whose visual sensory efficiency is such that visual recognition difficulties are likely. Norms: ages 6–10 years (Temple and Coleman 2000).

- Children with visual field defects should be encouraged to move their eyes over the stimuli.

- Children may present with visual anomalies whose impact on task performance is unclear. Contrasting results from tasks with similar visual input may be informative.

- If there is difficulty with phonological discrimination (see Section 4), hearing should be checked.

- Abnormalities of motor skills may affect performance on tasks where there is manual response. Oral–motor difficulties may affect the quality of language production, though not vocabulary or grammar. For children with motor difficulties, tasks should be interpreted with these in mind.

- For those with seizures, interictal performance may fluctuate reflecting abnormal subclinical activity. Repeat testing may be important to substantiate intertask contrasts in performance.

- The child may have reduced self-confidence, elevated anxiety, and a tendency to give up before failure in performance is too conspicuous. Continual encouragement and praise may be required to ensure that when testing ends it is because the child is unable to perform further, rather than reluctant to try. Overt errors are therefore more informative than refusals. Children may be particularly sensitive to feedback given in facial expression.

3 Intelligence

Most neuropsychological appraisals begin with a general measure of intellectual function. This provides an idea of overall performance level. Discrepancies between verbal and performance intelligence quotient (IQ) or between subtest scores may also indicate neuropsychological abnormality. Impaired intellect affects the acquisition of many skills but may also take many different forms with relative patterns of strength and weakness within the profile.

3.1 The Wechsler scales

The Wechsler scales are the most widely used measures of intellectual assessment and are available in many languages. They are divided into three age bands:

- the Wechsler Preschool and Primary Scale of Intelligence (WIPPSI-R; Wechsler 1989) for ages 3–7;
- the Wechsler Intelligence Scale for Children (WISC-III; Wechsler 1992) for ages 6–16;
- the Wechsler Adult Intelligence Scale (WAIS-R) for ages 16 upwards.

The three versions are similar in design. Each has a set of subtests that are combined to derive a verbal IQ and a set of subsets that are combined to derive a nonverbal performance IQ. A well practised tester and responsive, alert child may finish eight subtests within an hour, but a slower child may take double this time. Where there is time pressure a short version of the WISC-R using four subtests, two from each scale, has sometimes been employed: Block Design and Object Assembly from the performance scale and Vocabulary and Similarities from the verbal scale. More recently, the Wechsler Abbreviated Scale of Intelligence (WASI; Psychological Corporation 2000) has been produced, which contains four subtests to be used in similar fashion.

The Wechsler scales provide scores to derive IQ but the breakdown of scores across subtests also provides clues about more specific problems. The subtest scatter is informative clinically. However, perfectly normal Wechsler IQ and subtest scores can be produced by children who nevertheless have neuropsychological deficits. The scales do not address all skills. They are weak at detecting executive problems and memory difficulties. When a child has dramatically varying subtest scores it may be meaningless to derive an average IQ.

3.1.1 WISC-III (Wechsler 1992)

There are five subtests in the verbal scale and five subtests in the performance scale.

Verbal scale

- The Information subtest contains factual questions about general knowledge of the world. Low scores may be attained by a child with language difficulties. Where the score is below those of other verbal subtests, the possibility of memory impairment should be considered. Older children with reading difficulties may also score more poorly than on other verbal subtests, if more limited exposure to reading books has limited their general knowledge. Children with particular difficulties with number or time series (e.g. months of the year) will also score poorly as many initial questions require numerical responses or knowledge of time series.

- The Vocabulary subtest requires the child to define words spoken aloud. The scoring criteria are very explicit.

- The Similarities subtest requires the child to specify the similarity between pairs of items. The production of contrasting or incorrect information from the outset should be considered as possible failure to grasp task instructions. For children with memory, attentional, or language difficulties, it may also be necessary to re-emphasize task instructions if the child drifts off task.

- The Arithmetic subtest is unhelpful diagnostically in determining the form of any problem with arithmetic. Children with language difficulties and those with developmental dyscalculia will score poorly. For a child with suspected arithmetical difficulties, it is not appropriate to include this subtest in the derivation of IQ, since it reflects a specific problem potentially out of line with basic intellectual skill. For such children the other four verbal subtests should be prorated to derive verbal IQ.

- The Comprehension subtest asks the child about behaviours in real-life situations. Whilst it is a test of verbal comprehension, it also measures knowledge of society and compliance with social expectations. Non-compliant responses are sometimes produced that lower the language comprehension score but do not reflect language difficulties. Later questions are as much tests of general knowledge as of language comprehension. In a child who does not have arithmetical difficulties the comprehension subtest should be excluded and the other four verbal subtests should be prorated to derive verbal IQ.

Performance scale

- Picture Completion is usually a quick test and is the only performance subtest for which rapid, coordinated responses with hands are not required. Weak skills usually indicate perceptual difficulties.

- Picture Arrangement requires the sequencing of pictures to make a story. It is the most verbally loaded of the performance subtests. A lower score on this subtest than others can sometimes indicate executive difficulties.

- Block Design is a timed constructional task where patterns are built from coloured cubes. Weak skills usually indicate visuospatial problems, though sensorimotor problems will also lower scores through speed delays. Block design can be accomplished using a verbal strategy.

- Object Assembly is a jigsaw construction task. It is harder than block design to perform well using a verbal strategy. Weak scores are usually indicative of visuospatial problems, though again sensorimotor difficulties will lower scores through speed delays.

- Coding can be lowered by such a diverse range of neuropsychological impairments that it should be avoided for inclusion in calculating IQ. Prorate the four other tests.

3.1.2 WIPPSI-R (Wechsler 1989)

Similar to the WISC but norms 3–7 years. Mazes replace Picture Arrangement in the performance scale.

3.1.3 WASI (Psychological Corporation 2000)

This includes two verbal and two nonverbal subtests. It can be given in about half an hour. Norms 6–89 years. The two-subtest form using Vocabulary and a new subtest, Matrix Reasoning, can be given in about 15 minutes, and generates a full intelligence quotient (FIQ) only. Initial reports indicate that it works well. Useful for initial screening and screening controls for research.

3.2 Other scales

3.2.1 Bayley scales II (Bayley 1993)

An extensively used classical test providing an early general indication of cognitive skills, motor development and behaviour. Norms 1–42 months. A 10-minute screener, the Bayley Infant Neurodevelopmental Screener (BINS) for neuropsychological abnormality in infancy is also available. Norms 3–24 months (Aylward 1995).

3.2.2 McCarthy scales (McCarthy 1972)

This is a diverse assessment with 18 subtests. A subset of these generates a general cognitive index with mental age equivalents, 1–12 years. Norms 2–8 years.

3.2.3 British Ability Scales (BASII; Elliott *et al.* 1996)

This is a battery of subtests often used as an alternative to the Wechsler in the UK, but for cross-comparative work with other countries use the WISC-III.

3.2.4 Kaufman Assessment Battery for Children (K-ABC; Kaufman and Kaufman 1983)

This is popular in North America. Norms 2–12 years. It is better for low functioning young children than the WIPPSI-R. Estimations of IQ are derived from a Sequential Processing Scale, which assesses the processing of stimuli in series, and a Simultaneous Processing Scale, which assesses the integration of multiple stimuli. It has less emphasis on factual knowledge and language than the WISC. Scales should not be interpreted in relation to left–right hemispheres.

3.2.5 Raven's Progressive Matrices (Raven 1998)

Nonverbal measure of intellectual skill that tests inductive reasoning about patterns and designs. There are three forms:

- Coloured (CPM) for ages 5–11;

- Standard (SPM) for ages 6–16;
- Advanced (APM) for over 18 years.

The CPM or SPM are useful for the assessment of children with language difficulties. The test can be done using both verbal and nonverbal strategies, and performance is impaired to a similar degree by both right and left hemisphere damage, so impaired performance is not diagnostic of laterality. It is also a useful measure where groups of children are being screened together, e.g. in screening controls for research. Untimed SPM can take 40 minutes. Where used for screening controls, every second item may be given and scores doubled.

3.2.6 The Leiter International Performance Scale–Revised (LIPS-R; Roid and Miller 1996)

This is a monster of a test in both cost (UK £1847 in 2003) and apparatus. It is a widely used test of nonverbal intelligence for those with language difficulties or learning disabilities and its predecessor discriminated well between children with such difficulties. The revised version adds subtests addressing Attention and Memory to the core areas of Reasoning and Visualization. Some UK clinicians report that it is more complex and time-consuming than the original, suitable for fewer children. Others find it works well. Norms 2–20 years.

4 Language

At least 2% of children have language disorders with a male–female ratio of approximately 3 : 1. Language disorders affect all day-to-day communications with family, school, and friends. Whilst there are different ways in which language could be partitioned, some kind of decomposition of the skills involved is required for any meaningful assessment. One way to segment language skills is to divide them along two dimensions.

- The first dimension is the distinction between skills in understanding language and skills in expressing language—an input–output dimension.
- The second dimension relates to the unit of language being assessed. Here skills can be assessed in relation to increasingly large units:

    —phonological, lexical, and semantic;

    —grammatical and syntactic;

    —narrative and pragmatic.

If the difficulty is not generalized, contrasting performance across these dimensions may enable identification of the aspect of language that is the most problematic. The two dimensions are represented in a simplified schematic model of the language system in Fig. 23.1. The units of language being assessed are represented by distinct components in the model, with phonological skills being part of both phonological analysis and speech production. Narrative and pragmatic skills are not represented.

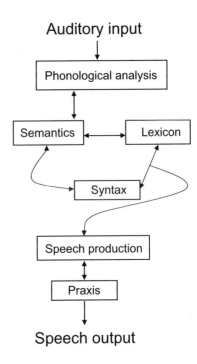

Fig. 23.1 A simplified schematic model of a language system.

The input–output dimension is represented by the flow. Feedback is present in many areas. This model does not preclude connectionist representations of any of its components. Some might argue that the whole language system is a connectionist mass but such modelling is insufficiently differentiated to be of much clinical utility.

4.1 Reception of language

4.1.1 Phonological skills

◆ Auditory Discrimination Test (ADT; Wepman and Reynolds 1994). This updated test remains a quick and easy screener for ability to discriminate similar sounding words. Norms 5–8 years.

◆ Rhyme subtest and Alliteration subtest of the Phonological Assessment Battery (PhAB; Frederickson *et al.* 1997). Norms 5–15 years.

◆ Rhyme detection subtest of the Phonological Abilities Test (PAT; Muter *et al.* 2000). Norms 4–7 years.

4.1.2 Lexical and semantic skills

◆ *Receptive vocabulary* is widely measured on the Peabody Picture Vocabulary Test (PPVT-III; Dunn and Dunn 1997), norms from 2 years, and the British Picture Vocabulary Scale (BPVS II; Dunn *et al.* 1997), norms 3–15 years. A word is spoken aloud and the child selects the matching picture from an array of four. These tests have the merit of speed, though the updated BPVS has abandoned a short form and is therefore less brief than its predecessor. They are useful in delineating a child's vocabulary even if the child has performed poorly at explicitly defining words, e.g. on the WISC-III Vocabulary subtest. If a child has a good BPVT/PPVT despite poor vocabulary subtest, then they have a good vocabulary and knowledge of words but they have difficulty in activating or using this knowledge to generate definitions. If both the BPVS/PPVT and the Vocabulary subtest are weak, the child may not have semantic representations for the words. This may be a selective difficulty in building up vocabulary stores of words or it may be part of a more general memory impairment (e.g. Julia in Temple 1997; Casalini *et al.* 1999).

◆ *Lexical decision* shows whether a child has a mental representation of a word's name even if he or she cannot indicate its meaning. There is no standardized task for children but nonwords may be derived from the BPVS/PPVT by altering the stimuli by one letter. These nonwords may be randomly presented with the words for a lexicality decision, which would enable determination of whether a child at least recognizes and therefore has a mental representation for the words' names.

◆ Single-word section of the Reynell Developmental Language Scales (RDLS III) Comprehension Scale (Edwards *et al.* 1997). Norms 1–7 years.

◆ Word classes and semantic relationships subtests of the Clinical Evaluation of Language Fundamentals (CELF-III; Semel *et al.* 2000). Norms: word class, 6–21 years; semantic relationships, 9–21 years.

4.1.3 Morphological, grammatical, and syntactic skills

◆ The Test for the Reception of Grammar (TROG; Bishop 1983) has sentences or phrases that are read aloud and the child selects the matching picture from an array of four. Useful screener. Includes blocks on varied morphological and syntactic skills.

◆ Token test (Lass *et al.* 1975). Traditional measure. Requests of increasing, though varied, grammatical complexity. Also involves memory.

◆ The concepts and directions subtest of the CELF-III has a similar format (Semel *et al.* 2000). Norms 6–21 years. For younger children the basic concepts and linguistic concepts subtests of the CELF preschool are also relevant. Norms 3–6 years.

◆ The RDLS III Comprehension scale has several sections, which give general measures (Edwards *et al.* 1997). Norms 1–7 years.

◆ For more detailed delineation of grammatical difficulty, there is no published instrument that is effective in relation to current theories. A number of tasks in the psycholinguistics literature are used in a research context to investigate the comprehension of explicit morphological or syntactic features.

4.1.4 Narrative, pragmatic, and metalinguistic skills

Although narrative and pragmatic skills are important there are few systematic instruments for their investigation.

- Listening to Paragraphs subtest of the CELF-111 (Semel *et al.* 2000). Norms 6–21 years.
- Inferencing section of the RDLS III (Edwards *et al.* 1997). Norms 1–7 years.
- Understanding Ambiguity: An Assessment of Pragmatic Meaning (Rinaldi 1996). Assesses understanding of idioms, words, and phrases with multiple meanings. Norms 10+. Also assesses contradictions between emotional prosody and phrase content. Norms 8–13 years.
- Children's Communication Checklist (CCC; Bishop 1998).

4.2 Expression of language

4.2.1 Phonological skills

- Children's Test of Non-Word Repetition (CN-REP; Gathercole and Baddeley 1996). Impairments in the reception of phonology will affect repetition but where receptive phonological skills are intact (see above), difficulties with phonological analysis, synthesis or production become evident on non-word repetition. Norms 4–8 years.
- Rhyme production, word completion and phoneme deletion subtests of the PAT (Muter *et al.* 2000). Norms 4–7 years.
- Samples of spontaneous speech in conversation or in response to picture or story description are also a useful data source to determine the quality of speech sounds within speech production (see narrative production in Section 4.2.4).

4.2.2 Lexical and semantic skills

- Picture naming assesses semantic knowledge and lexical access.
  —The Word Finding Vocabulary Scale (Renfrew 1977). Norms 3–9 years.
  —Expressive Vocabulary subtest of the K-ABC (Kaufman and Kaufman 1983). Photographs. Norms 2–4 years.
  —The BASII Naming subtest (Elliot *et al.* 1996). Coloured pictures. Norms 2–7 years.
  —The Boston Naming test (Kaplan *et al.* 1983). Norms 6–11 years (Halperin *et al.* 1989; Spreen and Strauss 1998). Phonological and semantic cues may be useful in discriminating genuine retrieval difficulties from failures to establish effective representations for the words. Test can be given without cues.
  —For more research-oriented questions and the exploration of category-specific effects the pictures of Snodgrass and Vanderwart (1980) are often employed. Data from normal children with these stimuli are provided by Cycowicz *et al.* (1997) with full responses reported, enabling comparative error analysis.
- Few tests look at the production of verbs.
  —Verbs and phrases in the Expressive Scale, RDLS III (Edwards *et al.* 1997). Norms 1–8 years.
  —An Object and Action Naming Battery (Druks and Masterson 2000). Norms 3–5 years.

◆ Non-pictorial naming.

   —Riddles subtest of the K-ABC (Kaufman and Kaufman 1983). Naming from descriptions. Useful for children with perceptual problems or agnosia. Norms 3–12 years.

4.2.3 Morphological, grammatical, and syntactic skills

There are few published psychometric tests that look in a systematic way at the production of specific linguistic forms and morphological structures. However, there are many studies within the psycholinguistic literature from which such tasks can be taken.

◆ Four sections of the RDLS III (Edwards *et al.* 1997) are also relevant: inflections: plurals, third person; past tense; clausal elements; auxiliaries: negatives, question tags. Norms 1–7 years.

◆ Word structure sections of the CELF-preschool and CELF-III (Semel *et al.* 2000). Norms 3–21 years.

The use of morphology, grammar, and syntax in narrative can be determined from analysis of narrative production (see Section 4.2.4).

4.2.4 Narrative skills

◆ Conversational speech can be taped for analysis of vocabulary used, mean length of utterance, and range of morphological, grammatical, and syntactic structures employed.

◆ Picture description. A set picture is presented for description to generate narrative, which can be analysed in a similar way to conversational speech. A variety of pictures are deployed, the most traditional being the Cookie Theft from the Boston Aphasia Battery (Goodglass and Kaplan 1972). A common stimulus enables cross-child comparison.

◆ Story description may elicit more extensive language for analysis. The picture-story book with no words entitled *Frog where are you?* (Mayer 1969) has been used with children with William's syndrome, and has potential to be used more extensively. *The bus story* (Renfrew 1991) is an alternative. Norms 3–8 years.

◆ Narrative can also be generated in response to a specific challenge requiring explanation. Possibilities that have been used in the past include how to use a telephone and how to organize a party. These tasks also have executive components.

4.2.5 Pragmatic and metalinguistic skills

◆ The Test of Word Knowledge (TOWK; Wiig and Secord 1992) enables assessment of figurative language and multiple meanings. Norms 5–18 years.

4.2.6 Motor speech

◆ Test of verbal dyspraxia (Blakeley 1980).

◆ The Apraxia Profile (Hickman 1997). Norms 3–13 years.

4.3 **Reading**

The incidence of specific developmental reading difficulties is reported as 6% in a population study in the UK (Lewis *et al.* 1994). There is now strong evidence for a biological basis to these disorders. Impairments in literacy are also common following neurological injury or disease in childhood. Children with reading difficulties commonly experience decline in self-confidence at school from which behaviour problems may follow. They may also be slower than normal in producing written work, and time dispensations in formal examinations are now common in both school and university. Most current theories identify two distinct components to reading.

- The *phonological* reading route is used to sound out unfamiliar words or nonwords. Children with impaired development of this route have *phonological dyslexia*. This may be identified by a lexicality effect in which nonwords are read much more poorly than words.

- In contrast, the *lexico-semantic* reading route contains word-specific information. All words can be read by this route and it is the only route by which to read irregular words that violate common pronunciation rules. Children with impaired development of the lexico-semantic reading route have *surface dyslexia*. This may be identified by a regularity effect in which regular words are read better than irregular words, and by the presence of regularization errors in which an irregular word is read incorrectly, though in a phonologically correct way (e.g. sweat → sweet). These errors result from overreliance on the phonological reading route.

Castles and Coltheart (1993) estimated that 85% of dyslexics show a dissociation between the two reading routes and, of these, 46% have a surface dyslexic pattern and 64% have a phonological dyslexic pattern. The other 15% showed no dissociation. For further discussion see Temple (1997).

4.3.1 Letter knowledge

The letters of the alphabet should be presented individually in both lower and upper case forms for both naming and sounding.

4.3.2 Reading age

This indicates general reading level. Further testing is required to determine the nature of the problem.

- Wechsler Objective Reading Dimension (WORD; Wechsler 1993). Measures general reading skills, spelling and reading comprehension Norms 6–16 years.

- Schonell single-word reading test (Schonell and Schonell 1956). Quick, single-word reading test. Old but useful screener. Norms 5–13 years.

- BASII reading subtest (Elliot *et al.* 1996). Quick, single-word reading test. UK norms 5–14 years.

- Neale Analysis of Reading (NARA-II; Neale 1997). Good measure of text reading. Norms 4–14 years. Accuracy Reading Age can be compared to single-word measures above. Set of questions used to derive Comprehension Reading Age. Reading is also timed to derive a Speed of Reading Age. The suggested error analysis is best ignored as it yields little information of theoretical relevance. Useful test to delineate children whose reading accuracy is better than their understanding of what they read. Seen in some forms of hyperlexia in children with learning disabilities. Can also be a sign of general language comprehension difficulties, memory impairment, or executive difficulties with narrative interpretation. Further testing is needed to distinguish between these possibilities.

If comprehension is an issue, a parallel version of the NARA-II can be given in a nonstandard way in purely oral form, by reading the text passages to the child and then asking the questions. There are no norms but scores can be compared to reading comprehension to determine specificity of comprehension difficulty.

4.3.3 Single words

- *Regular and irregular words.* Contrasting performance on the reading of regular and irregular words is a key element in the classification of reading disorders. Psychometric instruments do not in general appraise this specifically. Several relevant lists are in circulation (e.g. Coltheart *et al.* 1979). However many of these are designed for adults and have a number of items not suitable for children.

- *Words and nonwords.* There are several balanced lists of words and nonwords employed in the research literature (e.g. Temple 1997). Alternatively, reading age for words, from the measures in Section 4.3.2, may be compared to a nonwords reading age derived from the Graded Nonword Reading Test (Snowling *et al.* 1996), norms 5–11 years, or the nonword reading subtest of the PhAB (Frederickson *et al.* 1997), norms 5–15 years.

- *Homophones.* Surface dyslexics have difficulty in indicating the meaning of homophones. Several unpublished lists are available to appraise this skill (e.g. Temple 1985).

4.3.4 Text reading

- NARA-II (Neale 1997). Widely used. Norms 4–14 years.

4.4 Spelling

4.4.1 Writing

Some children have poor writing skills, even though spelling is normal. They may be referred because of a spelling difficulty when, in reality, it is the act of writing that is problematic, often linked to constructional apraxia, in which case there may also be impaired drawing and poor layout of school work. If pervasive, the apraxia may extend to difficulties with dressing, buckles, buttons, and bicycle riding. Poor writing may make analysis of spelling more difficult as the component letters in words are difficult to derive.

4.4.2 Letters

Individual letter names and letter sounds should be dictated for written response.

4.4.3 Spelling age

- WORD (Wechsler 1993) Norms 6–16 years.
- The Schonell spelling list of single words (Schonell and Schonell 1956). Old but quick screener. Norms 5–13 years.
- Single Word Spelling Test (Sacre and Masterson 2001). UK norms 6–14 years.

4.4.4 Single words

- *Regular and irregular.* Lists employed for reading can also be given for written spelling, though with awareness that irregularity in reading and spelling are not identical and there are further ambiguities in the spelling of regular words.
- *Words and nonwords.* Lists employed for reading can also be given for written spelling.

4.4.5 Written narrative

Quality can be assessed informally by asking the child to write a story or a description. The objective should be to find a topic about which the child will be motivated to write.

5 Memory

The incidence of memory disorders in children is unknown and, until relatively recently, these disorders were seldom recognized. It is likely that the attention focused upon disorders of memory will increase substantially in the next few years with increasing reports of developmental amnesia or dysmnesia (e.g. Baddeley *et al.* 2001; Temple 1997, 2002; Casalini *et al.* 1999; Gadian *et al.* 2000). Memory impairment that affects semantic stores may thereby affect the development of language itself, and the latter may be the more conspicuous presenting feature. In other cases, language and intelligence may measure as normal despite severe classroom difficulties in keeping track of activities and remembering day-to-day events.

- Wide Range Assessment of Memory and Learning (WRAML; Sheslow and Adams 1990). Nine subtests yield measures of verbal and visual memory and learning. Norms 5–17 years.
- Children's Memory Scale (CMS; Cohen 1997). Parallel to the structure of the Wechsler Memory Scale for adults. Immediate and delayed visual and verbal memory. Also recognition memory, working memory, and learning of paired associates. 30 minutes to give. Norms 5–16 years.
- The Rivermead Behavioural Memory Test for Children (RBMT-C; Wilson *et al.* 1991). Aims to assess everyday memory. Not always as sensitive as the two previous measures but oriented towards more realistic situations. Norms 5–10 years.
- Working Memory Test Battery for Children (WMTB-C; Pickering and Gathercole 2001). Assesses the three components of the Working Memory Model of Baddeley and Hitch (1974). Norms 5–15 years.

◆ Warrington's Recognition Memory Battery (WRMB; Warrington 1984). Norms 9–11 years (Temple and Cornish 1993).

◆ Benton's Visual Retention Test—Revised (BVRT-R; Benton Sivian 1991). Norms from 8 years.

6 Nonverbal functions

Impaired spatial and perceptual skills may have subtle effects on day-to-day life, creating problems at home and school in geography, mathematics, aspects of science, games, drawing and art, layout of school work, and technical skills. The children may also appear clumsy despite good fine motor skills. Object recognition difficulties may become more marked in evening or dimmed light or with partial views. Face processing difficulties create severe interpersonal social problems.

6.1 Spatial and spatiomotor skills

Perceptual skills are also involved in many of the tasks below.

◆ Benton's line orientation. Children's norms (Benton *et al.* 1994).

◆ Mental rotation.

◆ Block design subtest of the WISC-III (Wechsler 1992).

◆ Object Assembly subtest of the WISC-III (Wechsler 1992).

◆ Developmental Test of Visual-Motor Integration, 4th edn (VMI; Beery 1997). Copying designs tasks. Short form norms 2–8 years. Long form to 14 years.

◆ BVRT-R (see Section 5). Also has a copying section. Norms from 8 years.

6.2 Perceptual skills

Work on perception has distinguished between the processes involved in determining the identity of an object and those involved in identifying its location and its movement. The majority of tasks used in the neuropsychological assessment of children have focused upon processes involved in establishing identity, with a small number concerned with location.

6.2.1 Judgements of location

◆ The Position Discrimination subtest of the VOSP (Warrington and James 1991). Norms 6–10 years (Temple and Coleman 2000).

◆ The Number Location subtest of the VOSP (Warrington and James 1991). Norms 6–10 years (Temple and Coleman 2000).

◆ Position in Space subtest of the Developmental Test of Visual Perception (DTVP-2; Hammill *et al.* 1995). Norms 4–10 years.

6.2.2 **Judgements of identity: object recognition**

Difficulties in naming are usually attributed to a language impairment in children but where the child is unable to provide clues to the item's meaning an object recognition disorder remains a possibility. For those who are not overtly agnosic, object recognition difficulties may be identified when degraded, rotated, or unusual views are utilized.

Recognizing pictured objects.

◆ Naming; see verbal tasks (Section 4.2.2).

◆ Picture description; see verbal tasks (Section 4.2.4).

◆ Specific categories. Using stimuli from Snodgrass and Vanderwart (1980).

Recognizing degraded stimuli/unusual views.

◆ Silhouettes subtest of the VOSP (Warrington and James 1991). Stimulus items are silhouettes of animals and objects ordered for task difficulty. Norms 6–10 years (Temple and Coleman 2000).

◆ Object Decision subtest of the VOSP (Warrington and James 1991). Stimulus items are silhouettes of rotated objects and nonsense figures. Norms 6–10 years (Temple and Coleman 2000).

◆ Progressive Silhouettes subtest of the VOSP (Warrington and James 1991). A series of silhouettes of the same object, progressively easier to recognize as they are rotated closer to the normal lateral view. Norms 6–10 years (Temple and Coleman 2000).

◆ Visual Closure subtest of the DTVP-2 (Hammill *et al.* 1995). Norms 4–10 years.

6.2.3 **Judgements of identity: face recognition**

Face recognition disorders in children have received only limited study but may be more pervasive than the volume of literature might suggest. Incidence is unknown. Cases to date have been assessed in relation to the model of Bruce and Young (1986); see Fig. 23.2. In some cases there is impairment in the structural encoding required to establish face recognition units and performance on all the face tasks below would be impaired (e.g. De Haan and Campbell 1991). In other cases, the difficulty is later in the system and affects only the access to the person identity information required for recognition. In such cases matching faces and initial encoding of new face recognition units is normal (e.g. Temple 1992). There are also children for whom face recognition of identity is intact but who have problems in recognizing facial expression.

◆ Matching faces.
  —Benton's Face Recognition Task. Children's norms (Benton *et al.* 1994). Can be done successfully using a verbal piecemeal strategy (e.g. in William's syndrome).

◆ Short-term memory for faces/encoding new face recognition units.
  —WRMB (Warrington 1984). Norms data 9–11 years (Temple and Cornish 1993).

◆ Recognition of famous faces.

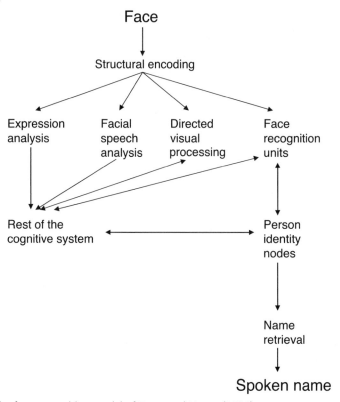

Fig. 23.2 The face recognition model of Bruce and Young (1986).

—Faces and places subtest of K-ABC (Kaufman and Kaufman 1983). Naming of fictional characters, famous people, and well known places. Most suitable for the US, though adaption feasible. Norms 2–12 years.

—For children, faces that are famous change rapidly with cultural and media shifts. Specific material usually has to be constructed taken from publications for children and with controls sampled for comparison.

—Photographs of family and friends can be borrowed from the family to detect serious levels of difficulty. In practice, difficulties are seldom as extreme as this.

♦ Facial expression.

—No standardized test for children but the Eckman faces are suitable for research in the area. The recent Facial Expressions of Emotion Stimuli Test (FEEST; Young *et al.* 2001) may be suitable for future collection of children's norms.

6.2.4 Visual neglect

Behavioural Inattention Test (BIT; Wilson *et al.* 1987). Normal data for the conventional subtests available from the author of this chapter. Publication forthcoming. Ages 6–10 years.

6.3 **Motor skills**

- Spatiomotor skills are involved in the VMI (Beery 1997) and BVRT-R (Benton Sivian 1991) discussed in Sections 5 and 6.1.

- Bruininks–Oseretsky Test of Motor Proficiency (Bruininks 1978). Large battery of eight subtests, assessing fine and gross motor skills, including speed and dexterity and bimanual coordination. Fine motor subtests straightforward, quick, and easy to give. Gross motor subtests more cumbersome. Norms 4–14 years.

6.4 **Drawing skills**

- Draw-a-Person (Naglieri 1987). Child draws a man, a woman, and his or her self. Norms 5–17 years.

- Goodenough–Harris Drawing Test (Goodenough and Harris 1963). Drawing of a person scored in relation to 73 characteristics. Quick to give. Slow to score. Norms 5–16 years.

7 **Executive functions**

Executive disorders are being reported in association with an increasing number of neuropsychological impairments in children, including autism (Ozonoff *et al.* 1991), attention deficit hyperactivity disorders (ADHD; Shue and Douglas 1992), conduct disorder (Pennington and Ozonoff 1996), Turner's syndrome (Temple *et al.* 1996), phenylketonuria (Welsh *et al.* 1990), Gilles de la Tourette syndrome (Baron-Cohen *et al.* 1994), and in survivors of acute lymphoblastic leukaemia (Waber *et al.* 1994). The cumulative incidence of these is unclear. Executive impairments have also been reported in children following frontal lobe lesions including closed head injury (e.g. Williams and Mateer 1992). Many of these assessments have used adult tasks adapted for children. There are many theoretical discussions about the partitioning of executive skills but the child literature has often identified a distinction between inhibitory processes and planning. Executive impairment may affect the child's ability to plan and organize his or her school work, sustain attention in task, respond rapidly and effectively to task instructions, restrain inappropriate responses and behaviours, and manage multiple goals.

- Concept formation and shifting.
  - —Wisconsin Card Sorting Test (WCST; Heaton *et al.* 1993). Norms 5–14 years (Spreen and Strauss 1998). Computer version (2nd research edn) also available.
  - —Brixton Spatial Anticipation Test (Burgess and Shallice 1997). (Modified for children.)
  - —Creature counting subtest of the Test of Everyday Attention for Children (TEA-Ch; Manly *et al.* 1998). Norms 6–16 years.
- Speeded responding.
  - —Ruff Figural Fluency Test (Ruff *et al.* 1987).

—Verbal fluency. Norms for Letter Fluency (FAS), ages 6–13 years (Gaddes and Crockett 1975) and for animals and foods, ages 6–12 years (Spreen and Strauss 1998).

—Fluency subtest of the PhAB (Frederickson *et al.* 1997). Norms 6–14 years.

♦ Inhibitory processes

—The Hayling Sentence Completion Test (Burgess and Shallice 1997). (Modified for children.)

—Luria's Hand Alternation Test (e.g. Baron-Cohen *et al.* 1994).

—The Stroop Test (Stroop 1935).

—Self-Ordered Pointing Task (Petrides and Milner 1982; Spreen and Strauss 1998).

—Walk Don't Walk and Opposite Worlds subtests of the TEA-Ch (Manly *et al.* 1998). Norms 6–16 years.

♦ Planning

—The Tower of London Task (Shallice 1982).

—Figure of Rey (Meyes and Meyes 1995). Norms 6 years up.

♦ Coordinating dual tasks

—Trail Making Test (Reitan and Wolfson 1985).

—Score DT subtest of the TEA-Ch (Manly *et al.* 1998). Children count scoring sounds on tape whilst monitoring a news story for mention of an animal name. Norms 6–16 years.

♦ Sustained attention

—Connors Continuous Performance Test Computer Program Version 3.0 (CPT; Connors 1994). Norms for accuracy and RTs 4 years and up. Also data for diagnosis of attention deficit disorders.

—BIT (Wilson *et al.* 1987). Normal data for the conventional subtests including letter and star cancellation, available from the author of this chapter. Publication forthcoming. Norms 6–10 years.

—Some subtests in the attention and executive function section of the Neuropsychological Assessment of Children (NEPSY; Korkman *et al.* 1997). Norms 3–12 years.

—Code Transmission subtest of TEA-Ch (Manly *et al.* 1988). Norms 6–16 years.

Further norms on a range of children's executive tasks are given in Elders (1997).

8 Arithmetic

The incidence of specific difficulties with arithmetic is 3–6% (Kosc 1974; Lewis *et al.* 1994). Impairments in arithmetical skill have practical significance in developing the ability to manage money and other information about quantities. McCloskey *et al.*'s

(1985) model of adult arithmetical skill has been a constructive backdrop for previous work differentiating some of the component modules of arithmetical skill and its disorders in development. This model distinguishes between skills associated with number processing, i.e. reading, writing, and understanding numbers, and those involved in calculation itself. Children with developmental dyscalculia may have particular difficulties in processing numbers (Temple 1989), learning facts such as tables (e.g. Temple 1991), or mastering the procedures of arithmetical operations (e.g. Temple 1991).

As a background screener for the degree of arithmetical disorder, the Numerical Operations section of the Wechsler Objective Numerical Dimensions Test (WOND; Wechsler 1996) may be employed. Norms 6–16 years. The Mathematics Reasoning scale is less helpful as it compounds multiple processes. For a breakdown of skills further processes should be explored as listed below. Some of these are addressed in a new battery from Butterworth (2003). Norms 5–14 years.

- Number processing
  —Reading arabic numbers and numeral words.
  —Writing arabic numbers and numeral words.
  —Transcoding arabic numbers to numeral words and vice versa.
  —Magnitude judgement. Which of a pair is larger?

- Calculation
  —Number facts: knowledge of signs, knowledge of tables—multiplication, addition, subtraction.
  —Procedural knowledge: steps, order, planning, decimals, fractions.

9 Prognosis

The prognosis for neuropsychological impairment in childhood is highly variable. The old adage that early injury leads to better recovery has been demonstrated to be untrue in many circumstances, with early injuries often having severe long-term effects. In developmental disorders, partial recovery sometimes follows a similar pattern to that of other family members who have experienced similar difficulties. In language, literacy, and arithmetic early detection and sustained remedial input are likely to affect the degree of long-term disability. Effective strategies may be taught to circumvent some problems with memory and executive skills. There is always hope of progress as development occurs but this is likely to be maximal where there is systematic neuropsychological assessment and focused teaching and remedial help to both acquire impaired skills and develop routes to circumvent problem areas by using other skills that are developing well.

10 Concluding comments

Neuropsychological tests for children are gradually becoming better integrated with contemporary theory. Large batteries addressing multiple skills of uncertain theoretical significance are being replaced by more specific tasks addressing explicit functions of neuropsychological significance. In the next decade the range of normative data for children on such tasks is likely to expand so that systematic analysis of specific developmental and acquired disorders in children becomes more straightforward.

Selective references

Aylward, G. (1995). *The Bayley Infant Neurodevelopmental Screener*. The Psychological Corporation, London.

Baddeley, A. and Hitch, G. (1974). Working memory. In *The psychology of learning and motivation*, Vol. 8 (ed. G.A. Bower), pp. 47–90. Academic Press, New York.

Baddeley, A., Vargha-Khadem, F., and Mishkin, M. (2001). Preserved recognition in a case of developmental amnesia: implications for the acquisition of sematic memory. *Journal of Cognitive Neuroscience*, 13, 357–69.

Baron-Cohen S., Cross, P., Crowson, M., and Robertson, M. (1994). Can children with Gilles de la Tourette syndrome edit their intentions? *Psychol. Med.* 24, 29–40.

Bayley, N. (1993). *Bayley Scales II*. The Psychological Corporation, London.

Beery, K.E. (1997). *The Visual-Motor Integration Test*, 4th edn. Pro-Ed, Austin, Texas.

Benton Sivian, A.L. (1991). *Benton Visual Retention Test*, 5th edn. The Psychological Corporation, New York.

Benton, A.L., Silva, A.B., Hamsher, K.D., Varnay, N.R., and Spreen, O. (1994). *Contribution to neuropsychological assessment*: a clinical manual, 2nd edn. Oxford University Press, New York.

Bishop, D.V.M. (1983). *Test for the Reception of Grammar*. D.V.M. Bishop, Manchester.

Bishop, D.V.M. (1998). Development of the children's communication checklist (CCC): a method for assessing qualitative aspects of communicative impairment in children. *J. Child Psychol. Psychiatry* 39, 879–91.

Blakeley, R.W. (1980). *Screening Test for Developmental Apraxia of Speech*. C.C. Publications, Tigard, Oregon.

Bruce, V. and Young, A. (1986). Understanding face recognition. *Br. J. Psychol.* 77, 305–27.

Bruininks, R. (1978). *Bruininks–Oseretsky Test of Motor Proficiency*. NFER-Nelson, Windsor, UK.

Burgess, P.W. and Shallice T. (1997). *The Hayling and Brixton Tests*. Thames Valley Test Company, Bury St Edmunds.

Butterworth, B. (2003). Dyscalculia Screener. NFER-Nelson, Windsor, UK.

Casalini, C., Brizzolara, D., Cavallaro, C., and Cipriani, P. (1999). 'Developmental dysmnesia': a case report. *Cortex* 35, 713–27.

Castles, A. and Coltheart, M. (1993). Varieties of developmental dyslexia. *Cognition* 47, 149–80.

Cohen, M. (1997). *Children's Memory Scale*. The Psychological Corporation, London.

Coltheart, M., Besner, D., Jonasson, J.T., and Davelaar, E. (1979). Phonological recoding in the lexical decision task. *Quart. J. Exp. Psychol.* 31, 489–508.

Connors, C.K. (1994). Conners Continuous Performance Test Computer Programme (CPT). The Psychological Corporation, London.

Crawford, J.R. and Howell, D.C. (1998). Comparing an individual's test score against norms derived from small samples. *Clin. Neuropsychologist* 12, 482–6.

Cycowicz, Y.M., Friedman, D., and Rothstein, M. (1997). Picture naming by young children: norms for name agreement, familiarity and visual complexity. *J. Exp. Child Psychol.* 65, 171–237.

De Haan, E. and Campbell, R. (1991). A fifteen year follow-up of a case of developmental prosopagnosia. *Cortex* **27**, 489–509.

Druks, J. and Masterson, J. (2000). *An Object and Action Naming Battery*. Psychology Press, Hove, East Sussex.

Dunn, L.M. and Dunn, L.M. (1997). *Peabody Picture Vocabulary Test—III*. American Guidance Service, Circle Pines, Minnesota.

Dunn, L.M., Dunn, L.M., Whetton, C., and Burley, J. (1997). *The British Picture Vocabulary Scale: Second Edition—BPVS II*. NFER-Nelson, Windsor, UK.

Edwards, S., Fletcher, P., Garman, M., Hughes, A., Letts, C., and Sinka, I. (1997). *Reynell Developmental Language Scales III*. NFER-Nelson, Windsor, UK.

Elders, S. (1997). The developmental neuropsychology of attention and executive function: normal and head injured children. Unpublished PhD Thesis. University of Newcastle-upon-Tyne.

Elliott, C.D., Murray, D.J., and Pearson, L.S. (1996). *The British Ability Scales—BASII*. NFER-Nelson, Windsor, UK.

Frederickson, N., Frith, U., and Reason, R. (1997). *Phonological Assessment Battery*. NFER-Nelson, Windsor, UK.

Gaddes, W.H. and Crockett, D.J. (1975). The Spreen–Benton aphasia tests: normative data as a measure of normal language development. *Brain Language* **2**, 257–80.

Gadian, D.G., Aicardi, J., Watkins, K.E., Porter, D.A., Mishkin, M., and Vargha-Khadem, F. (2000). Developmental amnesia associated with early hypoxic-ischaemic injury. *Brain* **123**, 499–507.

Gathercole, S. and Baddeley, A. (1996). *Children's Test of Non Word Repetition*. The Psychological Corporation, London.

Goodenough, F.L. and Harris, D.B. (1963). *Goodenough–Harris Drawing Test*. The Psychological Corporation, London.

Goodglass, H. and Kaplan, E. (1972). *The assessment of aphasia and related disorders*. Lea and Fediger, London.

Halperin, J.M., Healy, J.M., Zeitschiek, E., Ludman, W.L., and Weinstein, L. (1989). Developmental aspects of linguistic and mnestic abilities in normal children. *J. Clin. Exp. Neuropsychol.* **11**, 518–28.

Hammill, D.D., Pearson, N.A., and Voress, J.K. (1995). *Developmental Test of Visual Perception: Second edition—DTUP-2*. Stoelting Company, Wood Dale, Illinois and NFER Nelson, Windsor, UK.

Heaton, R.K., Chelune, G.J., Talley, J.L., Kay, G.G., and Curtiss, G. (1993). *Wisconsin Card Sorting Test manual: revised and expanded*. Psychological Assessment Resources, Odessa, Florida.

Hickman, L. (1997). *The Apraxia Profile*. The Psychological Corporation. San Antonio, Texas.

Kaplan, E.F., Goodglass, H., and Weintraub, S. (1983). *The Boston Naming Test*, 2nd edn. Lea and Febiger, Philadelphia.

Kaufman, A.S. and Kaufman, N.L. (1983). *Kaufman Assessment battery for Children*. American Guidance Service, Circle Pines, Minnesota.

Korkman, M., Kirk, U., and Kemp, S. (1997). *NEPSY*. The Psychological Corporation, London.

Kosc, L. (1974). Developmental dyscalculia. *Journal of Learning Disabilities* **7**, 164–77.

Lass, N.J., De Paolo, A.M., Simcoe, J.C., and Samuel, S.M. (1975). A normative study of children's performance on the short form of the Token Test. *J. Commun. Dis.* **8**, 193–8.

Lewis, C., Hitch, G., and Walker, P. (1994). The prevalence of specific arithmetic difficulties and specific reading difficulties in 9- to 10-year-old boys and girls. *J. Child Psychol. Psychiatry* **35**, 283–92.

Manly, T., Robertson, I.H., Anderson, V., and Nimmo-Smith, I. (1998). *The Test of Everyday Attention for Children*. Thames Valley Test Company, Bury St Edmunds.

Mayer, M. (1969). *Frog, where are you?* Dial Books for Young Readers, New York.

McCloskey, M., Caramazza, A., and Basili, A. (1985). Cognitive mechanisms in number processing and calculation: evidence from dyscalculia. *Brain Cognition* **4**, 171–96.

Meyes, J.E. and Meyes, K.R. (1995). *Rey Complex Figure Test and Recognition Trial.* The Psychological Corporation, London.

Muter, V., Hulme, C., and Snowling, M. (2000). *Phonological Abilities Test (PAT).* The Psychological Corporation, London.

Naglieri, J.A. (1987). *Draw-a-Person.* The Psychological Corporation, London.

Neale, M. (1997). *Neale Analysis of Reading: second revised British edition.* NFER Nelson, Windsor, UK.

Ozonoff, S., Pennington, B.F., and Rogers, S.J. (1991). Executive function deficits in high-functioning autistic individuals: relationship to theory of mind. *J. Child Psychol. Psychiatry* **32**, 1081–105.

Pennington, B.F. and Ozonoff, S. (1996). Executive functions and developmental psychopathology. *J. Child Psychol. Psychiatry* **37**, 51–87.

Petrides, M. and Milner, B. (1982). Deficits on subject-ordered tasks after frontal- and temporal-lobe lesions in man. *Neuropsychologia* **20**, 249–62.

Pickering, S. and Gathercole, S. (2001). *Working Memory Test for Children (WMTB).* The Psychological Corporation, London.

Psychological Corporation (2000). *Wechsler Abbreviated Scale of Intelligence.* The Psychological Corporation, San Antonio, Texas.

Raven, J.C. (1998). *Raven's Progressive Matrices.* NFER Nelson, Windsor, UK.

Reitan, R.M. and Wolfson, D. (1985). *The Halstead–Reitan Neuropsychological Test Battery.* Neuropsychological Press, Tucson, Arizona.

Renfrew, C.E. (1977). *Word Finding Vocabulary Scale.* Speechmark Publishing Ltd, Bicester.

Renfrew, C.E. (1991). *The bus story—a test of continuous speech.* Speechmark Publishing Ltd, Bicester.

Rinaldi, W. (1996). *Understanding ambiguity: an assessment of pragmatic meaning.* NFER Nelson, Windsor, UK.

Roid, G.H. and Miller, L.J. (1996). *Leiter International Performance Scale—Revised.* Stoelting Company, Wood Dale, Illinois and NFER Nelson, Windsor, UK.

Ruff, R.M., Light, R.H., and Evans, R.W. (1987). The Ruff Figural Fluency Test: a normative study with adults. *Dev. Neuropsychol.* **3**, 37–51.

Sacre, L. and Masterson, J. (2001). *Single Word Spelling Test.* NFER Nelson, Windsor, UK.

Sattler, J.M. (2001). *Assessment of children: cognitive applications*, 4th edn. Jerome M. Sattler, Inc, San Diego, California.

Schonell, F.J. and Schonell, E.F. (1956). *Schonell reading and spelling: diagnostic and attainment testing.* Oliver and Boyd, Edinburgh.

Semel, E., Wiig, E.H., and Secord, W. (2000). *Clinical Evaluation of Language Fundamentals—3rd edition (CELF Preschool & CELF-111).* The Psychological Corporation, London.

Shallice, T. (1982). Specific impairments in planning. *Phil. Trans. R. Soc. Lond.* B **298**, 199–209.

Sheslow, D. and Adams, W. (1990). *Wide Range Assessment of Memory and Learning (WRAML).* The Psychological Corporation, London.

Shue, K.L. and Douglas, V.I. (1992). Attention deficit hyperactivity disorders and frontal lobe syndrome. *Brain Cognition* **20**, 104–24.

Snodgrass, J.G. and Vanderwart, M. (1980). A standardised set of 260 pictures: norms for name agreement, image agreement, familiarity and visual complexity. *J. Exp. Psychol.: Hum. Learning Memory* **6**, 174–215.

Snowling, M., Stothard, S., and McLean, J. (1996). *Graded Nonword Reading Test*. Thames Valley Test Company, Bury St Edmunds.

Sparrow, S.S. and Davis, S.M. (2000). Recent advances in the assessment of intelligence and cognition. *J. Child Psychol. Psychiatry* **41**, 117–31.

Spreen, O. and Strauss, E. (1998). *A compendium of neuropsychological tests*. Oxford University Press, Oxford.

Stroop, J.R. (1935). Studies of interference in serial verbal reactions. *J. Exp. Psychol.* **18**, 643–62.

Temple, C.M. (1985). Developmental surface dysgraphia a case report. *Appl. Psycholinguistics* **6**, 391–406.

Temple, C.M. (1989). Digit dyslexia: a category-specific disorder in developmental dyscalculia. *Cogn. Neuropsychol.* **6**, 93–116.

Temple, C.M. (1991). Procedural dyscalculia and number fact dyscalculia: double dissociation in developmental dyscalculia. *Cogn. Neuropsychol.* **8**, 155–76.

Temple, C.M. (1992). Developmental memory impairment: faces and patterns. In *Mental lives: case studies in cognition* (ed. R. Campbell), pp. 199–215. Blackwell, Oxford.

Temple, C.M. (1997). *Developmental cognitive neuropsychology*. Psychology Press, Hove, East Sussex.

Temple, C.M. (2002). Developmental amnesias and acquired amnesias of childhood. In *Handbook of memory disorders*, revised edn (ed. A. Baddeley, B. Wilson, and M. Kopelman), pp. 521–42. John Wiley and Sons, New York.

Temple, C.M. and Coleman, N. (2000). Children's performance on the Visual Object and Space Perception Battery (VOSP). *Clin. Neuropsychol. Assess.*, **3**, 193–208.

Temple, C.M. and Cornish, K. (1993). Recognition memory for words and faces in school children: a female advantage for words. *Br. J. Dev. Psychol.* **11**, 421–6.

Temple, C.M., Carney, R.A., and Mullarkey, S. (1996). Frontal lobe function and executive skills in children with Turner's syndrome. *Dev. Neuropsychol.* **12**, 343–64.

Waber, D.P., Isquith, P.K., and Kahn, C.N. (1994). Metacognitive factors in the visuo-spatial skills of long term survivors of acute lymphoblastic leukaemia: an experimental approach to the Rey Osterrieth complex figure test. *Dev. Neuropsychol.* **10**, 349–67.

Warrington, E.K. (1984). *Recognition Memory Battery*. NFER Nelson, Windsor, UK.

Warrington, E.K. and James, M. (1991). *The Visual Object and Space Perception Battery*. Thames Valley Test Company. Bury St Edmunds.

Wechsler, D. (1989). *Wechsler Preschool and Primary Scale of Intelligence—Revised*. The Psychological Corporation, San Antonio, Texas.

Wechsler, D. (1992). *The Wechsler Intelligence Scale for Children—III*. The Psychological Corporation, New York.

Wechsler, D. (1993). *Wechsler Objective Reading Dimensions* (WORD). The Psychological Corporation, London.

Wechsler, D. (1996). *Wechsler Objective Numerical Dimensions (WOND)*. The Psychological Corporation, London.

Welsh, M.C., Pennington, B.F., Ozonoff, S., Rouse, B., and McCabe, E.R.B. (1990). Neuropsychology of early-treated phenylketonuria: specific executive function deficits. *Child Dev.* **61**, 1697–713.

Wepman, J.M. and Reynolds, W.M. (1994). *Wepman's Auditory Discrimination*, 2nd edn. Stoelting Co., Wood Dale, Illinois.

Wiig, E.H. and Secord, W. (1992). *Test of Word Knowledge (TOWK)*. The Psychological Corporation, London.

Williams, D. and Mateer, C.A. (1992). Developmental impact of frontal lobe injury in middle childhood. *Brain Cognition* **20**, 196–204.

Wilson, B.A., Cockburn, J., and Halligan, P. (1987). *Behaviour Inattention Test.* Thames Valley Test Company, Bury St Edmonds.

Wilson, B., Ivani-Chalian, R., and Aldrich, F. (1991). *The Rivermead Behavioural Memory Test for children aged 5–10.* Thames Valley Test Company, Bury St Edmonds.

Young, A., Perrett, D., Calder, A., Sprengelmeyer, B., and Ekman, P. (2001). *Facial Expressions of Emotion: Stimuli Test.* Thames Valley Test Company, Bury St Edmonds.

Chapter 24

Treatment and rehabilitation of paediatric/developmental neuropsychological disorders

Stephen Whitfield

1 The role of the paediatric neuropsychologist

The role of the paediatric neuropsychologist differs from that of clinical neuropsychologists working with adults both in terms of: (1) the perspective adopted, i.e. that the child is a growing individual so that a developmental view must be adopted when considering the results of clinical assessment and implementing treatment programmes, and (2) the context within which treatment/rehabilitation takes place. In terms of context, the paediatric neuropsychologist is generally much more involved in multidisciplinary working with health, social services, and education personnel than would be the case when working with adults. Treatment is also frequently carried out by others and in non-health (particularly educational) environments.

In the area of intervention/treatment the paediatric neuropsychologist contributes in an advisory, monitoring, and/or therapeutic role.

- The advisory role will include educating and informing the child (where appropriate and practicable), parents, therapists, teachers, and peers of the nature of the child's condition or injury and its likely impact upon his/her development and future education/occupation.
- Monitoring will include the evaluation of any intellectual or behavioural changes brought about by a disorder or injury and its clinical (e.g. radiation treatment) or pharmacological management (e.g. antiepileptic medication side-effects).
- The therapeutic role will include the management/treatment of behaviour disorders, memory complaints, emotional and adjustment problems, etc.

The psychological approaches used will include neurobehavioural and cognitive-behavioural methods; application of psychometric, developmental, and observational assessment techniques; rehabilitation methodology; and counselling. Contexts for interventions will include all aspects of the child's environment including home, school/college (or work), and leisure situations.

2 Specific issues in paediatric treatment and rehabilitation

2.1 Neuroplasticity

For children predictive factors would be the extent of damage (the more localized the damage, the greater the chance of a plastic response) and age at time of injury. Theoretically, plastic reorganization should be more easily achieved in the younger (under 2 years) brain where less development has taken place. Animal studies have shown some evidence to support this view, but it is not supported by research with human infants. Consequently, the process is either not a spontaneous one or it has critical periods during which injury will not stimulate neuronal modification. If the latter is true, the evidence so far suggests that the least favourable time for a plastic response is probably the period from the end of gestation to the first month of life, while the most favourable period is the age band of 1 to 2 years. At present neural transplantation has no role in childhood disorders.

2.2 Localization, lateralization, and modularity

Traditional approaches to adult neuropsychological assessment have emphasized localization or lateralization of cognitive functioning. This view has never been appropriate in young children where abnormal cerebral development or acquired injury could interrupt the establishment of localized or lateralized functions.

The view of cognitive abilities that emphasizes 'modularized' skills is more appropriate to the mature brain of adults. Cognitive—developmental views see a generalized and interdependent progression in skills throughout childhood, which explains the different patterns of deficit seen in adults and children following similar insults (see Section 3). The most important aspect of the paediatric neuropsychologist's approach is to relate neuropsychological observations to the developmental stage of the child.

2.3 Recovery

In the earliest stages of recovery the regular monitoring of the extent of postinjury confusion and disorientation is essential to ensure that therapeutic interventions with cognitive requirements are matched to orientation level.

- There is no UK-derived assessment for children. One can modify the Children's Orientation and Amnesia Test (Ewing-Cobbs *et al.* 1990).
- Questions relating to orientation to person, place, and time are most commonly used, with return of orientation usually occurring in this same order.

2.4 Rehabilitation

There is no evidence that rehabilitation efforts during the early stages of recovery alter its course or that sensory stimulation reduces the depth or duration of coma. However, physical health can deteriorate without appropriate medical and nursing support during this time. Children are also prone to the development of maladaptive behaviours during this period, which require management to prevent them entering the child's behavioural repertoire. A hospital or rehabilitation setting may prevent all the above.

Rehabilitation is distinct from recovery (the spontaneous process of return of pre-injury skills) and habilitation (the passive adaptation of environments to disabilities). The aim of rehabilitation is to reduce the 'mismatch between the skills a person possesses and the actual demands of the environment' (Dixon and Bäckman 1999). Its methodology is to use 'restorative' or 'compensatory/adaptive' strategies. This distinction is of less value in children as early insult denies many early learning experiences that the 'restorative' approach would utilize in rehabilitating adults. Consequently, the 'compensatory/adaptive' approach has primacy in younger children.

Restoration focuses upon reducing disability, whereas compensation and adaptation focus upon the reduction of handicap (World Health Organization 1980). The differences in these approaches can be summarized as follows.

- Restorative approaches are based upon recovering a lost skill.
- Compensation approaches aim to revive and/or modify a latent skill or develop a new skill to substitute for the lost one.
- Adaptation focuses upon modifying environments to reduce the mismatch between skills and demands or on altering the parents', teachers', and child's expectations to meet the changed circumstances.

Restorative and compensatory approaches are appropriate to higher levels of meta-awareness; adaptation to the lowest levels. As orientation returns, the strategies used will need to be adapted to incorporate the former as well as the latter.

2.5 Adjustment

2.5.1 Adjustment to a developmental disorder

A child with a developmental disorder may have little difficulty in adjusting to the neuropsychological consequences of the disorder as he or she will have always lived with it and will not have a model of 'normality'. The difficulty lies in trying to alert others to view the world from the child's perspective. This may not only yield empathic understanding of 'oddities' in the child's behaviour, but may also be useful in generating creative behavioural management solutions.

2.5.2 Adjustment to an acquired brain injury

Conversely, a child with an acquired brain injury in the later stages of recovery may feel a sense of loss for those things that he or she was able to do prior to the injury, but cannot do postinjury. This not infrequently leads to anxiety, frustration, and depression that can manifest themselves as oppositionality and aggression. Behavioural management will not be successful without addressing the underlying emotional adjustment issues involved.

Sharing with older children and their parents the rehabilitation team's analysis of their predicament and prognosis together with their full involvement in rehabilitation programme goal-setting can, in appropriate cases, be highly efficacious in reducing these feelings and moving forward the process of adjustment. After a period in which the child and parents have largely been recipients of medical treatment, they can find this emphasis on involvement empowering. However, such an approach is dependent upon an adequate degree of self-awareness, which may not be present in the early stages of recovery, in severe attentional or executive disorders, or where the child has been left with significant generalized learning difficulties. The same criteria would apply to those children who might benefit from cognitive-behavioural therapy.

2.5.3 Adjustment for parents and families

Parental adjustment encompasses a whole range of emotions including fear, detachment, helplessness, denial, anger, anxiety, depression, and guilt. Information, though needed by parents, may not be heard or may be rejected if given at the wrong time. Anger directed at professional staff, or even the child, is evidence of poor adjustment at that time, but not necessarily of poor overall adjustment.

Families have resources that they have to allocate to deal with life events with each member contributing their share to the collective whole. Multiple demands on these resources decrease that which can be devoted to any particular situation. Continuous demands, as produced by the long-term care of a family member, deplete the resources of the entire family. The additional demands of poverty, divorce, work pressures, young children, elderly parents, etc. draw even further on these finite resources.

Parents do not experience their child as a collection of cognitive abilities, but as a functioning individual within a social and personal historical context. Adjustment will be facilitated if the paediatric neuropsychologist does not describe the child's deficits, but integrates findings into an explanation of the neurological disorder in the context of the child's world and his or her past and future.

3 Neuropsychological dysfunction

Disturbance to central nervous system (CNS) development in the prenatal period primarily results in structural abnormalities (e.g. dysplasias, spina bifida, agenesis of the corpus callosum). Postnatal interruptions affect the elaboration of connections within the brain, processes that continue into early adolescence. The nature and severity of the insult determine, as for adults, outcome in a dose-response fashion. However, in children, the developmental stage attained at the time of insult/onset interacts with the nature of the insult to produce a complex pattern of deficits, unlike the more proscribed impairments found in adults.

Childhood CNS disorders are more likely to have a generalized effect (traumatic brain injury, infections, etc.). Focal disorders (tumour, stroke) are relatively rare. Consequently, specific impairments such as apraxias and aphasias are less common, while attention, memory, and executive disorders are most prevalent (see box, p. 430).

Functional impairments associated with specific conditions

Perceptual and spatial disorders

- Turner's syndrome
  - —Impairments in visual Gestalt perception and integrative spatial construction
  - —Most significant in children with karyotype 45XO
- William's syndrome
  - —Problems with drawing, copying, and block design
  - —Attention to detail rather than overall picture

Memory disorders

- Epilepsy
  - —Memory problems primarily associated with temporal lobe epilepsy (TLE) due to close anatomical association with hippocampus
  - —Lateralized impairments to verbal and nonverbal memory associated in some studies with side of TLE focus

Language disorders

- Auditory agnosia in Landau–Kleffner syndrome
- Pragmatic disorders in autism and Asperger's syndrome

Executive disorders

- Autism
- Phenylketonuria
- Gilles de la Tourette's syndrome
- Treatment of acute lymphoblastic leukaemia
- Turner's syndrome

4 Neuropathological disorders

4.1 Acquired brain injury

The types of acquired brain injuries are summarized in the box on p. 431.

Types of acquired brain injury

Traumatic

- Road traffic accidents (RTA) result in a combination of focal and diffuse injury
- Falls
- Non-accidental injury
  - —Cause of the majority of severe head injuries in children under 1 year, 10% of injuries in the under-fives. 50% will have permanent cognitive sequelae
  - —High incidence of repeated assaults/damage
  - —Higher incidence during teenage years probably as a result of parent–child conflicts
- Projectile injury

Hypoxic–ischaemic

- Near drowning
- Neonatal hypoxia—most commonly problems with labour and delivery.
- Anaesthetic accidents
- Prolonged status epilepticus
- Cerebrovascular accidents

Other medical

- CNS infections
- Tumours and their treatment
- Acute encephalopathies
- Metabolic disorders

4.1.1 Prognosis

The extent of cognitive sequelae and subsequent prognosis for intellectual recovery are dependent upon the nature and severity of the injury and the age at time of injury.

Suitable indices of severity of injury are the depth and duration of coma and length of posttraumatic amnesia (PTA).

- *Depth of coma* is most commonly assessed by the Glasgow Coma Scale (Jennett and Teasdale, pp. 258–63) or the paediatric version (Simpson *et al.* 1991). The lower the score, the poorer the prognosis for recovery.
- *Duration of coma.* Less than 20 minutes, mild; 20 minutes to 6 hours, moderate; 6–48 hours, severe; over 48 hours, very severe.

◆ *Length of PTA*. Under 60 minutes, mild; 1–24 hours, moderate; 1–7 days, severe; 1–4 weeks, very severe; over 4 weeks, extremely severe.

PTA is more difficult to assess in children as they may become confused between actual memories and information provided by parents/visitors.

The 'nature' of the injury relates to primary brain damage (whether focal, diffuse, or both) combined with results of any secondary factors (oedema, raised intracranial pressure, hypoxic/ischaemic injury, haematoma).

Contrary to the Kennard principle (commonly interpreted as 'if you are going to have brain damage, have it early'), experimental and clinical work now indicates that injuries sustained at a young age, before the brain has had time to mature, lead to greater cognitive sequelae than those occurring in the adult years (Johnson and Rose 1996). Functional deficits may not be obvious until the area of the brain concerned begins to mature. For the prefrontal lobes this happens between about 8 and 15 years. These delayed effects are sometimes referred to as 'sleeper' phenomena.

4.1.2 Cognitive sequelae

The most common cognitive sequelae to an acquired head injury are impairments to orientation and attention, memory (in children this includes access to long-term memory, which will be less well developed than in adults), new learning, and executive skills.

4.1.3 Behavioural sequelae

These are present in 30% of children with mild to severe traumatic brain injury (TBI) and 73% of children with multiple functional impairments. They occur most commonly after frontal and temporal lobe damage. They arise in part from cognitive impairments such as poor insight into their own behaviour and poor application of environmental feedback.

Disinhibition presents severe problems of social acceptability, which can be aided by a set of rules to apply in common settings, e.g. do not shout out in class. This approach is only successful if memory skills have returned to a level that permits its retention. Behavioural contracts can be successful with less severe cases.

4.1.4 The rehabilitation of neuropsychological functions

Cognitive rehabilitation   This consists of the application of strategies (largely behavioural) to improve cognitive and affective functioning following acquired brain injury. The methodology tends to be split between direct training of cognitive processes and functional skills training. The evidence is that functionally based cognitive rehabilitation in everyday life settings is more successful than rehabilitation exercises detached from the child's normal living environment. Success appears to be independent of the particular method used.

Attention training   There is no solid research basis that proves the effectiveness of retraining approaches.

Memory rehabilitation The effectiveness of retraining has not been proven. Compensatory aids are useful in improving function. The use of external memory aids to assist recall is only successful if the child remembers that they have a problem with their memory! Without this they go unused. Thus, they are more useful for those with mild rather than severe problems. The use of aids has to be built up with frequent reminders in 'real-life' situations. Similar considerations apply to the use of internal (verbal mnemonics) aids.

As procedural memory is frequently retained when explicit memory is impaired, this is often incorporated into compensatory strategies, e.g. inclusion of pre-injury procedural learning into new behaviours that are repeatedly practised using errorless learning approaches.

Rehabilitation of executive functions There has been some success in training for specific tasks, e.g. self-organization skills. Compensatory aids, e.g. diaries, electronic organizers, copies of school timetables, home–school books, picture sequences, etc., completed under guidance can be useful in training these skills. However, only limited generalization is seen in the training of problem-solving skills.

4.1.5 Neurobehavioural management

On emergence from coma, restlessness, wandering, and destructiveness occur. Acute phase problems with behaviour usually resolve with reduction in PTA. However, environmental control is important with avoidance of high-level stimulation, minimalization of staff changes, uncluttered treatment areas, acoustically quiet environments, etc.

In the early post-acute phase, whilst orientation is poor, memory is thrown back upon procedural learning rather than the more explicit systems. If not prevented, errors become established that are not open to correction using cognitively based interventions. In particular, this makes the child prone to the development of maladaptive behaviours and requires preventive management emphasizing errorless learning approaches. This stage may continue for months if the child's recovery is slow.

While cognitive difficulties persist (orientation, attention, and memory in particular), the use of contingency management will prove less effective than antecedent control techniques in the treatment of behavioural excess or deficit.

Focal impairments to the frontal lobes in the teenage years generally lead to one of two behavioural phenotypes manifesting as:

- irritability, anxiety, obsessionality, false euphoria, over sexualized behaviour, poor social responses, increased risk-taking behaviour (though unimpaired social or moral reasoning), and poor self-monitoring. The fundamental problem appears to be one of failure to inhibit responses.

- apathy, poor initiation, failure to maintain activity, and pseudo-depression.

Both groups benefit from a structured approach with a regular timetable, clear rules, and contingencies. Behavioural approaches are helpful. Management based upon reasoning, dependent as it is upon the ability to self-reflect, is seldom effective. It is preferable to create overlearned responses to simple everyday situations that utilize the tendency towards stimulus-driven behaviour. This approach is of proven effectiveness. Such an approach will allow basic anger management techniques to be trained with well-oriented children.

The psychosocial environment of the child during recovery is an important additional source of behavioural difficulties. Parental reactions to the child's injury may lead to overprotection, overindulgence, loss of confidence, guilt, anger, stress, anxiety or depression, all of which can have an effect upon behaviour. Social factors of peer rejection, loss of status (academic or sporting), and social isolation may add to this.

Neuropsychiatric disorders appearing after TBI include the following.

◆ *Disorders of thought and perception.* Their manifestations are aggression, agitation, conduct disorders, or disinhibition. Their neuropathology is still unclear. Paediatric neuropsychiatric evaluation is required.

◆ *Disorders of mood and affect.* The head-injured child is vulnerable to emotional and psychiatric disorders (double the vulnerability of peers at 2 years post-injury) emerging as lowered self-esteem and depression linked to poor adaptive skills. Daily variation is common and can be investigated by a paediatric neuropsychologist through standard behavioural recording. However, one should be aware that problems might arise from cyclical neuropsychiatric disturbance as well as environmental stimuli or contingencies.

4.1.6 Rehabilitation settings

The majority of children with an acquired brain injury will have early post-acute rehabilitation provided within their local community following discharge from hospital. A planning conference to coordinate professional inputs and resources will generally take place within 1 or 2 weeks of discharge. A key worker is generally identified to act as a case manager, though this should not be confused with head injury case management services, usually appointed following the settlement of a claim for compensation. Though postacute head injury teams exist in some health authorities, they seldom consist of staff dedicated to this role. In consequence, the head-injured child has to compete for resources with other children. Alternatively, some areas will use staff from adult head injury services to provide services. This is problematic in that staff may have little experience or knowledge of childhood disorders, child development, or paediatric interventions.

A small number of children, usually with more severe and complex needs, will be catered for within specialist paediatric head injury facilities.

The role of the paediatric neuropsychologist in rehabilitation is to provide a framework within which other therapeutic interventions may take place. He or she should ensure that the cognitive demands placed upon the child are within their present level of cognitive functioning, while bearing in mind that this will alter as the process of recovery takes place.

4.1.7 Education

Unlike adults who may become unemployed following head injury, there is a statutory duty to educate all children whatever their degree of disability. This means that the educational system has a central role to play in the rehabilitation of head-injured children, as schools will be the principal environments to which the children will return. Advice given to teachers should be precisely geared to the individual child rather than general based upon a particular syndrome or condition. The latter will reflect too great a variability across children to allow the teacher to formulate specific educational programmes for the child.

Unfortunately, few local education authorities have specific policies on providing for the educational needs of brain-injured children. The situation in the UK has several disadvantages.

◆   The system established in England and Wales (with minor variations in Scotland and Northern Ireland) for the drawing up of statements of special educational needs embodies a view of static educational needs. This model is unsuited to the situation of head-injured children who have (at least during the early postacute phase and not uncommonly during later 'spurts' in recovery) frequently changing needs. Though the review system for such statements can be utilized to accommodate changes, the time period for implementing changes can be protracted.

◆   There is a danger that the recovering child will have a placement suited to their apparent level of cognitive functioning at the time of assessment, but increasingly inappropriate as recovery takes place.

◆   If physical needs are significant, placements may be offered based on the location of resources such as physio- and occupational therapy, nursing, etc., rather than based upon the appropriateness of educational environment.

The paediatric neuropsychologist must have a role as an advocate for the child in seeking appropriate provision.

4.1.8 Family needs

The early stages of postacute recovery are important ones in beginning the process of adjustment to the changed circumstances of the child. Adjustment is an essential step to the success of rehabilitation.

◆   Parents may become 'stuck' and become focused upon the physical aspects of recovery (will she be able to walk?) when cognitive recovery may be the more important determinant of successful rehabilitation.

◆   Information is critical to parental adjustment and the paediatric neuropsychologist is best placed within a multidisciplinary team to objectively outline (after comprehensive assessment) what has happened to their child's brain and what the cognitive prognosis is likely to be.

- The paediatric neuropsychologist has an importance similar to that of other key figures in the child's world, e.g. teachers, classmates, friends on the social side, social workers, educational psychologists, and solicitors.
- Siblings frequently get left out whilst the focus is on the injured child. They too will suffer shock and sometimes guilt at their resentment of the attention being given to their brother or sister. Embarrassment at the reaction of friends can lead to anger and frustration. Counselling and play therapy can assist adjustment.

4.2 Brain tumours

Sixty per cent are astrocytomas or gliomas; 20–25% primitive neuroectodermal tumours. Neuropsychological sequelae include problems with:

- fine-motor coordination;
- perceptual–motor skills;
- visual constructional abilities;
- memory.

In turn these lead to decrements in IQ. The functional consequences are in academic and vocational skills. Memory problems can affect daily living and self-care.

However, these sequelae seem principally to be a consequence of radio- and, to a lesser degree, chemotherapy treatments, not of surgery. Age at diagnosis and treatment and the type and location of the tumour are also important factors in long-term outcome. Academic difficulties should be anticipated and teachers informed in order to adjust expectations in the classroom. Neuropsychologists have a role as information providers and interpreters and in the monitoring of post-treatment changes.

4.3 Epilepsy

The distribution of IQ in children with epilepsy is close to that of the general population. However, some epilepsy syndromes are associated with specific cognitive sequelae.

- Moderate to severe learning difficulties are observed in the majority of children with Lennox–Gastaut and West's syndrome.
- There are many other abnormalities of brain development or acquired disorders that include epilepsy in their symptomatology. These would include: developmental disorders, e.g. tuberous sclerosis and Angelman syndrome; CNS infections; acquired brain injuries; metabolic disorders; Rett syndrome; and neurofibromatosis.
- Epilepsy is a co-symptom of severe learning difficulties (9–31%), autism (11–35%), and cerebral palsy (18–35%).

Other factors associated with cognitive or functional problems in epilepsy are the following.

- Intellectual decline in epilepsy (not associated with other underlying conditions) is usually associated with antiepileptic drug (AED) toxicity.

- A history of status epilepticus is associated with decreased functioning.
- Children with early onset to their seizure disorder, poor response to anticonvulsant medication, and mixed seizure types tend to perform more poorly on IQ measures. However, these factors could disguise a common factor in the existence of pre-existing neurological impairments prior to seizure onset.
- Specific impairments likely to be associated with epilepsy are poor sustained attention and reduced short-term memory performance. A confounding factor again is AED toxicity.
- Subclinical electrical activity of even brief duration can produce educational difficulties referred to as transitory cognitive impairments (TCI). The mediating factor here is most probably disruption to attention.
- Some studies suggest that left temporal lobe epilepsy is associated with decreased performance on verbal memory tasks and right temporal lobe epilepsy related to reduced visual memory function. Others suggest bilateral memory impairments.
- Hippocampal damage from frequent seizures is associated with decreased new learning.

Despite a near-normal distribution in IQ, children with epilepsy are more at risk of educational underachievement. This is not yet understood, but is *not* associated with seizure type, duration, severity, or AED used in treatment. Self-esteem and emotional variables such as locus of control appear important.

Behavioural and psychiatric problems are also more prevalent in children with epilepsy. There is no specific symptomatology. Difficulties arise from a combination of neurological (brain damage, seizure activity in areas of brain associated with affective functioning, variations in neurotransmitter function) and psychosocial factors (lowered self-esteem, externalized locus of control, stigmatization, lowered expectations, reactions to parental overprotection, and lack of independence). The degree of neuropsychological dysfunction predicts behavioural and neuropsychiatric dysfunction, i.e. brain dysfunction not epilepsy is causative. AED treatment is also a factor with phenobarbitone associated with the most difficulties and carbamazepine and sodium valproate with the least, but dosage and multiple drug therapy are also important factors. It is important to include assessment and treatment of affective and behavioural functioning in management.

The paediatric neuropsychologist's role is as part of a multidisciplinary approach addressing medical treatment, educational management, and emotional and social adjustment—specifically, the monitoring of cognitive and behavioural change and the provision of information and management advice to the child, his/her parents, and teachers.

4.4 **Hydrocephalus**

Hydrocephalus is a secondary condition arising from a number of primary disorders. It is the primary disorder that is the dominant factor in outcome. It is associated in all aetiological groups with:

- gross and fine motor problems and visuomotor and spatial difficulties;
- greater impairment to language content than to structure (particularly in children with shunts);
- list-learning problems—results in regard to other aspects of memory are unclear other than that children with shunted hydrocephalus perform more poorly than other groups.
- problems with focused attention;
- deficits in executive skills where children with shunted hydrocephalus require an increased number of trials to reach the correct answers in problem-solving tasks;
- behavioural difficulties—children with shunted hydrocephalus have higher rates of behaviour disorder than those without.

Functional difficulties are apparent in school work (associated with visuospatial, executive, and learning problems) and everyday living (language, attention, and behaviour) The paediatric neuropsychologist's role is in the interpretation of cognitive and behavioural findings and in the provision of information and management advice appropriate to the needs of the referred child.

4.5 Meningitis

This is an infectious disease involving inflammation of the meningeal membrane with either a viral or bacterial cause. The latter is more likely to lead to disability. Of children with early childhood bacterial meningitis, 40% suffer additional acute neurological problems (sensory impairments, hydrocephalus, seizures, etc.), but only 20% of those who survive have persistent difficulties. In addition, many have cognitive, behavioural, and educational sequelae. The pattern of these is diverse covering motor, perceptual, language, attentional, and executive skills. Overall IQ is probably little affected.

The pattern and extent of deficits is thought to be dependent upon the age at the time of infection, time since insult, and developmental stage at time of assessment.

- Age at the time of infection is significant in that that pre-infection learning is retained, but new learning is significantly impaired.
- During the time following the insult compensation may have taken place, which will in turn influence the deficit observed.
- The developmental stage at time of assessment determines the expectations of the child's abilities at that stage and thus helps determine the extent of the deficits.

Initially, gross motor problems dominate; subsequently fine motor problems. Perceptual and language difficulties occur during the primary years, while, in the secondary phase, impairments to higher-order language and executive skills are most frequently reported.

Once again, the picture is of a multifactorial processes affecting outcome with psychosocial and environmental issues important contributory factors. This would suggest

that rehabilitative efforts could have significant benefits in this condition. The paediatric neuropsychologist's role is to inform parents and educators of the implications of observed deficits and to formulate suitable management approaches to behaviour and adaptive learning. The changing pattern of deficits suggests the need for neuropsychological oversight throughout childhood.

4.6 Metabolic and neurodegenerative disorders

These disorders arise from built-in errors of metabolism leading to a build-up of neurotoxins and consequent neurodegeneration. Cognitive deterioration is often difficult to detect in children due to the active interaction between normal development and the degenerative process. The earlier the onset, the more difficult this becomes with the lack of a clear premorbid period of 'normal' development. Decline in IQ can be misleading as it may represent a failure to maintain a rate of intellectual growth in keeping with one's peers, a period of 'plateaued development', or a 'real' loss of skills.

Initial identification of any decline should be by developmental history taking and educational reports (nursery, primary, and secondary) combined with cognitive assessment. Monitoring should be by periodic assessments combined with educational reports specifically asking if the child is keeping up with peers or has lost skills.

- Lost skills should be identified to ensure that their absence is not solely situation-specific or that they have not been subsumed into more complex behaviours.

- Educationalists may fear that a child is declining when they may simply not be keeping up with their peers—thus there is no absolute decline, only a relative one. Comparison of raw scores rather than scaled scores on normative tests will reveal the true state of affairs.

The pattern of decline observed is dependent on the periods between assessments. The shorter the period, the more obvious the continuing development of the child alongside the degenerative process. Longer periods give greater emphasis to the decline.

Childhood neurodegenerative diseases largely affect white rather than grey matter and consequently are enhanced by the factor of age at onset as it relates to the degree of both myelination and intellectual development that has already taken place. The specific neuropsychological and consequent functional sequelae of these multitudinous disorders are dependent upon the precise condition (see Shapiro and Balthazor 2000).

The paediatric neuropsychologist has a central role in the interpretation of this information, the provision of feedback to medical colleagues, and the support of parents and teachers coming to terms with a progressive intellectual decline in childhood.

4.7 Neurofibromatosis

Type one neurofibromatosis has known cognitive and behavioural sequelae; type two does not. The sequelae associated with type one are as follows.

- Mean IQ is lowered and mild-to-moderate learning difficulties are slightly more common than in the general population. About half of patients have reduced academic attainments.

- The range of neuropsychological impairments observed in different individuals includes attention deficits, speech and language difficulties, difficulties in visuospatial processing, and motor coordination problems. There is no specific neuropsychological profile.

- The increased presence of tumours (15–50% of cases) and their treatment may lead to further cognitive sequelae.

Educational provision should be matched to the individual's difficulties. There are no specialist approaches specific to neurofibromatosis type one or two. The extent of emotional problems appears to be related to the degree of physical disfigurement. Behavioural difficulties centre around attention deficits, hyperactivity, impulsivity, and distractability.

5 Neurodevelopmental disorders

5.1 Attention deficit hyperactivity disorders (ADHDs)

These are characterized by a triad of inattention, overactivity, and impulsivity. They can occur with or without 'hard' neurological signs. Symptoms persist into adolescence in two out of three cases. The problems associated with ADHD include:

- poor educational attainments;
- peer/friendship difficulties;
- conflict with parents;
- (in adolescence) engagement in high-risk behaviours—one in three has conduct disorder in adolescence.

These problems can result in reduced self-esteem and sometimes depression. The prognosis is poorer in the presence of a comorbid conduct disorder.

In carefully selected children stimulant medication can show significant benefits on attentional tasks and in everyday functioning. A multiple treatment approach would include:

- information provision;
- use of stimulant medication;
- family and school management advice;
- self-instructional training;
- (in some cases) dietary monitoring.

This approach improves long-term treatment efficacy.

The child clinical or paediatric neuropsychologist's role is the following.

- Diagnosis of children with the disorder. In particular, diagnosis must be based on the persistence of symptoms across settings. ADHDs are usually identified through

use of structured questionnaires such as the Achenbach Child Behaviour Checklists (Achenbach 1991).

◆ On-going monitoring of cognitive and behavioural changes using measures of focused and sustained attention and behavioural observation schedules such as those by Conners (1996).

◆ Provision of information, behavioural management advice, and self-control training to be used as adjunctive therapy with medication.

5.2 Specific learning difficulties (SpLDs)

This term is applied by educators to a number of 'disorders' (reading, writing, arithmetic, and spelling) having some similarities in symptomatology to conditions seen in persons with an acquired brain injury. The nature of the underlying pathologies and their relationships to observed neuropsychological impairments continue to be investigated (Hynd and Hiemenz 1997), but these are considered to be 'necessary, but not sufficient' elements for the manifestation of the condition with significant contributions from environmental and pedagogical factors.

There is a range of proven educational approaches in use by specialist teachers working in this field selected according to a child's particular pattern of strengths and weaknesses. The paediatric neuropsychologist would be best advised to seek referral to such local services.

5.3 Nonverbal learning disability (NVLD)

NVLD is a postulated condition of multiple aetiology including neuropathological disorders. Its characteristics are:

◆ bilateral tactile–perceptual difficulties particularly affecting the left side;

◆ impaired visual recognition and discrimination;

◆ problems with visuospatial organization;

◆ bilateral psychomotor coordination difficulties, again more marked on the left side;

◆ problems with managing novel information.

Auditory–verbal processing is preserved as are simple motor skills, auditory perception, rote learning, selective and sustained attention for auditory–verbal information, basic expressive and receptive language, reading, and spelling. Rourke (1989) outlines a wide range of secondary and tertiary neuropsychological, academic, and socioemotional deficits arising from NVLD.

The model is specifically a cognitive–developmental one linking neurological impairment to neuropsychological deficit by way of the 'white-matter hypothesis' that emphasizes the need for integrity of white matter function for normal child development. Rourke reasons that in the right hemisphere white matter is important for development and maintenance of function; in the left hemisphere it is only important for

development. Consequently, the right hemisphere is seen as particularly reliant upon cerebral integrity in order to continue functioning effectively. As one would expect from a cognitive–developmental model, the implication is that the degree of white matter damage, the nature of the lesion, and the developmental stage at the time of cerebral insult determine symptom severity.

There is no proven treatment for the condition. Management is through utilization of language-based strengths at home and in school. Visually based information needs to be supported with verbal description. Large tasks need to be broken down into smaller, more easily assimilated steps. Abstract material requires discussion and verbal labelling of concepts. There is limited evaluation of the success of such interventions.

Selective References

Achenbach, T. (1991). *Integrative guide for the 1991 Child Behaviour Checklist/4–18, YSR and TRF profiles.* University of Vermont Department of Psychiatry, Burlington, Vermont.

Anderson, V., Northam, E., Hendy, J., and Wrennall, J. (2001). *Developmental neuropsychology: a clinical approach.* Psychology Press, Hove, East Sussex.

Conners, C. (1996). *Conners Abbreviated Symptom Questionnaire.* Psychological Assessment Resources, Odessa, Florida.

Dixon, R.A. and Bäckman, L. (1999). Principles of compensation in neurorehabilitation. In *Cognitive rehabilitation* (ed. D.T. Stuss, G. Winocur, and I.H. Robertson), pp. 59–72. Cambridge University Press, Cambridge.

Ewing-Cobbs, L., Levin, H.S., Fletcher, J.M., Miner, M.E., and Eisenberg, H.M. (1990). The Children's Orientation and Amnesia Test: relationship to severity of acute head injury and to recovery of memory. *Neurosurgery* 27, 683–91.

Hynd, G.W. and Hiemenz, J.R. (1997). Dyslexia and gyral morphology variation. In *Dyslexia: biology, cognition and intervention* (ed. C. Hulme and M. Snowling), pp. 38–58. Whurr Publishers Ltd, London.

Jennett, B. and Teasdale, G. (1981). *The management of head injuries.* F.A.Davis and Co., Philadelphia.

Johnson, D. and Rose, D. (1996). *Brain injury in childhood—is younger better?*, Disability Awareness No. 13. Disability Management Research Group, Astley Ainslie Hospital, Edinburgh.

Rourke, B.P. (1989). *Nonverbal learning disabilities.* Guilford Press, New York.

Shapiro, E. and Balthazor, M. (2000). Metabolic and neurodegenerative disorders. In *Pediatric neuropsychology: research, theory and practice* (ed. K.O. Yeates, M.D. Ris, and H.G. Taylor), pp. 171–205. Guilford Press, New York.

Simpson, D.A., Cockington, R.A., Hanieh, A., Raftos, J., and Reilly, P.L. (1991). Head injuries in infants and young children: the value of a paediatric coma scale. *Child's Nerv. Syst.* 7, 183–90.

Temple. C. (1997). *Developmental Cognitive Neuropsychology.* Psychology Press, Hove, East Sussex.

World Health Organisation (WHO) (1980). International classification of impairments, disabilities and handicaps. WHO, Geneva.

Yeates, K.O., Ris, M.D., and Taylor H.G. (eds.) (2000). *Pediatric neuropsychology: research, theory and practice.* Guilford Press, New York.

Part 5

Neuropsychopharmacology

Chapter 25

Neuropsychopharmacology

C.M. Bradshaw

1 Introduction

An understanding of the principles of neuropsychopharmacology is important for the practising clinical neuropsychologist because a large proportion of neurological and psychiatric patients receive medication that can affect higher functions, both for good and for ill.

Improved understanding of the cellular mechanisms underlying the therapeutic and adverse effects of psychoactive drugs has shed considerable light on the neural bases of normal and abnormal neuropsychological function. As yet, however, there are no validated pharmacological treatments for specific neuropsychological dysfunctions (dysmnesias, dysphasias, etc.). Rational pharmacotherapy (i.e. treatment based on the actions of drugs on known pathological processes) exists for some neurological conditions (e.g. Parkinson's disease, some forms of epilepsy), but the utility of nearly all the drugs presently used to treat 'functional' psychiatric disorders has been discovered by fortuitous clinical observation.

Establishing the efficacy of drug treatment in psychiatry poses significant problems due to the complex and variable symptomatology and time-courses of the disorders, imperfect measuring instruments, and the frequently weak effects of the drugs in question, which are often confounded by side-effects (see Section 4). For the design of controlled clinical trials, their advantages, and pitfalls, see Harrison-Read and Tyrer (1995).

2 Synaptic transmission in the central nervous system (CNS)

2.1 General principles

Chemical synaptic transmission involves the following steps.

- *Precursor accumulation.* Precursors of transmitters are often amino acids that are present in the circulating blood. They are actively transported into neurons by a membrane 'pump'.

- *Transmitter synthesis.* Precursor molecules are converted into transmitter molecules by a sequence of enzyme-catalysed reactions.

- *Storage.* Transmitter molecules may be retained within vesicles in presynaptic terminals by a membrane 'pump'.

- *Release.* Ejection of transmitter molecules from the presynaptic terminal is triggered by the passage of an action potential down the axon, causing depolarization of the terminal membrane. Channels in the terminal membrane are opened, permitting influx of calcium ions, which cause the vesicles to discharge their contents into the synaptic cleft.

- *Receptor stimulation.* The binding of a transmitter molecule to a receptor initiates a sequence of events, culminating in a change in the electrical excitability of the postsynaptic cell.

- *Inactivation.* Transmitter molecules may be removed from the synapse by the action of enzymes on pre- and postsynaptic membranes, or by transport into presynaptic terminals (re-uptake). After re-uptake, transmitter molecules may be re-stored in vesicles or destroyed by enzymes.

2.2 Neurotransmitters and neuromodulators

2.2.1 Glutamate

Glutamate is an amino acid that mediates excitatory transmission in many central pathways. Corticofugal glutamatergic neurons are believed to play a key role in cognitive functions subserved by 'corticostriatal loops'. Excessive release of glutamate may cause overexcitation of postsynaptic neurons, which may die as a consequence (*excitotoxicity*). This may account for neuronal loss in the area surrounding a cerebral infarct, and also for neuronal loss in convulsive seizure disorders.

2.2.2 γ-Aminobutyric acid

γ-Aminobutyric acid (GABA) is the principal inhibitory amino-acid transmitter in supraspinal pathways, e.g. inhibitory efferent pathways from the basal ganglia and the cerebellar cortex. GABA also mediates the inhibitory effects of intracortical neurons. Suppression of GABAergic transmission can lead to convulsions.

2.2.3 Acetylcholine

Acetylcholine is the transmitter at skeletal neuromuscular junctions, parasympathetic (and some sympathetic) effector junctions, and all autonomic ganglia. It mediates both excitatory and inhibitory effects in the CNS. It is synthesized from choline by the action of choline acetyltransferase. Synaptically released acetylcholine is metabolized by acetylcholinesterase located on pre- and postsynaptic membranes. Cholinergic neurons arising in the basal forebrain project to the hippocampus and neocortex. Degeneration of these neurons is thought to underlie some of the cognitive deficits of Alzheimer's disease.

2.2.4 Dopamine

Dopamine is a catecholamine synthesized from the amino acid tyrosine. Tyrosine hydroxylase converts tyrosine to L-dopa, which is converted to dopamine by L-aromatic

amino-acid decarboxylase. Synaptically released dopamine is inactivated by re-uptake into presynaptic terminals followed by re-storage or degradation by monoamine oxidase (MAO). The cell bodies of dopaminergic neurons reside in circumscribed nuclei in the brainstem, their unmyelinated axons projecting to many parts of the neuraxis. The three principal dopaminergic pathways are:

◆ the *nigrostriatal pathway* (substantia nigra → corpus striatum), whose degeneration underlies the pathophysiology of Parkinson's disease;

◆ the *mesolimbic/mesocortical pathway* (midbrain ventral tegmental area → limbic structures and cerebral cortex), whose hyperfunction has been postulated to occur in schizophrenia;

◆ the *tuberoinfundibular pathway* (hypothalamus → pituitary stalk), which regulates the secretion of some adenohypophyseal hormones.

2.2.5 Noradrenaline (norepinephrine)

Noradrenaline is a catecholamine that is synthesized from tyrosine via the intermediate compounds L-dopa and dopamine. Synaptically released noradrenaline is inactivated by re-uptake into terminals followed by re-storage or degradation by MAO. Noradrenaline is the transmitter at most sympathetic effector junctions. The cell bodies of central noradrenergic neurons reside in nuclei in the pons and medulla, their axons projecting to most parts of the neuraxis. Noradrenergic pathways include:

◆ *dorsal noradrenergic bundle* (ceruleocortical pathway: locus ceruleus → neocortex and hippocampus);

◆ *ventral noradrenergic bundle* (tegmental nuclei → hypothalamus);

◆ *descending noradrenergic pathways* (tegmental nuclei → spinal cord and medullary autonomic nuclei).

Central noradrenergic transmission may contribute to the 'fine tuning' of some higher functions (e.g. improving signal/noise ratio in some sensory pathways) and the maintenance of arousal. Central noradrenergic hypofunction may be a contributory factor in depressive illness, while noradrenergic hyperfunction may be involved in some anxiety states.

2.2.6 5-Hydroxytryptamine (5-HT, serotonin)

5-HT is an indoleamine synthesized from tryptophan via the intermediate precursor 5-hydroxytryptophan. Synaptically released 5-HT is inactivated by re-uptake into terminals followed by re-storage or degradation by MAO. The cell bodies of 5-HTergic neurons reside in the raphe nuclei of the brainstem, their axons projecting to most parts of the neuraxis. 5-HTergic pathways include:

◆ ascending pathways from the dorsal and median raphe nuclei;

◆ descending raphe–spinal pathways.

The projections from the dorsal and median raphe nuclei show considerable overlap. However the median nucleus provides most of the 5-HTergic afferents to the hippocampus, while the dorsal nucleus provides most of the input to the striatum. 5-HTergic dysfunction has been proposed as a pathophysiological factor in depressive illness, obsessive–compulsive disorder, and anxiety disorders. There is evidence for 5-HTergic hypofunction in impulse-control disorders.

2.2.7 Neuropeptides

Neuropeptides are large molecules, made up of sequences of amino acids. Many 'families' of neuropeptide have been identified (e.g. hypothalamic hormone-releasing and release-inhibiting factors, tachykinins, opioid peptides). They are generally *co-localized* with 'classical' neurotransmitters, and act at specific receptors on pre- and postsynaptic membranes. One of the postulated roles of neuropeptides is to modulate the action of co-localized 'classical' transmitters. Neuropeptides have been implicated in pain transmission (substance P), anxiety (cholecystokinin), and the rewarding effects of drugs of abuse (enkephalin) (Hökfelt *et al.* 2000).

2.3 Receptors

There are two main receptor 'superfamilies', distinguished by the effector mechanisms to which they are coupled:

- *ionotropic (ion-channel-coupled) receptors*, in which the transmitter (or drug) molecule binds directly to a site on an ion channel and thereby regulates the movement of ions in or out of the postsynaptic cell;
- *metabotropic (G-protein-coupled) receptors*, in which binding of the transmitter or drug molecule to the receptor initiates a cascade of events within the postsynaptic cell, culminating in a change in the permeability of the membrane to particular ionic species.

Ionotropic receptors mediate rapid changes in electrical excitability, whereas metabotropic receptors mediate slower responses. In the case of metabotropic receptors, attachment of the transmitter molecule to the binding site alters the state of a protein in the postsynaptic membrane ('G-protein'), which in turn alters the activity of an enzyme. Two principal enzymes are associated with metabotropic receptors:

- adenylyl cyclase, which converts adenosine 5′-triphosphate (ATP) to cyclic adenosine 5′-phosphate (AMP);
- phospholipase-C, which converts phosphatidylinositol to inositol trisphosphate and diacylglycerol.

The products of these reactions are *second messengers* (in distinction from the neurotransmitter, the 'first messenger'); they activate a protein kinase that regulates ion channel opening. A transmitter may act at many types of receptor coupled to different effector mechanisms, giving scope for great variety of postsynaptic effects (Table 25.1).

Table 25.1 The major CNS neurotransmitters and some of their receptors*

Receptor[†]	Type[‡]	Effector[§]	Function
Glutamate			
AMPA	IR	Na^+/K^+ channels	Postsynaptic excitation
Kainate	IR	Na^+/K^+ channels	Postsynaptic excitation
NMDA	IR	$Ca^{2+}/Na^+/K^+$ channels	Postsynaptic excitation
mGlu group I	MR	PL (↑)	Postsynaptic excitation
mGlu groups II, III	MR	AC (↓)	Postsynaptic excitation
γ-aminobutyric acid (GABA)			
$GABA_A$	IR	Cl^- channel	Postsynaptic inhibition
$GABA_B$	MR	?	Postsynaptic inhibition
Acetylcholine			
Nicotinic	IR	$Ca^{2+}/Na^+/K^+$ channels	Postsynaptic excitation
Muscarinic M_1	MR	PL (↑)	Postsynaptic excitation
Muscarinic M_2	MR	AC (↓)	Postsynaptic excitation/inhibition (?)
Muscarinic M_3	MR	PL (↑)	Postsynaptic excitation
Muscarinic M_4	MR	AC (↓)	Postsynaptic excitation/inhibition (?)
Dopamine			
D_1	MR	AC (↑)	Postsynaptic inhibition (?)
D_2	MR	AC (↓)	Postsynaptic excitation/inhibition (?) somatodendritic autoreceptor
D_3	MR	?	Postsynaptic excitation/inhibition (?) somatodendritic autoreceptor
D_4	MR	?	Postsynaptic excitation/inhibition (?)
Noradrenaline (norepinephrine)			
α_1-adrenoceptor	MR	PL (↑)	Postsynaptic excitation
α_2-adrenoceptor	MR	AC (↓), K^+/Ca^{2+} channels	Somatodendritic autoreceptor, terminal autoreceptor, postsynaptic excitation (?)
β_1-adrenoceptor	MR	AC (↑)	Postsynaptic inhibition
β_2-adrenoceptor	MR	AC (↑)	Non-neuronal (glial, vascular) responses
5-hydroxytryptamine (5-HT; serotonin)			
$5\text{-}HT_{1A}$	MR	AC (↓)	Somatodendritic autoreceptor, postsynaptic inhibition (?)
$5\text{-}HT_{1B/D}$	MR	AC (↓)	Terminal autoreceptor, postsynaptic inhibition (?)
$5\text{-}HT_{2A}$	MR	PL (↑)	Postsynaptic excitation/inhibition (?)

Table 25.1 (*Continued*)

Receptor†	Type‡	Effector§	Function
5-HT$_{2C}$	MR	PL (↑)	Postsynaptic excitation/inhibition (?)
5-HT$_3$	IR	Na$^+$/K$^+$ channels	Postsynaptic excitation
5-HT$_4$	MR	AC (↑)	Postsynaptic excitation/inhibition (?)
5-HT$_5$, 5-HT$_6$	MR	AC (↓) ?	?
5-HT$_7$	MR	AC (↑)	?

* Note that the list is not exhaustive, and that the functions mediated by many of the receptors are poorly understood.

† AMPA, DL-α-amino-3-hydroxy-5-methyl-isoxazole proprionate; NMDA, *N*-methyl-D-aspartate.

‡ IR, ionotropic receptor; MR, metabotropic receptor.

§ AC, adenylyl cyclase system; PL, phospholipase-C system. ↑ and ↓ indicate stimulation and inhibition, respectively.

Transmitters and drugs that stimulate receptors and evoke physiological responses are *agonists*. *Antagonists* evoke no response of their own but prevent the action of agonists.

2.4 Regulation of neurotransmitter function

Many neurons regulate their own function via *autoreceptors* (receptors on the membrane of a neuron that respond to that neuron's own transmitter). *Somatodendritic autoreceptors* reside on the cell body and dendrites and *terminal autoreceptors* on the presynaptic terminals. Autoreceptors usually serve a negative feedback role, receptor stimulation resulting in suppression of neuronal activity.

Neurotransmitter function is also regulated by *receptor adaptation*. Excessive receptor stimulation leads to a decrease in the number of available receptors (downregulation), with a consequent loss of sensitivity to the transmitter and other agonists (desensitization). Conversely, low levels of receptor stimulation (e.g. following atrophy of afferent fibres) result in homeostatic receptor proliferation (upregulation), with consequent enhancement of sensitivity.

3 Pharmacokinetic principles

The magnitude of a drug's effect is related to its concentration at its site of action. For centrally acting drugs, this is not directly measurable, and plasma concentration provides the only practical measure of tissue concentration. This is satisfactory for drugs that gain easy access to the brain. However, many drugs enter the brain with difficulty, because of the blood–brain barrier (see Section 3.4).

3.1 Absorption, distribution, and elimination

The single-dose kinetics of a drug describe the rise in plasma concentration as the drug is absorbed into the circulation, and the subsequent fall in concentration as the drug is

distributed to the tissues and eliminated by metabolism and/or excretion (Fig. 25.1(a)). The rate of elimination of a drug relative to its concentration in the plasma is known as *clearance*. The clearance of most drugs is fairly constant over a wide range of concentrations; i.e. a constant fraction of the total amount of drug present in the plasma is eliminated per unit time (*first-order kinetics*). The *plasma half-life* ($t_{1/2}$) is the time taken for the plasma concentration to fall by 50%. Active metabolism of a drug may result in a short $t_{1/2}$. However, this does not necessarily imply a short duration of

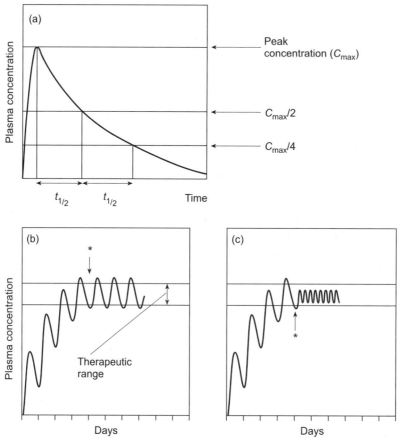

Fig. 25.1 (a) Single-dose kinetics. Ordinate, plasma concentration of the drug; abscissa, time measured from the time of administration. Note that plasma concentration falls to half its peak concentration in one half-life ($t_{1/2}$). A further half-life results in a further halving of the plasma concentration. (b) Change in plasma concentration following repeated dosing at intervals of approximately $t_{1/2}$. Steady-state mean plasma concentration is attained after approximately 4 half-lives (arrow at *). Note that the peaks and troughs of the steady-state concentration may fall outside the therapeutic range. (c) Administration of smaller doses more frequently (indicated by the arrow at *) results in smaller fluctuations in plasma concentration (see text for details).

action, e.g. the benzodiazepine flurazepam has a $t_{1/2}$ of about 2 hours but its effects are prolonged due to the production of an active metabolite, desalkylflurazepam, whose $t_{1/2}$ is 30–100 hours.

The rate of absorption is influenced by the route of administration. The most common routes are:

♦ *intravenous* (IV) infusion, which results in a very rapid rise in concentration because the obstacles to absorption posed by lipid membranes in the gut and the capillaries are bypassed;

♦ *intramuscular* (IM) injection, which results in somewhat slower absorption into the circulation;

♦ *oral* administration, which results in the slowest absorption, and is also less reliable than parenteral routes because the rate of absorption may be affected by such factors as the presence of food in the stomach. An orally administered drug, having been absorbed into the circulation, is first transported to the liver via the hepatic portal vein. Liver enzymes may destroy a substantial proportion of the absorbed drug (*first-pass metabolism*).

3.2 Multiple dosing and steady-state concentration

To produce a sustained therapeutic effect, a drug must be continuously present in the body in an adequate concentration. The purpose of repeated dosing is to maintain the concentration within the therapeutic range. If the drug concentration is not allowed to fall to zero between doses, mean plasma concentration rises progressively with repeated dosing, eventually approaching a steady state (Fig. 15.1(b)). However, in the case of a drug with a narrow therapeutic range, the interdose fluctuations in concentration may result in unacceptable side-effects soon after a dose and therapeutically insufficient concentrations before the next dose is administered. One solution to this problem is to give smaller doses more frequently (Fig. 25.1(c))—however, this may place an unacceptable burden of inconvenience on the patient. More satisfactory alternatives are available for some drugs in the form of sustained-release or depot preparations.

3.3 Sustained-release and depot preparations

Sustained-release preparations provide a gradual release of the drug from particles during their passage through the gut. They allow once-daily dosing rather than the three or four doses per day that may be needed with conventional oral preparations. Depot preparations provide a slow release from an oily vehicle administered by deep IM injection. Injections given at 2- or 4-week intervals may be used in place of multiple daily oral doses.

3.4 Blood–brain barrier (BBB)

This is a property of capillaries in the cerebral circulation that prevents passage of fat-insoluble molecules into the brain tissue.

3.5 Drug interactions

The presence of one drug in the body may alter the effect of another drug. There are two main types of interaction:

- *pharmacodynamic interactions*, e.g. drugs A and B competing for the same receptor site;
- *pharmacokinetic interactions*, e.g. drug A altering the activity of an enzyme that metabolizes drug B.

4 Therapeutic effects and side-effects

Most centrally acting drugs have multiple effects. However, different concentrations of a drug may be needed to exert its desired (therapeutic) effect and its undesired effects (side-effects).

- The *therapeutic range* is the concentration range in which therapeutic effects are obtained without intolerable side-effects.
- The *therapeutic index* is the ratio of the maximum tolerated concentration to the minimum effective concentration.

4.1 Cognitive side-effects

Cognitive side-effects of psychoactive drugs are readily quantifiable in placebo-controlled single-dose laboratory experiments, but are difficult to pin down in clinical settings. Many psychiatric and neurological conditions associated with cognitive dysfunction may be mistaken for side-effects of the drug. Side-effects seen in single-dose studies may be poor predictors of side-effects in chronic treatment. Some side-effects dissipate during continuous use, whereas others emerge only after months of regular treatment.

In most cases, cognitive side-effects of psychoactive drugs are not specific to particular classes of drug, although strongly sedative drugs and drugs that affect extrapyramidal motor functions have especially pronounced effects on test performance that requires fine movements or rapid responding. Memory test performance tends to be more vulnerable than linguistic and visuospatial performance. (For the effects of particular drug classes on cognitive functions, see Section 5.) Although cognitive side-effects do complicate the interpretation of neuropsychometric assessment data, it should be remembered that psychiatric symptoms (mood disturbance, psychosis, etc.) may distort test results to an even greater degree than the drug used to treat them.

4.2 Drug withdrawal

Adverse effects are sometimes seen in drug withdrawal. During continued use, *tolerance* may occur to the therapeutic and/or side-effects of the drug. This may arise from:

- a change in tissue sensitivity (neuroadaptation, pharmacodynamic tolerance); and/or
- a change in the rate of elimination of the drug (*pharmacokinetic tolerance*).

After drug withdrawal there may be a rebound of physiological processes that have been suppressed by the drug, and reversal of the tolerance that may have developed during repeated treatment. An example of the former is the occurrence of seizures upon rapid withdrawal of a drug with anticonvulsant properties. An example of the latter is the fatal overdose that may occur when an opiate addict takes his 'usual' dose after a period of abstinence.

5 Classes of centrally acting drugs

5.1 Antipsychotic drugs

Antipsychotics (neuroleptics) are currently classified as (i) *typical* (*classical*), and (ii) *atypical*, on the basis of their pharmacological profiles.

5.1.1 Typical antipsychotics

These include the chemical classes:

- *phenothiazines* (e.g. chlorpromazine, trifluoperazine, thioridazine);
- *thioxanthines* (e.g. flupenthixol, clopenthixol);
- *butyrophenones* (e.g. haloperidol, droperidol);
- *diphenylbutylpiperidines* (e.g. pimozide, fluspiriline).

Mode of action   Typical antipsychotics are D_2 dopamine receptor antagonists. This fact is one of the cornerstones of the dopamine theory of schizophrenia. D_2 receptors mediate postsynaptic effects of dopamine in the three major dopaminergic pathways. Blockade of D_2 receptors in the neocortex and limbic structures (mesolimbic/mesocortical projection) probably underlies the therapeutic action of typical antipsychotics, whereas blockade of D_2 receptors in the striatum (nigrostriatal projection) and pituitary stalk (tuberoinfundibular pathway) is responsible for many of their side-effects (see 'Side-effects', this section). These drugs differ widely in therapeutic potency. The average prescribed daily dose correlates highly with affinity for D_2 receptors (Seeman *et al.* 1976).

Receptor cloning techniques have revealed a 'family' of D_2-like receptors (D_2, D_3, D_4) with different regional distributions. D_3 and D_4 receptors are more abundant in the limbic system and neocortex than in the striatum. Typical antipsychotics have higher affinity for D_2 than for D_3 and D_4 receptors. At therapeutic doses typical antipsychotics occupy $>80\%$ of D_2 receptors (Seeman 1992).

Therapeutic uses   Typical antipsychotics are effective in managing acute psychotic episodes and as maintenance therapy for relapse prevention in chronic schizophrenia. They are better able to ameliorate positive psychotic symptoms (hallucinations, delusions) than negative symptoms (avolition, anhedonia, poverty of thought). They are also used to suppress manic excitement and (in combination with antidepressants) to treat psychotic depression.

Pharmacokinetics Typical antipsychotics are well absorbed following oral or parenteral administration, peak plasma concentration being attained 1–4 hours after oral administration. The $t_{1/2}$ of most typical antipsychotics is between 10 and 30 hours. They undergo first-pass metabolism. Hepatic metabolism of some drugs (e.g. chlorpromazine) increases during chronic treatment (*enzyme induction*), resulting in falling plasma concentrations. Treatment with depot preparations may require months to attain steady-state plasma levels, and the drug may be detected months after discontinuation.

Side-effects Typical antipsychotics, particularly the high-potency butyrophenones, are liable to induce extrapyramidal side-effects (EPSs: akathisia, dystonia, and 'parkinsonian' symptoms—rigidity, bradykinesia, and tremor). EPSs probably arise from dopamine receptor blockade in the striatum. They are treated by co-administration of centrally acting anticholinergic drugs (e.g. benztropine), which may correct the imbalance of dopaminergic and cholinergic influences on striatal function occasioned by D_2 receptor blockade. Phenothiazines have some anticholinergic action and are therefore less liable to induce EPSs than butyrophenones. About 10% of patients undergoing chronic treatment with typical antipsychotics experience a delayed side-effect, *tardive dyskinesias* (involuntary orofacial movements and choreoathetoid movements of the extremities). Patients suffering from Lewy-body dementia show greatly enhanced sensitivity to the EPS-inducing effects of antipsychotics (Ballard *et al.* 1998).

Single acute doses of typical antipsychotics reduce vigilance and impair psychomotor performance. In patients undergoing chronic treatment, it is difficult to disentangle the effects of the drug from the effects of the illness. Cognitive performance may actually improve as a result of antipsychotic medication, relative to the impairment seen in unmedicated schizophrenics (King 2003).

Typical antipsychotics increase prolactin secretion due to D_2 receptor blockade in the tuberinfundibular system. In sensitive males this may cause impotence and galactorrhoea.

A rare, idiosyncratic, life-threatening side-effect is the *neuroleptic malignant syndrome*, characterized by fever, muscular rigidity, autonomic instability, and coma.

5.1.2 Atypical antipsychotics

These include clozapine, olanzapine, risperidone, and quetiapine.

Mode of action These drugs have a lower affinity for D_2 receptors than typical antipsychotics. Clozapine has high affinity for many receptors (D_3 and D_4 dopamine receptors, 5-HT$_2$ receptors, muscarinic cholinoceptors, α_1- and α_2-adrenoceptors), making it difficult to attribute its therapeutic efficacy to any one mechanism. Most other atypical antipsychotics share clozapine's high affinity for 5-HT$_2$ receptors. It has been suggested that dual antagonism of dopamine and 5-HT receptors may underlie the therapeutic effect of these drugs (Meltzer 1995).

Therapeutic uses Clozapine is as effective as the typical antipsychotics in treating positive schizophrenic symptoms. Good symptom control may be achieved in some patients whose illness is refractory to typical antipsychotics. It is claimed that negative schizophrenic symptoms respond more favourably to clozapine than to typical antipsychotics (Meltzer *et al.* 1993).

Pharmacokinetics Atypical antipsychotics are rapidly absorbed from the gut and undergo extensive first-pass metabolism. Their $t_{1/2}$ values are approximately 7 (quetiapine), 15 (clozapine), and 30 hours (olanzapine). Risperidone $t_{1/2}$ is 3 hours but the $t_{1/2}$ of its antipsychotic metabolite, 9-hydroxyrisperidone is about 24 hours. Olanzapine can be given once daily, but twice-daily dosing is recommended for the others.

Side-effects Atypical antipsychotics are less liable to induce EPSs than typical antipsychotics, possibly due to their relatively low affinity for D_2 receptors in the striatum (Horacek 2000). Clozapine produces a potentially life-threatening blood disorder, agranulocytosis, in 1–2% of patients. Its use is therefore restricted to patients whose symptoms do not respond well to other antipsychotics—regular blood counts are implemented during treatment. Other adverse effects of clozapine include sedation, nocturnal hypersalivation, and anticholinergic effects (blurred vision, urinary retention, constipation). Other atypical antipsychotics, which have lower affinity for muscarinic cholinoceptors, are less liable to induce anticholinergic side-effects.

5.2 Antidepressants and mood-stabilizing drugs

Two major classes of antidepressant are:

◆ *monoamine oxidase inhibitors (MAOIs)*;

◆ *monoamine uptake inhibitors.*

A few drugs with clinical antidepressant efficacy do not belong to either category (see Szabadi and Bradshaw 2003). The most widely prescribed mood stabilizer is lithium. Carbamazepine and valproate also have mood-stabilizing effects (see Section 5.4).

5.2.1 MAOIs

Mode of action MAOIs block the enzyme MAO that normally destroys monoamine transmitters within presynaptic terminals. This increases the availability of the transmitter, and thus increases postsynaptic receptor stimulation. MAO exists in two forms, A and B. In the brain, noradrenaline and 5-HT are deaminated mainly by MAO-A, and dopamine by MAO-B. The 'traditional' MAOIs, phenelzine, tranylcypromine, and isocarboxasid, block both forms irreversibly. Clorgyline is selective for MAO-A and deprenyl for MAO-B. Deprenyl is not an effective antidepressant, suggesting that dopaminergic mechanisms do not play a major role in depressive illness. Unlike the aforementioned MAOIs, moclobemide is a reversible inhibitor of MAO-A (RIMA). Reversible MAO-A inhibition conveys some advantage in terms of safety (see 'Side-effects', this section).

When administered chronically, MAOIs induce downregulation of central 5-HT$_2$ and 5-HT$_{1A}$ receptors and β-adrenoceptors. The functional significance of this is controversial. The overall effect of chronic MAOI treatment on monoaminergic transmission is mainly facilitatory, as receptor downregulation merely attenuates the increased postsynaptic receptor stimulation caused by increased transmitter availability (Blier *et al.* 1991).

Therapeutic uses MAOIs are seldom the first choice of antidepressant due to their potential for adverse effects (see 'Side-effects'). They are useful in some anxiety disorders (panic disorder, posttraumatic stress disorder, social phobia, etc.; see Krishnan 1998).

Pharmacokinetics MAOIs are rapidly absorbed. They undergo extensive first-pass metabolism, and have short half-lives (Mallinger and Smith 1991).

Side-effects Orthostatic hypotension is a common side-effect. MAOIs potentiate the effects of sympathomimetic amines, including tyramine (a constituent of some foods, e.g. cheese) and amphetamines, and may induce hypertensive crises. RIMAs are safer in this respect, because high concentrations of sympathomimetic amines are able to displace the RIMA from the MAO molecule, allowing effective metabolism of the amines. MAOIs are never combined with selective serotonin re-uptake inhibitors (SSRIs) as this can result in the potentially lethal *serotonin syndrome* (agitation, autonomic instability, progressing to convulsions and coma).

5.2.2 Monoamine uptake inhibitors

Mode of action Re-uptake into presynaptic terminals is the principal inactivation mechanism for monoamine transmitters. Uptake blockade therefore potentiates monoaminergic transmission. Chronic administration of uptake inhibitors results in downregulation of β-adrenoceptors, α_2-adrenoceptors, 5-HT$_2$ receptors, and presynaptic 5-HT$_{1A}$ receptors. These changes may reflect homeostatic adaptation to increased postsynaptic stimulation. Electrophysiological evidence indicates that monoaminergic transmission continues to be enhanced during chronic treatment with uptake inhibitors (Blier *et al.* 1991).

Monoamine uptake inhibitors are classified as:

- tricyclic antidepressants (TCAs; e.g. imipramine, desipramine, amitriptyline, dothiepin), which inhibit both noradrenaline and 5-HT uptake and block muscarinic cholinoceptors and α_1-adrenoceptors;

- selective serotonin re-uptake inhibitors (SSRIs; e.g. fluoxetine, fluvoxamine, sertraline, paroxetine, citalopram), which specifically block 5-HT uptake;

- selective noradrenaline re-uptake inhibitors (NARIs; e.g. maprotiline, reboxetine);

- serotonin–noradrenaline re-uptake inhibitors (SNRIs; e.g. venlafaxine), which block both 5-HT and noradrenaline uptake, but lack the anticholinergic and adrenolytic effects of TCAs.

Therapeutic uses TCAs are effective treatments for moderate/severe depressive illness. However, SSRIs (and more recently NARIs and SNRIs) have become more popular, because they have fewer side-effects and are safer in overdose than TCAs. TCAs and SSRIs are prescribed for chronic pain. SSRIs are prescribed for panic disorder, obsessive—compulsive disorder, and impulse-control disorders (Kavoussi and Coccaro 1998; den Boer *et al.* 2000).

Pharmacokinetics   TCAs are readily absorbed from the gut. They have relatively long half-lives (8–36 hours), allowing once-daily dosing. SSRIs are also eliminated slowly, allowing once-daily dosing. Fluoxetine has a particularly long $t_{1/2}$ (85 hours) and its active metabolite has an even longer one. It is recommended that 5 weeks be allowed for effective 'wash-out' before replacement with potentially interactive drugs (MAOIs). Venlafaxine and its active metabolite have shorter half-lives (4–10 hours). Venlafaxine is usually given in divided doses or as an extended-release preparation.

Side-effects

- *TCAs.* The affinity of TCAs for muscarinic cholinoceptors accounts for the cluster of side-effects (anticholinergic effects) brought about by suppression of parasym-pathetically mediated functions: dry mouth, constipation, blurred vision, urinary hesitancy/retention, erectile impotence. Tachycardia may reflect both anticholiner-gic action and peripheral noradrenaline uptake blockade, and postural hypoten-sion may reflect α-adrenoceptor blockade. Increased sweating probably reflects central noradrenaline uptake blockade, as peripheral muscarinic receptor blockade would be expected to suppress sweating. TCAs are notoriously sedative, which may reflect blockade of central α_1-adrenoceptors and histamine receptors. TCAs may cause cognitive dysfunction, especially memory impairment, which may reflect central cholinoceptor blockade.

- *SSRIs* have fewer side-effects and a wider therapeutic range than TCAs (Szabadi and Bradshaw 2003). In combination with MAOIs they can cause the serotonin syndrome (see 'Side-effects' in Section 5.2.1). Sexual dysfunction, a common com-plaint, is attributable to central 5-HT potentiation. Nausea is common, but usually disappears during continued use. Early reports of increased risk of suicide in patients treated with SSRIs have not been confirmed (Warshaw and Keller 1996). In therapeutic doses, SSRIs do not cause significant cognitive side-effects.

- *NARIs* and *SNRIs* have the expected side-effect profile of drugs that potentiate cen-tral and peripheral noradrenergic transmission, including mild hypertension and increased alertness.

5.2.3 Lithium

Mode of action   Lithium is administered as a salt (lithium carbonate), in which lithium exists as a monovalent cation. It can replace other cations in ion transport systems, allowing it to enter neurons and blood cells. It has numerous effects on monoaminer-gic transmission, including facilitation of tryptophan uptake, increased 5-HT and noradrenaline release, prevention of postsynaptic dopamine receptor supersensivity, and inhibition of the cyclic AMP and phosphoinositol second-messenger systems. The relationship between these effects and clinical mood stabilization is uncertain (Lenox and Manji 1998).

Therapeutic uses Lithium is the first-line treatment for manic—depressive illness. Lithium can augment the effects of TCAs and SSRIs in treating refractory depression. It has also been advocated for the management of impulsive aggression (Kavoussi and Coccaro 1998).

Pharmacokinetics Lithium is rapidly absorbed from the gut and has a $t_{1/2}$ of about 20 hours. Because of its low therapeutic index (see 'Side-effects'), divided doses are recommended, even in the case of extended-release preparations, in order to avoid toxic side-effects (Baldessarini 1996).

Side-effects Lithium has a low therapeutic index, and regular monitoring of serum concentration is standard practice. Serum concentrations of 0.8–1.2 mEq l^{-1} are cited as the therapeutic range, but there is considerable variation between individuals. The signs of lithium toxicity are vomiting, diarrhoea, coarse tremor, ataxia, dysarthria, agitation or lassitude, and cognitive impairment. Untreated, it can progress to seizures and coma. Within the therapeutic range, many patients experience side-effects, including memory problems, thirst, polyuria, and fine tremor. Thyroid functions may also be suppressed. There are few objective data about the cognitive side-effects of lithium, although in this writer's experience memory impairment and general reduction of mental acuity are not uncommon in patients treated with lithium.

5.3 Anxiolytics and hypnotics

Barbiturates are no longer used as anxiolytics or sedatives. Benzodiazepines, β-adrenoceptor antagonists, and 5-HT$_{1A}$ receptor agonists are considered here. Antidepressants are also used to treat some anxiety disorders (see Section 5.2).

5.3.1 Benzodiazepines

Mode of action Benzodiazepines bind to specific sites on the GABA$_A$ receptor–ionophore complex. GABA's inhibitory action is mediated by the opening of Cl$^-$ channels in postsynaptic membranes. Benzodiazepines have no effect of their own on the Cl$^-$ channel, but potentiate GABA's channel-opening action. This action of benzodiazepines differs from that of barbiturates which act directly on the ionophore to promote Cl$^-$ influx (Haefely 1990). Potentiation of GABA's effect on brainstem monoaminergic nuclei may underlie both the anxiolytic and sedative actions of benzodiazepines.

Therapeutic uses Benzodiazepines are effective in relieving the symptoms of generalized anxiety disorder. Their popularity waned in the 1980s when problems of dependence were first recognized. However, more recent studies have generally failed to find compelling evidence for addiction to benzodiazepines in routine clinical use

(Miller *et al.* 1995). In the UK they are recommended for prescription for limited periods only (2–4 weeks) in severe anxiety. They are also used as night-time sedatives, as anticonvulsants, in alcohol withdrawal (to reduce withdrawal distress and prevent seizures), and as intravenous anaesthetics for minor surgery.

Pharmacokinetics   A range of benzodiazepines is available with pharmacokinetic profiles to suit their different uses. An ideal hypnotic has a rapid onset of action, and should not produce a 'hangover' the following day. Temazepam, which is rapidly absorbed and has a $t_{1/2}$ of about 8 hours, is appropriate for this purpose. Patients with generalized anxiety disorder require sustained anxiolysis, such as that afforded by the long $t_{1/2}$ of diazepam. Diazepam's slow elimination is also advantageous in the management of withdrawal from alcohol or other benzodiazepines.

Side-effects   Benzodiazepines are among the safest centrally acting drugs when taken in overdose. Their principal side-effect is sedation, resulting in impaired psychomotor performance and slow information processing (Tonne *et al.* 1995). Higher doses induce dysarthria and ataxia. Anterograde amnesia may follow intravenous administration (King 1992).

5.3.2 β-Adrenoceptor antagonists

Mode of action   These drugs (e.g. propranolol) block the effects of noradrenaline mediated by β-adrenoceptors, including tachycardia and tremor. By preventing these somatic manifestations of anxiety they may break the 'vicious cycle' of physiological and psychological responses that is postulated by some theories of anxiety (Granville-Grossman and Turner 1966).

Therapeutic uses   β-adrenoceptor antagonists suppress somatic anxiety symptoms (excluding sweating and xerostomia, which are cholinoceptor- and α-adrenoceptor-mediated). They are helpful in managing situational anxiety, e.g. in performing artists or public speakers.

Pharmacokinetics   Propranolol's $t_{1/2}$ is about 4 hours. A slow-release preparation is available.

Side-effects   β-adrenoceptor blockade can induce hypotension and dizziness, and may provoke asthmatic attacks in susceptible individuals. Lethargy is the most common CNS side-effect.

5.3.3 5-HT$_{1A}$ receptor agonists

Mode of action   Buspirone (the only drug of this class available for prescription) is an antagonist at somatodendritic 5-HT$_{1A}$ autoreceptors, and a partial agonist at post-synaptic 5-HT$_{1A}$ receptors. It also blocks dopamine receptors. Under conditions of 5-HTergic hypofunction (which is postulated to occur in anxiety states), buspirone's net effect is to promote 5-HTergic function.

Therapeutic uses Buspirone is mainly used in generalized anxiety disorder, although it may also have antidepressant potential (den Boer *et al.* 2000). Unlike the benzodiazepines, the onset of buspirone's anxiolytic action is usually delayed by about 2 weeks.

Pharmacokinetics Buspirone undergoes first-pass metabolism and has a short $t_{1/2}$, but its major metabolite, 1-PP, is eliminated more slowly from the brain.

Side-effects Buspirone is much less sedative than the benzodiazepines. Adverse effects on cognition are seldom encountered. Nausea is the most commonly reported side-effect.

5.4 Antiepileptic drugs (anticonvulsants)

Mode of action The pathophysiological basis of all epileptic seizures is assumed to be the abnormal synchronous discharging of neurons. All anticonvulsants share the ability to suppress neuronal excitability, either by enhancing inhibitory neurotransmission or by suppressing excitatory transmission (see Table 25.2).

Therapeutic uses Among the 'established anticonvulsants':

- *phenytoin* and *carbamazepine* are effective in primary generalized convulsive seizures, and complex partial seizures, but not in primary absence seizures. Phenytoin's use has declined beause of its unfortunate pharmacokinetics and side-effect profile (see the following subsections);
- *valproate* is effective in most forms of epilepsy, and is widely prescribed for complex partial seizures (with and without secondary generalization) and absence epilepsy;
- *ethosuximide* is especially effective in absence seizures;
- *phenobarbitone* and *benzodiazepines* (e.g. clonazepam, clobazam) are rarely used as monotherapies, but still have adjunctive roles in refractory epilepsy; *clonazepam* and *diazepam* are used in status epilepticus.

The 'newer anticonvulsants' (Table 15.2) are mainly prescribed as adjunctive medication (occasionally as monotherapy) for epilepsy inadequately controlled by established anticonvulsants. They are mainly used to treat partial seizures with or without secondary generalization.

In addition to their use in epilepsy, carbamazepine and valproate are used as mood stabilizers and in the management of impulsive aggression (Kavoussi and Coccaro 1998).

Pharmacokinetics

- Unlike other anticonvulsants, phenytoin's pharmacokinetics are nonlinear (zero-order kinetics), i.e. metabolism of phenytoin is saturable at therapeutic concentrations, resulting in a decline in clearance and a rise in $t_{1/2}$ with increasing doses. Since small changes in phenytoin dose can produce large changes in plasma concentration, regular monitoring of plasma concentration is essential.
- Carbamazepine is slowly absorbed following oral administration, and has a $t_{1/2}$ of about 10 hours.

Table 25.2 Commonly prescribed antiepileptic drugs and their putative mechanisms of action

Drug	Indication	Neuronal effect	Mechanism
'Established anticonvulsants'			
Phenytoin	All seizures (first-line or adjunctive)	Reduces excitation	Inhibition of voltage-/use-dependent Na^+ channels
Carbamazepine	All seizures except absences (first-line or adjunctive)	Reduces excitation	Inhibition of voltage-/use-dependent Na^+ channels
Valproate	All seizures (first-line or adjunctive)	Reduces excitation	? Inhibition of voltage-/use-dependent Na^+ channels
		? Increases inhibition	? Facilitation of GABA synthesis
Phenobarbitone	All seizures (adjunctive, for refractory epilepsy)	Increases inhibition	Facilitation of Cl^- channel opening
Clonazepam, clobazam	All seizures (adjunctive)	Increases inhibition	Potentiation of GABA-induced Cl^- channel opening
Ethosuximide	Absence seizures (first-line or adjunctive)	Reduces excitation	Inhibition of voltage-dependent Ca^{2+} channels
'Newer anticonvulsants'			
Lamotrigine	Mainly partial seizures (adjunctive or first-line)	Reduces excitation	Inhibition of voltage-/use-dependent Na^+ channels
Vigabatrin	Mainly partial seizures (adjunctive)	Increases inhibition	Inhibition of GABA catabolism by GABA transaminase
Topiramate	Mainly partial seizures (adjunctive)	Reduces excitation	Blockade of AMPA glutamate receptors, inhibition of Na^+ channels
		Increases inhibition	Potentiation of GABA-induced Cl^- channel opening
Gabapentin	Mainly partial seizures (adjunctive)	? Reduces excitation	? Inhibition of voltage-dependent Ca^{2+} channels
Levetiracetam	Mainly partial seizures (adjunctive)	Not known	Not known
Felbamate	Mainly partial seizures (adjunctive)	Reduces excitation	? Blockade of NMDA glutamate receptors, inhibition of Na^+ channels
Tiagabine	Mainly partial seizures (adjunctive)	Increases inhibition	Inhibits GABA uptake

* Valproate is rapidly absorbed and has a $t_{1/2}$ of about 15 hours.
* Ethosuximide's absorption is also rapid, but its $t_{1/2} > 30$ hours.

With the exception of *tiagabine* and *gabapentin*, which have short $t_{1/2}$s (6 hours), most of the 'newer anticonvulsants' have half-lives of >8 hours, and are suitable for twice-daily administration.

A major problem in prescribing anticonvulsants is *pharmacokinetic interaction* (e.g. one drug altering the metabolism of another).

* Carbamazepine enhances the metabolism of (and therefore reduces plasma levels of) phenytoin and valproate.
* Valproate inhibits the metabolism of phenobarbitone and lamotrigine.
* Vigabatrin, levetiracetam and gabapentin are relatively free of pharmacokinetic interactions (Elwes and Binnie 1996).

Side-effects

* *Phenytoin* has a low therapeutic index. Acute toxic effects include cerebellar and vestibular dysfunction (ataxia, intention tremor, nystagmus, imbalance). Hirsutism and thickening of the gums are troublesome long-term side-effects.
* *Carbamazepine* and *valprate* can induce liver dysfunction, which necessitates immediate discontinuation of treatment.

All anticonvulsants can induce sedation and cognitive impairment. *Barbiturates, benzodiazepines*, and *phenytoin* are especially culpable. However, *valproate* and *carbamazepine* may also adversely affect cognitive functions at therapeutic plasma concentrations (Kalviainen *et al.* 1996). *Lamotrigine, gabapentin*, and *vigabatrin* may be less sedative than other anticonvulsants. There have been occasional reports of confusion, aggression, and psychosis associated with *lamotrigine* and *vigabatrin*.

5.5 Antiparkinsonian drugs

The main symptoms of Parkinson's disease (PD), rigidity, bradykinesia, and tremor, arise from atrophy of the brainstem catecholaminergic nuclei. Atrophy of the dopaminergic nigrostriatal pathway results in $>90\%$ loss of dopamine from the striatum in advanced PD. Typical antipsychotics, which block D_2 dopamine receptors, induce EPSs which include some features of PD (drug-induced parkinsonism). Drug treatment of PD aims to:

1 restore dopaminergic function, or

2 restore the balance of dopaminergic/cholinergic function in the basal ganglia.

Treatment of drug-induced parkinsonism is discussed in Section 5.1.

5.5.1 L-dopa and other 'dopamine-enhancing' drugs

Mode of action   L-dopa is converted into dopamine by L-aromatic amino acid decarboxylase, an enzyme that is present in both 5-HTergic and catecholaminergic neurons.

Amantadine releases dopamine and blocks dopamine uptake. Bromocriptine, lisuride, and pergolide are postsynaptic D_2 receptor agonists. Selegiline is an MAO_B inhibitor. All these drugs are assumed to promote dopaminergic function in the striatum.

Therapeutic uses L-dopa is the most effective treatment for PD. Other 'dopamine-enhancing' drugs are prescribed as adjuncts to L-dopa therapy. Dopamine-enhancing therapy is generally unsuccessful in counteracting drug-induced parkinsonism, presumably because high concentrations are needed to displace the antagonist from receptor sites. Bromocriptine is useful in treating hyperprolactinaemia (e.g. due to pituitary tumours), because prolactin secretion is regulated by the dopaminergic tuberoinfundibular pathway.

Pharmacokinetics L-dopa is rapidly absorbed from the gut. However >90% of the administered dose is metabolized by peripheral L-aromatic amino-acid decarbolylase. This problem is overcome by administering an inhibitor of this enzyme (e.g. carbidopa) together with L-dopa. This prevents the conversion of L-dopa to dopamine in the periphery but, as carbidopa cannot cross the BBB, the therapeutically useful metabolism of L-dopa in the brain is not affected.

Side-effects Nausea is troublesome early in L-dopa therapy. Dyskinesias constitute a more serious problem for about 50% of patients during prolonged treatment. Behavioural side-effects include mood disturbance (depression or mania), insomnia, delirium, and, occasionally, psychosis. Hypersexuality may result from limbic/hypothalamic dopaminergic hyperfunction. The *on/off effect* refers to episodes of relapse into akinesia and rigidity, which occur with increasing frequency during prolonged L-dopa therapy. D_2 receptor agonists are useful in managing 'off' periods.

5.5.2 Anticholinergic drugs

Mode of action Procyclidine, benztropine, and related drugs block muscarinic cholinoceptors. By suppressing cholinergic function in the striatum they may restore the dopaminergic/cholinergic balance that is disturbed by dopamine insufficiency in PD.

Therapeutic uses Anticholinergic drugs are used in the initial stages of PD, and in cases where dopamine-enhancing treatments produce intolerable side-effects. They are routinely used to treat drug-induced parkinsonism and other EPSs (see Section 5.1).

Pharmacokinetics Anticholinergic drugs are well absorbed following oral administration. Treatment is usually by divided daily doses. Intramuscular injection is used for rapid relief of dystonias.

Side-effects Peripheral anticholinergic effects are common. Sedation may occur. In view of the putative role of central cholinergic pathways in cognition, cognitive impairment might be expected. However, there do not appear to be any data on the long-term neuropsychological effects of these drugs. Dependence/abuse is a problem in some patients.

5.6 Psychostimulants

Mode of action   Cocaine and amphetamine enhance catecholaminergic neurotransmission: cocaine inhibits uptake; amphetamine releases catecholamines (it also has some uptake-blocking and MAO-inhibiting actions). Dopamine potentiation in the mesolimbic pathway probably underlies the euphoriant/reinforcing effects. Noradrenaline potentiation in the periphery accounts for many of the adverse effects.

Therapeutic uses   Historically, amphetamine was used as an antidepressant and anorectic. Its alerting effect, exploited by pilots and radar operators in World War II, is the basis of its use in narcolepsy. It has been used to suppress behavioural stereotypies and hyperactivity in attention-deficit-hyperactivity disorder; this use has largely been usurped by the less dependence-prone methylphenidate.

Pharmacokinetics   Amphetamine is rapidly absorbed from the gut, and has a $t_{1/2}$ of about 10 hours. Intravenous infusion produces a very rapid onset of action ('rush'). Cocaine is well absorbed via the nasal mucosa ('snorting') and alveolar surface (smoking). Inhalation of the aerosol of particles produced by heating cocaine base ('crack') produces a very rapid rise to peak plasma concentration, resulting in an intense subjective effect. The $t_{1/2}$ of cocaine is about 1 hour.

Side-effects   The vigilance-enhancing effects of small doses of psychostimulants represent the peak of a Yerkes–Dodson 'inverted-U' function. Higher doses produce disorganization of cognitive performance and a disadvantageous speed/accuracy tradeoff. Psychotoxic effects include anorexia, anxiety, hallucinations, paranoid ideation, and behavioural stereotypies. Peripheral adverse effects, reflecting noradrenergic potentiation, include tachycardia, hypertension, tremor, and pupil dilatation (mydriasis). *Tolerance* to the psychostimulants may be partly pharmacokinetic (facilitated elimination). *Sensitization* ('reverse tolerance') to repeated doses occurs in some users, possibly reflecting enhanced dopaminergic function. The *withdrawal syndrome* includes fatigue, somnolence, dysphoria, anhedonia, and hyperphagia.

5.7 Opiates

Mode of action   Morphine, diamorphine (heroin), and related drugs are agonists at opioid receptors (μ-, δ-, and κ-receptors). Their action is blocked by opioid antagonists (e.g. naloxone). Stimulation of μ-receptors in the brain and κ-receptors in the spinal cord mediates their analgesic effects. Stimulation of μ-receptors in the mesolimbic dopaminergic pathway probably underlies their euphoriant/reinforcing effects.

Therapeutic uses   Opiates are the most effective treatment available for acute pain due to tissue damage and the pain of cancer. They are less effective in relieving neuropathic pain and 'chronic pain'. Opiates are occasionally used to suppress cough and to produce a firmer stool following ileostomy or colostomy.

Pharmacokinetics Opiates are well absorbed from the gut, but undergo extensive first-pass metabolism. Parenteral administration is commonly used both therapeutically and illicity. Morphine's $t_{1/2}$ is about 2 hours. As its therapeutic index is quite low, continuous intravenous infusion is sometimes employed in order to maintain a stable plasma concentration in the management of intolerable pain. Methadone, which is used in replacement therapy for opiate addiction, has a $t_{1/2}$ of 12–16 hours.

Side-effects Respiratory depression, nausea, vomiting, and constipation are significant adverse effects during therapeutic use. CNS side-effects include euphoria, sedation, and pupil constriction (miosis). Delirium/hallucinosis occurs occasionally—this has been attributed to σ-receptor stimulation. Pharmacodynamic *tolerance* develops to the euphoriant and analgesic effects. The *withdrawal syndrome* includes restlessness, craving, anxiety, mydriasis, lacrimation and piloerection ('goose-flesh').

5.8 Hallucinogens and other drugs affecting perception

These include:

- 'indoleamine-like' hallucinogens (e.g. lysergic acid diethylamide (LSD), psilocybin);
- 'catecholamine-like' hallucinogens (e.g. mescaline, methylenedioxymethamphetamine (MDMA, 'ecstasy'));
- dissociative anaesthetics (e.g. ketamine, phencyclidine (PCP));
- cannabinoids (e.g. Δ^9-tetrahydrocannabinol (THC)—the principal active ingredient of cannabis resin).

Mode of action LSD and related drugs have both agonist and antagonist actions at 5-HT receptors. Their principal action is thought to be stimulation of somatodendritic 5-HT autoreceptors. Mescaline and related drugs combine sympathomimetic ('amphetamine-like') action with LSD-like effects; facilitation of dopaminergic/noradrenergic mechanisms contribute to their mechanism of action. MDMA releases 5-HT and has a selective neurotoxic effect on 5-HTergic neurons. PCP binds to specific sites (*sigma receptors*) within the ionophore linked to glutamate (*N*-methyl-D-aspartate; NMDA) receptors. It thus interferes with glutamatergic transmission mediated by these receptors. THC binds to specific metabotropic receptors ('*cannabinoid receptors*') structurally related to opioid receptors. The relationship between these actions and the perceptual and cognitive effects of these drugs is unknown.

Therapeutic uses Mescaline- and LSD-like drugs have no legitimate therapeutic use. Ketamine is used as an analgesic/anaesthetic. THC (in the form of cannabis) is used illegally not only for recreational purposes, but also as an anxiolytic and, notably by some multiple sclerosis sufferers, as an analgesic. THC has antinauseant and anti-emetic effects that have been used to counteract the side-effects of cancer chemotherapy.

Pharmacokinetics Mescaline- and LSD-like drugs are well absorbed from the gut. Their half-lives are in the range of 3–6 hours. However, depending on the dose, the psychological effects may last for 24 hours or more. PCP's $t_{1/2}$ can be as long as 3 days, but in treating overdose victims excretion can be facilitated by acidification of the urine. Ketamine is administered intravenously as an anaesthetic; its $t_{1/2}$ is about 2 hours. THC, which is usually self-administered by inhaling the smoke of cannabis resin, has an elimination $t_{1/2}$ of about 30 hours. However its metabolites are eliminated much more slowly, and can be detected in the plasma and urine weeks after cannabis use.

Psychological and somatic effects   These drugs alter perception in all modalities. Enhanced subjective sensory acuity, perceptual distortion, and illusions are more common than frank hallucinosis. LSD- and mescaline-like drugs have little effect on arousal, whereas PCP and ketamine induce drowsiness. THC in modest recreational doses impairs attention and information-processing performance. Mood is affected somewhat unpredicably by all drugs in this class. Euphoria may give way to dysphoria and outright panic within a single 'trip'.

Mescaline and related drugs induce emesis, probably by an action on the chemosensitive 'trigger zone' in the brainstem. Tachycardia and mydriasis reflect the sympathomimetic effects of these drugs (see above).

Long-term effects of habitual use of hallucinogens are controversial. Delayed 'flashbacks' are sometimes reported by LSD users. These may reflect persistent, rather than episodic, perceptual disturbance (Abraham *et al.* 1996). MDMA's neurotoxic effects may be irreversible. Regular use of THC may lead to an 'amotivational syndrome' and sexual dysfunction. However there is little evidence that this is not fully reversible following discontinuation.

The tar from cannabis resin is more carcinogenic than that of tobacco.

5.9 Drug treatment of Alzheimer's-type dementia

The major neuropathological features of Alzheimer's disease (AD) are:

- extracellular *plaques* containing β-amyloid protein;
- intraneuronal neurofibrillary tangles;
- neuronal loss.

Among the most severely affected pathways are the cholinergic projections from the basal forebrain to the hippocampus and neocortex, whose atrophy has been held responsible for the cognitive decline in AD (Whitehouse 1998). Several drugs that enhance cholinergic function are available for treating AD.

Mode of action   The postsynaptic action of acetylcholine is curtailed by acetylcholinesterase, an enzyme present on pre- and postsynaptic membranes. Acetylcholinesterase inhibitors (AChIs) block the degradation of acetylcholine and thereby enhance central cholinergic function.

Therapeutic uses   Clinically available AChIs include donepezil and rivastigmine. (Tacrine, the first clinically used drug of this class, has hepatotoxic effects in about 40%

of patients, and is no longer prescribed.) These drugs have been shown to slow the progressive cognitive decline and deterioration of 'activities of daily living' (Rogers *et al.* 1998) and to alleviate 'non-cognitive' symptoms (hallucinations, anorexia, wandering) (Cummings 2000). There are reports of their utility in dementias other than AD (e.g. Lewy body disease; Liberini *et al.* 1996).

Pharmacokinetics   Donepezil's $t_{1/2}$ is about 100 hours, allowing a once-daily dosing regimen. Rivastigmine is eliminated more rapidly, and divided doses are recommended.

Side-effects   AChIs produce 'cholinergic side-effects', including abdominal discomfort, nausea, diarrhoea, and sweating. Anorexia has also been reported.

Acknowledgment

I am grateful to my colleague Professor E. Szabadi for helpful discussions and practical suggestions for improving the draft of this chapter.

Selective references

Abraham, H.D., Aldridge, A.M., and Gogia, P. (1996). The psychopharmacology of hallucinogens. *Neuropsychopharmacology* **14**, 285–98.

Baldessarini, R.J. (1996). Drugs and treatment of psychiatric disorders: depression and mania. In *Goodman and Gilman's The pharmacological basis of therapeutics*, 9th edn (ed. J.G. Hardman, L.E. Limbird, P.B. Molinoff, R.W. Ruddon, and A. Goodman Gilman) pp. 431–60. McGraw-Hill, New York.

Ballard, C.G., Grace, J., McKeith, I.G., and Holmes, C. (1998). Neuroleptic sensitivity in dementia with Lewy bodies and Alzheimer's disease. *Lancet* **351**, 1032–3.

Blier, P., de Montigny, C., and Chaput, Y. (1991). A role for the serotonin system in the mechanism of action of antidepressant treatments: preclinical evidence. *J. Clin. Psychiatry* **51**, 14–20.

Cooper, J., Bloom, F.E., and Roth, R.H. (2003). *The biochemical basis of neuropharmacology*, 8th edn. Oxford University Press, New York.

Cummings, J.L. (2000). Cholinesterase inhibitors: a new class of psychotropic compounds. *Am. J. Psychiatry* **157**, 4–15.

den Boer, J.A., Bosker, F.J., and Slapp, B.R. (2000). Serotonergic drugs in the treatment of depressive and anxiety disorders. *Hum. Psychopharmacol.* **15**, 315–36.

Elwes, R.D.C. and Binnie, C.D. (1996). Clinical pharmacokinetics of newer antiepileptic drugs. *Clin. Pharmacokinetics* **30**, 403–15.

Granville-Grossman, K.L. and Turner, P. (1966). The effects of propranolol on anxiety. *Lancet* **i**, 788–90.

Haefely, W. (1990). The GABA$_A$-benzodiazepine receptor: biology and pharmacology. In *Handbook of anxiety*, Vol. 3: *The neurobiology of anxiety* (ed. G.D. Burrows, M. Roth, and R. Noyes), pp 165–88. Elsevier, Amsterdam.

Harrison-Read, P. and Tyrer, P. (1995). The application and evaluation of drug treatment in psychiatric practice. In *Seminars in clinical psychopharmacology* (ed. D.J. King), pp 59–102. Gaskell, London.

Hökfelt, T., Broberger, C., Xu, Z-Q.D., Sergeyev, V., Ubink, R., and Diez, M. (2000). Neuropeptides—an overview. *Neuropharmacology* **39**, 1337–56.

Horacek, J. (2000). Novel antipsychotics and extrapyramidal side effects: theory and reality. *Pharmacopsychiatry* **33** (suppl. 1), 34–42.

Kalviainen, R., Aikia, M., and Riekkinen, P.J. (1996). Cognitive adverse effects of antiepileptic drugs. *CNS Drugs* 5, 358–68.

Kavoussi, R. and Coccaro, E.F. (1998). Psychopharmacological treatment of impulsive aggression. In *Neurobiology and clinical views on aggression and impulsivity* (ed. M. Maes and E.F. Coccaro), pp. 197–211. Wiley, New York.

King, D.J. (1992). Benzodiazepines, amnesia and sedation: theoretical and clinical issues and controversies. *Hum. Psychopharmacol.* 7, 79–87.

King, D.J. (2003). Neuroleptics and the treatment of schizophrenia. In *Seminars in clinical psychopharmacology* (ed. D.J. King). Gaskell, London.

King, D.J. (ed.) (2003). *Seminars in clinical psychopharmacology*. Gaskell, London.

Krishnan, K.R.R. (1998). Monoamine oxidase inhibitors. In *Textbook of psychopharmacology*, 2nd edn (ed. A.F. Schatzberg and C.B. Nemeroff), pp 239–49. American Psychiatric Press, New York.

Lenox, R.H. and Manji, H.K. (1998). Lithium. In *Textbook of psychopharmacology*, 2nd edn (ed. A.F. Schatzberg and C.B. Nemeroff), pp. 379–430. American Psychiatric Press, New York.

Leonard, B.E. (1997). *Fundamentals of psychopharmacology*, 2nd edn. Wiley, Chichester.

Liberini, P., Valerio, A., Memo, M., and Spano, P.-F. (1996). Lewy-body dementia and responsiveness to cholinesterase inhibitors: a paradigm for heterogeneity of Alzheimer's disease? *Trends Pharmacol. Sci.* 17, 155–60.

Mallinger, A.G. and Smith, E. (1991). Pharmacokinetics of monoamine oxidase inhibitors. *Psychopharmacol. Bull.* 27, 493–502.

Meltzer, H.Y. (1995). Role of serotonin in the action of atypical antipsychotic drugs. *Clin. Neurosci.* 3, 64–75.

Meltzer, H.Y., Cole, P., Way, L., *et al.* (1993). Cost-effectiveness of clozapine in neuroleptic-resistant schizophrenia. *Am. J. Psychiatry* 150, 1630–8.

Miller, N.S., Gold, M.S., and Stennie, K. (1995). Benzodiazepines: the dissociation of addiction from pharmacological dependence/withdrawal. *Psychiatric Ann.* 25, 149–52.

Rogers, S.L., Doody, R.S., Mohs, R.C., and Friedhoff, L.T. (1998). Donepezil improves cognition and global function in Alzheimer's disease: a 15-week, double-blind, placebo-controlled study. *Arch. Intern. Med.* 158, 1021–31.

Seeman, P. (1992). Dopamine receptor sequences: therapeutic levels of neuroleptics occupy D_2 receptors, clozapine occupies D_4. *Neuropsychopharmacology* 7, 261–84.

Seeman, P., Lee, T., Cha-Wong, M., *et al.* (1976). Antipsychotic drug dose and neuroleptic/dopamine receptors. *Nature* 261, 717–19.

Szabadi, E. and Bradshaw, C.M. (2003). Affective disorders: 1. antidepressants. In *Seminars in clinical psychopharmacology* (ed. D.J. King). Gaskell, London.

Tonne, U., Hiltunen, A.J., and Vikander, B. (1995). Neuropsychological changes during steady-state drug use, withdrawal and abstinence in primary benzodiazepine-dependent patients. *Acta Psychiatrica Scand.* 91, 299–304.

Warshaw, M.G. and Keller, M.B. (1996). The relationship between fluoxetine use and suicidal behavior in 654 subjects with anxiety disorders. *J. Clin. Psychiatry* 57, 158–66.

Whitehouse, P.J. (1998). The cholinergic deficit in Alzheimer's disease. *J. Clin. Psychiatry* 59 (suppl.), 19–22.

Part 6

Underlying medical disorders

Chapter 26

The neuropsychology of vascular disorders

Clive Skilbeck

1 Introduction

The term 'vascular disorders' covers a range of conditions, including cerebrovascular disease (e.g. stroke, vascular dementia) and specific blood vessel problems, such as aneurysm with associated subarachnoid haemorrhage (SAH) or arteriovenous malformation (AVM). An apparently discrete event, such as stroke, is often associated with a prior history of transient ischaemic attacks (TIAs) and pre-existing risk factors (e.g. hypertension).

Due to the wide range of conditions subsumed under 'vascular disorders', there are a number of roles for the clinical neuropsychologist. These range from involvement at the acute, diagnostic stage (e.g. in evaluating cognitive functioning early in the course of a vascular dementia) through to an extended participation in the rehabilitation process following stroke. In assessment terms, the clinical neuropsychologist may be monitoring the cognitive abilities of a patient with hypertension over a prolonged period, be charting the process of recovery after neurosurgery in SAH, or be providing data on the rate and extent of cognitive decline in vascular dementia. Increasingly, clinical neuropsychologists are active in the rehabilitation process, offering interventions both for the cognitive deficits they have documented and for psychological problems such as anxiety and depression that accompany vascular disorders.

2 Pre-stroke conditions: hypertension

Hypertension is raised blood pressure: High systolic pressure is a major risk factor for stroke (hypertension has been estimated as the cause of intracerebral haemorrhages in 25–94% of cases; Allen *et al.* 1988).

2.1 Diagnosis

Unfortunately, hypertension often appears virtually symptom-free for a considerable period of time and so the most efficient method for its detection is routine screening.

2.2 Neuropsychological presentation

People aged 70 years or older who are hypertensive (but who have not suffered stroke) will show a wide range of cognitive difficulties, including a variety of memory and learning deficits, compared with people of the same age who have normal blood pressure. Similarly, high blood pressure in patients at age 50 years has been shown to correlate with the cognitive deficits noted (using the neuropsychological tasks of digit span, trail making, and verbal fluency) in these same patients when they were tested approximately 20 years later (Kilander *et al.* 2000). There is evidence that, the longer the period of uncontrolled hypertension, the more marked are the resulting cognitive impairments (e.g. Dufouil *et al.* 2001).

2.3 Psychosocial aspects

These are minor in the absence of significant adverse physical effects upon the patient. Similarly, patient compliance with the medication regimen and recommended lifestyle changes can be problematic when no short-term threat to health is obvious.

2.4 Treatment and outcome

If blood pressure is raised during mid-life, then there is a greater risk of cognitive impairment in late-life (Kivipelto *et al.* 2001). A significant reduction in the probability of subsequent stroke is achieved when hypertension has been successfully treated and blood pressure is reduced and controlled. There is a potential role for the clinical neuropsychologist in providing advice to hypertensive patients who wish to reduce their risk of stroke by stopping smoking and adopting a healthier diet and lifestyle. Issues of cognitive rehabilitation are dealt with in Section 4.7.

3 Pre-stroke conditions: transient ischaemic attacks (TIAs)

As the name suggests, TIAs are temporary (lasting less than 24 hours) neurological deficits arising from an ischaemic episode.

3.1 Diagnosis

This is made on clinical grounds and in the light of the patient's history.

3.2 Neuropsychological presentation

Given that TIAs usually occur against a history of a generally deteriorating cerebrovascular supply, a wide range of cognitive deficits may be observed. There is evidence that severity of cognitive impairment correlates significantly with the patient's longest TIA episode. Early adverse cognitive effects from TIA include a slowed speed of information processing (e.g. reduced Wechsler Adult Intelligence Scale-III (WAIS-III) Digit Symbol age-scale score) and new learning (e.g. relatively poor Rey Auditory Verbal Learning Test scores).

3.3 Psychosocial aspects

These are usually relatively minor, but expressed anxiety by the patient can be utilized to reinforce adherence to medical advice. If TIAs persist they are likely to acquire occupational relevance, as job performance suffers with developing cognitive impairment.

3.4 Treatment and outcome

One of the reasons why TIAs are important is because they carry an annual 10% risk of subsequent stroke for the patient. Hart *et al.* (2001) found that a simple four-item questionnaire on TIA was an excellent predictor of subsequent stroke in a study involving over 15 000 participants and a 20-year follow-up. For the large majority of patients, aspirin or short-term anticoagulation therapy is recommended. Results of a national UK 5-year study (Gibbs *et al.* 2001) indicated that the prescription of antiplatelet and anticoagulant agents significantly reduced the subsequent occurrence of stroke. In cases where major stenosis (narrowing) of the carotid artery is noted, referral for carotid endarterectomy surgery may be appropriate, although an uncertain cognitive prognosis is frequently the result (Lunn *et al.* 1999). The issue of cognitive rehabilitation is treated in Section 4.7.

4 Stroke

Stroke is a disruption of the vascular supply to the brain, of rapid onset with neurological symptoms persisting longer than 24 hours, caused by haemorrhage from an artery or from its occlusion through progressive narrowing of the vessel (atherosclerosis) or a blockage (embolism). Haemorrhage accounts for only about 10–15% of strokes and is particularly associated with coma, neck stiffness, and vomiting.

4.1 Risk factors

These include age, cardiac disease, TIAs (Section 3), hypertension (Section 2), and diabetes mellitus (Allen *et al.* 1988). For example, from age 60 years the risk of suffering a stroke doubles each decade. Smoking is a risk factor for those under 65 years old, as is gender (30% higher risk in men).

4.2 Diagnosis

Initially, the diagnosis of stroke is usually a clinical decision, based upon medical examination and symptoms, although it may be confirmed by a subsequent computerized tomography (CT) or magnetic resonance imaging (MRI) scan.

4.3 Neuropsychological presentation

This is extremely variable—impairment in any cognitive ability can be observed, depending upon the site of the stroke and its severity. The length of the period of cerebrovascular disease pre-stroke will also influence the cognitive picture.

- Motor deficits in the limbs contralateral to the side of stroke may be acquired, in severe cases constituting hemiplegia.
- When the stroke involves the hemisphere in which the patient's primary language centres are located, aphasic problems often result.
- The 'classic' cognitive disturbance in right hemisphere stroke is perceptual deficit, particularly left-sided neglect: the patient behaves as if the left side of visual space

does not exist. Patients are unaware of it and so neglect incoming information from this side. For example, this lack of awareness can lead to the patient bumping into/falling over furniture on their left side and (in severe cases) ignoring food on the left-hand side of their plate during meals.

◆ Although most of the early reports of this disorder stressed the right hemisphere-left visual space relationship, right side neglect following left hemisphere stroke is now well recognized (although occurring less frequently, and less severely).

The visual impairment demonstrated is *perceptual*—the deficit occurs at the cortical level, in the presence of adequate primary sensory and motor input from peripheral receptors (it is not merely the consequence of a visual field defect).

4.4 Neuropsychological examination

Again, the specific content of this will depend partly upon the site of stroke, although, given the likelihood of significant pre-existing cerebrovascular disease, a wide range of cognitive functions should be assessed. Skilbeck (1992) provided a general review of the assessment of cognitive functions in stroke. There are a number of reasons for carrying out a neuropsychological assessment, including the provision of prognostically useful information and the obtaining of a baseline against which to judge spontaneous recovery or the effectiveness of cognitive rehabilitation. The assessment may also make a contribution towards the decision relating to the most appropriate post-acute care setting for the patient.

4.4.1 Assessing intelligence

◆ In the absence of significant oral and/or written language impairment, the National Adult Reading Test (NART; Nelson 1982) offers the best estimation of premorbid intellectual level.

◆ The Wechsler Adult Intelligence Scale-Revised (and its successor, the Wechsler Adult Intelligence Scale-III (WAIS-III; Wechsler 1997a)) is the most often used instrument to assess intelligence quotient (IQ), although obtaining a meaningful verbal IQ may be impossible if the stroke involves the language-dominant hemisphere and produces significant dysphasia. Similarly, marked manual motor deficit as a consequence of stroke often renders the WAIS-III inappropriate for the assessment of performance IQ.

◆ When either marked language or motor impairment is apparent post-stroke, then Raven's Matrices can be particularly useful in assessing intellectual level, as it only requires either a simple pointing or a minimal verbal response, and time to respond is not included in scoring the test. A number of versions of this test are available, to cover a large age range (Raven 1977).

4.4.2 Assessing perceptual functions

Examination of perceptual functions may employ a number of instruments. The most appropriate include assessment for unilateral visual neglect, given that the reported rate of this disorder after right hemisphere stroke is very high (up to 85% immediately and approximately 40% at least 1 week after stroke). Examples are the Rivermead Perceptual Assessment Battery (RPAB; Whiting *et al.* 1985) and the Behavioural Inattention Test (BIT; Wilson *et al.* 1987). Star Cancellation tasks, such as that offered by the BIT, have been shown to be amongst the best predictors of functional outcome after stroke. The BIT was specifically devised to test for visual neglect, as was the recently developed Balloons Test (Edgeworth *et al.* 1998). The latter not only assesses unilateral visual neglect, but also allows computation of an index of general visual inattention. It comprises two subtests. Subtest A incorporates the phenomenon of perceptual 'Pop-out', providing a measure in which the attentional processing demands for serial search are minimal. Subtest B requires effortful serial search, thereby requiring a much greater attentional resource. Patients showing unilateral visual neglect are significantly more impaired on subtest B than subtest A.

However, even very simple, brief testing, such as asking the patient to draw a clock face or a daisy, can also elicit contralateral visual neglect. When attempting to write in the numbers around the clock face, the right hemisphere stroke patient with neglect tends to ignore its left side, resulting in all of the numbers being crammed into the right-hand side (between positions '12' and '6'). When drawing a daisy the same patient will usually omit the petals on the left side of the flower or produce only rudimentary versions of them. An excellent and comprehensive consideration of the clinical and theoretical aspects of unilateral neglect phenomena was provided by Robertson and Marshall (1993).

4.4.3 Assessing memory

Assessment of memory functioning after stroke can involve a number of approaches, from brief screening instruments through to test batteries. While memory screening tests often show a number of disadvantages, including poor/no data on their reliability and validity, some provide useful clinical information.

- The Mini-mental State Examination (MMSE; Folstein *et al.* 1975) remains amongst the most useful.
- The Rivermead Behavioural Memory Test (RBMT; Wilson *et al.* 1999) is a particularly appropriate test of everyday memory functioning.
- Examples of batteries for memory examination are the Adult Memory and Information Processing Battery (AMIPB; Coughlan and Hollows 1985) and the Wechsler Memory Scale-III (WMS-III; Wechsler 1997b).

4.4.4 Assessing language

Studies suggest that approximately 20% of patients will be dysphasic at 1 month post-stroke, reducing slightly to about 15% by the 6-month follow-up. Information on disordered language is obtained from intellectual assessment, though specialized and comprehensive instruments such as the Boston Diagnostic Aphasia Examination and the Western Aphasia Battery may be employed by speech therapists or neuropsy-chologists working with stroke patients. Walker (1992) provided a very good overview of language dysfunction and its assessment.

4.5 Importance of cognitive deficits

Continuing cognitive impairment post-stroke has implications for a person's activities of daily living (ADL). For example, someone with significant persisting memory diffi-culties may not remember to switch the cooker off after preparing food, may forget to buy needed food items when shopping, and may not recall phone messages. Post-stroke perceptual problems will often preclude the person from taking responsibility for personal self-care such as shaving, food preparation, or leaving the house unaccom-panied. The assessment methods outlined in Section 4.4 will help to form a judgement of the person's abilities and functional competence after stroke.

- A recent study by Jehkonen *et al.* (2000) noted that the presence of visual neglect following right hemisphere stroke, identified using the BIT, was associated with poor real-life activities at follow-up 12 months post-stroke.
- A number of studies have shown significant correlations between scores on the RPAB and ADL performance, with some RPAB scores on admission to rehabilita-tion being good predictors of discharge home.
- Admission scores from memory tests and Raven's Coloured Matrices have also proved useful in predicting discharge from hospital and ADL competence.
- In addition, the findings from cognitive assessment after stroke provide good predictors of subsequent driving ability (e.g. Klavora *et al.* 2000), which is an important finding given that older adults are at greater risk of causing a road traffic accident after stroke.

In addition, post-stroke cognitive problems can help in coming to an opinion regarding physical prognosis. Wang *et al.* (2000) found that cognitive impairment was a significant independent factor in predicting survival for at least 2 years post-stroke.

4.6 Psychosocial aspects

Many studies have investigated depression following stroke, usually concluding that it is a frequent problem. In a rare population study, involving 850 patients, Wade *et al.* (1985) noted a 20% depression rate in both patients and their carers 6 months post-stroke, and there is evidence that the frequency of patient depression may rise as high as 33% by 1 year after stroke. In addition to its direct negative effects upon the individual stroke patient's well-being, depression also has adverse effects upon cognitive function-ing, producing 'dementia of depression'. The question of the cause of this depression is unresolved, there being conflicting evidence to implicate the site and size of the stroke and the occurrence of cognitive sequelae. A high level of depression in carers is not sur-prising given the major physical, functional, and cognitive impairments that many stroke patients are left with. The position of spouses as carers is made more difficult given that they are likely to be of similar age to their patient partner. A limited range of mood and 'quality of life' instruments has been used with stroke patients and their relatives, including Hospital Anxiety and Depression Scales, Frenchay Activities Index, Nottingham Health Profile, and the Sickness Impact Profile (Skilbeck 1996; Ellis-Hill and Horn 2000).

4.7 Treatment and outcome

One of the best predictors of death or long-term disability following stroke is urinary incontinence (Wang *et al.* 2001; Allen *et al.* 1988). In addition, Baird *et al.* (2001) found that recovery could be predicted from the extent of the ischaemic damage noted on MRI and a stroke scale score, these measures being obtained within 36 hours of the stroke. Medical treatment for stroke is limited.

- Vascular surgery to remove the blockage is not supported by research studies, and endarterectomy to prevent stroke may significantly raise the mortality rate.

- However, recent research (Hillis *et al.* 2000) has demonstrated the role of hypoperfusion in determining acquired cognitive deficits in acute stroke. Reducing hypertension has also been shown to reduce the probability of recurrent stroke.

- Although the possible treatment of stroke using transplanted neuronal tissue has yet to investigated adequately, there are studies (e.g. using basal ganglia stroke patients) reporting relevant research and arguing for the feasibility of this approach. In addition, there is now good evidence that a significant element in the spontaneous recovery of functioning post-stroke is associated with a complex pattern of brain reorganization (Cramer and Bastings 2000).

- Some very recent research using *transcranial magnetic stimulation* (TMS; Trompetto *et al.* 2000), in which magnetic pulses are delivered to the motor cortex and adjacent areas via the scalp surface, suggests that reorganization of motor tissue post-stroke may be enhanced using TMS.

4.7.1 Rehabilitation

Rehabilitation after stroke is still primarily directed towards physical, rather than cognitive, functioning. In a recent major review of the relevant studies, Majid *et al* (2000) concluded that there was insufficient evidence to decide whether or not cognitive rehabilitation of memory deficits following stroke is effective, although there is strong support from meta-analysis studies for rehabilitation effectiveness with a range of language and perceptual deficits. With regard to the latter, work by Robertson has demonstrated the therapeutic value of ipsilateral motor stimulation in treating unilateral visual neglect. Skilbeck (2000) provided a review of the range of strategies available to treat cognitive deficits in people suffering stroke, dividing them into internal and external approaches.

- Internal approaches aim to directly reduce the level of cognitive deficit using remedial training on the affected function, examples being the use of mnemonics with memory impairments and scanning training in visual neglect.

- External approaches concentrate upon the use of aids to ameliorate the effects of cognitive deficits, such as the employment of electronic diaries and 'reminder' systems. Older adults have been shown to cope surprisingly well with the involvement of PCs and electronic aids in the re-training of, or compensation for, their cognitive impairments.

4.7.2 Treating mood disorder

Mood disorder following stroke represents a major challenge for services. It is important in itself, although there is evidence that its successful resolution also carries the bonus of enhanced ADL gains (Chemerinski *et al.* 2001). Psychological intervention for post-stroke depression is underresearched, though a recent review (Kneebone and Dunmore 2000) suggests that cognitive behaviour therapy may be the current treatment of choice. Recent examination of pharmacological approaches to treatment of depression after stroke, using double-blind studies, have supported the use of nortryptyline and fluoxetine, with some evidence that the former may be more effective in improving both cognitive abilities and ADL functioning as measured by the Functional Independence Measure (Robinson *et al.* 2000).

5 Vascular dementia

Vascular dementia is defined as a generalized, significant reduction in cognitive functioning that is cerebrovascular in origin. The term 'vascular' dementia has tended to replace the traditional and more specific characterization of 'multi-infarct' dementia.

5.1 Diagnosis

As with other dementias, the most frequent identification is carried out using the WAIS-R (or WAIS-III), comparing the IQ figures obtained with the predicted premorbid IQs for the patient generated using the NART. Significant discrepancies between the two methods of IQ estimation, favouring the premorbid figures, can lead to the label 'dementia'. In addition, other neuropsychological test data, such as evidence that memory/learning abilities are significantly poorer than would be predicted from estimated premorbid cognitive level, may also be used in the decision.

5.2 Neuropsychological presentation

In the most frequently observed dementia, namely, Alzheimer's disease (AD), neuropsychological examination early in the condition frequently produces a characteristic profile of subtest results in which the age-scale scores for Vocabulary and Information within the Verbal scale will be higher than for Similarities and Digit Span. Similarly, within the Performance scale, the Picture Completion age-scale score is usually higher than the scores observed for Block Design and for Digit Symbol. Of course, the timing of the emergence of this pattern of subtest scores, and how marked it is, depend upon the stage of dementia when testing is undertaken and upon its speed of progression.

Whilst the above pattern of IQ subtest scores is also noted in vascular dementia, its appearance is much more variable. This is because the development of vascular dementia is more idiosyncratic, the particular cognitive deficits emerging according to the location and number of infarcts of a significant size at the time of assessment. It may be worth distinguishing two versions of vascular dementia.

- The first is this less predictable pattern of cognitive deficits that is dependent upon infarct location and number.
- The second is more generalized, producing an IQ subtest profile that is more predictable and similar to that noted in AD. Its basis is prolonged cerebrovascular disease, without major stroke, in which the gradual reduction of the blood supply to the cerebral cortex, principally through the narrowing of vessels, produces cognitive loss.

5.3 Psychosocial aspects

Whilst in some ways the psychosocial issues raised in vascular dementia are the same as those in AD, there are some differences. The principal amongst these is the question of insight. Frequently (and sometimes mercifully) in AD, quite early in the progression of the illness patients lose insight into their condition and their failing cognitive and ADL abilities. This loss of insight seems to occur less often for patients with a vascular dementia, unless there is significant ischaemic damage to frontal areas. An understandably higher level of distress usually accompanies preservation of insight for the patient, and sometimes for relatives. As with AD, the general picture is one of progressive cognitive decline, which requires much of the coping responses of both patient and relatives. Commensurate with the preservation of insight, depression in vascular dementia has been found to be resistant to treatment (Li *et al.* 2001).

5.4 Treatment and outcome

The rate of cognitive decline is dependent upon perfusion decline. Risk factors that accelerate the latter include TIAs and hypertension, so the use of aspirin and/or anti-hypertensive agents is recommended. Cognitive rehabilitation efforts are modelled on those referred to in Section 4.7, although the realistic successful outcome may be one of slowing down, or temporarily ameliorating, the process of cognitive impairment, rather than arresting or reversing its effects.

6 Subarachnoid haemorrhage (SAH)

The term 'haemorrhagic stroke' is usually applied to bleeding into the substance of the brain, whereas SAH refers to a blood vessel rupturing and bleeding into the subarachnoid space. However, the separation of these two causes of cerebrovascular haemorrhage is not always clear cut. About 80% of SAHs arise from the rupture of an aneurysm (sac extruded from the wall of an artery). Aneurysms can vary widely in their shape and size, although the majority are small ('berry'). In approximately 15% of SAH no cause is found (Bonita and Thompson 1985), with the remaining 5% of cases involving blood vessel malformations (arteriovenous malformations; AVM) or other causes.

Most aneurysms arise sporadically, although a familial link is identified in a minority of cases, and it is worth noting that SAH affects a younger population (average age 50–55 years) than 'stroke' and has a higher incidence in women (60%). The overall incidence in the general population is 1–2 per 10 000 per year (Deane *et al.* 1996).

6.1 Diagnosis

Patients often present to the Accident and Emergency Department of their local hospital complaining of severe headache of sudden onset, although in a minority of cases initial loss of consciousness occurs. Diagnosis of SAH is confirmed via CT scan and angiography.

6.2 Neuropsychological presentation

This varies widely, according to site of SAH and severity of the haemorrhage. Eighty-five per cent of aneurysms are found on the anterior cerebral artery distribution. The next most common are middle cerebral artery aneurysms, with the posterior cerebral circulation having the lowest occurrence. As might be predicted, those patients with an SAH involving an anterior artery often show some changes in personality, with increased irritability. Research studies in the past have provided inconsistent evidence of severe memory deficits following anterior communicating artery (ACA) SAH and it may be that at one time the neurosurgical intervention to clip the aneurysm itself used to produce some additional damage (to small perforator blood vessels).

The pattern of neuropsychological impairments observed generally follows that expected from cerebral functional geography with, for example, left hemisphere aneurysms of the anterior or middle cerebral arterial supply producing deficits in verbal expression and memory.

6.3 Psychosocial aspects

SAH often produces a very poor psychological (as opposed to cognitive) response. Depression of mood is frequently seen, with a minority seeking pharmacological treatment. A key factor in post-SAH mood problems appears to be the unexpected nature of the event—for nearly all patients there are no warning signs of the impending haemorrhage. As far as they were aware they were healthy, and many are young or middle-aged. The psychological shock of the SAH, with its serious health implications and probable 'brain surgery', also results in marked anxiety in patients. In a number of ways, the picture presented by some patients is similar to that noted in post traumatic stress disorder.

6.4 **Treatment and outcome**

Except in the cases where the SAH is of unknown origin, specific treatment for the aneurysm will be undertaken. Most often this requires neurosurgical intervention to clip the aneurysm, thereby ablating it, sometimes with the additional procedure of wrapping the vessel for extra security. Successful surgical treatment provides a permanent solution. It is also sometimes possible to avoid surgical intervention completely by using a coil. In this procedure a coil is passed, via the cerebrovascular arterial supply, to the site of the aneurysm and into it. This results in clotting, which seals off the aneurysm. This procedure is only suitable for a minority of aneurysms (generally small and narrow-necked). A coil intervention is associated with a better neuropsychological presentation and recovery, probably because neurosurgical intervention is not required and because coiling can only be used only with smaller (i.e. less destructive) aneurysms.

Cognitive recovery at 6 months post-SAH provides a good guide to the final outcome although, unlike stroke, significant cognitive gains can be noted to at least the 12-month follow-up point. The occurrence of vasospasm or hydrocephalus following SAH are poor prognostic signs for the final cognitive recovery achieved by the patient. Whilst there are few longer-term outcome studies, the available research suggests that a majority of patients show some permanent cognitive impairments as a consequence of SAH (e.g. Tidswell *et al.* 1995).

Despite reassurances from neurosurgeon and neuropsychologist, a sizeable minority of patients harbour the belief that an SAH may happen again (which is only realistic in cases where a person has multiple aneurysms). This can result in patients post-SAH being very reluctant to leave their house at all, or only doing so if accompanied. An almost phobic anxiety about being away from their house or being in public places may result. Symptoms of depression and anxiety tend to remit over the first few months after the haemorrhage, although a significant mood disturbance may persist for 6–12 months post-SAH. For these patients, intervention by a clinical neuropsychologist is recommended. Longer-term psychological difficulties tend to result from either marked persisting cognitive deficit (usually involving memory and/or language functions) or from permanent personality change.

7 **Specific cerebrovascular conditions: CADASIL**

Cerebral autosomal dominant arteriopathy with subcortical infarcts and leukoencephalopathy (CADASIL) is a rare condition that produces cerebrovascular problems in early adulthood or middle age (Desmond *et al.* 1999).

7.1 **Diagnosis**

In approximately 75% of cases, the disease presents as TIAs or young stroke, with migraine also being a frequent (40%) presenting symptom.

7.2 **Neuropsychological presentation**

If detected and assessed early, mild general cognitive difficulties are expected similar to those observed with TIAs. If initial assessment is undertaken following a first stroke, then greater cognitive deficit is observed, the pattern being determined by the site of the stroke. A stepwise progression of the disease usually occurs, resulting in dementia for approximately 50% of patients. The cognitive natural history of CADASIL is, therefore, very similar to that of multi-infarct dementia, although the progression begins at an earlier age. A very rare study (Harris and Filley 2001) involved case studies across three generations of one family, noting a range of cognitive deficits with relatively well preserved language functions.

7.3 **Psychosocial aspects**

Depression is a presenting symptom in approximately 10% of patients and with a prevalence of mood disorder of about 30%. Frequent coping problems are to be expected, given the disease's relatively early onset, its predictable progression, and the lack of any effective treatment.

7.4 **Treatment and outcome**

There is no effective treatment to halt, or reverse, the progression of CADASIL. For most patients the picture is one of deteriorating cognitive and physical functions. For example, more than 50% will be unable to walk unaided after the age of 60 years. Psychological intervention, in addition to addressing any mood disorder in the patient, should include family support, given the genetic basis of CADASIL, and may need to be episodic over a prolonged period.

8 **Summary**

From the neuropsychological point of view, vascular disorders are best regarded as specific features of the general process of cerebrovascular disease. Early signs of this process are represented by persisting hypertension and TIA, which are associated with usually mild, though developing cognitive impairment. Strokes are major events, involving physical, cognitive, and psychosocial sequelae. The pattern of deficits noted is dependent upon the site and size of the lesion caused by the stroke. Significant coping and adjustment problems are caused for patient and carers by stroke, which are somewhat different than those presented to people suffering SAH. The latter often occurs in middle-aged, rather than older, adults and for these patients there is a need to judge their recovery against additional criteria, including those linked to employment. The term 'vascular dementia' encompasses both the step-wise deterioration in functioning arising out of multi-infarct dementia and the more general progression of cognitive impairment produced by cerebrovascular disease.

Selective References

Allen, C.M.C., Harrison, M.J.G., and Wade, D.T. (1988). *The management of acute stroke.* Castle House, Kent.

Baird, A.E., Dambrosia, J., Janket, S., Eichbaum, Q., *et al.* (2001). A three-item scale for the early prediction of stroke recovery. *Lancet* 357 (9274), 2095–9.

Bonita, R. and Thompson, R.N. (1985). Subarachnoid haemorrhage: epidemiology, diagnosis, management and outcome. *Stroke* 16, 591–4.

Chemerinski, E., Robinson, R.G., Arndt, S., and Kosier, J.T. (2001). The effect of remission of post-stroke depression on activities of daily living in a double-blind randomised treatment study. *J. Nerv. Ment. Dis.* 189, 421–5.

Coughlan, A. K. and Hollows, S. E. (1985). *The Adult Memory and Information Processing Battery.* St James's University Hospital, Leeds.

Cramer, S.C. and Bastings, G.P. (2000). Mapping clinically relevant plasticity after stroke. *Neuropharmacology* 39, 842–51.

Deane, M., Piggott, T., and Dearing, P. (1996). The value of the short form 36 score in the outcome assessment of subarachnoid haemorrhage. *Br. J. Neurosurg.* 10, 187–91.

Desmond, D.W., Moroney, J.T., Lynch, T., Chan, S., Chin, S.S., and Mohr, P. (1999). The natural history of CADASIL: a pooled analysis of previously published cases. *Stroke* 30, 1230–3.

Dufouil, C., deKersaint, G.A., Besancon, L., Alperovitch, A., *et al.* (2001). Longitudinal study of blood pressure and white matter hyperintensities: the EVA MRI cohort. *Neurology* 56, 921–6.

Edgeworth, J.A., Robertson, I.H., and McMillan, T.M. (1998). *Manual for the Balloons Test.* Thames Valley Test Company Limited, Bury St Edmunds.

Ellis-Horn, C.S. and Horn, S. (2000). Change in identity and self-concept: a new theoretical approach to recovery following a stroke. *Clin. Rehab.* 14, 279–87.

Folstein, M.F., Folstein, S.E., and McHeugh, P.R. (1975). Mini-mental state: a practical method for grading the cognitive state of outpatients for the clinician. *J. Psychiatric Res.* 12, 189–98.

Gibbs, R.G., Newson, R., Lawrenson, R., Greenhalgh, R.M., and Davies, A.H. (2001). Diagnosis and initial management of stroke and transient ischaemic attack across UK health regions from 1992–1996: experience of a national primary care database. *Stroke* 32, 1085–90.

Harris, J.G. and Filley, C.M. (2001). CADASIL: neuropsychological findings in three generations of an affected family. *J. Int. Neuropsychol. Soc.* 7, 768–74.

Hart, C.L., Hole, D.J., and Smith, G.D. (2001). The relation between questions indicating transient ischaemic attack and stroke in 20 years of follow-up in men and women in the Renfrew/Paisley study. *J. Epidemiol. Commun. Hlth* 55, 653–6.

Hill, R.D. and Backman, L. (ed.) (2000). *Cognitive rehabilitation in old age.* Oxford University Press, New York.

Hillis, A.E., Barker, P.B., Beauchamp, N.J., Gordon, B., and Wityk, R.J. (2000). MR perfusion imaging reveals regions of hypoperfusion associated with aphasia and neglect. *Neurology* 55, 782–8.

Jehkonen, M., Ahonen, J.P., Dastidar, P., Koivisto, A.M., *et al.* (2000). Visual neglect as a predictor of functional outcome one year after stroke. *Acta Neurol. Scand.* 101, 193–201.

Kilander, L., Nyman, H, Boberg, M., and Lithell, H. (2000). The association between low diastolic blood pressure in middle age and cognitive function in old age. A population-based study. *Age Ageing* 29, 243–8.

Kivipelto, M., Helkala, E.L., Hanninen, T., Laakso, M.P., *et al.* (2001). Midlife vascular risk factors and late-life mild cognitive impairment: a population-based study. *Neurology* 56, 1683–9.

Klavora, P., Heslegrave, R.J., and Young, M. (2000). Driving skills in elderly persons with stroke: comparison of two new assessment options. *Arch. Phys. Med. Rehabil.* 81, 701–5.

Kneebone, I.I. and Dunmore, E. (2000). Psychological management of post-stroke depression. *Br. J. Clin. Psychol.* **39**, 53–65.

Li, Y.S., Meyer, J.S., and Thornby, J. (2001). Longitudinal follow-up of depressive symptoms among normal versus cognitively impaired elderly. *Int. J. Ger. Psychiatry* **16**, 718–27.

Lunn, S., Crawley, F., Harrison, M.J., Brown, M.M., and Newman, S.P. (1999). Impact of carotid endarterectomy upon cognitive functioning. A systematic review of the literature. *Cerebrovasc. Dis.* **9**, 74–81.

Majid, M.J., Lincoln, N.B., and Weyman, N. (2000). Cognitive rehabilitation for memory deficits following stroke. *Cochrane database systematic reviews 2000*, Vol. 3: CD002293.

Nelson, H. (1982). *The national adult reading test.* NFER-Nelson, Windsor, UK.

Raven, J.C. 1977. *Manuals for Raven's progressive and coloured matrices.* Lewis and Co, London.

Robertson, I.H. and Marshall, J.C. (eds). (1993). *Unilateral neglect: clinical and experimental studies.* LEA, Hove.

Robinson, R.G., Schultz, S.K., Castillo, C., Kopel, T., *et al.* (2000). Nortryptyline versus fluoxetine in the treatment of depression and in short-term recovery after stroke: a placebo-controlled, double-blind study. *Am. J. Psychiatry* **157**, 351–9.

Skilbeck, C.E. (1992). Neuropsychological assessment in stroke. In *A handbook of neuropsychological assessment* (ed. J.R. Crawford, D.M. Parker and W.W. McKinley), pp. 339–62. LEA, Hove, UK.

Skilbeck, C.E. (1996). Psychological aspects of stroke. In *Handbook of the clinical psychology of ageing* (ed. R.T. Woods), pp. 283–301. Wiley, Chichester.

Skilbeck, C. E. (2000). Strategies for the rehabilitation of cognitive loss in late life due to stroke. In *Cognitive rehabilitation in old age* (ed. R.D. Hill, L. Backman, and A.S. Neely), pp. 270–90. Oxford University Press, New York.

Tidswell, P., Dias, P.S., Sagar, H.J., *et al.* (1995). Cognitive outcome after aneurysm rupture: relationship to aneurysm site and perioperative complications. *Neurology* **45**, 875–82.

Trompetto, C., Assini, A., Buccolieri, A., Marchese, R., and Abbruzzese, G. (2000). Motor recovery following stroke: a transcranial magnetic stimulation study. *Clin. Neurophysiol.* **111**, 1860–7.

Wade, D.T., Langton-Hewer, R., Skilbeck, C.E., Bainton, D., and Burns-Cox, C. (1985). Controlled trial of home-care service for acute stroke patients. *Lancet* Feb 9, **1** (8424), 323–6.

Waldstein, S.R. and Elias, M.F. (ed.) (2001). *Neuropsychology of cardiovascular disease.* LEA, New Jersey.

Walker, S. (1992). Assessment of language dysfunction. In *A handbook of neuropsychological assessment* (ed. J. R. Crawford, D.M. Parker, and W.W McKinlay), pp. 177–221. LEA, Hove, UK.

Wang, S.L., Pan, W.H., Lee, M.C., Cheng, S.P., and Chang, M.C. (2000). Predictors of survival among elders suffering strokes in Taiwan: observation from a nationally representative sample. *Stroke* **31**, 2354–60.

Wang, Y., Lim, L.L., Levi, C., Heller, R.F., and Fischer, J. (2001). A prognostic index for 30-day mortality after stroke. *J. Clin. Epidemiol.* **54**, 766–73.

Wechsler, D. (1997a). *Manual for the Wechsler Adult Intelligence Scale-III.* Psychological Corporation, New York.

Wechsler, D. (1997b). *Manual for the Wechsler Memory Scale-III.* Psychological Corporation, New York.

Whiting, S., Lincoln, N. Bhavnani, G., and Cockburn, J. (1985). *The Rivermead Perceptual Assessment Battery: manual.* NFER-Nelson, Windsor.

Wilson, B.A., Clare, W., Cockburn, J.M., Baddeley, A.S., Tate, R., and Watson, P. (1999). *The Rivermead Behavioural Memory Test-extended version: manual.* Thames Valley Test Co, Fareham, UK.

Wilson, B., Cockburn, J., and Halligan, P. (1987). *The Behavioural Inattention Test: manual.* Thames Valley Test Co, Fareham.

Chapter 27

Neuropsychological presentation and treatment of head injury and traumatic brain damage

Nigel S. King and Andy Tyerman

1 Introduction

1.1 Clinical neuropsychology and head injury

Clinical neuropsychologists play a vital role in assessment and rehabilitation after head injury. Drawing upon both specialist neuropsychological knowledge and their general training, clinical neuropsychologists provide a number of key functions:

- carrying out detailed assessments of cognition, emotion, behaviour, and social competence;
- devising and implementing training programmes;
- liaising with educational agencies/employers to advise on the resumption of educational/vocational life;
- advising on the management of due to cognitive deficits; disabilities
- providing and advising about long-term care;
- providing psychotherapeutic input to address the emotional impact of injury and disabilities
- facilitating personal, family, and social adjustment (British Psychological Society 1989).

As such, clinical neuropsychologists contribute throughout the course of recovery after head injury across acute, rehabilitation, and community settings.

In the acute setting clinical neuropsychologists are usually based in regional neurosciences centres, working closely with neurosurgical and nursing staff during the acute admission. They will often see patients for more detailed assessment as out-patients at a 'post-acute' stage when the attention has shifted more to cognitive and other psychological changes. Until recently, clinical neuropsychologists working in rehabilitation in the UK were based primarily within regional in-patient neurological rehabilitation centres or in specialist units in the independent sector for the management of severe behavioural difficulties. However, over the last decade there has been a growth in clinical neuropsychology posts within generic physical disability teams, in specialist community brain injury rehabilitation services, and in specialist centres for cognitive and vocational rehabilitation after brain injury.

1.2 Epidemiology

The annual number of hospital admissions in Great Britain involving head injury is high (250–300 per 100,000 of the population). Of these, it is likely that 75–85% are mild head injuries and 5–8% severe or very severe injuries. The range of outcomes is huge, from complete recovery to persistent coma or death.

Serious disability from head injury occurs in an estimated 150 per 100,000 of the population in England and Wales with an estimated 210 totally disabled and 1500 severely or profoundly disabled every year. One family in 300 is thought to have a member with persisting disability following a head injury. A large proportion of head injury involves young males aged 18–25. Whilst rates vary with severity and geography, the most common causes of injury are road traffic accidents (RTAs) (~45%), falls (~30%), occupational accidents (~10%), recreational accidents (~10%), and assaults (~5%).

The disabilities associated with severe and very severe head injuries are extremely varied encompassing both physical disability (i.e. motor and sensory deficits) and psychological changes (e.g. cognitive impairment, altered emotional response, and loss of behavioural control). These often impact not only on the injured person but also on the family and wider psychosocial networks. The vast majority of rehabilitation services are therefore targeted on the more severely injured.

1.3 Severity of head injury

The severity of a head injury is usually measured by:

- length of posttraumatic amnesia (PTA)—the period of time between receiving a head injury and regaining continuous day-to-day memory for events;
- depth of unconsciousness—usually measured immediately after resuscitation, using the Glasgow Coma Scale (GCS; Table 27.1);
- length of unconsciousness (i.e. GCS < 9); and/or
- presence of neurological signs (e.g. paresis, damage revealed by neuroimaging techniques).

The most widely accepted classification of severity is detailed in Table 27.2.

2 Mild and moderate head injury

2.1 Pathophysiology

For the majority of mildly and moderately head-injured patients there are no measurable pathophysiological changes. In some cases however temporary electroencephalographic

Table 27.1 Glasgow Coma Scale

Response	Score
Eye opening subscale (score 1–4)	
Opens eyes on his/her own	4
Opens eyes when asked to do so in a loud voice	3
Opens eyes to pain	2
Does not open eyes	1
Verbal response subscale (score 1–5)	
Carries on a conversation correctly and tells examiner where he is, the year, and month	5
Seems confused or disoriented	4
Talks so the examiner can understand him/her but makes no sense	3
Makes sounds that the examiner cannot understand	2
Makes no noise	1
Motor response subscale (score 1–6)	
Follows simple commands	6
Pulls examiner's hand away on painful stimuli	5
Pulls a part of his body away on painful stimuli	4
Flexes body appropriately to pain	3
Decerebrate posture	2
Has no motor response to pain	1
Total score	3–15

Table 27.2 Severity of head injury

Severity	Glasgow Coma Scale score	Length of unconsciousness	Posttraumatic amnesia
Mild	13–15	<15 min	<1 hour
Moderate	9–12	15 min–6 hours	1–24 hours
Severe	3–8	>6 hours[†]	1–7 days
Very severe	N/a*	*	1–4 weeks
Extremely severe	N/a*	*	>4 weeks

* N/A, Not applicable.

[†] N.B. As many patients in extended coma are sedated and electively ventilated, it is often not possible to determine the duration of unconsciousness.

(EEG) abnormalities, reduced cerebral blood flow, or temporary macroscopic lesions (revealed by computerized tomography (CT) or magnetic resonance imaging (MRI)) are present. These predominate in the frontal or temporal cortical areas and usually resolve within 3 months. Where apparently minor injuries are associated with neurological signs or complications, it is usually not appropriate to make a classification of 'mild' head injury. Such injuries should be classified according to the extent of neurological signs and/or complications.

2.2 Clinical presentations and natural course

Many with mild or moderate injuries experience few or no symptoms and make a full recovery within a few days. Approximately 50% will, however, experience post-concussion symptoms (PCS)—headaches, dizziness, fatigue, irritability, poor concentration, nausea, sensitivity to light, sensitivity to noise, poor memory, sleep disturbance, tinnitus, slowed thinking, blurred/double vision, anxiety, depression, or frustration. These are caused by organic and/or psychological factors. For the majority, full recovery from PCS occurs from within a few days to 3 months. However 6–8% have persisting PCS at and beyond 1 year postinjury. Slow and/or incomplete recovery is associated with the following:

- ≥40 years old;
- premorbid psychopathology;
- previous head injury;
- premorbid alcohol/substance misuse;
- female gender.

When PCS persist major psychosocial disabilities can result.

2.3 Neuropsychological deficits

The most common neuropsychological impairments following mild and moderate head injuries involve impaired speed of information processing and divided attention (as measured by tests such as the Paced Auditory Serial Addition Task (PASAT) and Stroop Test). These types of impairments correlate well with severity of PCS and tend to mirror symptomatic recovery (i.e. recovery within 3 months of injury). Impairments in reaction time, verbal short-term and long-term memory (as measured by paragraph recall tests), and visuospatial short-term and long-term memory (as measured by figure recall tests) can also be present. These correlate less well with severity of PCS but also usually resolve within 3 months.

2.4 Related emotional disorders

The events that cause head injury are often precisely those where psychological trauma might also be expected. Posttraumatic stress (PTS) symptoms are therefore quite common and these often include phobic avoidance of situations where the injury occurred (e.g. driving). While organic amnesia following head injury is thought to offer some protection against PTS, the incidence of posttraumatic stress disorder (PTSD) following RTA and mild head injury is similar to that of the equivalent non-head-injured population (~20%). Frustration, depression, and anxiety due to the psychosocial disabilities caused by persisting PCS are common. A vicious cycle can easily develop where anxiety, depression, or frustration exacerbates PCS and leads to reduced coping. This causes further distress and further exacerbation of PCS. They may also be exacerbated by uncertainty over the relative contribution of psychological and organic factors, particularly when symptoms persist and become chronic.

2.5 Treatment/rehabilitation

Early assessment within 1–4 weeks of discharge is optimal and should include the following:

- assessment of the severity of head injury (e.g. by assessing the length of PTA);
- investigation of the extent and nature of PCS (e.g. using the Rivermead Post Concussion Symptoms Questionnaire);
- assessment of anxiety and depression symptoms (e.g. using the Hospital Anxiety and Depression Scale (HADS); Beck Depression Inventory (BDI); Beck Anxiety Inventory (BAI));
- investigation of the extent and nature of any posttraumatic stress symptoms (e.g.using the Revised Impact of Event Scale (IES)).

Intervention would normally focus on the provision of information, reassurance, education, support, and regular monitoring of progress. The information should address:

- the normality of PCS;
- good prognosis;
- regulating and pacing activities in line with the severity of PCS (e.g. taking short breaks when PCS feel worse rather than trying to push on through until longer breaks become unavoidable);
- graduated return to work and premorbid activities;
- education about the potential for developing the vicious cycle where stress and PCS becoming mutually exacerbating.

The overall aim is to minimize the effects of anxiety, worry, and stress on PCS by preventing the development of the vicious cycle. One single hour-long assessment and intervention session can be an effective intervention for the majority of cases. Specialist psychological and medical interventions are appropriate for persisting problems with posttraumatic stress, headaches, dizziness, anxiety, depression, return to work difficulties, irritability, tinnitus, or neuropsychological impairment.

2.5.1 Effectiveness

Studies evaluating the effectiveness of interventions for patients with mild and moderate head injuries are sparse. Randomized control trials in this area, however, have demonstrated that early intervention involving education, reassurance, support, and monitoring of progress can reduce the incidence and severity of persisting postconcussion symptoms. There is little hard evidence, however, to inform management guidelines when symptoms persist and become chronic.

3 Severe, very severe, and extremely severe head injuries

There are two main types of severe injury—open head injury and closed head injury.

- *Open head injury* occurs when the skull and protective linings of the brain are damaged so that brain is exposed.
- *Closed head injury* occurs when the skull and protective linings of the brain are not penetrated.

Closed head injury is by far the most common form of head injury in peacetime.

3.1 Pathophysiology

There are two kinds of damage to the brain following severe forms of head injury— primary damage and secondary damage.

3.1.1 Primary damage

Primary damage includes diffuse white matter damage, contusion (bruising), and haemorrhage.

- *Diffuse white matter damage* is due to the widespread rupturing of axons caused mainly by the brain impacting against itself as it moves within the skull. This is usually the most prevalent form of damage.
- *Contusion* is usually most pronounced in the undersurfaces of the frontal and temporal poles where the shearing forces of the brain impacting upon the sharpest and most confined parts of skull are maximal. Contusion can also occur both under the direct point of impact of the injury and directly opposite it (contrecoup injury).
- *Haemorrhage* occurs when the blood vessels supplying oxygen to the brain are ruptured.

3.1.2 Secondary damage

Secondary damage includes injury due to haematoma (collections of blood), cerebral haemorrhage leading to anoxic damage or death, subarachnoid haemorrhage, swelling, infection, hydrocephalus (buildup of cerebrospinal fluid), and anoxic damage due to breathing difficulties or low blood pressure.

3.2 Clinical presentation and natural course

For the majority of severely injured patients improvement takes place slowly over months and years. It is usually best to use the word 'improvement' rather than 'recovery' after more severe injuries, as recovery implies complete restoration of function which may well not occur. Permanent cognitive impairments are probable with severe injuries, although for some they will be quite subtle and only evident under stress, in busy environments, or on formal testing. Cognitive impairments are rarely absent after very severe and extremely severe injuries.

The rate and extent of recovery is impossible to predict early on and the process is not fully understood. It may involve the following:

- disrupted neurotransmitters regaining some of their original efficiency;
- damaged neurons repairing themselves/axonal sprouting;
- resolution of brain swelling and contusion, leading to restoration of neuronal efficiency;
- possibly some degree of neural plasticity for very widely distributed functions (e.g. language).

Typically, the majority of recovery occurs in the first 2 years after injury such that significant difficulties evident at 2 years rarely resolve completely thereafter. However, further small amounts of natural recovery can occur up to and beyond 5 years for extremely severe injuries. Adaptation to long-term disability is therefore an ongoing process and can result in improved function many years post-injury, especially when early rehabilitation has been limited.

3.3 Neuropsychological impairments

When physical disabilities (such as paresis, ataxia, dysarthria, dyspraxia, or reduced motor speed) are present, they are often the main concern for the patient during the first months after injury. Cognitive impairments, however, tend to have greater impact on long-term disability and handicap. These occur predominantly in the areas of attention, speed of information processing, explicit memory, and executive functioning. They reflect the most common areas of damage in the frontal and temporal cortical areas and with diffuse axonal shearing.

3.3.1 Attention (see Chapter 5)

- Impairments in speed of information processing are one of the most common deficits following severe head injury. These are often evident on tests such as the PASAT, Adult Memory and Information Processing Battery (AMIPB), Stroop Test, or Wechsler Adult Intelligence Scale III (WAIS-III) Digit Symbol Coding subtest. They may also be evident on tests requiring speed, e.g. WAIS-III Performance subtests or the Trail Making Test.
- Specific deficits in divided, selective, or sustained attention may be evident on tests such as the Test of Everyday Attention, WAIS-III Picture Completion subtest, and the Trail Making Test.
- Verbal active attention span is often impaired as evidenced by backward digit span deficits.

◆ Visuospatial attention span deficits may also be evident on tests such as the Corsi Block Tapping Test.

These deficits can cause reported problems with concentration, distractability, tasks requiring more effort, memory, fatigue, irritability, reduced speed of thinking, and increased error rates.

3.3.2 Memory (see Chapter 9)

Short- and long-term memory deficits are common for both verbal and visuospatial material.

◆ Verbal memory deficits are often indicated by impaired performance on paragraph recall tests and list learning tests (e.g. Wechsler Memory Scale III (WMS III) Paragraphs, WMS III Paired Associate Learning Test, AMIPB Story Recall and List Learning Tests).

◆ Visuospatial memory deficits are commonly indicated on measures such as Figure Recall Tests (e.g. Rey Complex Figure, AMIPB Figure Recall).

Remote memory and procedural/implicit memory functions are usually spared. Memory difficulties, therefore, usually involve new, explicit learning rather than previously learned material, overlearned procedures, and autobiographical memory. Some of the most commonly reported memory difficulties include not being able to remember conversations, appointments, reading material, peoples' names, new routes, or where things have been put. The patient may also report being told that they repeat themselves a lot.

3.3.3 Executive function (see Chapter 17)

Executive impairment following severe head injury is common. It is not unusual, however, for there to be little such evidence on formal testing—neuropsychological assessment is by its very nature highly structured and is conducted in a distraction-free setting. Therefore, judgements on executive impairments must often be inferred from behavioural observations, qualitative aspects of test performance, and reported observations by those close to the patient or other health-care professionals. The patient's own reports are of the utmost importance but difficulties with insight can often mean that they themselves are unaware of such deficits. Psychological denial of problems is a natural coping mechanism but can be mistaken for dysexecutive problems in some cases. Similarly, reports from those close to the patient may minimize difficulties due to their own psychological denial, in addition to the natural tendency to underplay the significance of difficulties early post-injury in the aftermath of major trauma.

◆ Deficits in cognitive flexibility, mental set shifting, and perseveration may be indicated on tests such as the Trail Making Test, Wisconsin Card Sorting Test, Stroop Test, Verbal Fluency Test, or the Card Sorting subtest of the Behavioural Assessment of Dysexecutive Syndrome (BADS).

◆ Verbal concept formation and verbal abstract thinking deficits may be evident on tests such as the WAIS-III Similarities subtest and on Proverbs tasks (e.g. from the WAIS-III Comprehension subtest).

- Planning and problem-solving deficits may be evident on tests such as the Six Elements, Zoo Search and Motor Action Program subtests of the BADS and by the quality of performance on tests such as the WAIS-III Block Design subtest and the copy task of figure recall tests.
- Insight difficulties may be highlighted through large discrepancies between patient and others' reports of problems. Assessment of insight may be aided by separate administration of standard problem schedules with patients and family members as part of routine assessment.
- Specific questionnaires may also highlight cognitive, behavioural, and emotional problems associated with executive impairments (e.g. Dex questionnaire from the BADS).

Observed problems in executive functioning might include, fragmented speech, a reduced abstract reasoning, fixed and concrete thinking, poor initiation, egocentricity, a reduced creativity, tangential speech, reduced insight or difficulties with organizing thoughts, social regulation, decision-making, problem-solving and adapting to new situations.

3.3.4 Language (see Chapter 14)

Pure language and dysphasic impairments following uncomplicated head injury are less common than attentional, memory, and executive impairments. Indeed, some language-based tests are used as 'hold' measures to help estimate premorbid levels of intellectual functioning, due to their resistance to the effects of brain injury of a generalized nature (e.g. National Adult Reading Test, WAIS-III Vocabulary subtest). Problems with word finding, sentence construction, and paraphasias, however are common language-based impairments.

3.3.5 Visual perception (see Chapter 11)

Visual perceptual impairments following uncomplicated head injury are rare. A small but significant proportion may have visuoconstructional difficulties but visual agnosias are not often seen. However patients may be slow in their processing of visual material.

3.3.6 Summary of cognitive impairments

A wide range of cognitive impairments is therefore seen after severe head injury. It can often be difficult to predict their specific impact upon an individual's life after head injury as such deficits typically form part of a complex interaction of cognitive and other disabilities. Management and the resultant long-term impact of cognitive impairment are also mediated by level of insight, the use of compensatory strategies, and the extent of concomitant behavioural and emotional difficulties.

3.3.7 Neurobehavioural problems

An extensive array of behavioural change is often reported after severe head injury including increased irritability, disinhibition, impulsivity, emotional lability, mood swings, and aggressive outbursts. Deficits in executive functioning (leading to lack of insight, egocentricity, poor social regulation, and low initiation) often mean that a head-injured patient's personality is seen as significantly changed, by both themselves and by others. In addition, problems arising from other impairments, such as fatigue, low drive, frustration, irritability, and reduced emotional and behavioural control, may lead to a very significant sense of changed personality. The wide range of behavioural changes observed therefore reflect an interaction of primary neurological damage and secondary psychological reactions to head injury and its effects.

3.4 Related emotional disorders

Short- and long-term emotional sequelae of severe head injury include the following.

- Post-traumatic stress reactions (PTS) relating to the events that caused or followed the head injury (e.g. RTA, assaults, etc). While unconsciousness and organic amnesia from severe injury can protect against PTS, this is not always the case. The prevalence of PTS, however, is almost certainly much less than in mild or moderate head injury.

- Anger, frustration, depression, and anxiety are common emotional responses to the disabilities that patients confront. For some these may be an early reaction to the trauma of neurological illness/injury; the loss of skills, roles, and control over one's life; the slow pace of progress; and the uncertain extent of future recovery. Reduced impulse control may also exacerbate the control of anger, irritability, and aggression. However, early in rehabilitation, many may appear unconcerned about their predicament due to limited insight into the extent of cognitive and emotional/behavioural changes, together with unrealistic expectations of a full recovery.

- Major distress in adjusting to and coming to terms with the losses and changes arising as a result of a head injury e.g. breakup of relationships, inability to return to work, shattered aspirations and ambitions, and changes in personality and sense of identity.

These responses often develop over many years as changes and disabilities become emotionally 'accepted' by the patients as being permanent.

3.5 Social and family consequences

The complex array of disability after head injury often has far-reaching social consequences.

- Those with the most severe injuries may require assistance in daily living. This may include practical assistance in personal and domestic care for those with severe physical disability and guidance or supervision for those with marked cognitive or personality changes. Others may be independent in daily care but unable to travel independently. They may need help from the family in making decisions or managing their financial affairs.

- Many will not be able to return to former training or employment. Reduced cognitive and motor speed, limited concentration, unreliable memory, headaches, and/or fatigue combine to render many uncompetitive in the workplace. Specific physical, cognitive, and emotional/behavioural difficulties may restrict or preclude a return to occupations where such skills are vital.

◆ Leisure pursuits are often compromised by motor, sensory, and cognitive difficulties. Friendships and social opportunities often decline progressively over subsequent years. This may be due to a combination of loss of confidence, low mood, intolerance to noise, or difficulty in contributing to conversations on the part of the patient, and embarrassment and unease on the part of others in response to unpredictable behaviour and loss of refinement in social skills.

The social impact for the patient is often paralleled by major impact upon the family. High levels of stress and distress for primary carers are common, tending to increase rather than decrease over time after very and extremely severe injuries. Marital relationships often become strained with increased discord and high rates of marital breakdown after more severe injuries. For couples who remain together, there is often a reduction in emotional intimacy and a lower frequency and satisfaction in sexual relations. Spouses may struggle to cope with competing needs of work, home, partner, and children, whilst parents may find themselves locked into a long-term caring role for their adult children, with major concerns about the future. The impact on children and siblings can also be marked but tends to be more variable. Many families face far-reaching changes in roles and relationships and disruption to overall family functioning. As life revolves around the needs of the patient, so the occupational, leisure, and social lives of family members often falter.

3.6 Treatment/rehabilitation (see Chapter 4)

The focus of neuropsychological rehabilitation varies according to the nature and severity of injury, the patients' psychosocial context, the clinical setting (e.g. acute, post-acute, or community), and time since injury. Early rehabilitation optimizes outcome, but late rehabilitation can also improve function significantly. Two key principles, however, underpin rehabilitation.

◆ The engagement and maintainance of patient (and family) involvement with rehabilitation services by the provision of an emotionally supportive environment and relationships within which empathic expert help can be easily accessed.

◆ A primary focus of increasing the patient's (and their family's) understanding of head injury, the patient's strengths and weaknesses, and the means by which impairments may be best managed.

These principles become increasingly important as the patient moves beyond acute settings to post-acute and community settings where engagement with services may be impeded by poor insight, lack of understanding, psychological denial, emotional disorder, or challenging behaviour.

In addition there are at least four important elements in the process of early rehabilitation:

- engaging the patient (and their family) in the rehabilitation process;
- facilitating the setting of realistic rehabilitation targets and goals;
- facilitating the achievement of targets and goals via coordinated interventions;
- evaluating, reviewing, and modifying targets and goals over time.

Successful engagement of a patient (and their family) is often linked intrinsically to the collaborative development of realistic targets and goals. It is common for the patient (and their family), initially, to have unrealistic expectations about the extent and pace of targets that are achievable (e.g. complete cognitive recovery or return to full time work within weeks of injury). These commonly need to be negotiated to allow for more time, a greater number of intervening targets, or the inclusion of additional forms of support. Formal goal planning procedures may help this process, although there is no evidence as yet that they affect outcomes.

The principles that guide the setting of goals and targets should include the following:

- the maintenance and development of appropriate levels of cognitive stimulation while avoiding cognitive overloading;
- education and minimization of the vicious cycle of cognitive impairments leading to reduced coping, leading to distress, leading to exacerbated cognitive impairments, etc.;
- the emphasis of cognitive rehabilitation through compensatory strategies and prostheses rather than through cognitive restoration and 'brain function therapy'(i.e. de-emphasizing the analogy that the brain operates like a muscle and discouraging inappropriate attempts to train unaffected brain areas to take over damaged areas);
- the provision of emotional support and specific psychological interventions for the emotional sequelae associated with head injuries for both the patient and their family;
- facilitating patients' and families' adjustment to changes in personality, identity, and psychosocial functioning;
- liaison with education and vocational systems to advise on and plan return to previous work or education.

Coordination and review of interventions are essential so that there is continuous feedback between professionals, patient, and family. This helps interventions to remain focused on mutually agreed goals and for targets and goals to be refined and modified as the patient progresses or circumstances change.

The use of groups for cognitive rehabilitation, education, and emotional support should not be underestimated. These allow peer support, sharing of cognitive and emotional coping responses, and an opportunity to provide formal education in an efficient way. They can be a very powerful and supportive means for developing insight into impairments and for exploring ways of minimizing disability.

Cognitive rehabilitation strategies that benefit patients with severe head injury are usually pragmatic in nature. Neuropsychological assessment, however, is vital for informing what strategies should be attempted, what modifications might be beneficial, what might cause strategies to be unsuccessful, how to develop new strategies, and what kind of advice and education is appropriate. The following list highlights frequent examples of management strategies for common areas of difficulty-general cognitive function; memory; executive function; behaviour difficulties; social skills. The list is not exhaustive and there is significant overlap between these areas.

3.6.1 General cognitive strategies

- Developing habits, routines, and overlearned procedures to:
  - —maximize the use of implicit and procedural memory functions;
  - —provide structure;
  - —minimize cognitive load.
- Developing a tidy living and working environment where belongings are kept in the same, intuitively obvious, places and can easily be found. This helps to minimize demand on memory and problem-solving skills and make maximum use of spared implicit memory.
- Taking many small breaks when impairments become apparent rather than 'pushing on' until forced to take a break due to 'cognitive overload'.
- Rearranging working environments to minimize background noise, 'busyness', unexpected events, and time pressures. This helps to reduce restrictions arising from attentional deficits, slow speed of information processing, and cognitive inflexibility.
- Graduated return to premorbid activities and minimization of nonessential activity to reduce cognitive overload and fatigue. This maximizes the chances of successful completion of activities.
- Identifying specific times or specific types of activity where fatigue, irritability, anxiety, or frustration occur and facilitating appropriate changes in these areas.
- Training the patient to allow extra time for tasks where temporal judgement or speed of information processing is reduced.
- Using a diary systematically as:
  - —an *aide-mémoire*;
  - —a means of structuring time;
  - —an orientation 'anchor';
  - —an aid to overcoming initiation difficulties; or
  - —a reminder of key messages, conclusions, and 'self-statements' from therapy.

3.6.2 Strategies for managing memory (see Chapter 10)

- Using a dictaphone/tape recorder to record meetings, lectures, etc., i.e. as an *aide-mémoire*.

- Using a watch with an alarm or a paging device as a cue to look at a diary or to perform particular tasks. (This may also increase immediate arousal levels sufficiently to overcome initiation impairments.)

- Systematically using written or photo journals for episodic memory deficits (memory for events).

- Using notes, calendars, and lists as external cues and reminders. These may also help with initiation difficulties.

- Introducing a noticeboard or white board in a prominent place in the home to prompt patients about specific actions, as well as daily/weekly schedules.

- Systematizing storage of household items with explicit labelling (e.g. colour coding). (Such strategies are especially important for safety of toxic substances for patients with visual agnosia.)

- Using errorless learning when teaching new skills to minimize the need to 'unlearn' mistakes, i.e. prompting and cueing in such a way that no errors are made during a training process.

- Developing internal memory strategies via repetition, association, chunking, visualization of verbal material, verbalization of visual material, or maximizing the relevance and depth of understanding of material. It should be noted, however, that the degree of cognitive effort required for such 'internal' memory strategies often exceeds their utility for patients with memory and executive impairments. They can, however, be useful for specific tasks like remembering names of people or studying for an exam where external strategies are inappropriate.

- Using principles from behavioural psychology such as shaping, modelling, chaining, and contingent reinforcement to maximize learning of new skills.

3.6.3 Strategies for executive difficulties (see Chapter 18)

- Providing problem-solving skills training to help develop an explicit and systematic approach to solving difficulties, e.g.
  —defining the problem to be overcome;
  —generating different strategies to overcome the problem;
  —highlighting the pros and cons of each strategy;
  —deciding the best strategy based on the pros and cons;
  —implementing the strategy;
  —evaluating the outcome.

- Using an alarmed stopwatch to help monitor the amount of time taken on given tasks to help planning and temporal judgement impairments.

- Using self-talk and self-instruction (verbal mediation) to help overcome initiation problems and as a reminder of self-statements for aiding social regulation.

- Breaking tasks down into their component steps with written instructions to reduce disabilities from planning deficits.
- Introduce repeating routine/cycles to reduce unnecesary decision-making (e.g. weekly menus, shopping lists, set times for visiting the gym, etc.).

3.6.4 Strategies for behavioural management

- Identifying a small range of people to provide behavioural feedback to help modify inappropriate social behaviours. This should be done with careful and sensitive collaboration between the patient and those providing the feedback. (It is important to stress that the feedback should be immediate, concrete, supportive, and constructive and aimed at very specific behaviours only.)
- Using a handheld counter to aid the self-monitoring of specified inappropriate social behaviours.
- Using video feedback to improve insight into specific inappropriate behaviours. As patients may be surprised or upset by being confronted visibly with inappropriate behaviours this should always:
  —be discussed and negotiated carefully with the patient;
  —be undertaken in a controlled and supportive atmosphere;
  —be conducted with sufficient time allocated for debriefing immediately afterwards.
- Using principles from behavioural psychology to help shape, model, and increase the frequency of appropriate social behaviours.

3.6.5 Strategies for social skills

- Teaching conversation skills for slowing, pacing, and allowing 'thinking time' during interactions to help minimize word finding, sentence construction, and concentration difficulties in conversation.
- Teaching social skills so that the patient is comfortable asking for things to be repeated during conversation when attention, memory, or language deficits have caused them to lose track.
- Encouraging others to use short sentences and high-frequency words and to allow enough time for the patient to reply to questions when word finding, attentional, receptive language, or expressive language impairments are present.
- Encouraging those close to patient to use closed, multiple-choice type questions rather than open-ended questions when decision-making and initiation of ideas are impaired.

3.6.6 Intervention for related emotional disorders

Psychological interventions for emotional disorders following head injury have largely been developed from the adult mental health field of clinical psychology and adapted to the specific challenges of this population. The most common forms of intervention include both individual and group therapies in the following areas:

- cognitive behavioural psychotherapy (CBT) with exposure and/or cognitive restructuring for post-traumatic stress symptoms;

- CBT for anger management;

- CBT for anxiety and depression;

In utilizing such interventions it is vital that the neuropsychological context and constraints are accommodated in the therapeutic process.

Alongside these types of interventions, there is a need for specialist 'neurorehabilitation counselling' to assist clients in their understanding and coping with the effects of head injury during the course of recovery. This is likely to involve provision of the following:

- general information and explanation about head injury;

- feedback about specific impairments;

- explanation of treatment rationale; negotiation of treatment goals;

- general advice and emotional support;

- promotion of insight, awareness, and coping strategies;

- progress review.

While the above list outlines some of the most commonly used interventions, it is in no way exhaustive. Also, it is essential that emotional disorders after head injury are addressed within the overall context of the head injury and patients' aspirations, hopes, social network, and overall psychosocial circumstances. 'Atomizing' their emotional experiences to a series of disorders or symptoms will not adequately address the complexity of emotional needs. Indeed, this principle must underpin all forms of rehabilitation for head-injured patients.

3.6.7 Facilitating personal and family adjustment

Many persons with severe head injury face major challenges of adjustment as they are unable to resume their former work, family, and social roles. The process of psychological adjustment is compounded by executive difficulties, especially lack of insight and reduced capacity for self-appraisal and problem-solving, often combined with lack of emotional and behavioural control. Without specialist help many struggle to make the necessary adjustments to their residual disability and continue to strive for an unrealistic degree of recovery. Others make decisions that do not take due account of restrictions arising from head injury, leading to repeated failure and loss of confidence and self belief.

Specialist 'neuropsychotherapy' may assist the person in addressing these issues and finding a positive way forward. This commonly involves the following:

♦ clarifying the long-term effects of the injury;

♦ reviewing strengths and weaknesses;

♦ making sense of and reconciling changes in the person and their lives;

♦ identifying, clarifying, and prioritizing unresolved issues;

♦ supported problem-solving in finding a new direction through which to start to re-build their lives.

Return to education or employment represents for many a major decision that can either facilitate positive adjustment or provoke a downward spiral of failure. For those unable to return to previous employment, a programme of specialist vocational rehabilitation may be required to highlight vocational restrictions, prepare the person for a graded return to employment, and guide and support them in their vocational adjustment to a position more suited to their residual disability.

It is vital to include the family as fully as possible in the process of rehabilitation. Close liaison with the family is essential both to obtain feedback about difficulties and progress in the home and to explain rehabilitation strategies, which can then be reinforced by family members. However, the needs of families warrant attention in their own right as family members may themselves need specialist advice and support in understanding and coping with the impact of severe head injury both upon themselves and the family as a whole. A range of family services is required to facilitate family adjustment including family education, individual family support, and specialist marital and family counselling.

3.7 The effectiveness of rehabilitation and treatment

Studies evaluating the effectiveness of cognitive rehabilitation for patients with severe head injury are relatively sparse and frequently suffer from significant methodological constraints. There is some modest evidence that restorative techniques involving repeated practice of specific tasks in laboratory settings can be effective for improving some specific attention and language-based functions. There is little evidence, however, that any gains are generalized to everyday activities. Restorative strategies for other impairments have virtually no empirical support. In contrast, the current evidence regarding compensatory strategies indicates that these are effective in reducing everyday memory failures, minimizing anxiety, increasing self-concept and improving quality of interpersonal relationships. Behavioural approaches aimed at maximizing skill acquisition and monitoring, including performance feedback and reinforcement, have also demonstrated their efficacy. It is these types of rehabilitation that generalize best to everyday life situations.

The cognitive rehabilitation programmes that have the strongest outcomes tend to be those combining early intervention, compensatory strategies, and supported employment. Our clinical experience is that neuropsychological interventions (including educational, cognitive, behavioural, psychotherapeutic, and family components) are most effective when delivered as part of specialist interdisciplinary brain injury rehabilitation programmes, and there is evidence that such multifaceted post-acute rehabilitation programmes can significantly improve psychosocial outcome after severe head injury.

4 Summary and conclusions

Patients with head injury present with a complex interaction of cognitive, behavioural, and emotional changes, which often exert a major impact upon their lives and the lives of their family.

After mild and moderate head injury cognitive impairments are usually of mild severity and temporary. Speed of information processing is most frequently affected, but reaction time and short-term and long-term memory deficits are also common. Posttraumatic stress reactions are at least as prevalent as for those without head injury. Where post-concussion symptoms persist frustration, anxiety, and depression are common reactions to the disabilities caused by these. Anxiety can also result from uncertainty over the relative contribution of psychological and organic factors to problems and the uncertainty of ultimate prognosis.

After severe head injury cognitive impairments are often wide-spread, significant, and permanent. They are most often in some or more of the following domains:

- speed of information processing;
- divided, selective, and sustained attention;
- short- and long-term memory;
- executive function;
- expressive language (in terms of word finding and sentence construction).

Depression, anger, anxiety, and frustration often result from the disabilities caused by severe head injury, while posttraumatic stress reactions are less prevalent than in mild/moderate injuries. Irritability, anger, and aggression can be exacerbated by reduced impulse control. Difficulties in long-term adjustment are common, as are difficulties in marital, family, and social relationships.

Specialist neuropsychological interventions are required across acute, post-acute, and community settings if patients are to make and sustain their optimal recovery. For those with mild and moderate injury, early brief assessment and intervention can usually reduce further complications. Patients with severe head injury, however, whilst often responding positively to rehabilitation and making marked improvement over a period of years, are frequently left with substantial psychological disability and associated social restrictions. Patients often struggle to maintain the full benefits of rehabilitation once active therapeutic involvement has been phased out, particularly those with executive difficulties. Even after long periods when patients have appeared settled, they may struggle to adapt to changes in work, family, and social circumstances. As such, further intervention may be required from time to time throughout the whole of their life. Open-door access to specialist rehabilitation and support is therefore vital if patients and their families are to maintain optimal adjustment to the long-term effects of their injury.

Selective references

British Psychological Society (1989). *Services for adults patients with acquired brain injury*. British Psychological Society, Leicester.

Carney, N., Chestnnut, R.M., Maynard, H., Mann, N.C., Patterson, P., and Helfund, M. (1999). Effect of cognitive rehabilitation on outcomes for persons with traumatic brain injury: a systematic review. *J. Head Trauma Rehabil.* **14**, 271–307.

King, N.S. (1997). Mild head injury. Neuropathology, sequelae, measurement and recovery. *Br. J. Clin. Psychol.* **36**, 161–84.

Ponsford, J. (1995). *Traumatic brain injury: rehabilitation for everyday adaptive living*. Psychology Press, Lawrence Erlbaum, Hove.

Robertson, I. (1990). Does computerised cognitive rehabilitation work: a review. *Aphasiology* **4**, 381–405.

Rose, F.D. and Johnson, D.A. (1996). *Brain injury and after. Towards improved outcome*. John Wiley and Son, Chichester.

Tyerman A (1991). Counselling in head injury. In *Counselling and communication in healthcare* (ed. H. Davis and L. Fallowfield), pp. 115–28. John Wiley and Son, Chichester.

Tyerman A. (1999). Head injury: community rehabilitation. In *Rehabilitation of the physically disabled adult*, 2nd edn (ed. C.J. Goodwill, M.A. Chamberlain, and C.D. Evans), pp. 432–43. Stanley Thornes, Cheltenham.

Wade, D.T., King, N.S., Wenden, F.S., Crawford, S., and Caldwell, F.E. (1998). Routine follow-up after head injury: a second randomised controlled trial. *J. Neurol., Neurosurg., Psychiatry* **65**, 177–83.

Chapter 28

Neuropsychological presentation of Alzheimer's disease and other neurodegenerative disorders

Robin G. Morris and Claire L. Worsley

1 Introduction

This chapter outlines the neuropsychological presentation of neurodegenerative disorders, those in which an idiopathic degeneration of the brain takes place, resulting in cognitive dysfunction. The main disorders are considered with the exception of demyelinating disorders, which are dealt with in Chapter 29. Neurodegeneration is the primary cause of neuropsychological dysfunction in adults and, within this, Alzheimer's disease (AD) can be considered to be the most common form. Neurodegenerative disorders can affect neuropsychological functioning in several ways. Generalized dysfunction, or dementia, can be a prime feature from the start, as is frequently the case with AD following a prodromal period. Alternatively, the disorder is accompanied by certain types of cognitive dysfunction and, in a proportion of patients, this becomes generalized. Parkinson's disease falls into this category. Neurodegenerative disorders also vary in terms of the location of brain deterioration, and the balance between cognitive and motoric involvement is reflected generally in the relative involvement of cortical and subcortical structures—although this notion is simplistic because of the role of structures such as the basal ganglia in cognitive dysfunction (e.g. in Parkinson's disease) and the motor cortex in motor impairment (e.g. in motor neuron disease). Nevertheless, these distinctions are used as a basis for the sections that follow.

The first main section focuses on the relevance of understanding the neuropsychology of neuro-degenerative disorders to clinical practice. Section 3 concerns AD. An in-depth understanding of the cognitive neuropsychology of this illness is presented. The bulk of neuropsychological studies have focused on this disease and Section 3 presents what was described by Morris (1996) as the 'patch work of theories' that cover different aspects of cognitive impairment in AD. This is followed by Section 4 on other neuro-degenerative causes of dementia. Section 5 includes disorders where extrapyramidal motoric dysfunction is a main feature, but with additional neuropsychological impairments or dementia.

2 Clinical context

In clinical practice, the clinical neuropsychologist may be called upon to assess cognitive functioning in the full range of neurodegenerative disorders and the approach used may call for an understanding of each in turn. In broad terms three main areas of understanding can be identified:

♦ detection of neuropsychological impairment;

♦ identification of disability;

♦ monitoring change.

2.1 Detection of neuropsychological impairment

At the early stages of neurodegenerative disorders such as AD, determining whether cognitive dysfunction exists may require more than simple mental status examinations or dementia rating scales. A neuropsychological assessment can be used to detect impairment where it exists and, conversely, rule out this possibility in patients who may incorrectly perceive significant cognitive impairment. Detection has implications for early diagnosis and management (e.g. through pharmacological intervention). In other disorders, such as Parkinson's disease, where dementia only occurs in a proportion of patients, a neuropsychological approach can be used to determine whether this is the case or whether there only exists subtle cognitive impairment. Knowledge of the neuropsychological profile associated with each disorder helps guide the choice of assessment procedures.

2.2 Identification of disability

Even within specific neurodegenerative disorders there can be considerable variation in presentation, and understanding this can aid in the management of a patient. Knowledge of relative strengths and weaknesses can inform appropriate advice and intervention in a large range of areas, from assessing competence to drive to helping with possible compensatory strategies, such as in memory retraining.

2.3 Monitoring change

In terms of management and treatment, neuropsychological assessment can be used to provide a baseline from which to monitor further changes in function. This applies to early diagnosis, where subtle cognitive changes are difficult to interpret but, on follow-up, a deteriorating pattern can confirm neurodegenerative progression. In the context of pharmacological intervention, neuropsychological assessment can be used to determine treatment effects, although, currently, this tends to occur in research settings, rather than routine clinical practice. Whilst understanding the neuropsychological profile can help tailor neurorehabilitation approaches in neurodegenerative disorders, it should be acknowledged that changes in the quality of life and in the daily living skills of the patient may be more important outcome indicators than neuropsychological function in the narrow sense.

3 Alzheimer's disease

Alzheimer's disease (AD) is the most common neurodegenerative disorder resulting in neuropsychological dysfunction and the most well known of the 'cortical' dementias. As with some of the other types of dementia, a firm diagnosis *in vivo* cannot be made. Instead, certain diagnostic criteria are applied to determine with different degrees of certainty whether a person has AD. Hence, many of the findings relating to AD outlined below refer to patients with 'probable' AD.

Of all the different dementias, because of the ubiquity of this disorder, the clinical presentation and neuropathological basis of AD have been the most extensively studied, yielding a substantial understanding of the cognitive neuropsychological features (Morris 1996). The neurodegeneration affects all cognitive functions in the end, but at the early stages there are clear areas of relative preservation, as indicated in the following subsections.

The neurobiological changes can be summarized as follows:

◆ Gross atrophy, with widening sulci and ventricular enlargement, with the frontoparietal region and temporal lobes most affected.

◆ Senile or neuritic plaques that are widely distributed in the cortex, the hippocampus, and certain subcortical structures such as the putamen, locus cerulus, and hypothalamus. They tend to occur first in neocortical areas.

◆ Neurofibrillary tangles affect more areas but the main ones are the neocortex in general, the hippocampus, amygdala, and parahippocampal gyri. Subcortical regions are also affected and these include the thalamus, the mamillary bodies, the nucleus basalis of Meynert, the substantia nigra, and locus cerulus.

The density of these changes has been shown to correlate well with the degree of dementia and there is some regional specificity in terms of linking changes to specific impairments (Morris 1996). In addition, a range of neurotransmitter systems are implicated, including cholinergic, noradrenergic, and serotinergic systems.

These changes produce predictable neuropsychological impairments. A series of investigations have delineated the general pattern, but it should be noted that considerable heterogeneity exists and this may depend on the precise areas of damage in each patient. For example, metabolic asymmetries between the hemispheres have been observed and these are associated with varying degrees of either language or visuospatial impairment. Also, some patients present early on with executive dysfunction as the main feature, whilst others present with memory impairment. Such variability means that the notion of an AD general profile of cognitive dysfunction should be viewed with caution, although group studies have identified features that characterize AD in broad terms, as outlined below.

3.1 Prodromal features

The onset of AD is insidious, consistent with the neurodegenerative nature of the disease. Because of this, there is a prodromal phase in which neuropsychological impairment is present, but the patient has not yet been diagnosed as having AD. The nature of this impairment has been investigated by following up groups of normal people, testing their cognitive functioning, and then retrospectively inspecting the functioning of those who have subsequently 'developed' AD. Studies suggest that the prodromal period can last up to 20 years, with measurable decline 2–3 years before symptoms are manifested and 4–5 years before the criteria for AD can be met (Fox *et al.* 1998). The main feature is a subtle and isolated memory impairment (although the existence of isolated mild memory impairment should be viewed extremely cautiously as indicating future AD). The prodromal memory decline has been linked to hippocampal atrophy and decreased cerebral perfusion in mesiotemporal regions, including the hippocampus and the amygdala, as well as the cingulate gyrus (Jack *et al.* 1999).

3.2 Language

Language dysfunction is apparent even early on in AD, with an estimate that it is seen in 8–10% of patients as a major symptom (Kertesz 1994). One of the main features is problems with word retrieval, accompanied by a necessarily circumlocutious style of language production. As the dementia progresses, comprehension difficulties emerge and careful analysis of language production suggests that the syntax is simplified. Other signs of language dysfunction at this stage include a reduction in the overall content or meaning of the language produced, with paraphasic errors and verbal perseveration common features. At the end stage, the patient may only be able to produce simple phrases or words or repeat nonsense sounds, finally becoming mute (see Table 28.1).

The different aspects of language have been explored and generalizations can be made concerning the overall pattern. This can be split into the following areas:

♦ *Phonology* is generally preserved in AD, in the sense that patients are able to produce the sounds of words appropriately, at least until the advanced stages, including segmental sound combinations and prosody.

♦ *Syntax production* also shows some degree of preservation early on, in that syntactically correct language output is a common feature but, when analysed in detail, this may not be so for complex syntactical structures. In general, syntactical forms that are overlearned or 'automatic' show preservation.

♦ *Word retrieval difficulties* have been demonstrated across a range of tests. Prominent among these have been the various forms of word fluency tests in which a person has to generate a series of words according to a given rule. With the controlled oral word association test, in which a series of words has to be generated beginning with a certain letter, AD patients show substantial impairment. AD patients appear to be better differentiated from controls if they are required to produce words of a particular category (e.g. names of animals; Rosen 1980), but this may be because of the larger semantic or executive memory load. Confrontation naming can also be substantially impaired, with real objects less problematic than photographs or drawings, suggesting a perceptual as well as a word retrieval component. Additionally, breakdown of semantic memory contributes to problems with naming (see Section 3.7.3).

Table 28.1 Language impairment at the different stages of Alzheimer's disease

Prodromal stage
Mild word-finding difficulties
Early stage
Word-finding difficulties affect both naming and spontaneous language production
Circumlocutional discourse
Middle stage
Difficulties with comprehension relating mainly to more complex material
Simpler syntactical structures with vague and sometimes meaningless content
Paraphasias (often semantic)
Ideational perseveration
Late stage
Single words or phrases repeated in a meaningless fashion
Nonsense sounds produced and repeated
Mutism at the end stages

◆ Comprehension impairment is readily evident in AD. In relation to comprehension of material with different levels of syntactic complexity, there is a clear effect of difficulty in performance contributing to comprehension problems; although this may also partly be due to differences in semantics associated with these levels of complexity. An additional feature is that people with AD appear to lose an understanding of the truth values of statements, along with a loss of pragmatic use of language as a means of interacting with other people.

There is some consensus that the language disturbance in AD has a specific profile unlike the main patterns of aphasia. However, the profile can be said to be most like that of transcortical sensory aphasia, with relatively preserved fluency of articulation and repetition of words, but poor comprehension.

3.3 Reading

Reading impairment in AD can be understood in relation to a cognitive analysis of reading function. Here, the standard models suggest a lexical route that has direct access to language output, contrasting with a sublexical route that links up a visual analysis of a word through grapheme to phoneme conversion, the latter being involved in learning. A third route is through lexical analysis to the semantic system and then language production. In AD the main pattern (see also Mathias 1996; Morris and Worsley 2001) is as follows.

- Semantic processing contributes substantially to reading problems and deteriorates before lexical access. For this reason, reading comprehension shows more impairment than, for example, the ability to read single words out loud without necessarily understanding them.

- There is relative preservation in reading words with irregular spellings (e.g. cellist), as exemplified by performance on the National Adult Reading Test—Restandardized (NART-R). The irregular spellings force reliance on either the lexical or semantic route, the former showing relative preservation and hence supporting reading ability.

- There is also some evidence in some cases of AD for a form of surface dyslexia, whereby, as the semantic system deteriorates, patients can utilize the sublexical route with grapheme to phoneme conversion.

Because of preserved oral reading of single words, the NART-R has become an established method for estimating premorbid intelligence in AD. In normal older adults the NART-R has been found to be a good predictor of intelligence. It accounts for about two-thirds of the variance in performance on the Wechsler Adult Intelligence Scale (WAIS), considerably better than the combination of education and social class (Crawford *et al.* 1989). In AD, NART-R performance holds up well, although some decline does eventually take place (Patterson *et al.* 1994; see also Morris *et al.* 2000).

3.4 Writing and spelling

Impairment in writing in AD is an early sign, but also tends to correlate with the severity of dementia, reflecting many of the characteristics of language (including semantic) dysfunction in general. In addition to this, nonlinguistic aspects such as problems with praxis will contribute to writing deterioration. In terms of spelling, the same pattern as normal is seen, relating to the effect of lexical, phonological and orthographic variables when writing words to dictation. An example of this is the normal advantage of spelling regular words.

3.5 Attention

Four main aspects of attention have been investigated in AD and these are considered in turn.

- *Phasic attention*, which involves maintaining a state of readiness to respond for short periods, is unimpaired in early AD, as indicated by the normal facilitatory effect of warning tones in reaction time experiments (Nebes and Brady 1993).

- *Sustained attention*, perhaps surprisingly, is not impaired at the early stages of AD, as indicated by a vigilance task in which a target digit has to be detected in stream of digits over a long period (Lines *et al.* 1991).

- *Selective attention*, however, is impaired and this has been demonstrated using the Posner Spatial Attentional Shift Paradigm, where a key has to be pressed if stimulus appears either to the left or right of a computer screen. A warning arrow can either provide congruent or incongruent information about the position of the stimulus, either appropriately engaging attention or forcing the subject to disengage attention to the inappropriate location in order to respond. The most comprehensive study by Parasuraman *et al.* (1992) shows that the deficit in AD lies in disengaging attention. Auditory attentional impairments have also been shown using the Dichotic Listening task, in which patients with AD have been shown to fail to show the normal right ear advantage when recalling digits (Mohr *et al.* 1990)

- *Divided attention* is consistently impaired in AD (Morris 1996; Baddeley *et al.* 1991) as indicated in Section 3.6.

3.6 Executive function

3.6.1 Cognitive signs

The inability to coordinate and sequence mental activity and behaviour is a characteristic feature of AD, with only subtle impairment at the early stages, but considerable difficulties when the dementia is moderate. A variety of tests have been used to demonstrate executive impairment, and these include the Wisconsin Card Sorting Test, the Stroop Test, Verbal Fluency, and Random Generation of Digits (Becker *et al.* 1992). Core impairment on these tests is found relating to mental flexibility, initiation, and response inhibition. Low performance is also associated with impairment in other functions that support test performance, such as language or visuospatial functioning. Some studies have identified subgroups of AD in which executive impairment is more pronounced, but these tend to become more generalized as the dementia progresses (Becker *et al.* 1992; Baddeley *et al.* 1991).

3.6.2 Working memory

This term encompasses material that is held in memory up to approximately 30 seconds and frequently involves manipulation of the material, such as computation or reordering. Because the use of the material guides cognitive processing and the manipulation of the material requires mental coordination, this can be viewed as an aspect of executive function. In AD, working memory impairment is reflected in a reduction in memory span performance and substantial impairment on the Petersen and Petersen test. Experimental investigations of working memory in AD have used the working memory model as a framework. This splits up the supporting cognitive structures into:

- a *central executive system* (CES) that coordinates working memory processes;
- a *verbal storage mechanism*, the articulatory loop system (ALS);
- a *visuospatial store*, the visuospatial scratchpad (VSSP).

The CES The CES is thought to be impaired in the early stages of AD as indicated by problems in a variety of tasks that require divided attention. These include the Petersen and Petersen task, where three memory items (e.g. letters) have to be remembered following a very short period of distraction. Even very simple distracter tasks, such as tapping the testing table with a hand rhythmically, have been found to result in substantial forgetting on this task (Morris 1996). More formal studies have combined remembering strings of digits, up to the digit span of each patient, with either detecting tones or tracking a moving object on a VDU screen with a light pen. Combining these tasks results in very substantial mutual interference (Baddeley *et al.* 1991).

The ALS In contrast, in the early stages of AD, the ALS appears to be intact, as indicated by the manner in which various phenomena related to the ALS are unaffected. This includes the word length effect in which shorter words normally result in a reduction in memory span, explained in terms of the lesser amount of time taken to rehearse material within the ALS. There is also the phonological similarity effect in which words dissimilar in phonological characteristics also result in better memory. These effects remain robust in AD at the early stages, but show some decline as the dementia progresses (Morris 1994; Collette *et al.* 1999). They explain why memory span impairment is relatively mild in comparison to other working memory tasks.

The VSSP The functioning of the VSSP has been investigated less extensively, but the reduction in the spatial equivalent of memory span (the Corsi Block Span Test) and tests that require retention of visuospatial material for short intervals, such as delayed matching to sample, are consistently impaired early in AD (Morris 1996).

3.6.3 Behavioural features

Random and purposeless behaviour is a characteristic of the presentation as the dementia becomes more severe and there is some evidence that this is linked to the breakdown of well-established behavioural routines (such as scripts; Kidron and Freedman 1996).

In addition, AD is associated with impairments in executive control relating to switching behaviour. Various forms of perseveration are common in AD and operate at different levels. These include the following.

- *Continuous perseveration,* related to disturbances in motor output, is an unchecked repetition of movement with continuous facilitation of the same motor impulses.
- *Stuck in set perseveration,* which has been seen to reflect postfacilitation of motor responses in which there is a breakdown between intent and action, creates difficulties in switching from one response to another.
- *Recurrent perseveration* involves repeating an unintentional response after a delay in response to a new stimulus. It was found that 88% of an AD group produced recurrent perseverations in a test battery, but none in a matched normal older adult sample (Fuld *et al.* 1982).

Patients with AD also exhibit utilization behaviour in which reaching responses are made to objects in the environment in an inappropriate fashion.

3.7 Memory

Memory function has been seen as the *sine qua non* of AD and the prodromal expression of memory disorder seems to support this idea. The memory impairment in AD is perhaps one of the most disabling, starting at the early stages with memory lapses, proceeding to difficulties in keeping track of daily events, and ending with severe amnesia and disorientation. The structural decomposition of memory makes possible a more detailed analysis of how memory is impaired in AD. The main distinctions create categories of memory. The principal categories will now be considered separately.

3.7.1 Episodic memory

This is the ability to recall events within a specific spatial temporal context after a period varying from minutes to hours or days. Table 28.2 indicates the effects of breakdown in episodic memory at the different stages of AD. In the initial stages, the memory impairment is only mild and the insidious onset is associated with a general forgetfulness that can be attributed wrongly to other factors. The spatial and temporal disorientation tends to develop later, starting with situations in which the person is outside their everyday routine, but then becoming more pervasive as the dementia progress.

The main explanation for the ubiquitous nature of the memory impairment in AD is likely to be the degree of damage to memory structures such as those in the mesiotemporal lobe. These include not only the hippocampus, but also the immediately connected cortical structures such as the parahippocampal gyrus and the perirhinal and

Table 28.2 Memory impairment in the different stages of Alzheimer's disease

Prodromal stage

Very mild memory difficulties but not yet seen as part of cluster of features that would indicate AD

Early stage

Mild memory lapses are seen, e.g. not passing on messages, forgetting errands, becoming disoriented in unfamiliar surroundings, and tending to repeat things or not remember everyday conversations consistently. At this stage memory impairment can be falsely attributed to other factors by relatives or friends

Middle stage

Very significant effect on everyday life emerges, e.g. disorientation in familiar surroundings, forgetting familiar friends, and an inability to keep track of daily events or conversations. Repetition of what is said can become frequent because of lack of monitoring of conversation. Memory lapses can be hazardous, e.g. forgetting to turn off the cooker or bathroom taps

Late stage

Severe memory difficulties with no memory for day-to-day events, associated with loss of recognition of close relatives and wandering.

Marked positive signs may occur, such as confabulation and paramnesia entorhinal cortices. In AD, severe neurodegeneration of the hippocampus is seen, particularly in relation to the CA1 fields. In addition, neurofibrillary tangles (NFTs), a neuropathological marker of AD, are seen in large amounts in the entorhinal cortices. Of note, a hierarchical progression of vulnerability, mapped using histological analysis of NFTs has been identified, with changes first in the entorhinal cortex, followed by the CA1 field, and then association cortices (Arriagada *et al.* 1992; Geula 1998). There is also evidence, using structural magnetic resonance imaging (MRI), that hippocampal volume reduction is related to episodic memory loss rather than to other aspects of cognition (Wilson *et al.* 1996).

A range of methods for measuring memory can be used to detect episodic memory impairment in AD, including recalling stories, sentences, individual words, word pairs, and recognition for words, pictures, and faces. The memory impairment is ubiquitous across these different techniques for measuring memory performance. Nevertheless, certain features have been identified that suggest an interaction between problems with remembering and problems with processing material. For example, memory for lists of words can normally be improved by clustering together material in the same semantic categories to aid retrieval. This effect is diminished in early AD (Weingartner *et al.* 1983). In addition, memory can be improved using associative links with other material, as in the case of the 'Depth of Processing' manipulation in which a word that has to be remembered is prefaced with an orientating sentence (e.g. Swan. Is this a type of bird?). It has been shown that people with AD fail to benefit from this type of orientation (Martin *et al.* 1985).

Nevertheless, a series of studies have shown that there are ways of circumventing the semantic problems that prevent patients taking advantage of orientating techniques. These include semantic–praxis cues in which the patient pantomimes a movement or series of movements. For this to work, the same movements are produced as a cue at the retrieval stage. Alternatively, when trying to remember an object, a semantic category cue can be given (such as 'find the animal' when looking at a picture). When this is matched at retrieval with a related cue (such as 'what animal did you see in the picture?'). These findings are consistent with the notion that encoding and retrieval processes share similar mechanisms, so that attempts to reactivate the encoding mechanism can help ameliorate the effects of memory impairment (Backman and Herlitz 1996).

3.7.2 Remote memory

A common clinical impression is that memory for distant events, e.g. childhood experiences, is more preserved in AD. Generally, this is the case, but the overall result may be biased by the fact that this is true for autobiographical memories for older adults in general. The most distant memories are more likely to be recounted. Those in middle age are less well recalled, with an increment in relation to recent memories. In AD, this general function was explored by Fromholt and Larsen (1991) using single words to cue memory. The overall result is that performance falls across the lifespan, but the lower baseline level of 'midlife' memories means that a greater proportion appear to be lost. Recent memories are also lost differentially. The overall effect tends to orientate patients to their distant past, a common phenomenon in people with moderate or severe AD.

Techniques that have explored the ability to remember the names of or recognize the faces of famous people show a deficit that is relatively constant across time periods (Greene and Hodges 1996).

3.7.3 Semantic memory

This refers to the storage of facts, rules, concepts, and associations—unlike in episodic memory, the retrieval and processing of such material is not dependent on the context in which it was learned. Semantic memory also encompasses understanding what objects are and so being able to talk about them or recognize them when presented.

In AD, there is evidence for loss of semantic memory early and this may account for the clinically observed 'emptiness of thought' that develops as the dementia progresses. In the early stages, semantic memory loss can be demonstrated using various methods.

- AD patients show an impairment on various versions of the Verbal Fluency Test, the ability to produce a series of words that begin with a certain letter or are in a specific category.

- Patients also have difficulties in naming objects, explained only in part by impairments in visual perception. It has been shown that, with object naming, a typical error is to provide a name relating to the same category (e.g. calling a violin a trumpet) or to the superordinate category (e.g. using the term 'musical instrument').

- Finally, there are impairments in matching pictures of appropriate objects or matching the name of an object to the picture of it.

Because these errors occur for the same type of item across tasks, this points to a core deficit relating to the underlying representation of the object, the semantic representation (Hodges *et al.* 1990).

Recently, it has been shown that category-specific semantic loss exists in AD, with some patients showing difficulties with living and others with non-living things (Garrard *et al.* 1998; Gonnerman *et al.* 1997). It has been hypothesized that these differential impairments reflect the heterogeneity of the underlying neurodegeneration (Garrard *et al.* 1998). Here focal damage to the temporal lobe has been associated with impairment in representing living things, while frontoparietal damage has been linked to impairment in representing non-living things. An alternative view, put forward by Gonnerman *et al.* (1997), is that representation of living things tends to preserved early in AD because living things have a larger number of intercorrelated attributes, making them less vulnerable. In later stages of AD, the deterioration of features of the representation causes a collapse of this correlational structure and the pattern of deficit reverses.

Another aspect of semantic memory is the ability to retain knowledge relating to the rules of everyday activities or social interaction. Although, superficially, aspects of social skills can be remarkably preserved in the early stages of AD, there is evidence for loss of schema or script knowledge. For example, in studies of scripts, a patient might be asked to describe the typical events involved in 'visiting a doctor' or 'going to a film.' There is a tendency to produce only the most central aspects of a script and also to have difficulties in assigning particular activities to certain types of scripts.

3.7.4 Procedural memory

In contrast to episodic and semantic memory, there are aspects of cognitive functioning in which learning takes place, but does not involve specific encoding and retrieval of material in which there is an awareness of the product of the retrieval mechanism. This includes various priming phenomena and perceptual and motor learning, all of which have been labelled aspects of *procedural memory*. In AD a distinct pattern emerges with respect to this type of memory.

Priming   A widely used test of priming is the stem completion task in which individual words are first presented. Later on, the first few letter are shown, with the patient having to produce the word (e.g. 'elephant' followed by the stem 'ele'). This is done without reference to recalling the previous words. Patients with AD are significantly less like to come up with the previous words than normal controls, or those with Huntington's disease or 'pure' amnesia (Salmon *et al*. 1988). Whilst other types of methodologies confirm this finding as well (Salmon and Fennema-Nostetine 1996), there are instances where normal priming effects have been observed. For example, if the initial presentation of a word is accompanied by a sentence frame (e.g. Hammer: He hit the nail with a . . .) in order to enhance the semantic processing of the word, normal stem completion can be obtained. Additionally, in the homophone spelling bias test, a semantically related word will bias the spelling of a subsequently presented homophone. For example, if the word 'moon' is presented, then when the word 'Sun' or 'Son' is presented aurally it is more likely to be spelt 'sun'. This effect is robust in early AD (Fennema-Notestine *et al*. 1994).

Perceptual learning   A facet of perceptual learning is perceptual priming where processing the perceptual features of a stimulus affects the subsequent processing of the same stimulus. This includes repetition priming in which the patient is required to read geometrically transformed script or identify previously presented words, but now degraded. In both cases, early AD patients show normal priming with significantly more rapid processing after prior exposure. (e.g. Grober *et al*. 1992). A different aspect is the perceptual biasing that can occur within sensorimotor processing. For example, lifting a weight for a while can bias the perception of the weight of another object, making the person think it is lighter. Such experiments have been conducted with AD patients and show the normal illusion, despite lack of memory for the original biasing experience (Heindel *et al*. 1991). Similarly, AD patients have been shown to be successful in adapting to distorting prisms that shift the relative location of objects 20 degrees to the right or left (Paulsen *et al*. 1993).

Skill learning   Normal skill acquisition has been shown in AD at a simple level. For example, Eslinger and Damasio (1986) compared the learning ability of AD patients and older adult controls on the Pursuit Rotor Task, which requires a patient to maintain a stylus over a rotating metallic disc. Improvements in this skill can also be measured whilst varying the difficulty of the task by varying the speed of rotation (Heindel *et al.* 1988). The performance of the AD patients improved significantly across trials, at the same rate as that of the controls. Preserved learning is also seen on more complex visuospatial tasks. These include the method applied by Nissen and Bullemer (1987) in which one of a set of four keys has to pressed in response to one of four lights. Repetitive sequences of lights followed by the keying response show specific learning. This type of learning was found to be normal in AD.

3.8 Visuospatial functioning

Visuospatial functioning tends to be sensitive to impairment in AD because of the substantial neurodegeneration that occurs in the parietal and temporal regions. The former is likely to affect spatial or visuoconstructional function, whilst the latter may cause visual perceptual impairment.

Overall impairment can be readily shown by a variety of standard tests, such as the Benton Line Orientation and Face Recognition tests (Eslinger and Benton 1983) or figure ground identification (Mendez *et al.* 1990). Constructional impairments can be demonstrated using tasks such as the WAIS Block Design test, with patients who have moderate dementia frequently showing constructional dyspraxia.

There is also evidence that object recognition is impaired, but this is complicated by the breakdown of semantic memory, rather than representing a pure visual agnosic disturbance. Naming an object, for example, may be affected by problems with lexical retrieval, the semantic representation of the object, and the visuoperceptual aspect. However, the visuospatial aspect is supported by the finding that confrontation naming is increased when photographs or line drawing of objects are used rather than the objects themselves.

3.9 Summary

AD is the main form of dementia and in the early stages has a characteristic profile, but one that can vary between patients.

◆   The main prodromal feature of AD is memory impairment.

◆   The pattern of language impairment is most similar to that of transcortical sensory aphasia, but with relatively preserved phonology and syntax, and impaired word retrieval (including generation and naming) and comprehension. Reading is characterized by relative preservation of reading single words, but with poor comprehension affected by semantic memory impairment.

◆   Attentional dysfunction shows a mixed pattern, with phasic attention relatively normal but difficulties with selective (at the disengagement stage) or divided attention.

◆ Executive impairment is seen in relation to initiation, coordinating several tasks simultaneously, and in perseverative behaviour.

◆ Episodic memory impairment is substantial and across different modalities.

◆ Remote memory is impaired across the lifespan, and the propensity to recall old memories reflects the more established store of these memories premorbidly.

◆ Semantic memory is impaired and affects other functions, such as episodic memory and language functioning.

◆ Although lexical and semantic priming is impaired, perceptual learning and motor learning can be preserved.

◆ Visuospatial dysfunction is reflected in visuoperceptual and visuoconstructional deficits.

4 Non-Alzheimer neurodegenerative disorders causing dementia

It is now recognized that there a number of neurodegenerative dementias that differ from AD in terms of clinical features and neuropathology. These have been termed non-Alzheimer degenerative dementias (NADDs) and make up about one-fourth of the dementias that are not vascular in origin (Knopman 1993). The main NADDs are considered in Sections 4.1–4.5.

4.1 Frontotemporal dementia

Frontotemporal dementia (FTD) is a recently defined entity and is associated with neurodegeneration specifically of the frontal and anterior temporal lobes (Neary and Snowden 1996). The distinguishing features include:

◆ early signs of disinhibition;

◆ loss of personal and social awareness (relating, respectively, to personal hygiene and social behaviour);

◆ changes in affect;

◆ language disorder.

FTD can, in turn, be divided in turn into Pick's disease and frontal lobe degeneration of non-Alzheimer type.

4.1.1 Pick's disease

This is very rare, approximately 30 to 60 cases per 100 000 (Constandidis *et al.* 1985). The diagnosis is based on dementia with focal neuropsychological impairment, in turn relating to focal frontal and/or temporal atrophy, with the characteristic histological signs, including the Pick's bodies or Pick's cells. Patients with Pick's disease tend to present earlier and show early behavioural changes reminiscent of those of patients with frontal lobe damage, and disinhibition, but they also show language disorder, including reiterative phenomena such as stereotyped utterances or echolalia. In contrast, auditory comprehension is relatively preserved, with an absence of fluent jargon aphasia (Mendez *et al.* 1993). Visuospatial abilities and calculation have also been found to be relatively preserved, and agraphia, alexia, and apraxia are typically not seen. Although, cognitively, there can be substantial overlap with AD, greater functional impairment is seen in Pick's disease as measured by the Activities of Daily Living Scale (Binetti *et al.* 2000). Pick's disease may be the cause in patients who present with semantic dementia or progressive aphasia, in which case the focal damage is in the temporal lobe (Boller and Muggia 1999).

4.1.2 Frontal lobe degeneration of non-Alzheimer type (FLD)

This is the more common form of frontotemporal dementia and has also been given the title 'frontal lobe type dementia' (Neary *et al.* 1988). Neuropathologically, patients have cerebral atrophy affecting the frontal lobes, but also in the temporal lobes. The neuropathological markers, common in AD, namely, senile plaques and neurofibrillary tangles, are absent. The syndrome presents as changes in personality, disinhibition, and language deterioration.

FLD is characterized by personality and behavioural changes, with an aphasic impairment that is akin to dynamic aphasia. Memory functioning is relatively preserved (Hodges *et al.* 1999) and so is semantic memory. The cognitive feature is impairment in executive functioning, with problems relating to divided attention, mental flexibility, and monitoring output. There is also evidence, in relation to planning ability, that there is impairment in relation to plan development and execution, with a significantly higher number of rule violations on the Tower of London test (Carlin *et al.* 2000). Visuospatial and praxic functions are relatively spared.

4.2 Diffuse Lewy body disease (DLBD)

DLBD presents as a progressive dementia, but with psychiatric features, such as psychotic symptoms (mainly visual hallucinations and paranoid ideation) and depression. Additionally, a fluctuating confusional state may be seen and emerging extrapyramidal signs These are matched neuropathologically by the cytoplasmic inclusions that occur in both cortical and subcortical structures. The cognitive features are similar to those of AD, with impairments in attention, memory, and executive functioning, as well as patterns of aphasia and visuospatial disturbances (Luis *et al.* 1999; Perry *et al.* 1990). Comparative studies of DLBD suggest that attentional, visuoconstructive, visuospatial, and psychomotor performances are all more severely impaired than in AD (Salmon *et al.* 1996). The importance of examining the clinical features of DLBD is that diagnosis relies on distinguishing these from those of other neurodegenerative disorders such as AD or the dementia associated with Parkinson's disease.

4.3 Cortical basal degeneration (CBD)

This is a rare condition that is associated with basal ganglia and other subcortical degeneration, as well as frontal and parietal atrophy. In the early stages, motoric disorders are most apparent and these are of a frontal or extrapyramidal type (Rinne *et al.* 1994). Neuropsychological impairment tends to occur later on in the progression of the disease, with more mild dementia than in AD. The main features include memory and executive impairment (Litvan *et al.* 1998), but also include the characteristic apraxic disturbance, usually asymmetric and ideomotor in type (Massman *et al.* 1996).

4.4 Motor neuron disease (MND)

This progressive disorder is characterized by degeneration of the upper and lower motor neurons, with resulting neurological signs. Associated cognitive deficits have been delineated comparatively recently (Abrahams and Goldstein 2001). A small proportion (3%) also develop dementia, similar in type to that of FLD.

In the non-demented patients, the main features are as follows.

♦ Executive functioning is impaired, particularly on tests of fluency, where careful control in relation to motor/dysarthric impairments demonstrates these to be present.

♦ Memory has not been found consistently to be impaired.

♦ Language functioning is generally preserved, with care needed in assessment because of the associated dysarthria.

♦ Visuospatial functioning is also preserved when the tasks used do not rely on motor speed for effective performance.

♦ Emotional lability may be present and is associated with bulbar involvement.

4.5 Progressive focal neuropsychological deficits (PFND)

In addition to the main neurodegenerative causes of cognitive dysfunction, there is a range of patients with specific progressive neuropsychological deficits. These may overlap in aetiology with the main forms outlined above and also may represent early and isolated impairments that develop into dementia (Della Sala and Spinnler 1999). Patients with focal progressive impairment in different functions are often reported as single-case studies and include, aphasia (Della Sala and Spinnler 1999), semantic dementia (Hodges *et al.* 1999; Snowdon *et al.* 1989), aphemia (Tyrrel *et al.* 1991), Gerstmann syndrome (Strub and Geschwind 1974), and apraxia (see Della Sala and Spinnler 1999 for more examples of types).

5 Extrapyramidal neurodegenerative disorders

5.1 Parkinson's disease

Parkinson's disease, the most common 'extrapyramidal' neurodegenerative disorder, is associated with cognitive dysfunction in two senses.

♦ A proportion of patients meet the criteria for dementia. Consistent estimates of incident and prevalence have been difficult to obtain (approximately 15% of patients identified). Similarly, the pattern of dementia is varied, which may reflect the heterogeneous pathology, which varies in the degree of cortical and subcortical degeneration (Whitehouse *et al.* 1983).

♦ In the remaining patients, more subtle cognitive deficits exist and these tend to show a distinct pattern as indicated below.

Many studies have shown impairments in executive functioning and not only on standard psychometric tasks such as the Wisconsin Card Sorting Test, the Stroop Test, and Trail Making Test. More experimental tasks have shown a reduction in the speed of planning, even when isolating motor slowing (Morris *et al.* 1988), and also in shifting mental sets, such as indicated by performance on the Cambridge Neuropsychological Test Battery Intra–Extradimensional Shift task (Downes *et al.* 1989). Problems with cognitive initiation can be elicited using verbal fluency tests. Long-term memory is impaired and there is also evidence for impairment in procedural memory (Saint-Cyr *et al.* 1988). Language in general is not impaired, but there are difficulties in selected aspects, such as in word retrieval The degree to which visuospatial functioning is impaired is not entirely clear. Generally, patients do poorly in terms of test performance, but this may be because these tests either tend to have a motor component or high executive or attentional demands.

The neural basis for the cognitive impairment is not fully determined. Degeneration of the nigrostratial system is an obvious candidate for explaining executive dysfunction. Cortical dysfunction may also affect those cognitive functions more sensitive to diffuse damage, for example, executive and visuospatial functioning. This is supported by Hu *et al.* (2000) who reported that changes in cortical integrity measured using MRI spectroscopy correlated with decline in visuospatial functioning, even when covarying out motor impairment.

5.2 Progressive supranuclear palsy (PSP)

This neurological condition, also called Steele–Richardson–Olszewski's disease (Steele *et al.* 1964), is characterized by an extrapyramidal syndrome with axial rigidity, postural instability, and oculomotor disturbances, the latter including a supranuclear gaze palsy. Because of these and other neurological signs it can be difficult to gauge the level of neuropsychological impairment, and some have disputed whether dementia occurs even at the late stages (Steele 1972). Nevertheless, extensive neuropsychological testing has been conducted and the tests show deficits in a variety of functions, including reduced psychomotor speed, long-term memory, impaired visuoconstructional abilities, and problems with sustained and divided attention and executive functioning in general. Impairments are also seen in verbal reasoning tasks with a reduction in verbal fluency (Esmonde *et al.* 1996; see also Boller and Muggia 1999 for a detailed review).

♦ The progression of cognitive decline in PSP appears to be greater than in other extrapyramidal syndromes, such as Parkinson's disease (Soliveri *et al.* 2000), consistent with neurodegeneration affecting both cortical and subcortical regions.

- ◆ A characteristic feature is that executive functioning tends to be impaired, consistent with prefrontal dysfunction over and above that seen in other dementias (Grafman *et al.* 1995). This is consistent with damage to the frontostriatal loops, effectively deafferentating the prefrontal cortex.

- ◆ Another feature is that, in PSP, the slowing of information processing can be easily separated from the motor problems, in a way that is not necessarily the case with other neurodegenerative disorders, such as Parkinson's disease (Grafman *et al.* 1995).

5.3 **Huntington's disease**

This autosomal dominant neurodegenerative disorder with its insidious onset with motor disorders is accompanied by eventual dementia. The neurodegeneration includes mainly atrophy of the caudate nuclei and involvement of the frontal cortex, but the neuropsychological changes are more diffuse. Nevertheless, a characteristic pattern of impairment is seen.

- ◆ Memory function is impaired. Studies that compare the nature of the memory impairment with that of other disorders such as AD indicate relative preservation of recognition memory (Butters *et al.* 1985).

- ◆ In contrast to AD, skill learning is generally impaired (Heindel *et al.* 1989).

- ◆ In common with other extrapyramidal syndromes, language functioning is relatively preserved, with significant aphasia rarely seen. Despite this, subtle deficits can be observed, such as a reduction in the syntactical complexity of written and spoken language and word-finding difficulties relating both to fluency (Butters *et al.* 1986) and confrontation naming (Podroll *et al.* 1988).

- ◆ Spatial cognition is impaired with visuoconstructional difficulties demonstrated by impaired copying performance on the Rey Osterreith task (Browers *et al.* 1984), and also such tests as the WAIS-R Block Design and Object Assembly tests. This is not explained entirely by motor difficulties, since performance on visuospatial tests that do not require more responses is preserved.

6 **Conclusion**

The neuropsychological features of the principal neurodegenerative groups have been considered. The overlap in types of deficits between certain groups is apparent, but each group appears to have its own specific profile that can be related to the regions of the brain most affected. Knowledge of the specific profiles can be used diagnostically, but also to understand the resulting disabilities. Although assessment procedures can be tailored to suit individual patients, specific protocols can be developed to take into account the aetiology of the patient. Since many of these disorders occur in older adults, specific approaches may be needed, and the reader might refer to a number of reviews in this area for more information (e.g. Morris and McKiernan 1994; Morris *et al.* 2000; Woods 1999).

Selective references

Abrahams, S. and Goldstein, L.H. (2001). Motor neurone disease. In *Cognitive deficits in brain disorders* (ed. J.E. Harrison and A. Owen). Martin Dunitz, London.

Arriagada, P.V., Growdon, J.H., Hedley-Whyte, T., and Human, B.T. (1992). Neurofibrillary tangles but not senile plaques parallel duration and severity of Alzheimer's disease. *Neurology* 42, 631–9.

Backman, L. and Herlitz, A. (1996). Knowledge and memory in Alzheimer's disease: a relationship that exists. In *The cognitive neuropsychology of Alzheimer-type dementia* (ed. R.G. Morris), pp. 89–104. Oxford University Press, Oxford.

Baddeley, A.D., Della Sala, S., and Spinnler, H. (1991). The two component hypothesis of memory deficit in Alzheimer's disease. *J. Clin. Exp. Neuropsychol.* 13, 372–80.

Becker, J. T., Bajulaiye, O., and Smith, C. (1992). Longitudinal analysis of a two-component model of the memory deficit in Alzheimer's disease. *Psychol. Med.* 22, 437–45.

Binetti, G., Locascio, J.J., Corkin, S., Vonsatttel, J.P., and Growdon, J.H. (2000). Differences between Pick disease and Alzheimer disease in clinical appearance and rate of cognitive decline. *Arch. Neurol.* 57, 225–32.

Boller, F. and Muggia, S. (1999). Non-Alzheimer dementias. In *Handbook of clinical and experimental neuropsychology* (ed. G. Denes and L. Pizzamiglio), pp. 747–74. Psychology Press, Hove, East Sussex.

Brouwers, P., Cox, C., Martin, A., Chase, T., and Fedio, P. (1984). Differential perceptual spatial impairment in Huntington's and Alzheimer's dementias. *Arch. Neurol.* 41, 1073–6.

Butters, N., Wolfe, J., Martone, M., Granholm, E., and Cermak, L.S. (1985). Memory disorders associated with Huntington's disease: verbal recall, verbal recognition and procedural memory. *Neuropsychologia* 23, 729–43.

Butters, N., Wolfe, J., Granholme, E., and Martone, M. (1986). An assessment of verbal recall, recognition and fluency abilities in patients with Huntington's disease. *Cortex* 22, 11–32.

Carlin, D., Bonerba, J., Phipps, M., Alexander, G., Shapiro, M., and Grafman, J. (2000). Planning impairments in frontal lobe dementia and frontal lobe lesion patients. *Neuropsychologia* 38, 655–65.

Collette, F., Van der Linden, M., and Salmon, E. (1999). Executive dysfunction in Alzheimer's disease. *Cortex* 35, 57–72.

Constantinidis, J., Richard, J., and Tissot, R. (1985). Pick dementia: anatamoclinical correlations and pathophysiological considerations. *Interdiscipl. Topics Gerontol.* 19, 72–97.

Crawford, J.R., Stewart, L.E., Cocharan, R.H.B., *et al.* (1989). Estimating premorbid IQ from demographic variables: regression equations derived from a UK sample. *Br. J. Clin. Psychol.* 28, 275–8.

Della Sala, S. and Spinnler, H. (1999). Slowly progressive isolated cognitive deficits. In *Handbook of clinical and experimental neuropsychology* (ed. G. Denes and L. Pizzamiglio), pp. 775–807. Psychology Press, Hove, East Sussex.

Downes, J.J., Roberts, A.C., Sahakian, B.J., Evenden, J.L., Morris, R.G., and Robbins, T.W. (1989). Impaired extradimensional shift performance in medicated and unmedicated Parkinson's disease: evidence for a specific attentional deficit. *Neuropsychologia* 27, 1329–43.

Eslinger, P.J. and Benton, A. L. (1983). Visuoperceptual performance in aging and dementia: clinical and theoretical observations. *J. Clin. Neuropsychol.* 5, 213–20.

Eslinger, P.J. and Damasio, A.R. (1986). Preserved motor learning in Alzheimer's disease: implications for anatomy and behavior. *J. Neurosci.* 6, 3006–9

Esmonde, T., Giles, E., Gibson, M., and Hodges, J.R. (1996). Neuropsychological performance, disease severity, and depression in progressive supranuclear palsy. *J. Neurol.* 243, 638–43.

Fennema-Notestine, C., Butters, N., Heindel, W. C., and Salmon, D. (1994). Semantic homophone priming in patients with dementia of the Alzheimer type. *Neuropsychology* 8, 579–87.

Fox, N.C., Warrington, E.K., Seiffer, A.L., Agnew, S.K., and Rossor, M.N. (1998). Presymptomatic cognitive deficits in individuals at risk of familial Alzheimer's disease: a longitudinal perspective study. *Brain* **131**, 1631–9.

Fromholt, P. and Larsen, S.F. (1991). Autobiographical memory in normal aging and primary degenerative dementia. (dementia of the Alzheimer type). *J. Gerontol. (Psychol. Sci.)* **46**, 85–91.

Fuld, P., Katzman, R., Davies, P., and Terry, R. (1982). Intrusions as a sign of Alzheimer's dementia: chemical and pathological verification. *Ann. Neurol.* **11**, 155–9.

Garrard, P., Patterson, K., Watson, P.C., and Hodges, J.R. (1998). Category specific semantic loss in dementia of Alzheimer type: functional–anatomic correlations from cross-sectional analyses. *Brain* **121**, 633–46.

Geula, C. (1998). Abnormalities of neural circuitry in Alzheimer's disease: hippocampus and cortical cholinergic innervation. *Neurology* **51**, S18–S29.

Gonnerman, L.M., Andersen, E.S., Devlin, J.T., Kempler, D., and Seidenberg, M.S. (1997). Double dissociation of semantic categories in Alzheimer's disease. *Brain Language* **57**, 254–79.

Grafman, J., Litvan, I., and Stark, M. (1995). Neuropsychological features of progressive supra-nuclear palsy. *Brain and Cognition* **28**, 311–20.

Greene D.W. and Hodges, J.R. (1996). Identification of famous faces and famous names in early Alzheimer's disease: relationship to anterograde episodic and general semantic memory. *Brain* **119**, 111–28.

Grober E., Ausubel, R., Sliwinski, M., and Gordon, B. (1992). Skill learning and repetition priming in Alzheimer's disease. *Neuropsychologia* **30**, 849–58.

Heindel, W., Butters, N., and Salmon, D. (1988). Impaired learning of a motor skill in patients with Huntington's disease. *Behav. Neurosci.* **102**, 141–7.

Heindel, W.C., Salmon, D., Shults, C.W., Walicke, P.A., and Butters, N. (1989). Neuropsychological evidence for multiple implicit memory systems: a comparison of Alzheimer's, Huntington's, and Parkinson's disease patients. *J. Neurosci.* **9**, 582–7.

Heindel, W., Salmon, D., and Butters, N. (1991). The biasing of weight judgements in Alzheimer's and Huntington's disease: a priming or programming phenomenon? *J. Clin. Exp. Neuropsychol.* **13**, 189–203.

Hodges, J.R., Salmon, D.P., and Butters, N. (1990). Differential impairment of semantic and episodic memory in Alzheimer's and Huntington's diseases: a controlled prospective study. *J. Neurol., Neurosurg., Psychiatry* **53**, 1089–95.

Hodges, J.R., Patterson, K. Ward, R., Garrard, P., Bak, T., Perry, R., and Gregory, C. (1999). The differentiation of semantic dementia and frontal lobe dementia (temporal and frontal variants of frontotemporal dementia) from early Alzheimer's disease: a comparative neuropsychological study. *Neuropsychology* **13** (1), 31–40.

Hu, M.T.M., Taylor-Robinson, S.D., Chaudhuri, K.R., Bell, J.D., Labbe, C., Cunningham, V.J., Koepp, M.J., Hammers, A., Morris, R.G., Brooks, D.J., and Turnjanski, N. (2000). Cortical dysfunction in non-demented Parkinson's disease patients: a combined ^{31}phosphorus MRS and ^{18}FDG PET study. *Brain* **123**, 140–352.

Jack, C.R. Jr, Petersen, R.C., Xu, Y.C., O'Brien, P.C., Smith, G.E., Ivnik, R.J., Boeve, B.F., Waring, S.C., Tangalos, E.G., and Kokmen, E. (1999). Prediction of AD with MRI-based hippocampal volume in mild cognitive impairment. *Neurology* **52** (7), 1397–403.

Kertesz, A. (1994). Language deterioration in dementia. In *Dementia: presentation, differential diagnosis, and nosology* (ed. V.O.B. Emery and T. E. Oxman), pp. 123–38. John Hopkins University Press, Baltimore.

Kidron, D. and Freedman, M. (1996). Motor functioning. In *The cognitive neuropsychology of Alzheimer-type dementia* (ed. R.G. Morris), pp. 206–20. Oxford University Press, Oxford.

Knopman, D. (1993). The non-Alzheimer degenerative dementias. In *Handbook of neuropsychology*, Vol. 8 (ed. F. Boller and J. Grafman), pp. 295–313. Elsevier, Amsterdam.

Lines, C.R., Dawson, C., Preston, G.C., Reich, S., Foster, C., and Traub, M. (1991). Memory and attention in patients with senile dementia of the Alzheimer type and normal elderly subjects. *J. Clin. Exp. Neuropsychol.* **13**, 2691–702.

Litvan, I., Cummings, J.L., and Mega, M. (1998). Neuropsychiatric features of corticobasal degeneration. *J. Neurol., Neurosurg., Psychiatry* **65**, 717–21.

Luis, C.A., Mittenberg, W., Gass, C.S., and Duara, R. (1999). Diffuse Lewy body disease: clinical, pathological, and neuropsychological review. *Neuropsychol. Rev.* **9** (3), 137–50.

Martin, A., Browers, P., Cox, C., and Fedio, P. (1985). On the nature of the verbal memory deficits in Alzheimer's disease. *Brain Language* **25**, 232–41.

Massman, P.J., Kreiter, K.T., Jankovic, J., and Doody, R.S. (1996). Neuropsychological functioning in cortical-basal ganglionic degeneration: differentiation from Alzheimer's disease. *Neurology* **46**, 720–6.

Matthias, J. (1996). Reading disorder in Alzheimer-type dementia. In *The cognitive neuropsychology of Alzheimer-type dementia* (ed. R. G. Morris), pp. 149–65. Oxford University Press, Oxford.

Mendez, M.F., Mendez, M.A., Martin, R.N. *et al.* (1990). Complex visual disturbance in Alzheimer's disease. *Neurology* **40**, 329–43.

Mendez, M.F., Selwood, A., Mastri, A.R., and Frey, W.H. (1993). Pick's disease versus Alzheimer's disease: a comparison of clinical characteristics. *Neurology* **43**, 289–92.

Mohr, E., Cox, C., Williams, J., Chase, T.M., and Fedio, P. (1990). Impairment of central auditory function in Alzheimer's disease. *J. Clin. Exp. Neuropsychol.* **13**, 235–46.

Morris, R.G. (ed.) (1996). *The cognitive neuropsychology of Alzheimer-type dementia.* Oxford University Press, Oxford.

Morris, R.G. and McKiernan, F. (1994). Neuropsychological approaches to the assessment of dementia. In *Dementia* (ed. A. Burns and R. Levy), pp. 327–54. Chapman and Hall, London.

Morris, R.G. and Worsley, C.L. (2002). The neuropsychology of Alzheimer's disease. In *Encyclopedia of the human brain* (ed. V.S. Ramachandran), pp. 119–29. Academic Press, San Diego.

Morris, R.G., Downes, J., Sahakian, B., Evenden, J., Heald, A., and Robbins, T.W. (1988). Planning and working memory in Parkinson's disease. *J. Neurol., Neurosurg., Psychiatry* **51**, 757–66.

Morris, R.G., Worsley, C.L., and Matthew, D. (2000). Neuropsychological assessment in older people: old principles and new directions. *Advan. Psychiatric Treatment* **6**, 362–72.

Neary, D. and Snowden, J. (1996). Fronto-temporal dementia: nosology, neuropsychology, and neuropathology. *Brain Cognition* **31**, 176–87.

Neary, D., Snowden, J.S., Northen, B., and Gouldin, P. (1988). Dementia of frontal lobe type. *J. Neurol., Neurosurg., Psychiatry* **51**, 352–61.

Nebes, R.D. and Brady, C.B. (1993). Phasic and tonic alertness in Alzheimer's disease. *Cortex* **29**, 77–90.

Nissen, M.J. and Bullemer, P. (1987) Attentional requirements of learning: evidence from performance measures. *Cogn. Psychol.* **19**, 1–32.

Parasuraman, R., Greenwood, P.M., Haxby, J.V., and Grady, C.L. (1992). Visuospatial attention in dementia of the Alzheimer-type. *Brain* **115**, 711–33.

Patterson, K.E., Graham, N., and Hodges, J.R. (1994). Reading in dementia of the Alzheimer's type: a preserved ability? *Neuropsychology* **8**, 395–412.

Paulsen, J.S., Butters, N., Salmon, D.P., Heindel, W.C., and Swenson, M.R. (1993). Prism adaptation in Alzheimer's and Huntington's disease. *Neuropsychology* **7**, 73–81.

Perry, R.H., Irving, D., Blessed, G., Fairburn, A., and Perry, E.K. (1990). Senile dementia of Lewy body type. A clinically and neuropathologically distinct form of Lewy body dementia in the elderly. *J. Neurol. Sci.* **95**, 119–39.

Poldroll, K., Caspary, P., Lange, H.W., and Noth, J. (1988). Language functions in Huntington's disease. *Brain* **111**, 1475–503.

Rinne, J.O., Lee, M.S., Thompson, P.D., and Marsden, C.D. (1994). Corticobasal degeneration. A clinical study of 36 cases. *Brain* **117**, 1183–96.

Rosen, W.G. (1980) Verbal fluency in aging and dementia. *J. Clin. Neuropsychol.* **2**, 135–46.

Saint-Cyr, J., Taylor, A., and Lang, A. (1988). Procedural learning and neostriatal dysfunction in man. *Brain* **111**, 941–59.

Salmon, D.P., Galasko, D., Hansen, L.A., Masliah, E., Butters, N., Thal, L.J., and Katzman, R. (1996). Neuropsychological deficits associated with diffuse lewy body disease. *Brain and Cognition*, **31** (2), 148–65.

Salmon, D. and Fennema-Notestine, C. (1996). Implicit memory. In *The cognitive neuropsychology of Alzheimer-type dementia* (ed. R. G. Morris), pp. 105–27. Oxford University Press, Oxford.

Salmon, D., Shimamura, A., Butters, N., and Smith, S. (1988). Lexical and semantic priming deficits in patients with Alzheimer's disease. *J. Clin. Exp. Neuropsychol.* **10**, 477–94.

Snowdon, J. S., Goulding, P. J., and Neary, D. (1989). Semantic dementia: a form of circumscribed cerebral atrophy. *Behav. Neurol.* **2**, 167–182.

Soliveri, P., Monza, D., Paridi, D., Carella, F., Genitrini, S., Testa, D., and Girotti, F. (2000). Neuropsychological follow up in patients with Parkinson's disease, striatonigral degeneration-type multisystem atrophy, and progressive subnuclear palsy. *J. Neurol., Neurosurg., Psychiatry* **69**, 313–18.

Steele, J.C. (1972). Progessive supranuclear palsy. *Brain* **95**, 693–704.

Steele, J.C., Richardson, J.C., and Olszewski, J. (1964). Progressive supranuclear palsy. A heterogeneous degeneration involving the brain stem, basal ganglia and cerebellum, with vertical gaze and pseudobulbar palsy, nuclear dystonia and dementia. *Arch. Neurol.* **10**, 333–59.

Strub, R. and Geschwind, N. (1974). Gerstmann syndrome without aphasia. *Cortex* **10**, 378–87.

The Lund and Manchester Groups (1994). Clinical and neuro-pathological criteria for frontotemporal dementia. *J. Neurol., Neurosurg., Psychiatry* **57**, 416–18.

Tyrell, P.J., Kartsounis, L.D., Frackowiak, R.S.J., Findley, L.J., and Rossor, M.N. (1991). Progressive loss of speech output and orofacial dyspraxia associated with frontal lobe hypometabolism. *J. Neurol., Neurosurg., Psychiatry* **54**, 351–7.

Weingartner, H., Grafman, J., Boutelle, W., Kaye, W., and Martin, P. (1983). Forms of memory failure. *Science* **221**, 380–2.

Wilson, R.S., Sullivan, M., De Toledo-Morell, L., Stebbins, G.T., Bennett, D.A., and Morrell, F. (1996). Association of memory and cognition in Alzheimer's disease with volumetric estimates of temporal lobe structures. *Neuropsychology* **10**, 459–63.

Chapter 29

Neuropsychological presentation and treatment of demyelinating disorders

Peter A. Arnett

1 Introduction

By far the most commonly seen and studied demyelinating disorder in clinical neuropsychology is multiple sclerosis (MS). Most of this chapter will focus on MS. Other demyelinating disorders on which some neuropsychological data are available will be reviewed in Section 6.

Clinical neuropsychologists play a pivotal role in the assessment and treatment of MS patients. Prior to the advent of sensitive neuropsychological tests, when cognitive evaluations involving brief mental state examinations were primarily used, cognitive difficulties were thought to affect less than 5% of patients (Rao 1986). Prevalence estimates based on the use of neuropsychological tests now range from 40 to 60% (see Section 2.1). Because cognitive deficits in MS are associated with real-world functioning, neuropsychologists first evaluate the extent to which tested difficulties displayed by the patients may map on to real-world problems. Neuropsychologists can then help patients make modifications to their daily routines that allow them to circumvent their cognitive difficulties. Neuropsychologists can also help identify and treat the depression that is so common, but often overlooked, in MS patients.

1.1 The pathophysiology of MS

MS is a demyelinating disease of the central nervous system thought to be caused by an autoimmune process, a slow-acting virus, or a delayed reaction to a common virus (Brassington and Marsh 1998). It is characterized by multiple discrete plaques at demyelinated sites formed, in part, by proliferating astrocytes. Myelin sheaths within plaques are either destroyed or swollen and fragmented. Neural conduction is facilitated by myelin because an intact nerve is enclosed in myelin sheaths separated by gaps from which the nerve impulse jumps. The areas affected by MS thus interfere with or block neural transmission by limiting this process known as *saltatory conduction*. Axons and cell bodies of neurons often remain intact.

The size of plaques varies from about 1.0 mm to several cm. The resulting symptoms typically reflect functions associated with affected areas. Plaques can occur in the brain and/or spinal cord and their location is highly variable between patients. Within the cerebrum, plaques are most commonly found near the lateral and third ventricles. Frontal lobes are the next most commonly affected, even when the size of frontal lobes relative to the rest of the brain is considered. Plaques are also frequently observed in other major lobes of brain. In addition, plaques are commonly seen in the optic nerves, chiasm, or tracts, as well as the corpus callosum, brainstem, and cerebellum. The majority of plaques (about 75%) are observed in white matter, but some occur in grey matter and in the junction between grey and white matter. Some remyelination occurs with acute MS plaques.

1.2 The clinical presentation and natural course of MS

MS is probably acquired before puberty, but the actual disease onset occurs in most (two-thirds) patients between ages 20 and 40. Onset before age 15 is rare. Late onset after age 40 is commonly characterized by quicker progression and greater morbidity. The average life expectancy following onset is estimated at 30+ years, but the variability is great.

MS is more common in females than in males with a ratio of about 2:1. An environmental contribution is suggested by a generally higher prevalence in temperate zones away from the equator. There is a 30–40% concordance in identical twins but only 1–13% in fraternal twins, suggesting a genetic contribution.

1.2.1 Symptoms

Common symptoms include muscle weakness, urinary disturbance, and visual anomalies such as diplopia, loss of visual acuity, blurry vision, and visual field defects. Fatigue, problems with balance, and paraesthesias (usually numbness and tingling in the limbs, trunk, or face) are also common. In addition, significant cognitive difficulties and problems with depression are very common. The most common symptoms at MS onset are muscle weakness, paraesthesias, visual disturbances, and gait/balance problems. The mode of symptom onset is typically acute or subacute. Many MS symptoms are transient and unpredictable. For example, visual disturbances and paraesthesias may last for seconds or hours. Because of the short-lived and sometimes bizarre nature of symptoms, it is not uncommon for patients in the early stages before formal diagnosis to be diagnosed as having hysterical/somatization disorders.

1.2.2 Diagnosis

The diagnosis of MS is clinical. Patients must have had at least two discrete episodes of neurological change implicating the presence of lesions in at least two different sites in the central white matter. Attacks, relapses, or exacerbations that imply new disease activity are common. Several course scenarios have been identified (Lublin and Reingold 1996).

◆ *Relapsing–remitting* (RR). Most common and characterized by clearly defined disease relapses. Recovery can be full or with sequelae and residual deficit. No progression of disease between relapses.

- *Secondary-progressive.* Next most common type. First characterized by RR course then progression. Relapses and remissions may or may not occur.
- *Primary-progressive.* Next most common type. Unremitting disease progression from onset for most patients, but occasional stabilization and even improvement in functioning for others. No clear relapses.
- *Progressive–relapsing.* Least common type. Disease progression from onset. Acute relapses also occur from which patients may or may not fully recover.

The term 'chronic-progressive' formerly encompassed all progressive types.

Two categories of severity of outcome have also been identified.

- *Benign.* Patient remains fully functional 15 years post disease onset.
- *Malignant.* Rapidly progressing course leading to significant disability or death relatively soon after disease onset.

Most patients fall in between these two extremes.

2 Neuropsychological deficits in multiple sclerosis

2.1 Prevalence of neuropsychological deficits

Of MS patients 40–60% have cognitive deficits, but most (about 80%) patients with deficits are relatively mildly affected. Global cognitive deficits are uncommon. However, even mild cognitive problems in MS have been shown to relate to everyday activities (e.g. work, homemaking, personal care activities, social activities; Higginson *et al.* 2000).

2.2 The nature of the neuropsychological deficits

2.2.1 Intellectual functioning and academic skills

Intellectual functioning is affected significantly in about 20% of patients. Most patients score within the broad normal range. Little systematic research has been conducted on academic skills in patients with MS, but the skills are assumed to be intact in most patients.

2.2.2 Memory

Memory is one of the most commonly affected cognitive domains in MS. Problem encoding and/or retrieving both verbal and visual information are most common and are typically manifested as immediate- and delayed-recall memory deficits on neuropsychological testing. About 30% of patients have substantial problems, another 30% have moderate problems, and the remaining 40% have mild or no problems with this type of memory (Brassington and Marsh 1998). Working memory, the ability to maintain and manipulate information 'on-line', is also commonly impaired. Delayed-recall deficits are usually a function of deficient immediate recall, not forgetting. The learning curve across repeated trials is similar in slope to that of controls, but lower in magnitude. Percentage retention, recognition, and incidental memory following a delay and remote memory are usually intact. Clinically, memory problems often manifest as complaints of difficulty in remembering conversations, appointments, work tasks, etc.

2.2.3 Attention and concentration/speeded information processing

This is one of most commonly affected cognitive domains in MS. It is difficult to separate speeded information processing from attentional functioning because the latter is necessary for performing any speeded cognitive task. In clinical evaluations it is important to be aware of the possibility that memory problems in MS may, in part, be a function of deficits in these domains. MS patients show the greatest difficulty on tasks requiring rapid and complex information processing, such as those requiring swift application of working memory operations, attentional switching, or rapid visual scanning. About 20–25% of MS patients have substantial difficulty with this cognitive domain. Simple attention span is usually intact, but mild impairments are sometimes found. Clinically, attention/speeded processing problems commonly manifest as difficulty in tracking and keeping up with and focusing on details of conversations, work tasks, television programmes, etc.

2.2.4 Verbal/linguistic deficits

Aphasias are rare in MS, but mild confrontation-naming difficulties are sometimes seen. Deficits in verbal fluency are common. It is important in clinical evaluations to determine if the latter deficits are associated with memory retrieval difficulties common to MS (Fischer *et al.* 1994). Because fluency tasks require rapid production of information, patients' poor performance on them may also be related to their speeded-processing deficits. In addition, the slowed speech common to MS should be considered as a possible contributor to patients' verbal fluency, as well as speeded processing/attentional deficits. Twenty to 25% of patients have substantial problems on verbal fluency tasks (e.g. Rao *et al.* 1991). Fluency problems may manifest clinically as word-finding problems impairing the flow of patients' conversations.

2.2.5 Visuospatial deficits

Of individuals with MS, 10–20% show substantial difficulty with higher-order visuospatial skills involving angle matching or face recognition. It is unclear whether higher-order visual deficits are a function of primary visual disturbances involving blurred vision and diplopia (Rao *et al.* 1991). Clinical manifestations may involve accounts of running into things frequently while walking (e.g. doorways) or driving (e.g. curbs) because of visual miscalculations.

2.2.6 Executive skills

Executive skills are reasonably commonly affected in MS. Deficits in cognitive flexibility, concept-formation, verbal abstraction, problem-solving, and planning are found. Of individuals with MS, 15–20% show substantial difficulties in this cognitive domain.

These deficits may manifest clinically as difficulty in planning day-to-day activities (e.g. job tasks, meals, grocery shopping), verbal disinhibition, and tangential speech, as well as problems in organizing ideas and shifting appropriately from one topic to another in conversation.

2.3 Measurement of neuropsychological deficits in MS

2.3.1 Brief screening batteries/repeatable batteries

An efficient way of approaching neuropsychological testing in MS is to conduct a brief screening evaluation to determine if further testing is warranted. MS patients impaired in one domain of cognitive functioning are not necessarily impaired in others (Rao *et al.* 1991). Thus, neuropsychological assessments that evaluate major areas of cognitive functioning typically impaired in MS are critical because performance on a test in one domain provides little information about the likelihood of deficits in other domains. Rao and colleagues have developed the Brief Repeatable Battery of Neuropsychological Tests in Multiple Sclerosis (BRB; Rao 1990) comprised of tests most sensitive to the cognitive impairments typically seen in MS. Most tests also include 15 alternate forms to allow for repeat testing. The battery includes a six-trial version of the Verbal Selective Reminding Test, 10/36 Spatial Recall, Oral Symbol Digit Modalities Test, 2s and 3s PASAT, and Word List Generation (verbal fluency). Comprehensive norms for BRB can be found in Boringa *et al.* (2001).

- ◆ BRB takes 20–30 minutes to administer.
- ◆ The two-subtest (Vocabulary, Matrix Reasoning) form of the Wechsler Abbreviated Scale of Intelligence (WASI; Wechsler 1999) is also recommended and takes 15 minutes. The latter provides a reliable and valid estimate of full-scale intelligence quotient (IQ) and has excellent norms.
- ◆ Adding the Chicago Multiscale Depression Inventory (CMDI; Nyenhuis *et al.* 1998), as recommended by Beatty *et al.* (1995), and the Fatigue Severity Scale (FSS; Krupp *et al.* 1988) is also suggested. Together, the latter two measures take about 10 minutes and are self-administered, so that they could be completed in a waiting room before actual testing.

Thus, in only 35–45 minutes of actual patient contact time, a reasonably comprehensive neuropsychological screen can be obtained and more extensive testing conducted if deficits are detected. Table 29.1 summarizes the brief neuropsychological batteries considered here and also the comprehensive batteries discussed in Section 2.3.2.

2.3.2 Comprehensive batteries

Intellectual functioning and academic functioning *Intellectual functioning* is best measured using the four-subtest (Vocabulary, Similarities, Matrix Reasoning, Block Design) form of WASI. It allows for derivation of reliable and valid full-scale, verbal, and performance IQ estimates. The entire Wechsler Adult Intelligence Scale,

Table 29.1 Recommended brief and comprehensive neuropsychological batteries for assessing multiple sclerosis patients

Brief screening battery

Intellectual functioning

Two-subtest form of the Wechsler Abbreviated Scale of Intelligence (WASI)

Memory

Verbal Selective Reminding Test (6-Trial Version) with delayed recall and recognition

10/36 Spatial Recall with delayed recall and copy

Attention and concentration/speeded information processing

Symbol Digit Modalities Test (SDMT), oral version

Paced Auditory Serial Addition Test (PASAT), 2s and 3s versions

Verbal–linguistic

Controlled Oral Word Association test (COWA)

Affective/emotional fatigue

Chicago Multiscale Depression Inventory (CMDI)

Fatigue Severity Scale

Standard comprehensive battery

Orientation

Information and Orientation subtest from Wechsler Memory Scale, 3rd Edition (WMS-III)

Intellectual functioning

Four-subtest form of the Wechsler Abbreviated Scale of Intelligence (WASI)

Academic functioning

Wide Range Achievement Test, 1993 Edition

Memory

Verbal Selective Reminding Test (6-trial version) with delayed recall and recognition

10/36 Spatial Recall with delayed recall and copy

Logical Memory subtests from WMS-III

Family Pictures subtests from WMS-III

Word Lists subtests from WMS-III

Information subtest from Wechsler Adult Intelligence Scale, 3rd Edition (WAIS-III)

Attention and concentration/speeded information processing

Digit Span subtest from WMS-III

Spatial Span subtest from WMS-III

Letter-Number Sequencing subtest from WMS-III

SDMT, oral version

PASAT, 2s and 3s versions

Table 29.1 (*continued*)

Verbal/linguistic
COWA
Boston Naming Test
Visuospatial
Judgement of Line Orientation
Executive
Tower subtest from Delis–Kaplan Executive Function System (D–KEFS)
Card Sorting subtest from D-KEFS, free-sorting condition only
Affective/emotional, fatigue
CMDI
Hospital Anxiety and Depression Scale
Fatigue Impact Scale
Disability
Multiple Sclerosis Functional Composite
Optional tests for comprehensive battery
Visual Reproduction subtests from WMS-III
California Verbal Learning Test-II

3rd edition (WAIS-III; Wechsler 1997*a*) is not necessary in most cases. However, individual subtests are useful for measurement of specific functional areas and are highlighted below. Block Design results must be interpreted with caution because the motor manipulation and visual demands required for it and many other Performance subtests make it difficult to use reliably and validly in MS patients with sensorimotor disturbance.

Academic functioning Best evaluated using the Wide Range Achievement Test (WRAT3; Wilkinson 1993). Significantly worse performance on subtests when compared to full-scale IQ can suggest the possibility of a learning disability contributing to the pattern of cognitive test performance observed.

Memory The Wechsler Memory Scale, 3rd edition (WMS-III; Wechsler 1997*b*) provides a detailed view of multiple aspects of memory. The subtests most useful in characterizing MS memory problems include:

◆ Logical Memory I and II plus recognition;

◆ Word Lists I and II plus recognition;

◆ Family Pictures I and II.

All subtests have normed percentage retention scores. Patients with motor writing difficulties may find Visual Reproduction difficult, but such difficulty and its possible contribution to memory can be systematically evaluated with the 'Copy' part of the task. However, 10/36 Spatial Recall is generally preferred over Visual Reproduction, because many patients have significant motor-writing difficulties and 10/36 tests visual memory without any drawing component. The California Verbal Learning Test, 2nd edition (CVLT-II; Delis *et al.* 2000) can be a useful adjunct to WMS-III subtests when examination of executive and/or implicit aspects of memory is desired. The Letter–Number Sequencing and Spatial Span subtests of WMS-III are recommended as measures of working memory independent of speed. Remote memory is screened by the Information subtest of WAIS-III and orientation by the Information and Orientation subtest from WMS-III.

Attention and concentration/speeded information processing

- Speeded visual attention is best measured using the Symbol Digit Modalities Test (Smith 1982), one of the tests most sensitive to cognitive deficit in MS (Zakzanis 2000). It is also predictive of everyday function and sensitive to depression in MS. The oral form is preferred to the written one because it circumvents motor writing difficulties common to MS.

- The Paced Auditory Serial Addition Test (PASAT; Rao *et al.* 1989) is excellent for measuring speeded auditory attention combined with working memory. Caution is required when using PASAT in lower functioning patients, as its use can damage rapport with the patients because of their great difficulty in performing it.

- Poor performance on the Arithmetic subtest of WRAT3 may suggest primary arithmetic calculation difficulties, which may contribute to PASAT deficits.

- Digit Span forward and Spatial Span forward subtests from WMS-III are most useful as measures of simple attention span.

Verbal/linguistic deficits   Confrontation naming is best measured by the Boston Naming Test (Kaplan *et al.* 1983), which is sufficient as a screen for aphasia in most examinations. The Controlled Oral Word Association test (COWA; Spreen and Strauss 1998) is used for testing letter–word fluency and animal naming for category fluency (Spreen and Strauss 1998). Significantly better animal naming than letter–word fluency can suggest that letter–word fluency problems are, in part, a function of memory retrieval difficulties.

Visuospatial deficits   The Judgement of Line Orientation test (Benton *et al.* 1983) is usually sufficient for screening visuospatial ability.

Executive skills   The Wisconsin Card Sorting Test (WCST) is traditionally used to measure cognitive flexibility and concept formation in MS. However, a study by Beatty and Monson (1996) suggests that the California Card Sorting Test (CCST) may be better because it allows for differentiation of perseverative responding and concept formation, unlike the WCST. This is important because MS patients show impaired concept formation but not perseverative responding. The Delis–Kaplan

Executive System battery (D–KEFS; Delis *et al.* 2001) now includes a subtest analogous to CCST called the Card-Sorting Test which has excellent norms. Because of the lengthy administration time, however, only administration of the free-sorting condition is recommended. The Tower Test from D–KEFS is recommended for measuring planning ability. The Similarities subtest from WAIS-III is a good index of verbal abstraction.

2.4 Possible causes of cognitive deficits

Primary causes of cognitive deficits emanate from a direct consequence of the location and extent of brain damage. Thus, cognitive problems caused by primary influences are generally not reversible. There is clear evidence that overall cognitive impairment is associated with total white matter lesion burden in MS and some evidence that frontal lobe lesions are associated with deficits on executive tasks such as the Wisconsin Card-Sorting Test (WCST). The association between lesions in other brain areas and specific cognitive deficits is less clear (Brassington and Marsh 1998).

Secondary causes of cognitive impairment involve something associated with a disease such as depression, anxiety, or fatigue. Cognitive problems caused by these secondary influences are potentially reversible if secondary influence is successfully treated. Relative to primary causes, less attention is paid in the MS literature to these possible causes of cognitive dysfunction. Recent work shows that depression is associated with impairments in speeded attentional functioning, working memory, and executive functions, but this link is still controversial (Arnett *et al.* 2001). The key difference between this and prior studies is that Arnett *et al.*'s study defined depression according to mood symptoms only using the CMDI scale. Prior studies may not have found a relationship because of their use of depression measures that contain many neurovegetative symptoms of depression that overlap with MS symptoms. There is little evidence that self-reported fatigue or anxiety is significantly associated with cognitive deficits in MS, but these associations are relatively infrequently examined to date. However, recent work suggests that MS patients show greater decline in performance on cognitively demanding tasks over the course of an evaluation using other demanding cognitive tasks. This possibly suggests a greater susceptibility to cognitive fatigue during testing in MS (Krupp and Elkins 2000), something that should be taken into consideration when ordering tests in a battery.

2.5 The relationship between cognitive deficits and illness variables

Kurtzke's Expanded Disability Status Scale (EDSS; Kurtzke 1983) has been the most commonly used measure of disability in MS. Occasional studies have reported a relationship between EDSS scores and cognitive impairment, but the majority of studies have not found a relationship. Because of problems with EDSS as a measure of disability, the Multiple Sclerosis Functional Composite (Fisher *et al.* 1999) was developed.

It assesses three clinical dimensions:

- leg function/ambulation;
- arm/hand function;
- cognitive function.

It is now recommended for use in standard clinical evaluations.

Most studies have found MS disease duration to be unrelated, or only minimally related, to cognitive dysfunction (Fischer *et al.* 1994). However, it is important to note that these findings are based on cross-sectional studies. Bobholz *et al.*'s (1998) 8-year longitudinal study reveals a different picture in which MS patients declined significantly compared with controls on measures of verbal intelligence, verbal and visual memory, and visuospatial functions. Also, Kujala *et al.* (1997) showed in a 3-year longitudinal study that mild cognitive dysfunction in MS is a significant risk factor for further cognitive deterioration.

Compared with relapsing–remitting patients, chronic progressive patients generally show greater cognitive dysfunction. Nonetheless, relapsing–remitting patients were shown to be cognitively impaired relative to healthy matched controls even when they were in remission (Fischer *et al.* 1994). There is insufficient neuropsychological data on the new course type system (Section 1.2.2).

3 Related emotional disorders in multiple sclerosis

3.1 Depression

Depression is very common in MS with a lifetime prevalence of around 50% for major depression. Point prevalence rates vary between about 15% and 50%, depending on diagnostic approach. Studies using clinical interviews and diagnostic criteria report lower prevalence. Those using cut-offs from self-report measures report higher prevalence.

Depression has been shown to be treatable through brief and even telephone-based cognitive behavioural therapy (Mohr *et al.* 2000), as well as group therapy. In addition, cognitive–behavioural stress management training has been shown to reduce emotional distress in MS (Fischer *et al.* 1994). Nonetheless, depression/distress is historically undertreated in MS. Successful treatment of depression is associated with greater adherence to immunotherapy.

There is no consensus regarding the nature of depression in the literature. Some investigators have presented evidence that neurovegetative symptoms of depression are not valid indicators of depression because of their overlap with MS symptoms (e.g. sleep disturbance, fatigue, sexual dysfunction), while others have provided evidence to the contrary. This debate suggests that caution is warranted in interpreting neurovegetative symptoms of depression as depression symptoms in any individual MS patient.

The causes of depression in MS are unknown, but high levels of perceived stress, low levels of social support, and disease exacerbation/pharmacological treatment have been shown to be associated with increased emotional distress. Depression is associated with reduced quality of life and the employment of generally less effective (emotion-focused) coping strategies in MS. A premorbid history of depression is no more common than in non-MS patients. However, patients with a history of depression, before or after MS onset, may be at increased risk for future depressive and manic states.

3.2 Anxiety

Anxiety is possibly more common than depression in MS, but it has infrequently been studied. Data are limited, but the point prevalence of clinically significant anxiety is thought to be about 25%; lifetime prevalence is unknown. The cause of anxiety in MS is unknown, but it is prominent in the early stages of disease when diagnosis and prognosis are most uncertain. Decline in distress is associated with more definitive diagnostic statements by treatment professionals. Also, as noted above, several other factors have been shown to be associated with emotional distress in general in MS. There are no published studies treating specific anxiety disorders in MS. Comorbidity of anxiety and depression is more associated with thoughts of self-harm, social dysfunction, and somatic complaints than either alone (Feinstein *et al.* 1999).

3.3 Other emotional disorders

The only other emotional disorder occurring with any significant frequency in MS is bipolar disorder. The point prevalence is estimated at 0–2% and the lifetime prevalence at 13–16%. There are no published treatment studies of bipolar disorder in MS. Its cause is unknown.

3.4 Measurement of emotional disorders

- There is no consensus on how depression is best measured in MS because of neurovegetative symptoms. However, CMDI is recommended because it has been validated in MS and allows for breakdown of depression into mood, evaluative, and neurovegetative symptoms of depression in separate scales. Mood and evaluative scales are more likely to reflect depression in MS because they are not confounded with MS symptoms, whereas the neurovegetative scale is. Nonetheless, neurovegetative symptoms may reflect depression in some patients and so should not be dismissed. They should just be interpreted with caution. Clinical interview can be used to follow up initial screening with CMDI, if necessary.

- There is no consensus on how anxiety is best measured in MS, but the Hospital Anxiety and Depression Scale has been shown to be useful (Feinstein *et al.* 1999). This measure takes only about 5 minutes to complete and can be followed up with a clinical interview, if necessary.

- It is unclear how bipolar disorder is best measured in MS. Diagnostic interviews are the only reliable method reported to date.

4 Neuropsychological/cognitive rehabilitation in multiple sclerosis

Approaches to cognitive rehabilitation in MS have been suggested, but no approach has convincing empirical validation. A few empirical studies have tested specific approaches, but most interventions are characterized by small sample sizes, absence of control groups, and disappointing results in terms of their effect on cognitive functioning (Brassington and Marsh 1998). The failure to demonstrate specific effects of cognitive retraining has led some to suggest that pursuing compensatory strategies for MS patients may be more promising. However, cognitive retraining has not been sufficiently studied to rule out the possibility that it may work for some patients. Nonetheless, because compensatory strategies have been studied more extensively in other neurological populations (e.g. traumatic brain injury) and have been shown to be beneficial, it may be useful to apply them to MS patients (Fischer *et al.* 1994). These include strategies such as:

* using external aids (e.g. date books, wristwatches with alarms) for tracking and prompting for important information such as appointments, to-do lists, and medication times;
* keeping things that must be remembered in one place;
* putting calendars in prominent locations and having family members use them so that the affected individual can track family and her/his own activities better.

Although also not systematically studied to date, making workplace modifications that involve things such as reducing distractions and minimizing requirements for speed in the work area might be especially beneficial to persons with MS who suffer from attentional and speeded processing difficulties. Also, because even MS patients with memory difficulties typically show learning with repetition, providing opportunities for recording important meetings, lectures, etc. for later review/rehearsal may be helpful to some patients. Given how common speeded processing difficulties are in MS, making changes in patients' day-to-day environments that allow for adequate time to process information may improve their accuracy in performing day-to-day cognitive tasks (Demaree *et al.* 1999).

Most studies examining the effects of medication on cognitive functioning have reported null or minimal effects. An exception is a study by Fischer *et al.* (2000). One hundred sixty-six persons with relapsing forms of MS from the original double-blind, placebo-controlled trial of IFNβ-1a (Avonex) were compared at baseline and then after 2-year follow-up on a variety of neuropsychological tests. Compared with the placebo group, the IFNβ-1a group improved significantly more on the CVLT (trials 1–5 total), Tower of London, and Ruff Figural Fluency Test. In addition, significantly fewer IFNβ-1a group patients showed sustained PASAT decline by treatment end. Because the study sample was restricted to patients with relapsing MS between ages 18 and 55 and with a very restricted range of EDSS scores (1–3.5), however, caution is warranted in applying the results to patients not meeting such criteria.

The effect of treatment of depression on neuropsychological functioning in MS was studied systematically in only one study (Rodgers *et al.* 1996). Significant improvement in performance on tests of word-list learning and verbal abstraction corresponded to significant reduction in depression in a cognitive therapy treatment group. Although characterized by non-random assignment of patients to treatment groups, non-clinically depressed patients, and a relatively small *n*, results are promising and suggest that depression treatment (even in subclinical patients) could have beneficial cognitive effects in MS. Therefore, beyond improving the well-being of individuals with MS and making them more likely to adhere to important disease-modifying medication regimens (see above), successful treatment of depression may improve patients' cognitive functioning in some domains.

5 Other considerations for multiple sclerosis

Sleep problems are common in MS, but poorly understood. The high and debilitating levels of fatigue reported by MS patients may be related to sleep problems but this possible link is not well-established. It is recommended that fatigue be briefly screened using FSS or examined in more detail using the Fatigue Impact Scale (FIS; Fisk *et al.* 1994). The FIS allows for evaluation of physical, social, and cognitive fatigue in separate scales. A cut-off score of 75 for total score is recommended to identify those with significant functional limitations relating to fatigue. Providing breaks throughout the testing day may help minimize the possible impact of fatigue on test performance.

6 Other demyelinating diseases

Demyelinating diseases other than MS are comparatively rare, have been only minimally studied neuropsychologically, and are infrequently seen by clinical neuropsychologists. A brief discussion of two other demyelinating diseases follows.

6.1 Marchiafava–Bignami disease

This is characterized by focal demyelination in the medial zone of corpus callosum and is most commonly associated with chronic alcoholism. There are rare but well-documented cases reported in non-alcoholics. Degeneration of anterior and posterior commissures, centrum semiovale, middle cerebellar peduncles, subcortical white matter, and long association bundles is also sometimes seen. Symptom onset is usually insidious and non-specific with both focal and diffuse manifestations of cerebral disease common. Acute presentations involving deteriorating speech, gait, orientation, and consciousness are also seen. Psychiatric symptoms are frequently present including delusional states, paranoia, mania, and depression. Psychomotor slowing, apathy, and dysarthria are also seen. Neuropsychologically, non-specific dementia is most common. Callosal signs are also characteristic. For example, patients may be able to name objects placed in one hand or presented to one visual field, but not those in the other hand or field. Hemispheric disconnection signs also include unilateral apraxias and agraphias in the absence of aphasia, in addition to unilateral sensory (i.e. auditory, tactile, visual) simultaneous extinction. Alien hand syndrome is sometimes seen, most often on the left side or bilaterally.

6.2 Central pontine myelinolysis (CPM)

This involves destruction of myelin sheaths in the central portion of the basis pontis and is most often found in young to middle-aged adults. Myelinolytic lesions are not restricted to the brainstem and are observed in cerebral cortex, thalamus, basal ganglia, subcortical white matter, amygdala, centrum semiovale, internal capsule, cerebellum, and corpus callosum. CPM is associated with chronic alcoholism and/or malnutrition in most cases, but also with liver, kidney, and brain disease and organ transplants. More recently, it has been seen with AIDS, chemotherapy, and viral infections. The definitive cause is unknown, but rapid correction of hyponatraemia is suspected. Acute symptoms include altered levels of consciousness, seizures, lethargy, mutism, pseudobulbar palsy, and quadriparesis. The course of disease can be rapid, with death ensuing within days or weeks of symptom onset, but more patients have survived the acute phase of illness in recent years. Neuropsychological data to date are limited to case reports that indicate persistence of deficits beyond acute stage involving global intelligence and reasoning, learning and memory, visual- and fine-motor speed, and attention and concentration. Confusional states most likely associated with the underlying metabolic problem that causes CPM are not uncommon. Neuropsychiatric features including pressured and tangential speech, restlessness and agitation, and impaired insight and judgement have been reported as initial presenting symptoms of CPM.

Acknowledgements

Special thanks are owed to my colleagues in the field, Drs Stephen Rao, Michael Basso, William Beatty, John DeLuca, Lauren Krupp, and David Mohr, for their thoughts regarding the optimal battery of tests to be used for the neuropsychological assessment of MS patients. I also wish to express my gratitude to the MS participants and their significant others who have contributed their time in my studies to help me better understand the nature of MS.

Selective references

Arnett, P.A., Higginson, C.H., and Randolph, J.R. (2001). Depression in multiple sclerosis: relationship to planning ability. *J. Int. Neuropsychol. Soc.* **7**, 665–74.

Beatty, W.W. and Monson, N. (1996). Problem solving by patients with multiple sclerosis. *J. Int. Neuropsychol. Soc.* **2**, 134–40.

Beatty, W.W., Paul, R.H., Wilbanks, S.L., Hames, K.A., Blanco, C.R., and Goodkin, D.E. (1995). Identifying multiple sclerosis patients with mild or global cognitive impairment using the Screening Examination for Cognitive Impairment (SEFCI). *Neurology* **45**, 718–23.

Benton, A.L., Hamsher, K. deS., Varney, N.R., and Spreen, O. (1983). *Contributions to neuropsychological assessment.* Oxford University Press, New York.

Bobholz, J., Rao, S., Seidenberg, L., Sweet, J., Patterson, K., Bernardin, L., Binder, J.R., and Lobeck, L. (1998). Cognitive decline in MS: an 8-year longitudinal study. *J. Int. Neuropsychol. Soc.* **4**, 35.

Boringa, J.B., Lazeron, R.H.C., Reuling, I.E.W. *et al.* (2001). The Brief Repeatable Battery of Neuropsychological Tests: normative values allow application in multiple sclerosis clinical practice. *Multiple Sclerosis* **7**, 263–8.

Brassington, J.C. and Marsh, N.V. (1998). Neuropsychological aspects of multiple sclerosis. *Neuropsychol. Rev.* **8**, 43–77.

Cook, S.D. (ed.) (2001). *Handbook of Multiple Sclerosis*, 3rd edn. Dekker, New York.

Delis, D.C., Kramer, J.H., Kaplan, E., and Ober, B.A. (2000). *California Verbal Learning Test—second edition—adult version*. The Psychological Corporation, San Antonio, Texas.

Delis, D.C., Kaplan, E., and Kramer, J.H. (2001). *Delis–Kaplan Executive Function System (D–KEFS)*. The Psychological Corporation, San Antonio, Texas.

Demaree, H.A., DeLuca, J., Gaudino, E.A., and Diamond, B.J. (1999). Speed of information processing as a key deficit in multiple sclerosis: implications for rehabilitation. *J. Neurol. Neurosurg. Psychiatry* **67**, 661–3.

Feinstein, A., O'Connor, P., Gray, T., and Feinstein, K. (1999). The effects of anxiety on psychiatric morbidity in patients with multiple sclerosis. *Multiple Sclerosis* **5**, 323–6.

Fischer, J.S., Foley, F.W., Aikens, J.E., Ericson, D.G., Rao, S.M., and Shindell, S. (1994). What do we really know about cognitive dysfunction, affective disorders, and stress in multiple sclerosis? A practitioner's guide. *J. Neurol. Rehabil.* **8**, 151–64.

Fischer, J.S., Rudick, R.A., Cutter, G.R., and Reingold, S.C. (1999). The Multiple Sclerosis Functional Composite Measure (MSFC): an integrated approach to MS clinical outcome assessment. *Multiple Sclerosis* **5**, 244–50.

Fisk, J.D., Pontefract, A., Ritvo, P.G., Archibald, C.J., and Murray, T.J. (1994). The impact of fatigue on patients with multiple sclerosis. *Can. J. Neurol. Sci.* **21**, 9–14.

Higginson, C.I., Arnett, P.A., and Voss, W.D. (2000). The ecological validity of clinical tests of memory and attention in multiple sclerosis. *Arch. Clin. Neuropsychol.* **15**, 185–204.

Kaplan, E.F., Goodglass, H., and Weintraub, S. (1983). *The Boston Naming Test (2nd edn)*. Lea and Febiger, Philadelphia.

Krupp, L.B. and Elkins, L. (2000). Fatigue and declines in cognitive functioning in multiple sclerosis. *Neurology* **55**, 934–9.

Krupp, L.B., Alvarez, L.A., LaRocca, N.G., and Scheinberg, L.C. (1988). Fatigue in multiple sclerosis. *Arch. Neurol.* **45**, 435–7.

Kujala, P., Portin, R., and Ruutianinen, J. (1997). The progress of cognitive decline in multiple sclerosis: a controlled 3-year follow-up. *Brain* **120**, 289–97.

Kurtzke, J.F. (1983). Rating neurologic impairment in multiple sclerosis: an expanded disability status scale (EDSS). *Neurology* **33**, 1444–52.

Lublin, F.D. and Reingold, S.C. (1996). Defining the clinical course of multiple sclerosis: results of an international survey. *Neurology* **46**, 907–11.

Mohr, D.C., Van Der Wende, J., Dwyer, P., and Dick, L.P. (2000). Telephone-administered cognitive–behavioral therapy for the treatment of depressive symptoms in multiple sclerosis. *J. Consult. Clin. Psychol.* **68**, 356–61.

Nyenhuis, D.L., Luchetta, T., Yamamoto, C., Terrien, A., Bernardin, L., Rao, S.M., and Garron, D.C. (1998). The development, standardization, and initial validation of the Chicago Multiscale Depression Inventory. *J. Personality Assess.* **70**, 386–401.

Rao, S.M., Cognitive Function Study Group, National Multiple Sclerosis Society (1990). *Manual for the Brief Repeatable Battery of Neuropsychological Tests in Multiple Sclerosis*. National Multiple Sclerosis Society, New York.

Rao, S.M., Leo, G.J., Haughton, V.M., St. Aubin-Faubert, P., and Bernardin, L. (1989). Correlation of magnetic resonance imaging with neuropsychological testing in multiple sclerosis. *Neurology* **39**, 161–6.

Rao, S.M., Leo, G.J., Bernardin, L., and Unverzagt, F. (1991). Cognitive dysfunction in multiple sclerosis. I. Frequency, patterns, and prediction. *Neurology* **41**, 685–91.

Rodgers, D., Khoo, K., MacEachen, M., Oven, M., and Beatty, W.W. (1996). Cognitive therapy for multiple sclerosis: a preliminary study. *Altern. Ther.* **2**, 70–4.

Smith, A. (1982). *Symbol Digit Modalities Test. Manual (revised)*. Western Psychological Services, Los Angeles.

Spreen, O. and Strauss, E. (ed.) (1998). *A compendium of neuropsychological tests: administration, norms, and commentary*, 2nd edn. Oxford University Press, New York.

Wechsler, D. (1997*a*). *WAIS-III administration and scoring manual*. The Psychological Corporation, San Antonio, Texas.

Wechsler, D. (1997*b*). *WMS-III administration and scoring manual*. The Psychological Corporation, San Antonio, Texas.

Wechsler, D. (1999). *WASI manual*. The Psychological Corporation, San Antonio, Texas.

Wilkinson, G.S. (1993). *WRAT3 administration manual*. Wide Range, Inc, Wilmington, Delaware.

Zakzanis, K.K. (2000). Distinct neuropsychological profiles in multiple sclerosis subtypes. *Arch. Clin. Neuropsychol.* **15**, 115–36.

Chapter 30

The neuropsychology of infectious and inflammatory brain disorders

François Boller and Sandra Suarez

1 Introduction

Many infectious processes can involve cerebral tissues and cause cognitive disorders. The aetiology includes viral, bacterial, and parasitic agents. The precise pathology associated with these agents varies, consisting mainly of infection of the meninges (meningitis) and formation of abscesses. Several general considerations apply to conditions covered by this chapter.

- Following the introduction of antibiotics, infectious pathology was thought to have lost its importance at least in the most developed countries. Unfortunately, the appearance of acquired immune deficiency syndrome (AIDS) has put infections of the central nervous system (CNS) at the forefront again. In addition, the immunodeficiency induced by AIDS has made some uncommon infectious pathologies appear or reappear on the scene.

- Some of these conditions, particularly AIDS, demonstrate the need for an alternative way of defining dementia, differing from the 'classical' concepts inspired by Alzheimer's disease. AIDS-related dementia turns out to be one of the best examples of subcortical dementia.

- Finally, the general 'rules' of brain–behaviour relationships apply here as well. The cognitive sequelae of a CNS infection depend mainly on the localization and size of the lesions. The nature of the lesions determines the evolution of the process.

In recent years, there have been some changes in the role of the neuropsychologist in dealing with these patients. He or she can assist in the diagnosis, in establishing a precise aetiology, and also in specifying the extent of lesions in anatomical and, above all, functional terms. During rehabilitation, the neuropsychologist can not only monitor the changes that occur with time, but also in many cases help establish the rehabilitation plan and participate directly in its implementation.

2 Some viral infections causing dementia

2.1 AIDS dementia complex or mild cognitive–motor impairment of HIV-1 infection

Human immunodeficiency virus type 1 (HIV-1) infection is one of the most dangerous epidemics of our time. At the end of 2000, the World Health Organization's

(WHO) estimations were of 36.1 million people living with HIV/AIDS and 21.8 million deaths. More than 95% of infected people do not receive any treatment. HIV-1 infection, particularly in the late phase, may be complicated by mild or severe cognitive impairment. The stages of HIV infection are characterized by the Centers for Disease Control (CDC) classification systems (Centers for Disease Control 1986) and the revised version of CDC in 1992 (Centers for Disease Control and Prevention 1992).

2.1.1 HIV-1-associated dementia complex (ADC)

This form was first recognized as an AIDS-related illness by Navia *et al.* (1986), under the name of AIDS dementia complex (ADC). The presence of ADC was added to the definition of AIDS a year later. This pathology affects about 15% of HIV-1 patients (McArthur *et al.* 1993). It is a neurological complication of AIDS that seems to be associated with HIV CNS infection. ADC is characterized by (Bornstein *et al.* 1993):

◆ psychomotor slowing;

◆ memory impairment;

◆ disturbances in complex attentional tasks and executive functioning;

◆ behavioural manifestations.

Those symptoms meet the criteria of a subcortical dementia.

Typically, the patients show moderate cognitive disorders that evolve rapidly. Less frequently, the onset is abrupt. The intellectual changes lead invariably to a severe deficit, mainly because of inertia and general slowing.

◆ Language functions tend to be preserved except for a general reduction.

◆ Reasoning is clearly impaired, particularly when the task implies a series of related operations.

◆ Motor acts and sequences on command are slow and complex commands are often not followed or left unfinished.

One gets a general impression of a global decline of mental activity and of a deficit affecting all cognitive tasks. At the end stage, the majority of patients show a global cognitive deterioration as well as major motor disorders (particularly akinesia, tremor, and myoclonus). Neurological examination shows frontal signs in some patients. Affective indifference and mutism added to loss of sphincter control contribute to a situation of abandonment, passivity, and loss of contact with the environment. At times, unexpectedly lucid short sentences contrast with the general impression of a global dementia.

Data concerning the appearance and the evolution of ADC are still conflicting. Navia *et al.* (1986) report that the onset is most often insidious with a progressive evolution. Selnes *et al.* (1995) report that the onset is most often fast. The mean survival time is 6 months (Mc Arthur *et al.* 1993).

The relationship between cognitive dysfunction in HIV and physiopathological lesions remains unclear. Recent neuropathological and neuroimaging studies found no direct correlation between lesions and rate of cognitive impairment (Glass *et al.* 1993; Seilhean *et al.* 1993; Bell *et al.* 1996; Everall *et al.* 1994). Studies of demented AIDS patients have shown that the multinucleated giant cells and diffuse myelin pallor that occur in HIV encephalitis are observed in only 40–50% of patients (Glass *et al.* 1993; Bell *et al.* 1996). Prospective (Seilhean *et al.* 1993) and retrospective studies (Everall *et al.* 1994) showed no correlation between cortical neuronal loss and cognitive impairment. Moreover, brain atrophy, most prominent in the subcortical grey matter (Dal-Pan *et al.* 1992; Aylward *et al.* 1993), was a frequent finding in AIDS patients who do not manifest overt features of dementia (Raininko *et al.* 1992). One study found no relationship between subcortical atrophy and neuropsychological performance (Hestad *et al.* 1993). Another study showed a strong association between brain atrophy and clinical stage, but no association between atrophy and cognitive impairment (Di Sclafani *et al.* 1997). Whether atrophy is related to cognitive dysfunction or to clinical stage is unclear. This is crucial since it may mean that ADC is directly related to neuropathological mechanisms such as neocortical neuronal loss or, conversely, to reversible neuronal dysfunction.

2.1.2 Staging of ADC

A classification of the staging of ADC, according to the cognitive impairment and daily living abilities, was proposed by Price and Brew (1988; see Table 30.1).

Table 30.1 Staging scheme for AIDS dementia complex

Stage 0—normal

Normal mental and motor function

Stage 0.5—equivocal/subclinical

Either minimal or equivocal symptoms of cognitive or motor dysfunction characteristic of ADC or mild signs (snout response, slowed extremity movements) but without impairment of work or capacity to perform activities of daily living (ADL). Gait and strength are normal.

Stage 1—mild

Unequivocal evidence (symptoms, signs, neuropsychological test performance) of functional, intellectual, or motor impairment characteristic of ADC but able to perform all but the more demanding aspects of work or ADL. Can walk without assistance.

Stage 2—moderate

Cannot work or maintain the more demanding aspects of ADL but able to perform basic activities of self-care. The patient may require assistance in walking.

Stage 3—severe

Major intellectual incapacity (cannot follow news or personal events, cannot sustain complex conversation, considerable slowing of all output) or motor disability (cannot walk unassisted, requiring walker or personal support, usually with slowing and clumsiness of arms as well).

Stage 4—end stage

Nearly vegetative. Intellectual and social comprehension and responses are at rudimentary level. Nearly or absolutely mute. Paraparetic or paraplegic with double incontinence.

- Stage 0, normal mental and motor function;
- Stage 0.5, subclinical symptoms;
- Stage 1, mild cognitive deficit;
- Stage 2, moderate impairment;
- Stage 3, severe cognitive–motor deficit;
- Stage 4, higher deficit.

Another rapid classification, the 'Power-McArthur AIDS dementia test', has been proposed (Power *et al.* 1995). A score of 0 represents a major deterioration and 16 no cognitive troubles.

2.1.3 Diagnostic criteria for ADC

There are two classifications that provide diagnostic criteria for ADC:

- the DSM-IV (*Diagnostic and statistical manual of mental disorders*) classification of AIDS dementia (American Psychiatric Association 1994);
- the American Academy of Neurology (AAN) AIDS Task Force classification.

The DSM-IV classification

AIDS dementia diagnosis implies the observation of progressive dementia with both memory and executive impairment. DSM-IV diagnostic criteria include the following.

- Dementia associated with HIV infection of the CNS is typically characterized by forgetfulness, slowness, poor concentration, and difficulties with problem-solving.
- Behavioural manifestations most commonly include apathy and social withdrawal. Occasionally, delirium, delusions or hallucinations may accompany these.
- Tremor, impaired rapid repetitive movements, imbalance, ataxia, hypertonia, generalized hyperreflexia, positive frontal release signs, and impaired pursuit and saccadic eye movements may be present on physical examination.

The AAN AIDS Task Force classification of the HIV-1 cognitive/motor complex (Table 30.2). This is the most frequently used classification (Janssen *et al.* 1991). In this classification the term 'HIV-1 cognitive/motor complex' was introduced. In 1996, Marder *et al.* put into operation the AAN definition of the HIV-1 cognitive/motor complex; a test was considered impaired if standard deviation was greater than or equal to 2. The classification covered six cognitive fields:

- attention/concentration;
- speed of motor or cognitive processing;
- abstraction/reasoning;
- memory/learning;
- visuospatial skills;
- speech/language.

Table 30.2 HIV-1-associated cognitive/motor complex

HIV-1-associated dementia complex (ADC)

Probable (must have each of the following)

1   Acquired abnormality in at least two of the following cognitive abilities (present for at least 1 month):

—attention/concentration;

—speed of processing of information;

—abstraction/reasoning;

—visuospatial skills;

—memory/learning;

—speech/language.

2   Cognitive dysfunction causing impairment of work or activities of daily living, not attributable solely to severe systemic illness.

3   At least one of the following:

—acquired abnormality in motor function and/or performance verified by clinical examination (e.g. slowed rapid movements, abnormal gait, limb incoordination, hyperreflexia, hypertonia, or weakness);

—decline in motivation or emotional control or change in social behaviour. This may be characterized by any of the following: change in personality with apathy, inertia, irritability, emotional lability, or new onset of impaired judgement characterized by socially inappropriate behaviour or disinhibition.

4   Absence of clouding of consciousness during a period long enough to establish the presence of requisite abnormalities in point 1

5   If another potential aetiology (e.g. major depression) is present, it is not the cause of the above cognitive, motor, or behavioural symptoms and signs

Possible (must have one of the following)

1   Other potential aetiology present (must have each of the following):

—As above (see *Probable*), points 1, 2, and 3;

—Other potential aetiology is present but the cause of point 1 under *Probable* is uncertain.

2   Incomplete clinical evaluation (must have each of the following):

—As above (see *Probable*), points 1, 2, and 3;

—Aetiology cannot be determined (appropriate laboratory or radiological investigations not performed).

HIV-1-associated minor cognitive/motor disorder

Probable (must have each of the following)

1   Cognitive/motor/behavioural abnormalities (must have each of the following):

—At least two of the following acquired cognitive, motor, or behavioural symptoms (present for at least 1 month) verified by reliable history:

(a) impaired attention or concentration;

(b) mental slowing;

(c) impaired memory;

(d) slowed movements;

Table 30.2 (*continued*)

(e) incoordination;

(f) personality change, or irritability or emotional lability.

—Acquired cognitive/motor/behavioural abnormalities verified by clinical neurological examination or neuropsychological testing

2   Disturbance from cognitive/motor/behavioural abnormalities (see point 1) causes mild impairment of work of activities of daily living

3   Does not meet criteria for HIV-1-associated dementia complex or HIV-1-associated myelopathy

4   No evidence of another aetiology

Possible (must have one of the following)

1   Other potential aetiology present (must have each of the following):

—As above (see *Probable*) points 1, 2, and 3

—Other potential aetiology is present and the cause of the cognitive/motor/behavioural abnormalities in point 1 under *Probable* is uncertain

2   Incomplete clinical evaluation (must have each of the following):

—As above (see *Probable*) points 1, 2, and 3

—Aetiology cannot be determined (appropriate laboratory or radiological investigations not performed)

2.1.4 HIV-1-associated minor cognitive–motor disorder

The milder form, described as 'HIV-1-associated minor cognitive-motor disorder' by the AAN AIDS Task Force (Janssen *et al.* 1991), is characterized by impaired motor speed and working memory, but relatively spared attention, episodic memory, and visuoconstructive abilities (Dunbar *et al.* 1992; Stout *et al.* 1995; Selnes *et al.* 1995).

2.1.5 Diagnostic criteria

Two classifications are available:

◆   the DSM-IV addendum of mild cognitive impairment;

◆   the AAN AIDS Task Force definition of HIV-1-associated minor cognitive/motor disorder.

Some authors emphasize the similar subcortical pattern of cognitive impairment in AIDS patients with and without dementia (Suarez *et al.* 2000), and differentiate mild cognitive impairment, characterized by bradyphrenia, inattention, poor conceptualization, poor initiation, and memory impairment, from the cognitive impairment of ADC patients, in whom bradykinesia and impaired free recall are more severe. But the question of the continuity between minor cognitive/motor disorder and ADC is still debated. Data from a longitudinal study of the cognitive performance of HIV patients developing AIDS, showed that decreasing psychomotor speed was the only presymptomatic factor predictive of dementia (Selnes *et al.* 1995).

The DSM-IV addendum of mild cognitive impairment (Gutierrez *et al.* 1993)

♦ The impairment is severe enough to impair activities of daily living but not sufficiently severe to lead to a diagnosis of dementia.

♦ The neurocognitive disorder must present impairments of at least two of the following cognitive functions, which must be impaired for at least 2 weeks:

—memory;

—executive function;

—concentration abilities;

—motor abilities;

—language.

In the specific case of mild cognitive impairment of HIV-1 infected patients, the cognitive abilities most impaired are slower psychomotor speed, loss of executive control, and episodic memory pattern (disturbance of free and cued recall) (Suarez *et al.* 2000).

The AAN AIDS Task Force classification of HIV-1-associated minor cognitive/motor disorder (Table 30.2).

The impairments are not sufficient for the diagnosis of AIDS. The main difference between ADC and minor cognitive/motor disorder lies in the capacity to perform activities of daily living (Janssen *et al.* 1991). This impairment in daily living abilities must be assessed clinically and with daily living scales.

♦ Patients with minor cognitive/motor disorder are able to realize most daily living activities.

♦ Even if the majority of the patients can work, mild perturbations can be observed at work and in social activities.

♦ The patients are not dependent on other people. They can feed themselves, take care of their sanitation, use money, or drive a car.

♦ More complicated situations of daily living such as remembering a date or taking medication can occasionally be impaired.

The HIV-1-associated minor cognitive/motor disorder classification of the AAN was made operational by Marder *et al.* (1996).

2.1.6 Cognitive impairments in HIV-1 infected patients

2.1.6.1 Psychomotor slowing Several articles have emphasized the importance of psychomotor slowing in AIDS patients (with and without dementia) (Bornstein *et al.* 1993; Maruff *et al.* 1994; Portegies *et al.* 1993; Sacktor *et al.* 1996; Suarez *et al.* 2001). In a 9-year longitudinal study of HIV patients, Sacktor *et al.* (1996) showed that a sustained decline in psychomotor performance is predictive of dementia, AIDS, and death. Beeker and Salthouse (1999) showed that psychomotor and memory impairments are the most explicit signs of the global deterioration of the patients. Some authors suggest that psychomotor tests are the most sensitive to a CNS deterioration (Martin *et al.* 1992; Dunlop *et al.* 1993; Suarez *et al.* 2001). One study shows differences in the kinetics of memory and psychomotor improvements under highly active antiretroviral therapy and suggests that distinct neuropathological mechanisms might cause psychomotor and memory dysfunctions in AIDS (Suarez *et al.* 2001).

2.1.6.2 Executive function   Impairment in executive function may appear in the asymptomatic stage (Sahakian *et al.* 1995). Priming impairment may be related to the subcortical pathologies (Nielsen-Bohlman *et al.* 1997; Jasiukaitis and Fein 1999). A recent study, using an adapted version of the Stroop test, showed psychomotor slowing in HIV seropositive patients with an interference effect (Hinkin *et al.* 1999). Cognitive studies must use sensitive and specific tests, particularly in the earliest stages of HIV-1 infection. There is a need to improve the specificity and sensitivity of neuropsychological measurements currently used to detect cognitive impairment in HIV-1 infected patients, especially in the medically asymptomatic stage (Clemente-Millana and Portellano 2000).

2.1.6.3 Working memory   HIV is associated with executive and attentional functions, which may be impaired. Tests of working memory that require the interaction of these components may be particularly sensitive to cognitive dysfunction that arises from HIV infection. Stout *et al.* (1995) showed impairment in the Reading Span Test (reverse) and the Digit Span subtest from the Wechsler Memory Scale-Revised (WMS-R) for symptomatic HIV positive subjects (relative to HIV negative control subjects). Asymptomatic and mildly symptomatic HIV positive groups exhibited a trend towards impairment on these tests (Stout *et al.* 1995). The impairment of working memory is demonstrated by tests that involve a manipulation of information but not by tests involving simple storage such as the direct Reading Span Test. Sahakian *et al.* (1995), using a spatial working memory test, showed that the impairment is relative to the complexity of the test. Seropositive subjects were impaired only for more difficult versions of the test. Similar results were found with the 'Tower of London' test. These deficits in planning and spatial working memory suggest a frontal impairment (Owen *et al.* 1990) and support a hypothesis that frontostriatal dysfunction occurs in HIV-1 infected individuals prior even to the expression of clinical symptoms (Sahakian *et al.* 1995).

2.1.6.4 Episodic memory   Many studies about verbal memory suggest subcortical memory impairment. Among seropositive patients, 35.5% have acquisition and retention impairments, although recognition is better preserved (Becker *et al.* 1995). Peavy *et al.* (1994) showed that symptomatic seropositive patients make more mistakes than seronegatives in acquisition and retention verbal memory, using the California Verbal Learning Test. Seropositive patients used the semantic organization of the words to be remembered as a strategy to a lesser extent than the seronegatives. The profile of verbal memory deficits exhibited by the subgroup of impaired HIV positive subjects was similar to that of patients with Huntington's disease, a prototypical subcortical dementia with impaired free recall with intrusions, and different from that of patients with Alzheimer's disease, a prototypical cortical dementia. Another study, using the Grober and Buschke test (a verbal memory test that differentiates amnesia due to temporal-lobe-related storage deficit from free recall deficit) showed that AIDS patients with mild cognitive impairment had an early disturbance of free and cued recall compared with asymptomatic seropositive patients. The memory pattern of ADC patients, as compared to mildly cognitively impaired patients, was marked by significantly impaired free recall, but undisturbed total recall (Suarez *et al.* 2000). Such a pattern of impaired free recall but preserved cued recall is typical of memory impairment resulting from subcortical–frontal dysfunction (Pillon *et al.* 1994). HIV positive patients with subcortical verbal memory troubles had a generally lower CD4 lymphocyte count, which suggests that, in contrast to working memory, verbal memory impairment may appear later in the disease (Becker *et al.* 1995).

2.1.7 Evolution of cognitive impairment under highly active antiretroviral therapy

Since the introduction, in mid-1996, of highly active antiretroviral therapy (HAART), a protease inhibitor-containing combination therapy, the rates of hospitalizations (Baum *et al.* 1999), morbidity, and mortality (Palella *et al.* 1998; Mocroft *et al.* 1999) have been declining among patients with advanced HIV infection along with the incidence of major opportunistic infections (Palella *et al.* 1998; Ledergerber *et al.* 1999). HAART improves prognosis for patients with HIV encephalopathy (Chang *et al.* 1999; Tozzi *et al.* 1999), despite the low capacity of antiretroviral therapy to cross the blood–brain barrier (Dore *et al.* 1999; Enting *et al.* 1998). Nevertheless, cognitive disturbances are still an important predictive factor of fatal outcome (20% in cognitively impaired patients), and more severe psychomotor slowing and lower CD4 count are associated with higher mortality (Suarez *et al.* 2001).

- Sacktor *et al.* (1999) showed that combination antiretroviral therapy including protease inhibitors is associated with improved psychomotor speed performance (Grooved Pegboard nondominant hand test and the Symbol Digit Modalities Test) in HIV positive homosexual men with abnormal neuropsychological testing.

- Suarez *et al.* (2000), using a short battery of neuropsychological tests to identify minor to severe cognitive impairments, showed an improvement of psychomotor speed, verbal anterograde memory, and executive functions related to the duration of HAART (Suarez *et al.* 2001).

- Studies since the introduction of HAART utilization have shown an improvement of psychomotor speed (Price *et al.* 1999; Sacktor *et al.* 1999).

Even in HAART-treated patients, psychomotor slowing is still associated with higher mortality (Suarez *et al.* 2001).

Since HAART has increased survival, the question of disability and, consequently, quality of life has become paramount for the survivors (McArthur 1997; Dore *et al.* 1999). Improvement in quality of life of persons with neurological AIDS complications should receive a high priority.

2.2 Neurological cytomegalovirus (CMV) infection

CMV encephalitis is quite common in immunodepressed patients. Different symptoms can appear in neurological CMV.

♦ When the virus attacks the spinal cord and roots (myelitis, myeloradiculitis, and polyneuropathy), a rapid loss of bladder function, saddle anaesthesia, and weakness of the legs with a variable degree of pain and paralysis are seen.

♦ On the other hand, the symptoms of dementia (encephalitis) may develop over just a few weeks time, sometimes associated with cranial nerve abnormalities affecting vision (retinitis), hearing, and balance.

This disorder is generally rapidly fatal over a period of just 4–8 weeks. Patients with CMV retinitis are at increased risk of developing diffuse CMV encephalitis (McCutchan 1995). CMV encephalitis has no clinical specificity, but is generally either diffuse or focal CMV. A microglial nodular encephalitis can also occur, characterized by confusion and delirium, which do not occur in ventriculoencephalitis (Grassi *et al.* 1998). The presence of apathy and psychomotor slowing may lead to a confusion with AIDS dementia, the main differential diagnosis (Holland *et al.* 1994).

Clinical signs of focal CMV encephalitis depend on their localization. The diagnosis will be done by revealing the presence of the CMV in the spinal fluid or in the brain matter. Neuropsychological examination should be performed with special care in patients with CMV retinitis because they are also at increased risk of developing diffuse CMV encephalitis and more subtle levels of cognitive impairment can be detected (McCutchan 1995). Current medical treatment options are monotherapy of ganciclovir, foscarnet, or cidofovir. Ganciclovir and foscarnet have improved the prognosis of multifocal neuropathy and polyradiculopathy (Anders and Goebel 1999). However, the encephalitis response rates to standard treatments are unfortunately low (Anders and Goebel 1999; Cinque *et al.* 1998). Neurological sequelae, such as mental retardation, are frequent.

2.3 Herpes simplex encephalitis

This is a life-threatening disease, caused by the herpes virus, with a high mortality rate (about 30%) in the acute phase as well as significant morbidity among its survivors. Lesions consist of an acute necrosis of the cortical and subcortical cerebral tissue of the temporal and orbitofrontal regions. Survivors may present cognitive sequelae with most often impairment in retrograde memory, executive function, and language functioning. Personality and behavioural changes are also observed. The long-term outcome of herpes simplex encephalitis is better after acyclovir treatment (cognitive recovery and functional independence for activities of daily life). The time from first symptoms to antiviral medical treatment appears to be the best predictor of outcome.

The most common long-term symptoms (McGrath *et al.* 1997) are:

◆ short-term memory impairment;

◆ anosmia;

◆ dysphasia;

◆ personality and behavioural abnormalities;

◆ epilepsy.

One study has shown that dysnomia and impaired new learning are among the long-term cognitive sequelae of herpes simplex encephalitis treated early with acyclovir (Gordon *et al.* 1990). The original description of category-specific semantic memory impairment (selective impairment and selective preservation of certain categories of visual stimuli) by Warrington (1975) and Warrington and Shallice (1984) involved patients with herpes simplex encephalitis.

2.4 Progressive multifocal leukoencephalopathy (PML)

PML is a rare, usually fatal, demyelinating disease of the brain caused by the JC virus (JCV). Patients with PML often present with rapidly progressive focal findings of cognitive impairment, hemiparesis, and visual field defects. Symptoms depend on the location of the demyelinating lesion, which is usually (but not always) posterior. Symptoms may progress to include aphasia, ataxia, cranial nerve deficits, cortical blindness, quadriparesis, profound dementia, and coma. Findings are usually localized to the white matter, and death frequently occurs within 6 months of presentation.

There is a continuous expansion of the multifocal brain lesions caused by the JC virus. This condition is characterized by rapid evolution going within a few weeks from a picture of multiple functional impairment to dementia, delirium, seizures, coma, and death. It is typically seen in patients with impaired immunological competence following, for instance, severe granulomatous pathology, tumours, or leukaemia. It can also be associated with AIDS. HAART improves prognosis in terms of survival in PML associated to HIV-1 infection (Gasnault 1999; Clifford 1999). However, 'despite the addition of cidofovir to HAART, no significant benefit is observed in the neurological outcome, particularly in patients with an early worsening' (Gasnault *et al.* 2001).

2.5 Subacute sclerosing panencephalitis

Subacute sclerosing panencephalitis, extensively studied by Van Bogaert, is a rare pathology of the CNS, associated with increase of antibody titres for measles. It produces, in children and adolescents, a rapidly progressive dementia with disorders of language and personality changes. Electroencephalographic (EEG) abnormalities are associated with seizures and myoclonus (Jayawant *et al.* 2000). The disease is usually lethal.

3 Bacterial causes of dementia

3.1 Neurosyphilis

Neurosyphilis is a bacterial infection caused by the spiral-shaped bacteria, *Treponema pallidum*. The epidemiology of the condition has followed a U-shaped curve. It was one of the leading causes of institutionalization for dementia until a few decades ago, but has become quite uncommon since the introduction of antibiotics. The present pandemic of AIDS has made syphilis (and its neurological complications) a more frequent occurrence but it is still most uncommon in non-AIDS patients (Masmoudil *et al.* 1996).

The psychiatric and neurological symptoms of neurosyphilis can mimic virtually any psychiatric or neurological disorder (Russouw *et al.* 1997). The complex of dementia characterized by cognitive slowing, amnesia, confabulations, and delirium is known under the name 'general paresis of the insane' (GPI). GPI occurs as a tertiary manifestation of syphilis, which follows by 5 to 30 years the original infection, following a meningoencephalitis. Its early stages are characterized by what appears to be a 'frontal' syndrome. There is insidious onset of memory defect (forgetfulness), impairment in reasoning, and reduction in clinical faculties. One also notices behavioural changes consisting of depression or 'odd' behaviour, irritability, and lack of interest in personal care. As pointed out by Adams *et al.* (1997), classical writing has stressed the development of delusional systems, most dramatically in the direction of megalomania. In fact, the representation of psychiatric disorders in the popular imagination is inspired by that notion. The clinical reality, however, shows this to be an exceptional event. The symptoms are partially responsive to treatment (Farina *et al.* 1994).

3.2 Neurotuberculosis (tuberculous meningoencephalitis)

Tuberculous meningoencephalitis, another pathology that has decreased considerably in the last decades in the industrialized world, is a more frequent occurrence in developing nations and among the least protected individuals in all countries. Its symptoms include subtle personality changes with confusion and amnesia evolving later into clear-cut disorientation and alterations of consciousness that may lead to coma and, if no adequate treatment is provided, death (Williams and Smith 1954). The cognitive and behavioural symptoms, usually related to cerebral vasculitis, occur within a context of increased intracerebral pressure, normal pressure hydrocephalus (NPH), sub-acute or chronic meningitis, involvement of cranial nerves, and, occasionally, focal signs due to haemorrhagic infarcts or to tuberculomas. Even in cases of improvement, now practically guaranteed by appropriate and timely therapeutic intervention, cognitive sequels, particularly amnesia, are frequent. Here again, this pathology has reappeared on a fairly large scale as a complication of infection with HIV, leading some authors to refer to it as the new neurotuberculosis (Sanchez-Portocarrero *et al.* 1999).

4 Parasite infections

4.1 Cerebral toxoplasmosis (toxoplasmal abcesses)

Toxoplasma gondii, an obligate intracellular protozoan, is recognized as a major cause of neurological morbidity and mortality among patients with advanced HIV disease. The complaint is suggestive of a focal neurological process. The symptoms are often vague and non-specific. Headache, usually dull and constant, is present in about 50% of patients presenting with toxoplasma encephalitis (TE). On the basis of therapeutic responses (but in the absence of biopsy), it has been suggested that it would be prudent to initiate empirical anti-toxoplasma treatment for all HIV patients with mass lesions and to assess clinical and radiological response (Wadia *et al.* 2001).

4.2 Malaria

Cerebral malaria complicates about 2% of cases of infection by *Plasmodium falciparum*. It occurs mainly in children in hyperendemic areas, in pregnancy, and in individuals who are immunosuppressed. Cerebral malaria has a mortality rate of up to 50%, and also a considerable long-term morbidity, particularly in children.

- CNS manifestations of malaria include intracranial haemorrhage, cerebral arterial occlusion, and transient extrapyramidal and neuropsychiatric manifestations.
- Hemiplegia, aphasia hemianopsia, and other focal neurological signs may occur, but are uncommon.
- A self-limiting, isolated cerebellar ataxia, presumably caused by immunological mechanisms, in patients recovering from falciparum malaria has been recognized in Sri Lanka.
- Malaria is a common cause of febrile seizures in the tropics, and it also contributes to the development of epilepsy in later life (Roman and Senanayake 1992).

Cerebral malaria is considered to be a form of disseminated vasculomyelinopathy, a hyperergic reaction of the CNS to the antigenic challenge of *Plasmodium falciparum* infection (Toro and Roman 1978). However it has been argued that cerebral involvement could be the mere result of the cumulative effect of the malfunction of other organs (Enwere 2000). With *Plasmodium vivax* infections, there may be drowsiness, confusion, and seizures without invasion of the brain by the parasite (Adams *et al.* 1997).

4.3 Lyme disease (*Borrelia burgdorferi*)

Lyme disease is a tick-borne disease, caused by *Borrelia burgdorferi*. It usually presents as a solitary, enlarging, ring-like erythematous lesion that may be surrounded by annular satellite lesions. Usually, influenza-like symptoms are associated. Weeks to months later, neurological symptoms appear in 15% of cases, in the form of an aseptic meningitis or a fluctuating meningoencephalitis. Still later, if the patient remains untreated, arthritis or, more precisely, synovitis develops in about 60% of cases.

A small percentage of Lyme patients develop mild to moderate encephalopathic symptoms months to years after diagnosis and treatment. Their symptoms typically include fatigue, memory loss, sleep disturbance, and depression. The deficit predominantly affects mnestic functions with deficits of verbal memory (retrieval is mostly affected but not recognition, suggesting intact capacity of storing, mental flexibility, verbal associative functions, and articulation), but patients perform adequately on tests of intellectual and problem-solving skills, sustained attention, visuoconstructive abilities, and mental speed (Krupp *et al.* 1991). A superficial resemblance to Alzheimer's disease has led several groups in the past to propose a common neuropathology, but this is almost certainly not the case (Gutacker *et al.* 1998). Cognitive dysfunction usually improves with adequate antibiotic treatment (Shadick *et al.* 1999), but persons with a history of Lyme disease have more musculoskeletal impairment and a higher prevalence of verbal memory impairment (Shadik *et al.* 1994).

4.4 Cryptococcosis (torulosis, European blastomycosis)

Cryptococcal meningitis is another condition that has increased markedly in incidence, occurring in 5–10% of patients with AIDS (Saag *et al.* 2000). This fungal meningitis, caused by *Cryptococcus neoformans*, is one of the more frequently seen meningitises in patients with immunodeficiency. Cryptococcal meningitis is a serious fungal infection when the condition is diagnosed early but, without treatment, it may be fatal within a few weeks (only a few patients have a slow progression, lasting for years). The presentation is commonly indolent and this may lead to a delay in diagnosis. Clinically, it presents, in the majority of patients, as a chronic or subacute meningitis or encephalitis. At first, the symptoms are vague: mild headache, fever, and nausea. As the infection progresses more symptoms will appear with headache, nausea, vomiting, and sometime mental changes. In other cases it presents with the symptoms of endocranial hypertension or, on rare occasions, as single or multiple focal mass lesions (cryptococcomas) or with a confusional state, dementia, cerebellar ataxia, or spastic paraparesis.

5 Fungal infections: cryptococcal meningitis

Cryptococcal meningitis is a life-threatening infection that can occur if there has been exposure to a fungus called *Cryptococcus neoformans*. This fungal meningitis is one of the more frequent seen in patients with immunodeficiency, it has increased markedly in incidence, occurring in 5 to 10 percent of patients with AIDS (Saag *et al.* 2000). It may be very slow in developing, so at first, very vague symptoms may appear: mild headache, fever, and nausea. As the infection progresses, more symptoms will appear: severe headache, nausea with vomiting, blurred vision and/or sensitivity to bright light, stiff neck, seizures, confusion, behavioural changes, and coma.

6 Spongiform encephalopathies, including Creutzfeldt–Jakob disease

Prion diseases are neurodegenerative conditions related to non-conventional transmissible agents, the prion proteins. The transmissible agent is a modified isoform of a glycoprotein, the prion protein PrP, which is normally produced by the host cells and encoded by a host gene. Unlike the other disease agents, the modified form of this protein appears to be able to induce the disease although lacking informational nucleic acids. It is characterized by its resistance to proteolysis. It aggregates in the host's brain interacting with cellular PrP and possibly causing its conversion to the modified form, thus producing the typical spongiform changes in brain tissue.

Creutzfeldt–Jakob Disease (CJD) is the most common type of the prion-linked spongiform encephalopathies. It presents between 55 and 70 years with rapidly progressive psychiatric and cognitive changes (Byrne 1997). In the early stages, one often finds confusion, delusions, and hallucinations, which usually evolve toward a frontal syndrome and/or focal signs such as aphasia and visuospatial disorders. The dementia is associated with early cerebellar ataxia, visual disturbances, and myoclonic jerks, often elicitable through sensory stimulation. Within weeks or at most a few months, these changes give way to stupor and coma. Most patients have a typical electroencephalogram showing pseudoperiodic sharp waves.

The disease is known to occur in sporadic (most of the cases), familial (around 15%), and iatrogenic form (treatment with human pituitary derived growth hormone, dura mater, or corneal grafts) and is usually fatal within a few months from onset. No therapy is available.

The families identified have mutations in the PrP gene, located on chromosome 20. Both iatrogenic and sporadic cases occur predominantly in genetically susceptible individuals (Chatelain *et al.* 1998). Heterozygote individuals seem to be at lower risk of developing prion disease.

Recently, a hot debate has grown around the presence of a new variant of prion disease in young people in the UK and a few other countries, and its possible relationship with bovine spongiform encephalopathy (BSE) and the safety of beef and bovine offal (Will *et al.* 1996). The features characterizing this new variant include a younger age of onset, absence of typical CJD electroencephalographic features, and a more prolonged course. Strains of transmissible spongiform encephalopathies have been distinguished, and the new variant strain seem to resemble BSE, suggesting that BSE may well be the source of the new disease. BSE has been transmitted to mice, domestic cats, and macaques.

Selective references

Adams, R.D., Victor, M., and Ropper, A.H. (1997). *Principles of neurology*, 6th edn. McGraw Hill, New York.

American Psychiatric Association (1994). *Diagnostic and statistical manual of mental disorders* (ed. A. Press). American Psychiatric Association, Washington, DC.

Anders, H.J. and Goebel, F.D. (1999). Neurological manifestations of cytomegalovirus infection in the acquired immunodeficiency syndrome. *Int. J. STD AIDS* **10** (3), 151–9.

Aylward, E., Henderer, J., McArthur, J., *et al.* (1993). Reduced basal ganglia volume in HIV-1-associated dementia: results from quantitative neuroimaging. *Neurology* **43**, 2099–104.

Baum, S., Morris, J., Gibbons, R., and Cooper, R. (1999). Reduction in human immunodeficiency virus patient hospitalizations and nontraumatic mortality after adoption of highly active antiretroviral therapy. *Mil. Med.* **164**, 609–12.

Becker, J., Caldararo, R., Lopez, O., Dew, M., Dorst, S., and Blank, G. (1995). Qualitative features of the memory deficit associated with HIV infection and AIDS: cross-validation of a discriminant function classification scheme. *J. Clin. Exp. Neuropsychol.* **17**, 134–42.

Beeker, J. and Salthouse, T. (1999). Neuropsychological test performance in the acquired immunodeficiency syndrome: independent effects of diagnostic group on functioning. *J. Int. Neuropsychol. Soc.* **5**, 41–7.

Bell, J., Donaldson, Y., Lowrie, S., *et al.* (1996). Influence of risk group and zidovudine therapy on the development of HIV encephalitis and cognitive impairment in AIDS patients. *AIDS* **10** (5), 493–9.

Bornstein, R., Nasrallah, H., Para, M., Whitacre, C., Rosenberger, P., and Fass, R. (1993). Neuropsychological performance in symptomatic and asymptomatic HIV infection. *AIDS* **7**, 519–24.

Byrne, E.J. (1997). Overview of differential diagnosis. *Int. Psychogeriatr.* **9** (suppl. 1), 39–50; 85–6 [discussion].

Centers for Disease Control (1986). CDC classification system for human T-lymphotropic virus type III/lymphadenopathy-associated virus infections. *Morb. Mortal. Wkly Rep.* **35**, 334–9.

Centers for Disease Control and Prevention (1992). 1993 revised classification system for HIV infection and expanded surveillance case definition for AIDS among adolescents and adults. *Morb. Mortal. Wkly Rep.* **41** (RR-17), 1–19.

Chang, I., Ernst, T., Leonido-Yee, M., *et al.* (1999). Highly active antiretroviral therapy reverses brain metabolite abnormalities in mild HIV dementia. *Neurology* **53**, 782–9.

Chatelain, J., Delanesrie-Laupretre, N., Lemaire, M., Cathala, F., Launay, J., and Laplanche, J. (1998). Cluster of Creutzfeldt–Jakob disease in France associated with the codon 200 mutation (E200K) in the prion protein gene. *Eur. J. Neurol.* **5**, 375–9.

Cinque, P., Cleator, G.M., Weber, T., Monteyne, P., Sindic, C., Gerna, G., van Loon, A.M., and Klapper, P.E. (1998). Diagnosis and clinical management of neurological disorders caused by cytomegalovirus in AIDS patients. European Union Concerted Action on Virus Meningitis and Encephalitis. *J. Neurovirol.* **4** (1), 120–32.

Clemente-Millana, L. and Portellano, J.A. (2000). Neuropsychological evaluation of the cognitive deficits in infection by human immunodeficiency virus type 1 (HIV-1). *Rev. Neurol.* **31** (12), 1192–201.

Clifford, D.B., Yiannoutsos, C., Glicksman, M., Simpson, D.M., Singer, E.J., Piliero, P.J., Marra, C.M., Francis, G.S., McArthur, J.C., Tyler, K.L., Tselis, A.C., and Hyslop, N.E. (1999). HAART improves prognosis in HIV-associated progressive multifocal leukoencephalopathy. *Neurology* **52**, 623–5.

Dal-Pan, G., McArthur, J., Aylward, E., *et al.* (1992). Patterns of cerebral atrophy in HIV-1-infected individuals—results of a quantitative MRI analysis. *Neurology* **42**, 2125–30.

Di Sclafani, V., Mackay, S., Meyerhoff, D., Norman, D., Weiner, M., and Fein, G. (1997). Brain atrophy in HIV infection is more strongly associated with CDC clinical stage than with cognitive impairment. *J. Int. Neuropsychol. Soc.* **3**, 276–87.

Dore, G., Correll, P., Li, Y., *et al.* (1999). Changes to AIDS dementia complex in the era of highly active antiretroviral therapy. *AIDS* **13**, 1249–53.

Dunbar, N., Perdices, M., Grunseit, A., and Cooper, D. (1992). Changes in neuropsychological performance of AIDS-related complex patients who progress to AIDS. *AIDS* **6**, 691–700.

Dunlop, O., Bjoklund, R., Abdelnoor, M., and Myrvang, B. (1993). Total reaction time: a new approach in early HIV encephalopathy? *Acta Neurol. Scand.* **88**, 344–8.

Enting, R., Hoetelmans, R., Lange, J., *et al.* (1998). Antiretroviral drugs and the central nervous system. *AIDS* **12**, 1941–55.

Enwere, G. (2000). Severe malaria with impaired cerebral function? *Lancet* **356**, 860.

Everall, I., Glass, J., McArthur, J., Spargo, E., and Lantos, P. (1994). Neuronal density in the superior frontal and temporal gyri does not correlate with the degree of human immunodeficiency virus-associated dementia. *Acta Neuropathol.* **88**, 538–44.

Farina, E., Cappa, S., Polimeni, M., Magni, E., Canesi, M., Zecchinelli, A., Scarlato, G., and Mariani, C. (1994). Frontal dysfunction in early Parkinson's disease. *Acta. Neurol. Scand.* **90**, 34–8.

Gasnault, J., Kousignian, P., Kahraman, M., Rahoiljaon, J., Matheron, S., Delfraissy, J.F., and Taoufik, Y. (2001). Cidofovir in AIDS-associated progressive multifocal leukoencephalopathy: a monocenter observational study with clinical and JC virus load monitoring. *J. Neurovirol.* **7** (4), 375–81.

Gasnault, J., Taoufik, Y., Goujard, C., Kousignian, P., Abbed, K., Boue, F., Dussaix, E., and Delfraissy, J.F. (1999). Prolonged survival without neurological improvement in patients with AIDS-related progressive multifocal leukoencephalopathy on potent combined antiretroviral therapy. *J. Neurovirol.* **5**, 421–9.

Glass, J., Wesselingh, S., Selnes, O., and McArthur, J. (1993). Clinical–neuropathologic correlation in HIV-associated dementia. *Neurology* **43**, 2230–7.

Gordon, B., Selnes, O.A., Hart, J. Jr, Hanley, D.F., and Whitley, R.J. (1990). Long-term cognitive sequelae of acyclovir-treated herpes simplex encephalitis. *Arch. Neurol.* **47** (6), 646–7.

Grassi, M.P., Clerici, F., Perin, C., D'Armino Monforte, A., Vago, L., Borella, M., Boldorini, R., and Mangoni, A. (1998). Microglial nodular encephalitis and ventriculoencephalitis due to cytomegalovirus infection in patients with AIDS: two distinct clinical patterns. *Clin. Infect. Dis.* **27**, 504–8.

Gutacker, M., Valsangiacomo, C., Balmelli, T., Bernasconi, M., Bouras, C., and Piffaretti, J. (1998). Arguments against the involvement of *Borrelia burgdorferi sensu lato* in Alzheimer's disease. *Res. Microbiol.* **149**, 31–7.

Gutierrez, R., Atkinson, J., and Grant, I. (1993). Mild neurocognitive disorder: a needed addition to the nosology of cognitive impairment (organic mental) disorders. *J. Neuropsychiatry Clin. Neurosci.* **5**, 161–77.

Hestad, K., McArthur, J., Pan, G.D., *et al.* (1993). Regional brain atrophy in HIV-1 infection: association with specific neuropsychological test performance. *Acta Neurol. Scand.* **88**, 112–18.

Hinkin, C., Castellon, S., Hardy, D., Granholm, E., and Siegle, G. (1999). Computerized and traditional Stroop task dysfunction in HIV-1 infection. *Neuropsychology* **13**, 306–16.

Holland, N.R., Paver, C., Mathews, V.P., Glass, J.D., Forman, M., and McArthur, J.C. (1994). Cytomegalovirus encephalitis in acquired immunodeficiency syndrome (AIDS). *Neurology* **3**, 507–14.

Janssen, R., Cornblath, D., Epstein, L., Foa, R., McArthur, J., and Price, R. (1991). Nomenclature and research case definitions for neurologic manifestations of human immunodeficiency virus-type-1 (HIV-1) infection: reports of a working group of the American Academy of Neurology AIDS Task Force. *Neurology* **41**, 778–85.

Jasiukaitis, P. and Fein, G. (1999). Differential association of HIV-related neuropsychological impairment with semantic versus repetition priming. *J. Int. Neuropsychol.* **5**, 434–41.

Jayawant, S., Feyi-Waboso, A., Wallace, S., Heath, J., Leary, M., Evans, R., and Ellis, J. (2000). Retinitis and dementia in a pregnant girl: an unusual case. *Eur. J. Paediatr. Neurol.* **4**, 177–9.

Krupp, L.B., Masur, D., Schwartz, J., *et al.* (1991). Cognitive functioning in late Lyme borreliosis. *Arch. Neurol.* **48** (11), 1125–9.

Ledergerber, B., Egger, M., Erard, V., *et al.* (1999). AIDS-related opportunistic illnesses after initiation of potent antiretroviral therapy: the Swiss HIV Cohort Study. *J. Am. Med. Assoc.* **282**, 2220–6.

Marder, K., Albert, A., Dooneief, G., *et al.* (1996). Clinical confirmation of the American Academy of Neurology algorithm for HIV-1-associated cognitive/motor disorder: The Dana Consortium on Therapy for HIV Dementia and Related Cognitive Disorders. *Neurology* **47** (5), 1247–53.

Martin, A., Heyes, M., Salazar, A., *et al.* (1992). Progressive slowing of reaction time and increasing cerebrospinal fluid concentrations of quinolinic acid in HIV-infected individuals. *J. Neuropsychiatry Clin. Neurosci.* **4**, 270–9.

Maruff, P., Currie, J., Malone, V., McArthur-Jackson, C., Mulhall, B., and Benson, E. (1994). Neuropsychological characterization of the AIDS dementia complex and rationalization of a test battery. *Arch. Neurol.* **51**, 689–95.

Masmoudil, K., Joly, H., Rosa, A., and Mizon, J. (1996). [Does general paralysis still exist in non-AIDS patients?] *Rev. Med. Interne* **17**, 576–8.

McArthur, J. (1997). NeuroAIDS: diagnosis and management. *Hosp. Practice* **15**, 73–84.

McArthur, J., Hoover, D., Bacellar, H., *et al.* (1993). Dementia in AIDS patients: incidence and risk factors. *Neurology* **43**, 2245–52.

McCutchan, J.A. (1995). Clinical impact of cytomegalovirus infections of the nervous system in patients with AIDS. *Clin. Infect. Dis.* (suppl. 2), S196–201.

McGrath, N., Anderson, N.E., Croxson, M.C., and Powell, K.F. (1997). Herpes simplex encephalitis treated with acyclovir: diagnosis and long term outcome. *J. Neurol., Neurosurg., Psychiatry* **63** (3), 321–6.

Mocroft, A., Madge, S., Johnson, A., *et al.* (1999). A comparison of exposure groups in the EuroSIDA study: starting highly active antiretroviral therapy (HAART), response to HAART, and survival. *J. Acq. Immune Defic. Syndr.* **22**, 369–78.

Navia, B., Jordan, B., and Price, R. (1986). The AIDS dementia complex: I. Clinical features. *Ann. Neurol.* **19**, 517–24.

Nielsen-Bohlman, L., Boyle, D., Biggins, C., Ezekiel, F., and Fein, G. (1997). Semantic priming impairment in HIV. *J. Int. Neuropsychol. Soc.* **3**, 348–58.

Owen, A., Downes, J., Sahakian, B., Polkey, C., and Robbins, T. (1990). Planning and spatial working memory following frontal lobe lesions in man. *Neuropsychologia* **28**, 1021–34.

Palella, F.J., Delaney, K., Moorman, A., *et al.* (1998). Declining morbidity and mortality among patients with advanced human immunodeficiency virus infection. HIV outpatient Study Investigators. *New Engl. J. Med.* **338**, 853–60.

Peavy, G., Jacobs, D., Salmon, D., *et al.* (1994). Verbal memory performance of patients with human immunodeficiency virus infection: evidence of subcortical dysfunction. *J. Clin. Exp. Neuropsychol.* **16**, 508–23.

Pillon, B., Michon, A., Malapani, C., Agid, Y., and Dubois, B. (1994). Are explicit memory disorders of progressive supranuclear palsy related to damage to striatofrontal circuits? Comparison with Alzheimer's, Parkinson's, and Huntington's diseases. *Neurology* **44** (7), 1264–70.

Portegies, P., Enting, R., Gans, J.D., *et al.* (1993). Presentation and course of AIDS dementia complex: 10 years of follow-up in Amsterdam, The Netherlands. *AIDS* **7**, 669–75.

Power, C., Selnes, O., Grim, J., and McArthur, J.M. (1995). HIV dementia scale: a rapid screening test. *J. Acq. Immune Defic. Syndr. Hum. Retrovirol.* **8**, 273–8.

Price, R.W. and Brew, B.J. (1988). The AIDS dementia complex. *J. Infect. Dis.* **158** (5), 1079–83.

Price, R., Yiannoutsos, C., Clifford, D., *et al.* (1999). Neurological outcomes in late HIV infection: adverse impact of neurological impairment on survival and protective effect of antiviral therapy. *AIDS* **13**, 1677–85.

Raininko, R., Elovaara, I., Virta, A., Valanne, L., Haltiaa, M., and Valle, S. (1992). Radiological study of the brain at various stages of human immunodeficiency virus infection: early development of brain atrophy. *Neuroradiology* **34**, 190–6.

Roman, G. and Senanayake, N. (1992). Neurological manifestations of malaria. *Arq. Neuropsiquiatr.* **50**, 3–9.

Russouw, H., Roberts, M., Emsley, R., and Truter, R. (1997). Psychiatric manifestations and magnetic resonance imaging in HIV-negative neurosyphilis. *Biol. Psychiatry* **1** (41), 467–73.

Saag, M., Graybill, R., Larsen, R., Pappas, P., Perfect, J., Powderly, W., Sobel, J., and Dismukes, W. (2000). Practice guidelines for the management of cryptococcal disease. Infectious Diseases Society of America. *Clin. Infect. Dis.* **30**, 710–18.

Sacktor, N.C., Bacellar, H., Hoover, D.R., Nance-Sproson, T.E., Selnes, O.A., Miller, E.N., Dal Pan, G.J., Kleeberger, C., Brown, A., Saah, A., and McArthur, J.C. (1996). Psychomotor slowing in HIV infection: a predictor of dementia, AIDS and death. *J. Neurovirol.* **2** (6), 404–10.

Sacktor, N.C., Lyles, R.H., Skolasky, R.L., Anderson, D.E., McArthur, J.C., McFarlane, G., Selnes, O.A., Becker, J.T., Cohen, B., Wesch, J., and Miller, E.N. (1999). Combination antiretroviral therapy improves psychomotor speed performance in HIV-seropositive homosexual men. Multicenter AIDS Cohort Study (MACS). *Neurology* **52** (8), 1640–7.

Sahakian, B., Elliott, R., Low, N., Mehta, M., Clark, R., and Pozniak, A. (1995). Neuropsychological deficits in tests of executive function in asymptomatic and symptomatic HIV-1 seropositive men. *Psychol. Med.* **25**, 1233–46.

Sanchez-Portocarrero, J., Perez-Cecilia, E., and Romero-Vivas, J. (1999). Infection of the central nervous system by Mycobacterium tuberculosis in patients infected with human immunodeficiency virus (the new neurotuberculosis). *Infection* **27**, 313–17.

Seilhean, D., Duyckaerts, C., Vazeux, R., *et al.* (1993). HIV-1-associated cognitive/motor complex: absence of neuronal loss in the cerebral neocortex. *Neurology* **43**, 1492–9.

Selnes, O., Galai, N., Bacellar, H., *et al.* (1995). Cognitive performance after progression to AIDS: a longitudinal study from the multicenter AIDS cohort Study. *Neurology* **45**, 267–75.

Shadick, N.A., Phillips, C.B., Logigian, E.L., Steere, A.C., Kaplan, R.F., Berardi, V.P., Duray, P.H., Larson, M.G., Wright, E.A., Ginsburg, K.S., *et al.* (1994). The long-term clinical outcomes of Lyme disease. A population-based retrospective cohort study. *Ann. Intern. Med.* **121** (8), 560–7.

Shadick, N.A., Phillips, C.B., Sangha, O., Logigian, E.L., Kaplan, R.F., Wright, E.A., Fossel, A.H., Fossel, K., Berardi, V., Lew, R.A., and Liang, M.H. (1999). Musculoskeletal and neurologic outcomes in patients with previously treated Lyme disease. *Ann. Intern. Med.* **131** (12), 919–26.

Stout, J., Salmon, D., Butters, N., *et al.* (1995). Decline in working memory associated with HIV infection. *Psychol. Med.* **25** (6), 1221–32.

Suarez, S.V., Stankoff, B., Conquy, L., Rosenblum, O., Seilhean, D., Arvanitakis, Z., Lazarini, F., Bricaire, F., Lubetzki, C., Hauw, J.J., and Dubois, B. (2000). Similar subcortical pattern of cognitive impairment in AIDS patients with and without dementia *Eur. J. Neurol.* **7** (2), 151–8.

Suarez, S.V., Baril, L., Stankoff, B., Khellaf, M., Dubois, B., Lubetzki, C., Bricaire, F., and Hauw, J.J. (2001). Outcome of patients with HIV-1-related cognitive impairment on highly active antiretroviral therapy. *AIDS* **2**, 195–200.

Toro, G. and Roman, G. (1978). Cerebral malaria. A disseminated vasculomyelinopathy. *Arch. Neurol.* **35**, 271–5.

Tozzi, V., Balestra, P., Galgani, S., *et al.* (1999). Positive and sustained effects of highly active antiretroviral therapy on HIV-1-associated neurocognitive impairment. *AIDS* **13**, 1889–97.

Wadia, R., Pujari, S., Kothari, S., Udhar, M., Kulkarni, S., Bhagat, S., and Nanivadekar, A. (2001). Neurological manifestations of HIV disease. *J. Assoc. Physcns India* **49**, 343–8.

Wang, J.T., Hung, C.C., Sheng, W.H., Wang, J.Y., Chang, S.C., and Luh, K.T. (2002). Prognosis of tuberculosis meningitis in adults in the era of modern antituberculosis chemotherapy. *J. Microbiol. Immunol. Infect.* **35**, 215–22.

Warrington, E.K. (1975). The selective impairment of semantic memory. *Quart. J. Exp. Psychol.* **27**, 635–57.

Warrington, E.K. and Shallice, T. (1984). Category specific impairment. *Brain* **107**, 829–53.

Will, R., Ironside, J., Zeidler, M., Cousens, S., Estibeiro, K., Alpérovitch, A., Poser, S., Pocchiari, M., and Hofman, A. (1996). A new variant of Creutzfeldt–Jakob disease in the UK. *Lancet* **347**, 921–5.

Chapter 31

The neuropsychology of endocrine disorders

David M. Erlanger

1 Introduction

A basic understanding of how endocrine dysfunction affects the central nervous system (CNS) is important for a majority of cases referred for assessment by clinical neuropsychologists. Beyond playing a role in assessment and management in the more obvious scenarios, such as pituitary adenoma and Graves's disease, increasing attention is being paid to the role of neuropsychology in the assessment and management of cognitive dysfunction due to illnesses with direct or indirect effects on the endocrine system and, secondarily, the CNS. In addition, patients referred for routine assessment of traumatic brain injury, attention deficit/hyperactivity disorder, or neurodegenerative disorder may have significant histories of thyroid dysfunction, diabetes, and other common conditions with known effects on the brain and cognitive function. In all such cases, neuropsychologists should be prepared to integrate their understanding of these factors into their clinical interview and the interpretation of their objective neuropsychological test findings.

Regardless of the referral question, clinical neuropsychologists have expertise in understanding how cognitive problems play out in real-life situations at work and at home. Problems with the endocrine system can have discrete, often remediable effects on motor function, learning, or even emotional functions. Monitoring and intervention in such cases by means of periodic assessment has the potential to lead to more cost-effective health care and improved quality of life (Ryan and Hendrickson 1998).

1.1 Guidelines for the assessment of metabolic history

The following are critical issues to keep in mind.

- Because they may not be aware of the relevance of the information, patients may neglect to mention an illness with no obvious association with cognition.
- Even though many treatments for some chronic clinical syndromes are provided in an outpatient setting, clinicians should be careful to include a thorough inpatient *and* outpatient medical history in their interview.
- Because chronic syndromes can be stable and well-controlled for years, history should extend to the initial onset of symptoms, regardless of how remote.

◆ Age may be an important consideration. Generally, perinatal and/or early childhood onset increases the possible relevance of such history to current cognitive dysfunction. Also, because of the associated reductions in levels of metabolic and endocrine function, an ageing brain may be more vulnerable and less responsive to intervention.

Obtaining an accurate history of metabolic imbalance may be a complex undertaking. Determining the date of onset is frequently ambiguous. Because the endocrine system and metabolism in general are subject to degeneration due to age, subclinical syndromes may exist for years before being identified, which may be associated with poorer response to therapeutic intervention. Also, because multiple systems may be affected, presenting symptoms may be physiological, psychiatric, cognitive, or a combination thereof. Psychiatric symptoms, in particular, frequently accompany the insidious onset of symptoms in most syndromes entailing dysregulation of the endocrine system. Similarly, physiological symptoms secondary to autonomic system dysfunction such as weight gain or sexual dysfunction may be useful indicators of the onset of illness retrospectively.

Once diagnosed, stabilization may entail ongoing consultation because, not infrequently, treatment of a hypofunctional system may result in hyperfunction of that same system (or vice versa), resulting in an ongoing process of adjustment. Therefore, in addition to noting the duration of the illness, severity should be ascertained according to the patient's individual history of metabolic control. Adolescent males with type I diabetes, for example, typically have more difficulty maintaining stable glucose levels due to lifestyle factors. Even remote periods of poor control may be worthy of consideration. Of even greater importance, episodes associated with extreme hormonal imbalance and acute metabolic crises such as hypoglycaemic shock are particularly relevant. A single such event may produce persistent symptoms, including cognitive sequelae.

Finally, metabolic control for the several days preceding neuropsychological assessment as well as on the day of the evaluation may affect neuropsychological test performance. This may be due to a direct effect of a hypometabolic condition on performance, or to a secondary effect of a psychiatric symptom such as anxiety or depression on the patient's interaction with the examiner and the test materials.

1.2 Guidelines for assessment

◆ With few exceptions, neuroendocrine dysregulation results in a worsening of cognitive functions due to disruptions in neurochemical messages in a manner both generalized and focal. The cognitive domains of attention, memory, and psychomotor speed are most commonly affected.

◆ Because follow-up may be of interest for individuals receiving treatment interventions such as hormone replacement therapy, neuropsychological instruments should be chosen based on the availability of alternate forms for repeat assessment.

◆ Because relatively subtle differences may be clinically meaningful, intelligence quotient (IQ) data will be useful to determine relative decreases from an individual's expected level of performance.

◆ Because of the frequent comorbidity of psychiatric symptoms, the use of mood inventories and mental status evaluations will facilitate assessment and allow recovery to be monitored multidimensionally (Erlanger *et al.* 1999).

1.3 Principles of operation of the endocrine system

The endocrine system produces its effects on bodily and mental functions by means of various hormones secreted by specific endocrine glands and transmitted via the bloodstream to proximate or remote sites. Table 31.1 lists the endocrine glands and hormones with particular relevance to cognitive functioning. Metabolic control of hormone levels is maintained by feedback loops or *axes* of related hormones. For example, the hypothalamic–pituitary–thyroid axis, or HPT axis, is comprised of thyrotrophin-releasing hormone (TRH), a hormone manufactured in the hypothalamus that induces the pituitary gland to produce thyroid-stimulating hormone (TSH), which stimulates the thyroid gland to produce triiodothyronine (T_3) and thyroxine (T_4), the principal thyroid hormones. These in turn provide feedback both directly and indirectly to the hypothalamus, thus regulating stable thyroid hormone levels. Disruption can occur at any location along the axis. It is in this way, for instance, that a pituitary tumour can affect thyroid functioning.

Individual hormones may perform a number of roles and have multiple types of receptors located throughout the body, including the brain. Two general categories of actions have been described.

◆ Those that affect the developing brain are known as *organizational* effects. For instance, congenital hypothyroidism can produce permanent functional and structural changes by altering the pattern of thyroid receptors present in the brain substrate.

◆ *Activational* effects, on the other hand, are the result of a chemical being present at any given moment. Like any chemical substance, a given hormone's activational effects on behaviour are due not only to the identity, dose, and duration of the hormone, but also to the brain substrate upon which it acts.

1.3.1 The hypothalamus

The hypothalamus is the principal autonomic centre of the brain, acting on the sympathetic and parasympathetic nervous systems to maintain homeostasis and to prepare the body to deal with emergencies. In addition, the hypothalamus is an integral component of the limbic system, mediating drives for hunger and thirst, sexual activity, and aggression. Finally, the hypothalamus directly regulates the vast majority of endocrine functions, largely by means of its regulatory effect on the pituitary gland.

Table 31.1 Principal endocrine glands and hormones

Anterior pituitary gland
Growth hormone causes growth of most bodily tissues and cells
Prolactin promotes breast development and milk secretion
Follicle-stimulating hormone is involved in reproductive and gonadal functioning
Luteinizing hormone causes ovulation in females and stimulates the gonads in both sexes
Adrenocorticotrophin stimulates the adrenal cortex to secrete adrenocortical hormones
Thyroid-stimulating hormone causes the release of thyroid hormones by the thyroid gland

Posterior pituitary gland
Vasopressin causes the kidneys to retain water and regulates blood vessels
Oxytocin facilitates childbirth and lactation

Thyroid gland
Thyroxine and triiodothyronine regulate the chemical processes in cells
Calcitonin causes the deposit of calcium in bones

Adrenal cortex
Cortisol contributes to the control of proteins, carbohydrates, and fats
Aldosterone regulates levels of sodium and potassium

Pancreas
Insulin promotes the storage of glucose into cells
Glucagon promotes the release of glucose into the bloodstream

Testes
Testosterone causes growth of male sex organs and secondary sex characteristics

Ovaries
Oestrogen causes growth of female sex organs and secondary sex characteristics
Progesterone nurtures the developing fetus and causes development of milk apparatus

Pineal gland
Melatonin regulates circadian rhythms and aspects of sexual behaviour

Parathyroid gland
Parathormone controls calcium ion concentrations in extracellular fluid

1.3.2 The pituitary gland

Immediately juxtaposed to the hypothalamus is the pituitary gland, or *hypophysis*. Known as the master endocrine gland, the pituitary affects the body's overall metabolism, the nervous system, and many aspects of behaviour both through the direct effect of its hormones and secondarily through its effects on other endocrine glands. Pituitary hormones are secreted primarily under stimulation by hormones generated in the hypothalamus, and are modulated by means of feedback loops and various neurotransmitter mechanisms. The anterior pituitary secretes a number of hormones vital to the body's metabolic function and capacity to deal with stress. Known as *trophic* hormones, these substances act to stimulate their target organs at distances from the pituitary. Chief among these are growth hormone (GH), adreno-corticotrophin hormone (ACTH), thyroid-stimulating hormone (TSH), the gonadotrophins known as follicle-stimulating hormone (FSH) and luteinizing hormone (LH), and prolactin.

2 Cognition and generalized dysfunction of the neuroendocrine system

Cognitive dysfunction secondary to irregular hypothalamic or pituitary operation may be due to a number of causes including trauma, vascular disease, and neoplasm. As would be expected given their role as the principal mediators of the autonomic nervous system, the resulting symptoms can produce an array of autonomic effects. Symptoms may include temperature dysregulation, obesity, aphagia, hypersomnia, and sexual dystrophy. Affective symptoms of fear and rage may also ensue.

Commonly, hypothalamic dysfunction may result from compression secondary to a pituitary adenoma or craniopharyngioma. Macroadenomas (>10 mm) frequently come to medical attention due to their prominent mass effect, producing symptoms such as headache and visual abnormalities. Symptoms may result from either *hyper*-secretion of a hormone as a result of the tumour and/or *hypo*secretion of other hormones secondary to the tumour's mass effect on the pituitary gland and hypothalamus. Hormonal declines due to mass effect follow a pattern. Hyposecretion of GH precedes that of LH and FSH, which precedes that of TSH, which precedes that of ACTH.

Cognitive deficits including amnesia and executive dysfunction have been noted following surgery and hormone replacement therapy (Grattan-Smith *et al.* 1992; Peace *et al.* 1997). However, these cognitive symptoms appear to be due to multiple factors such as surgical sequelae, pre- and postsurgical hormonal imbalance, tumour size, secondary hydrocephalus, and radiotherapy. Indeed, some patients with craniopharyngiomas manifest physiological changes such as extreme weight gain and visual disturbance to such an extent that neuropsychological test data may be difficult to interpret clearly.

In adults, a generalized hypopituitarism syndrome may result from pronounced age-related changes in multiple hormone systems including the gonadal, thyroid, pancreatic, and adrenal axes (Lamberts *et al.* 1997). Patients experience a range of symptoms such as decreased energy, loss of libido, and depressed mood and/or increased irritability. Women may experience irregular menses or amenorrhoea and men may experience impotence and fertility problems.

3 Disorders involving the thyroid hormones

The thyroid hormones T_3 and T_4 result from iodine processed in the presence of TSH, a product of the anterior pituitary gland. Although the primary action of thyroid hormones is typically described as the stimulation of heat production, their influence on metabolic processes throughout the organs and tissues is significant. Dysregulation of thyroid functioning is therefore a frequent concomitant of systemic illness.

The hormones and their receptors are widely distributed throughout the brain, affecting adrenergic function, striatal dopaminergic activity, and levels of substance P and serotonin.

3.1 Thyrotoxicosis and Graves's disease

An excessive presence of thyroid hormone is referred to as thyrotoxicosis. When associated with diffuse goitre, ophthalmopathy, and dermopathy due to an autoimmune disorder, hyperthyroidism is referred to as Graves's disease.

- Patients with Graves's disease typically present with symptoms similar to those of a generalized anxiety disorder: nervousness, poor concentration, apprehension, restlessness, and emotional lability.

- Other symptoms include heat intolerance, increased sweating, weight loss, muscle weakness, fatigue with dysomnia, and—in women—changes in menstrual flow. Increased metabolic rates may produce tachycardia autonomic tremor.

- The incidence is approximately 0.3 per 1000 in the USA. The condition peaks during the third and fourth decades of life and is seven to ten times more common in women than in men. The explanation for this gender difference and for the underlying cause of the disease is unknown.

3.1.1 Psychiatric symptoms

Although prominent psychiatric symptoms have been noted since the earliest descriptions by Parry (1825) and Graves (1835), researchers have generally found that psychiatric symptom presentations are understated. Whybrow et al. (1969), for instance, found Minnesota Multiphasic Personality Inventory (MMPI) profiles in thyrotoxic patients to be somewhat elevated, but inconsistent with hypomania. MacCrimmon et al. (1979) similarly found nonsignificant elevations on a number of MMPI scales (hypochondriasis, depression, hysteria, psychaesthenia, and schizophrenia). Although a number of researchers have found that psychiatric symptoms largely resolve when patients are returned to a euthyroid state (e.g. Paschke et al. 1990), in Stern et al.'s (1996) survey, 33.1% of respondents reported being prescribed psychotropic medication following diagnosis and treatment of Graves's disease even though only 7.7% of the sample reported any premorbid history of psychotropic medication.

3.1.2 Neuropsychological symptoms

In the thyrotoxic state, researchers have consistently found that patients manifest worsened performances on tests of attention, concentration, memory, and fine motor speed (e.g. Trzpacz et al. 1988). The findings consistently show that the presence of thyroid hormones acting on the noradregenergic system affects attention with dose correlating as an inverted U-shaped curve. Thus, Schlote et al. (1992) also found impaired psychomotor speed in overt but not subclinical cases. However, it is plausible that the effects are due to a more general disruption of the brain's thyroid economy as well. Such a hypothesis would help account for reports of poor performances on tests of conceptual thinking and organization. In contrast to generally improved psychiatric symptoms, there are a number of reports of ongoing worsened performances on neuropsychological tests of attention, fine motor speed, and memory long after a euthyroid state has been established (Perrild *et al.* 1986; Trzepacz *et al.* 1988; Bommer *et al.* 1990).

3.2 Congenital hypothyroidism

Children born with congenital hypothyroidism (CH) are typically identified at birth. In the USA, Whites are affected at a substantially higher rate than African-Americans (1 : 5000 versus 1 : 32 000). Due to the infant brain's vulnerability to the organizational effects of a lack of thyroid hormone, those who do not receive replacement therapy are at high risk for developing severe motor and sensory impairments, as well as mental retardation. Even in children receiving early intervention, meta-analysis demonstrates a relatively small but significant trend toward lower IQ (≈ 6.3 points) and poorer motor skills in treated CH children (Derksen-Lubsen 1996). Any delay in intervention leads to severe cognitive problems with 72% of patients in one study obtaining IQ scores more than one standard deviation below normal with nearly two-thirds of those in the borderline or impaired range (Mendorla *et al.* 1988). Untreated congenital hypothyroidism leads to a syndrome known as cretinism, characterized by mental retardation, deaf mutism, short stature, and myxoedema—a puffiness in the face, hands, and feet due to the infiltration of the tissues with mucopolysaccharides. In geographic areas with iodine-deficient diets, the severity of deficits correlates with the extent of the deficiency (Aghini-Lombardi *et al.* 1995; Sankar *et al.* 1994).

3.3 Adult hypothyroidism

Primary hypothyroidism in adults has an incidence approximately one-eighth that of hyperthyroidism. Hypothyroidism may also result from Hashimoto's thyroiditis, a condition similar to Graves's disease, in which the thyroid gland at first enlarges and subsequently atrophies. Another frequent cause is secondary to thyroid replacement therapy for Graves's disease.

- Clinical symptoms of hypothyroidism include intolerance to cold, puffy face, coarse, dry skin and hair, fatigue and somnolence, muscular sluggishness, bradycardia and reduced cardiac output, weight gain, development of a husky voice, constipation, oedematous body tissue, and arteriosclerosis.
- There is a significant gender bias, as it is four to seven times more common in females than males.

- The prevalence of hypothyroidism steadily increases with age, with subclinical hypothyroidism manifesting as lethargy and dysphoria, although these symptoms appear to resolve with treatment.
- Myopathies and delayed tendon reflexes may be evident on neurological exam.

3.3.1 Psychiatric symptoms

The most typical presenting picture is that of a depressed patient: dysphoria, apathy, fatigue, diminished libido, motor and psychomotor retardation, and even suicidal ideation. MMPI profiles of individuals are characteristic of other depressed populations, with elevated depressed and reduced mania scales. With thyroid replacement therapy, remission of psychiatric symptoms is common.

3.3.2 Neuropsychological symptoms

Classically, severe hypothyroidism or 'myxoedema madness' is considered a 'reversible dementia' with treatment by thyroid replacement therapy. However, variables mediating the extent of recovery following treatment are still being investigated. In extreme cases, coma can result from severe, prolonged hypothyroidism. Impairment in cognition has been noted in hypothyroidal patients since Gull's (1874) initial description.

Bradyphrenia, increased response latencies, and poor concentration and memory are typical presenting symptoms. There is a surprising lack of investigations into severe hypothyroidism despite its relative prevalence. Although a number of studies have identified cognitive deficits on tests of mental status, psychomotor speed, memory, semantic fluency, concentration, and design fluency during the acute stage, in the Osterweil et al. (1992) study, a lack of significant improvement on a number of tests following stabilization of thyroid levels suggested that deficits in effortful attention may persist. Also, two published case studies (Menemeier et al. 1993; Leentjens and Kappers 1995) found that replacement therapy did not reverse cognitive deficits, but may have prevented further deterioration. These and other studies suggest that the duration of thyroid dysfunction is an important factor, although such duration would have to be extreme because healthy individuals have up to a 100-day reserve available. Also, there is evidence that age may increase vulnerability to the effects of hypothyroidism on cognitive functioning.

Researchers of minimal and subclinical hypothyroidism have found that a normalization of cognitive functioning following treatment is to be expected. Monzani et al. (1993) and Baldini et al. (1997) both found improved memory performance in subclinical hypothyroid populations following return to a euthyroidal state.

4 Diabetes mellitus

Diabetes mellitus is a term applied to certain disorders that result in chronic elevations in blood glucose levels or *hyperglycaemia*.

◆ *Type I diabetes*. In the USA, approximately 500 000 persons have been diagnosed with juvenile-onset insulin-dependent diabetes mellitus (IDDM), also known as type I diabetes, with most children diagnosed in their early teens. In these individuals, beta cells within the pancreas are destroyed, curtailing the body's supply of insulin. Treatment is by means of intramuscular injection of insulin, with the primary goal of therapy being the maintenance of metabolic control by avoiding both hyper- and hypoglycaemic states.

◆ *Type II diabetes*. Non-insulin-dependent diabetes (NIDDM), or type II diabetes, is characterized by an insidious onset of symptoms due to hyposecretion of insulin and/or insulin resistance. Prevalence increases with age so that approximately 20% of the population over 65 years of age are affected (Winograd *et al.* 1990). For a majority of individuals diagnosed with NIDDM, metabolic control is frequently achieved through a combination of diet and/or oral hypoglycaemic agents.

4.1 **Psychiatric symptoms**

Both type I and type II diabetes may be accompanied by symptoms of depression, anxiety, and, infrequently, mania. More severe psychiatric symptoms are correlated with poorer compliance to therapeutic regimes and more severe course, although no clear cause and effect model has been established. Stressors include factors associated with living with chronic disease such as stress and concern with dietary regimen. Chronic pain associated with neuropathy is present for a sizeable subset of diabetics.

4.2 **Neuropsychological symptoms**

4.2.1 Type I diabetes

Cognitive deficits due to diabetes have been the subject of many investigations. For type I patients, age of onset has been shown to be related to cognitive deficits with impairments in visuospatial tasks in patients afflicted before the age of 4 years, probably due to higher rates of hypoglycaemic seizures and the increased vulnerability of the developing brain (Ryan 1988). Cognitive problems have also been identified on verbal recall and fluency tasks.

In adult type I diabetics, medical complications due to macro- and microvascular damage are common, increasing diabetics' risks for stroke, heart attack, retinopathy, and end-stage renal disease. Peripheral neuropathies with the potential to affect activities of daily living (ADLs) and instrumental activities of daily living (IADLs) are common as are paraesthesias and/or painful sensations in the distal limbs. Cognitively, this increased risk of stroke results in increased rates of vascular dementia in diabetics (McCall 1992). Long histories of poorly controlled glucose levels are associated with the vascular complications noted above, the peripheral neuropathies being most immediately pertinent to performance on neuropsychological tests entailing a psychomotor speed component. Poorly controlled glucose levels have also been associated with reduced mental flexibility, poor conceptual reasoning, and inefficient information processing.

4.2.2 Type II diabetes

Ironically, neurocognitive deficits in type II diabetics may be somewhat more pronounced—particularly in regard to memory function—despite these patients' shorter histories. Ryan and Williams (1993) hypothesized an age–hyperglycaemia interaction to account for these findings, noting that the ageing brain has been found to be increasingly vulnerable to mnestic dysfunction in other patient groups (e.g. alcholics). Moreover, as with type I patients, history of metabolic control has been found to be key to understanding who is most vulnerable (Assisi *et al.* 1996). Research has shown that improved metabolic control may improve cognitive functions in both type I and type II diabetics.

5 Disorders involving the reproductive hormones

In concert with chromosomal factors, the reproductive hormones are responsible for sexually dimorphic characteristics in behaviour, affect, and cognition. Through their influence on sexual differentiation during key developmental phases, the reproductive hormones play an important organizational role in neuronal development, with women's brains having, on average, larger corpus colossi and planum temporale. These differences correlate with women generally outperforming men on certain verbal tasks and having lower rates of language disorders such as dyslexia. In contrast, men display relative strengths in quantitative and visuospatial skills, particularly mental rotation (Maccoby and Jacklin 1974, Halpern 1992). Importantly, differences between groups of men and women on such cognitive tests are far smaller than the variability within each gender group. Nevertheless, individuals affected by disorders marked by excessive or diminished levels of reproductive hormones during key developmental periods manifest behaviours and characteristics determined by permanent structural changes in brain morphology. Due to the effects of physiological differences on an individual's self-concept, resultant syndromes may require some period of social and emotional adjustment in adolescence or later. Reproductive hormones may also play an activational role in producing transient changes in cognitive function in both healthy and afflicted individuals. However, these changes appear to be relatively minor and may depend to an extent on pre-existing organizational pathways for their effects.

5.1 Genetic, perinatal, and environmental abnormalities

5.1.1 Klinefelter's syndrome

Klinefelter's syndrome results from the presence of an additional X chromosome in the male. The syndrome is characterized by delayed maturation, hypogonadism and infertility, and androgen deficiency. Individuals manifest relative strengths in visuospatial abilities, and may rely more on the right hemisphere for processing both verbal and nonverbal information. Although lowered IQ has been found in a number of studies, this does not always appear to be the case (Netley and Rovet 1984).

5.1.2 Turner's syndrome

Turner's syndrome is due to a single X chromosome in females, resulting in short stature, webbing of the neck, and sexual infantilism. A number of deficiencies in brain structure have been identified, including decreased hippocampal, thalamic, caudate, and lenticular nuclei volumes, and decreased right temporal evoked potentials. Cognitively, individuals with Turner's syndrome manifest relative weaknesses in visuospatial ability and non-verbal memory, consistent with right hemisphere dysfunction (Schucard *et al.* 1994).

5.1.3 Congenital adrenal hyperplasia

Excessive levels of androgens are associated with congenital adrenal hyperplasia (CAH), an endocrine disorder beginning in the early prenatal environment. The condition is typically detected at birth and androgen levels are normalized. Clinically, CAH females manifest masculinization of the genitalia and clitoral hypertrophy. In males, an enlarged phallus typically results. In understanding the effects of androgens on the developing brain, researchers have focused on CAH females since identifying the effects of excessive androgens in CAH males is, by definition, a difficult proposition.

Research by Resnick *et al.* (1986) using a sample of adolescent CAH females revealed selectively better performances on tests of mental rotation and a hidden figures test compared to those of unaffected siblings. Similarly, Hampson *et al.* (1998) found an advantage in spatial capacity among preadolescent CAH females on a mental rotation test. Curiously, the researchers found that CAH boys scored significantly lower than control boys on a test of spatial relations, suggesting that overexposure to androgens may have a demasculinizing effect on males. More generally, CAH females may develop verbal IQ (VIQ)–performance IQ (PIQ) discrepancies favouring performance domain abilities (Nass and Baker 1991).

5.1.4 Androgen insensitivity

Patients with androgen insensitivity (AI) are genetic males who produce androgens but manifest partial to total insensitivity of androgen receptors. Depending on the degree of insensitivity they are born either with external female genitalia (and no female reproductive organs)—total AI—and are raised as girls, or ambiguous genitalia—partial AI—and are raised as either girls or boys. AI patients typically demonstrate a VIQ–PIQ discrepancy with decreased PIQ (Imperato-McGinley *et al.* 1991). However, lower PIQ subtest scores in these individuals may be due to either visuospatial deficits or attentional factors on speeded tests.

5.1.5 Idiopathic hypogonadotrophic hypogonadism (IHH)

At puberty, some males manifest a deficiency of gonadotrophin-releasing hormone (GnRH), resulting in smaller testes and decreased levels of androgens. Consistent with the organizational effects of androgens on the brain, IHH males have impaired visuospatial abilities and intact verbal skills (Hier and Crowley 1982).

5.2 The influence of gonadal hormones on adult behaviour

5.2.1 Androgens

Behaviourally, androgens have been associated with sexual drive and increased aggression in both genders. However, because aggressive encounters alter testosterone levels, no clear cause/effect relationship between the two variables has been established. Males receiving testosterone replacement therapy report enhanced well-being and increased energy. However, testosterone in males is converted or *aromatized* into oestrogens, obscuring the interpretation of these phenomena.

Optimal levels of androgens in both genders are necessary for normal visuospatial functioning. Moreover, androgens appear to have an activational effect on spatial abilities in females. However, high levels of testosterone in males have been associated with decreased spatial ability, suggesting a gender–hormone interaction (Gouchie and Kimura 1991). These capacities are best measured by means of route learning tasks and mental rotation tasks, although gross PIQ–VIQ discrepancies may also be evident. There is support from the animal literature for enhanced spatial ability in males. In a number of non-human species, spatial–navigational ability is sexually differentiated, with males learning to utilize routes more efficiently (Beatty 1984). Further, male mice castrated at birth exhibit reduced spatial efficiency in adulthood relative to controls (Williams *et al.* 1990).

5.2.2 Oestrogens and progesterone

Affective features have been associated with normal variation in ovarian hormones as well as with premenstrual syndrome (PMS), a cyclical disorder with depressive/mood-related and somatic symptoms occurring during the luteal phase of the menstrual cycle (Schmidt *et al.* 1998). Cognitively, increased verbal ability and decreased spatial ability have been identified during the high oestrogen phases, suggesting that oestrogen may differentially affect hemispheric functioning. Despite clinical reports, there has been little empirical support for variation in memory functioning according to the menstrual cycle that cannot be accounted for by the co-occurrence of mood symptoms.

In postmenopausal women, hormone replacement therapy (HRT) has been utilized for many years due to its association with reduced risk of stroke, heart disease, vascular dementia, and osteoporosis, although oestrogen replacement therapy (ERT) may be contraindicated for some women, especially those with a family history of breast cancer (see Colditz *et al.* 1995). A beneficial effect of HRT on verbal and nonverbal memory, and on cognition in general has been found across a number of studies. However, because decreases in memory functioning are increasingly compromised with age in both genders, such memory problems are unlikely to be due in their entirety to low circulating levels of oestrogen. Indeed, some large-scale studies have found no significant memory advantage for women with histories of ERT. Recent evidence suggests that cognitive advantages in ERT users may be due to enhanced activation of frontal lobe functioning, which could account for improved performance on cognitive measures in general, as well as on memory specifically via the associated executive functions (Berman *et al.* 1997).

5.2.3 Oestrogen and Alzheimer's disease

A potential role for female reproductive hormones in Alzheimer's disease (AD) is suggested by the disease's greater prevalence among women than men, even after adjusting for differences in life expectancy (Jorm *et al.* 1987). Likewise, several studies have found that women with AD perform worse than men with AD on various verbal tasks (Henderson and Buckwalter 1994; Ripich *et al.* 1995), despite a premorbid advantage on such tasks favouring women. A number of other clinical and experimental findings including body weight, neurophysiological processes, and genetic mechanisms further support the relevance of oestrogen to AD (see Henderson 1997 for a discussion).

Clinically, ERT has been utilized in the treatment of women with AD for many years. In a number of studies, ERT has been shown to be useful in improving cognition in general. However, improvements in memory function may be due to mood enhancement and an associated improvement in general cognition (Birge 1997). More importantly, several retrospective studies have found a reduced risk factor for dementia in women receiving ERT (Birge 1994; Henderson *et al.* 1994; Mortel and Meyer 1995). Similarly, prospective epidemiological studies have also suggested a significant reduction—more than 50% in some studies—in risk for AD in women receiving ERT (Henderson *et al.* 1994; Paganini-Hill and Henderson 1994; Morrison *et al.* 1996; Kawas *et al.* 1997; Tang *et al.* 1996; Yaffe *et al.* 1999). However, ongoing controlled studies are required to support these results.

6 Disorders involving the adrenal hormones

The adrenal glands are located at the superior poles of the kidneys. Each gland is divided into two distinct portions:

- the adrenal medulla, which secretes the hormones adrenaline (epinephrine) and noradrenaline (norepinephrine) and is functionally related to the sympathetic nervous system;
- adrenal cortex, which secretes the hormones known as corticosteroids, of which cortisol is of principal interest in regard to cognitive functions.

Another adrenal hormone, dehydroepiandrosterone (DHEA), has recently been studied for its possible effects on mood and memory and is discussed in Section 6.2. The adrenal glands also produce small amounts of certain androgens.

6.1 Cortisol

The hypothalamic–pituitary–adrenal axis is an integral component of the body's reactions to physiological stressors. Cortisol acts to increase blood glucose concentrations, which in turn mobilizes available energy stores, and helps the body to maintain home-ostasis through its regulatory effects on protein, carbohydrate, and lipid metabolism. The axis is controlled by a feedback loop as follows. Corticotrophin-releasing hormone (CRH) is produced by hypothalamic neurons both according to a circadian pattern and in response to physiological stress. CRH regulates the release of adrenocorti-cotrophin hormone (ACTH) from the pituitary. ACTH stimulates the adrenal glands, which in turn produce cortisol. Cortisol completes the feedback loop by its effect on the hypothalamus and other structures.

In normal subjects, administration of exogenous glucocorticoids may produce eupho-ria, hyperactivity, and increased appetite, leading to dependence and abuse. Short- and long-term administration of corticosteroids has been shown to produce mild impair-ments in verbal memory, although it is unclear if the dysfunction is due to disruption of attentional factors, memory processes, or both. However, mild increases in psychomotor speed and verbal fluency have also been reported, possibly due to a hyperactivation effect (Naber *et al.* 1996). Elevated cortisol levels are also found in individuals diagnosed with major depression, in whom memory and attention problems are frequently observed. However, elevations in serum cortisol cannot solely account for these cognitive problems.

6.1.1 Hypercortisolism

Cushing's syndrome refers to the clinical manifestation of increased concentrations of cortisol due to any number of disorders.

◆ Cushing's syndrome may be the result of a pituitary adenoma, a primary adrenal tumour, ectopic production of ACTH by a carcinoma of the lung, or, frequently, the long-term treatment of a variety of diseases with exogenous cortisol such as cortisone or prednisone.

◆ When cortisol evelations are secondary to a pituitary adenoma, the condition is known as *Cushing's disease*. Onset typically occurs between the ages of 20 and 40, but has also been reported in infants and elderly patients. Unlike Cushing's syn-drome, females are eight times more likely than males to develop Cushing's disease.

◆ Typical features associated with hypercortisolism include truncal obesity, plethoric (full) facies, hirsutism and baldness, osteoporosis, impotence or amenorrhoea, hypertension, and generalized muscular weakness.

Psychiatric symptoms Psychiatric symptoms are present in more than half of all cases of hypercortisolism and may include depression, anxiety, irritability, affective lability, decreased libido, and psychosis (i.e. 'steroid psychosis'). Because psychiatric symptoms may be the initial indications of Cushing's syndrome, dexamethasone-suppression testing is frequently used as a screening tool. However, as noted above, patients with major depression may have elevated cortisol levels with no evidence of endocrinopathy.

Neuropsychological symptoms A wide array of cognitive functions may be affected in more than two-thirds of all patients with Cushing's syndrome, including disruptions in orientation, concentration, memory, and comprehension (Whelan *et al.* 1980;

Starkman and Schteingart 1981) consistent with a pattern of diffuse bilateral frontal lobe dysfunction. However, correlations between ACTH or cortisol levels and cognitive performances were not found in one study of 25 patients with Cushing's syndrome (Mauri *et al.* 1993). Nevertheless, normalization of ACTH and cortisol levels was accompanied by a significant cognitive recovery for these patients.

Chronic elevations in cortisol in the elderly have been associated with deficits in explicit memory and selective attention (Lupien *et al.* 1994). Hippocampal atrophy has been associated with both chronic and short-term elevations in cortisol in patients with Alzheimer's disease and posttraumatic stress disorder, respectively (Davis *et al.* 1986; Bremner *et al.* 1995), consistent with the presence of concentrations of cortico-sterone receptors in the hippocampus (Ruel and DeKloet 1985).

6.1.2 Hypocortisolism

Addison's disease, a rare autoimmune disorder, accounts for approximately 75% of all cases of primary adrenocortical insufficiency. Insufficient production of cortisol results in increased levels of ACTH due to decreased feedback to the hypothalamus and anterior pituitary. The aetiology is typically an autoimmune adrenalitis due to tuber-culosis, malignancy, sarcoidosis, or infection but hypocortisolism may also result from bilateral adrenal haemorrhage after sepsis, trauma, surgery, or burns. Hypocortisolism may also result secondary to pituitary or hypothalamic dysfunction, resulting in diminished CRH and/or ACTH. Clinical features of hypocortisolism include pigmen-tation of the skin and mucous membranes, nausea, vomiting, weight loss, muscle weakness, fatigue, and dizziness. Psychiatric symptoms include depression, confusion, apathy, anhedonia, psychosis, paranoia, schizophrenic behaviours, and self-mutilation.

Neuropsychological sequelae of Addison's disease have been the subject of few studies. Reports document confusion and severe problems with short-term memory and attention in the acute stage, with improved cognition following treatment with adrenal replacement therapy. At present, it is unclear whether the psychiatric and cog-nitive symptoms are due to diminished cortisol, or increased CRH and ACTH acting on the CNS.

6.2 Dehydroepiandrosterone

The biological roles of dehydroepiandrosterone (DHEA) and its sulfate (DHEA-S) have recently been the subject of numerous investigations due to their decrease with normal ageing and correlation with age-related immune system decline (Thoman and Weigle 1989). Epidemiological data have demonstrated an association between low cir-culating DHEA and cardiovascular morbidity in males (Barrett-Connor *et al.* 1986) and breast cancer in females (Helzlsouer *et al.* 1992). DHEA and DHEA-S are also thought to affect behaviour and cognition by mediating γ-aminobutyric acid (GABA) receptors and by acting as a GABA antagonist, respectively.

In healthy subjects, DHEA appears to enhance general well-being, manifested as increased energy, deeper sleep, improved mood, greater relaxation, and better stress-handling capacity. Although some benefit in mnestic functions has been shown in depressed patients receiving DHEA, this has not been demonstrated in healthy populations.

7 Melatonin

The pineal gland is known by many as Descartes' hypothetical 'seat of the soul' and for its phyloanatomical history as a remnant of a 'third eye' in the posterior portion of the head in lower animals. In addition to its possible role in the seasonal regulation of human sexual behaviour and its role in regulating body temperature, the pineal gland has received scrutiny because of its synthesis of the hormone melatonin.

Melatonin is secreted cyclically, with low levels associated with daylight, and increases peaking toward midnight and then gradually returning to baseline by morning. Exogenous melatonin is currently sold as a treatment for jet lag due to its ability to re-set the body's circadian rhythms and induce sleepiness. Several studies have found significant variation in cognitive functioning, particularly in

Table 31.2 Selected neuropsychological tests/indices with demonstrated sensitivity to change in hormones

Androgens
Mental Rotations Tests: Vandenberg and Kuse 1978
Spatial Relations Test: Thurstone and Thurstone 1963
Card Rotation Test: Ekstrom *et al.* 1976

Ovarian hormones
Story Memory/Logical Memory: Wechsler Memory Scale, 1945/Wechsler Memory Scale, Revised, 1974
California Verbal Learning Test, Delis *et al.* 1987

Hypothyroidism
Trail Making Test
Wechsler Memory Scale, Revised, 1974
Symbol Digit Modalities Test: Smith 1982

Hyperthyroidism
Stroop Test: Stroop 1935
Finger Tapping: Reitan 1955

Hypercortisolism
Logical Memory, Visual Reproductions: Wechsler Memory, Revised, 1974
Digits Backwards, Digit Symbol: Wechsler Adult Intelligence Test, Revised, 1981

Type I diabetes
Trail Making Test, Part B
Grooved Pegboard Test: Klove 1963
PIQ: Wechsler Adult Intelligence Scale, Revised, 1981

Type II diabetes
Stroop Test: Stroop 1935
Grooved Pegboard Test: Klove 1963
Selective Reminding Test: Buschke and Fuld 1974

Table 31.3 Reference summary of neuroendocrine effects on behaviour and cognition

Hormone/condition	Primary hormonal axis	Primary axial hormones*	Ageing effects?	Psychological features	Principal cognitive findings†	Permanency of deficits?
Androgens (congenital adrenal hyperplasia, androgen insufficiency)	Hypothalamic–pituitary–gonadal	GnRH, LH, FSH, T, oestradiol, progesterone	Gradual decline in males	Libido, aggression	Inverted U-shaped curve with visuospatial in males; improved visuospatial in females	Improvement with replacement therapy
Ovarian hormones	Hypothalamic–pituitary–gonadal	GnRH, LH, FSH, T, oestradiol, progesterone	Rapid decline in females	Depression, anxiety	E_2 with verbal fluency and verbal memory; *Attention; visual memory; executive functions*	Possible improvement with replacement therapy
Hyperthyroidism (Graves's disease)	Hypothalamic–pituitary–thyroid	TRH, TSH, T_3, T_4	Decline	Anxiety, hypermania	Fine motor; attention; *memory*	Improvement with suppression therapy
Hypothyroidism (congenital hypothyroidism)	Hypothalamic–pituitary–thyroid	TRH, TSH, T_3, T_4	Decline	Depressive symptoms	General cognition; attention; learning; psychomotor speed	Limited improvement, especially of attention
Hypercortisolism (Cushing's disease/syndrome)	Hypothalamic–pituitary–adrenal	CRH, ACTH, cortisol	Possible increase	Anxiety, psychosis, hypermania	Memory; attention	Limited improvement, especially of memory
Hypocortisolism (Addison's disease)	Hypothalamic–pituitary–adrenal	CRH, ACTH, cortisol	Possible increase	Depression, poor motivation	General attention and motivation	Improvement with suppression therapy
DHEA	NA	DHEA, DHEA-S	Decline	DHEA: depression DHEA-S: anxiety	General cognition; *memory*	Improvement with replacement therapy
Type I diabetes (IDDM)	NA	Insulin, glucagon, somatostatin	Decline in insulin	Anxiety	Psychomotor speed; inefficient processing; *memory*	Improvement with replacement therapy
Type II diabetes (NIDDM)	NA	Insulin, glucagon, somatostatin	Decline in insulin	Anxiety	Psychomotor speed; inefficient processing; memory	Improvement except for memory
Melatonin	NA	Melatonin	None	NA	*Reduced speed of information processing*	NA

* GnRH, gonadotrophin-releasing hormone; LH, luteinizing hormone; FSH, follicle-stimulating hormone; T, testosterone; TRH, thyrotrophin-releasing hormone; TSH, thyroid-stimulating hormone; T_3, triiodothyronine; T_4, thyroxine; CRH, corticotrophin-releasing hormone; ACTH, adrenocorticotrophin hormone; DHEA, dehydroepiandrosterone; DHEA-S, dehydroepiandrosterone sulfate.

† Italic type indicates inconsistent or unreplicated findings.

reaction time tasks. However, there is no evidence that circulating melatonin has a direct effect on cognitive functioning. Instead, cognitive weaknesses appear to be due to reduced speed of information processing secondary to melatonin's hypothermic properties.

8 Summary

Hormones act on the brain and nervous system in general to produce an array of physiological, psychiatric, affective, and cognitive sequelae. Although the interplay of these symptoms may be complex, neuropsychologists are well prepared to assess and interpret these multidimensional findings, both in clinical and research settings. Neuropsychological assessment of neuroendocrine dysfunction is a relatively new area of research. Consequently, no 'gold standards' have been established regarding which instruments should be used in research and clinical applications. In order to provide specific guidance regarding test selection, Table 31.2 notes several measures found to be sensitive to dysfunction of specific hormonal axes. For ready reference, Table 31.3 summarizes the principal characteristics and cognitive findings relevant to neuropsychological assessment and the neuroendocrine system. Where known, response to intervention is indicated.

Selective references

Aghini-Lombardi, F.A., Pinchera, A., Anonangeli, L., *et al.* (1995). Mild iodine deficiency during fetal/neonatal life and neuropsychological impairment in Tuscany. *J. Endocrinol. Invest.* 18, 57–62.

Assisi, A., Alimenti, M., Maceli, F., Di Pietro, S., Lalloni, G., and Montera, P. (1996). Diabetes and cognitive function: preliminary studies. *Arch. Gerontol. Geriatr.* (suppl. 5), 229–32.

Baldini, I.M., Wita, A., Mauri, M.C., *et al.* (1997). Psychopathological and cognitive features in subclinical hypothyroidism. *Prog. Neuropsychopharmacol. Biol. Psychiatry* 21, 925–35.

Barrett-Connor, E., Khaw, K., and Yen, S.S.C. (1986). A prospective study of DS, mortality and cardiovascular disease. *New Engl. J. Med.* 315, 1519–24.

Beatty, W.W. (1984). Hormonal organization of sex differences in play fighting and spatial behavior. *Prog. Brain Res.* 61, 315–29.

Berman, F.B., Schmidt, P.J., Rubinow, D.R., *et al.* (1997). Modulation of cognition-specific cortical activity by gonadal steroids: a positron-emission tomography study in women. *Proc. Natl. Acad. Sci., USA* 93, 8836–41.

Birge, S.J. (1994). The role of estrogen deficiency in the aging central nervous system. In *Treatment of the postmenopausal woman: basic and clinical aspects* (ed. R.A. Lobo), pp. 153–7. Raven Press, New York.

Birge, S.J. (1997). The role of estrogen in the treatment of Alzheimer's disease. *Neurology* 48 (suppl. 7), S36–S41.

Bommer, M., Eversmann, T., Pickardt, R., Leohnardt, A., and Naber, D. (1990). Psychopathological and neuropsychological symptoms in patients with subclinical and remitted hyperthyroidism. *Klin. Wochenschr.* 68, 552–8.

Bremner, J.D., Randall, P., Scott, T.M., *et al.* (1995). MRI-based measurement of hippocampal volume in patients with combat-related posttraumatic stress disorder. *Am. J. Psychiatry* 152, 973–81.

Buschke, H. and Fuld, P.A. (1974). Evaluation of storage, retention, and retrieval in disordered memory and learning. *Neurology* 11, 1019–25.

Colditz, G.A., Hankinson, S.E., Hunter, D.J., *et al.* (1995). The use of estrogens, and progestins and the risk of breast cancer in postmenopausal women. *New Engl. J. Med.* 332, 1589–93.

Davis, K.L, Davis, B.M., Greenwald, B.S., *et al.* (1986). Cortisol and Alzheimer's disease. I. Basal studies. *Am. J. Psychiatry* **143**, 300–5.

Delis, D.C., Kramer, H.H., Kaplan, E., and Ober, B.A. (1987). *California Verbal Learning Test: Adult Version*, The Psychological Corporation, San Antonio.

Derksen-Lubsen, G. (1996). Neuropsychologic development in early treated congenital hypothyroidism: analysis of literature data. *Pediatr. Res.* **39**, 561–6.

Ekstrom, R.B., French, J.W., Harman, H.H., and Derman, D. (1976). *Manual for Referenced Cognitive Tests.* Educational Testing Service, Princeton.

Erlanger, D.M., Kutner, K.C., and Jacobs, A.R. (1999). Hormones and cognition; current concepts and issues in neuropsychology [review article]. *Neuropsychol. Rev.* **9**, 175–207.

Gouchie, C. and Kimura, D. (1991). The relationship between testosterone levels and cognitive ability patterns. *Psychoneuroendocrinology* **16**, 323–34.

Grattan-Smith, P.J., Morris, J.G.L., Shores, E.A., Bachelor, J., and Sparks, R.S. (1992). Neuropsychological abnormalities in patients with pituitary tumors. *Acta Neurol. Scand.* **86**, 626–31.

Gull, WW. (1874). On a cretinoid state supervening in adult life in women. *Trans. Med. Soc. London* **21**, 298–300.

Halpern, D.F. (1992). *Sex differences in cognitive abilities*, 2nd edn. Erlbaum, Hillsdale, New Jersey.

Hampson, E., Rovet, J.F., and Altmann, D. (1998). Spatial reasoning in children with congenital adrenal hyperplasia due to 21-hydroxylase deficiency. *Dev. Neuropsychol.* **13** (2), 299–320.

Helzlsouer, K.J., Gordon, G.B., Alberg, A., Bush, T.L., and Comstock, G.W. (1992). Relationship of prediagnostic serum levels of DHEA and DS to the risk of developing premenopausal breast cancer. *Cancer Res.* **52**, 1–4.

Henderson, V.W. (1997). Epidemiology of estrogen replacement therapy and Alzheimer's disease. *Neurology* **48** (suppl. 7), S27–S35.

Henderson, V.W. and Buckwalter, J.G. (1994). Cognitive deficits of men and women with Alzheimer's disease. *Neurology* **44**, 90–6.

Henderson, V.W., Paganini-Hill, A., Emanuel, C.K., *et al.* (1994). Estrogen replacement therapy in older woman: comparisons between Alzheimer's disease cases and on-demented control subjects. *Arch. Neurol.* **51**, 896–900.

Hier, D.B. and Crowley, W.F. (1982). Spatial ability in androgen-deficient men. *New Engl. J. Med.* **306**, 1202–5.

Imperato-McGinley, J., Pichardo, , M., Gautier, T., Voyer, D., and Bryden, M.P. (1991). Cognitive abilities in androgen-insensitive subjects: comparison with control males and females from the same kindred. *Clin. Endocrinol.* **34**, 341–7.

Jorm, A.F., Korten, A.E., and Henderson, A.S. (1987). The prevalence of dementia: a quantitative integration of the literature. *Acta Psychiatr. Scand.* **76**, 475–9.

Kawas, C., Resnick, S., Morrison, A., *et al.* (1997). A prospective study of estrogen replacement therapy and the risk of developing Alzheimer's disease: the Baltimore Longitudinal study of Aging. *Neurology* **48**, 1517–21.

Kløve, H. (1963). Clinical Neuropsychology. In *The Medical Clinics of North America* (ed. F.M. Foster), Saunders, New York.

Lamberts, S.W.J., van den Beld, A.W., and van der Lely, A. (1997). The endocrinology of aging. *Science* **278**, 419–24.

Leentjens, A. F.G. and Kappers, E.J. (1995). Persistent cognitive defects after corrected hypothyroidism. *Psychopathology* **28**, 235–7.

Lupien, S., Lecours, A.R., Lussier, I., *et al.* (1994). Basal cortisol levels and cognitive deficits in human aging. *J. Neurosci.* **14**, 2893–903.

Maccoby, E.E. and Jacklin, C.N. (1974). *The psychology of sex differences.* Stanford University Press, Stanford.

MacCrimmon, D.J. Wallace, J.E., Goldberg, W.M., and Streiner, D.L. (1979). Emotional disturbance and cognitive deficits in hyperthyroidism. *Psychosomat. Med.* 41, 331.

Mauri, M., Sinforiani, E., Bono, G., *et al.* (1993). Memory impairment in Cushing's disease. *Acta Neurol. Scand.* 87, 52–5.

McCall, A.L. (1992). The impact of diabetes on the CNS. *Diabetes* 41, 557–70.

Mendorla, G., Sava, L., Calaciura, F., Lisi, E., Castorina, S., and Vigneri, R. (1988). Personality traits and mental prognosis in patients with congenital hypothyroidism not treated from early life. *J. Endocrinol. Invest.* 11, 289–95.

Mennemeier, M., Garner, R.D., and Heilman, K.M. (1993). Memory, mood and measurement in hypothyroidism. *J. Clin. Exp. Neuropsychol.* 15 (5), 822–31.

Monzani, R., Del Guerra, P., Caraccio, N., *et al.* (1993). Subclinical hypothyroidism: Neurobehavioral features and beneficial effect of L-thyroxine treatment. *Clin. Invest.* 71, 367–71.

Morrison, A., Resnick, S., Corrada, M., Zonderman, A., and Kawas, C. (1996). A prospective study of estrogen replacement therapy and the risk of developing Alzheimer's disease in the Baltimore Longitudinal Study of Aging. *Neurology* 46, A435–6.

Mortel, K.F. and Meyer, J.S. (1995). Lack of postmenopausal estrogen replacement therapy and the risk of dementia. *J. Neuropsychiatry Clin. Neurosci.* 7, 334–7.

Naber, D., Sand, P., and Heigl, B. (1996). Psychopathological and neuropsychological effects of 8-days' corticosteroid treatment. A prospective study. *Psychoneuroendocrinology* 21, 25–31.

Nass, R. and Baker, S. (1991). Learning disabilities in children with congenital adrenal hyperplasia. *J. Child Neurol.* 6, 306–12.

Netley, C. and Rovet, J. (1984). Hemispheric lateralization in 47, XXY Klinefelter's syndrome boys. *Brain Cogn.* 3, 10–18.

North, W.G., Moses, A.M., and Share, L. (eds.) (1993). *The neurohypophysis: a window on brain function*. The New York Academy of Sciences, New York.

Osterweil, D., Syndulko, K., Cohen, S.N., Pettler-Jennings, P.D., Hershman, J.M., Cummings, J.L., Tourtellotte, W.W., and Solomon, D.H. (1992). Cognitive function in non-demented older adults with hypothyroidism. *J. Am. Geriatr. Soc.* 40, 325–35.

Paganini-Hill, A. and Henderson, V.W. (1994). Estrogen deficiency and risk of Alzheimer's disease in women. *Am. J. Epidemiol.* 140, 256–61.

Paschke, R., Harsch, I., Schloe, B., Vardarli, I., Schaaf, L., Kaumeier, S., Teuber, J., and Usadel, K.H. (1990). Sequential psychological testing during the course of autoimmune hyperthyroidism. *Klin. Wochenschr.* 68, 942–50.

Peace, K.A., Orme, S.M., Thompson, A.R., Padayatt, S., Ellis, A.W., and Belchetz, P.E. (1997). Cognitive dysfunction in patients treated for pituitary tumours. *J. Clin. Exp. Neuropsychol.* 19, 1–6.

Perrild, H., Hansen, J.M., Arnung, K., Olsen, P.Z., and Danielsen, U. (1986). Intellectual impairment after hyperthyroidism. *Acta Endocrinol.* 112, 185–91.

Reitan, R.M. (1955). Investigation of the validity of Halstead's measure of biological intelligence. *Archives of Neurological Psychiatry* 73, 28.

Resnick, S.M. Berenbaum, S.A., Gottesman, I., and Bouchard, T.J. (1986). Early hormonal influences on cognitive functioning in congenital adrenal hyperplasia. *Dev. Psychol.* 12, 524–33.

Ripitch, D.N., Petril, S.A., Whitehouse, P.J., and Ziol, E.W. (1995). Gender differences in language of AD patients: a longitudinal study. *Neurology* 45, 299–302.

Ruel, J.M. and DeKloet, E.R. (1985). Two receptor systems for corticosterone in rat brain: microdistribution and differential occupation. *Endocrinology* 117, 2505–11.

Ryan, C.M. (1988). Neurobehavioral disturbances: the pancreas. In *Medical neuropsychology: the impact of disease on behavior* (ed. R.E. Tart, D.H. Van Thiel, and K.L. Edwards), pp. 121–58. Plenum Press, New York.

Ryan, C.M. and Hendrickson, R. (1998). Evaluating the effects of treatment for medical disorders: has the value of neuropsychological assessment been fully realized? *Appl. Neuropsychol.* 5, 209–19.

Ryan, C.M. and Williams, T.M. (1993). Effects of insulin-dependent diabetes on learning and memory in adults. *J. Clin. Exp. Neuropsychol.* 15, 685–700.

Sankar, R., Rai, B., Pulger, T., *et al.* (1994). Intellectual and motor functions in school children from severely iodine deficient region in Sikkim. *Ind. J. Pediatr.* 61, 231–6.

Schlote, B., Nowotny, B., Schaaf, L., *et al.* (1992). Subclinical hyperthyroidism: physical and mental state of patients. *Eur. Arch. Psychiatry Clin. Neurosci.* 241, 357–64.

Schmidt, P.J., Nieman, L.K., Danaceau, M.A., Adams, L.F., and Rubinow, D.R. (1998). Differential behavioral effects of gonadal steroids in women with and in those without premenstrual syndrome. *New Engl. J. Med.* 338, 209–16.

Schucard, P.W., Schucard, J. L., Clopper, R.R., and Schacter, M. (1994). Electrophysiological and neuropsychological indices of cognitive processing deficits in Turner's syndrome. *Dev. Neuropsychol.* 8, 299–323.

Smith, A. (1982). *Symbol Digit Modalities Test*, Western Psychological Service, Los Angeles.

Starkman, M.N. and Schteingart, D.E. (1981). Neuropsychiatric manifestations of patients with Cushing's syndrome. *Arch. Intern. Med.* 141, 215–19.

Stern, R.A., Robinson, B., Thorner, A.R., Arruda, J.E., Prohaska, M.L., and Pranges, A.J. Jr (1996). A survey of neuropsychiatric complaints in patients with Graves' disease. *J. Neuropsychiatry Clin. Neurosci.* 8, 181–5.

Stroop, J.R. (1935). Studies of interference in serial verbal reactions. *Journal of Experimental Psychology* 18, 643–62.

Tang, M.X., Jacobs, D., Stern, Y., *et al.* (1996). Effect of oestrogen during menopause on risk and age at onset of Alzheimer's disease. *Lancet* 348, 429–32.

Tartar, R.E., Butters, M., and Beers, S.R. (2001). *Medical neuropsychology*, 2nd edn. Kluwer Academic/Plenum Publishers, New York.

Thoman, M.L. and Weigle, W.O. (1989). The cellular and subcellular bases of immunosenescence. *Advan. Immunol.* 46, 221–61.

Thurstone, L.L. and Thurstone, T.G. (1963). *Primary Mental Abilities*, Science Research Associates, Chicago.

Trzepacz, P.T., McCue, M., Klein, I., Levey, G.S., and Greenhouse, J. (1988). A psychiatric and neuropsychological study of patients with untreated Graves' disease. *Gen. Hosp. Psychiatry* 10, 49–55.

Vandenberg, S.G. and Kuse, A.R. (1978). Mental relations: a group test of three dimensional spatial visualization. *Perceptual and Motor Skills* 47, 599–601.

Whelan, T.B., Schteingart, M.N., Starkman, M.N., and Smith, A. (1980). Neuropsychological deficits in Cushing's syndrome. *J. Nerv. Ment. Dis.* 168, 753–7.

Whybrow, P.C. and Prange, A.J. Jr, and Treadway, C.R. (1969). Mental changes accompanying thyroid gland dysfunction. A reappraisal using objective psychological measurement. *Arch. Gen. Psychiatry* 20, 48–63.

Williams, C.L., Barnett, A.M., and Meck, W.H. (1990). Organizational effects of early gonadal secretions on sexual differentiation in spatial memory. *Behav. Neurosci.* 104, 84–97.

Winograd, D.L., Sensheima, P., Barrett-Connor, E.L., and McPhillips, T.B. (1990). Community-based study on the prevalence of NIDDM in older adults. *Diabetes Care,* 13 (suppl. 2), 3–8.

Yaffe, K., Sawaya, G., Lieberburg, I., and Grady, D. (1998). Estrogen therapy in postmenopausal women: effects on cognitive function and dementia. *J. Am. Med. Assoc.* 17, 1848–59.

Chapter 32

Neuropsychological assessment and treatment of epilepsy

Pamela J. Thompson

1 Introduction

Clinical neuropsychologists can make a unique contribution to the management of epilepsy. They are skilled in identifying cognitive strengths and weaknesses. Neuropsychological deficits are hidden and often overlooked with most attention focused on seizure control. If unnoticed, cognitive deficits can adversely impact on academic, social, and emotional development. The longer the cognitive impairment is undetected, the worse the outcome. A verbal learning deficit may be a sequela of left temporal lobe epilepsy. This may result in a child falling behind at school and failing examinations. Frequent failure results in loss of confidence. A failing child may also be the butt of jokes and bullying. Low self-esteem and depression may ensue.

Executive skills deficits may accompany frontal lobe epilepsy and, if these are undetected, patients' expectations may be set too high. An individual may be wrongly judged capable of independent living. Problems with reasoning and regulating behaviour may result in poor time management and self-care. Physical neglect and disturbed sleep patterns, which will adversely effect seizure control, may follow. Frequent drop attacks will increase the risk of injury. Frequent injuries may result in further brain damage. A neuropsychological assessment enables more realistic goal setting.

Clinical neuropsychologists are experienced in developing rehabilitation programmes. An undetected memory impairment will result in poor compliance. Forgotten tablets will result in increased seizure frequency. Training in memory support strategies will improve compliance. This reduces the need for an increase in medication.

Neuropsychological assessment may assist diagnosis. It is the main tool for detecting dementia and monitoring its course. This may be crucial in identifying certain epileptic syndromes. Test profiles may help to differentiate between partial and generalized epilepsies, which in turn may influence drug treatment. Possible adverse drug side-effects can be measured with cognitive tests and drug changes can be promptly made if difficulties are demonstrated.

The neuropsychologist is a well established member of the surgical multidisciplinary team. Cognitive test profiles may yield vital cerebral lateralizing and localizing data. Preoperative test scores provide evidence relating to postoperative cognitive complications. This enables patients to make better decisions regarding surgery.

2 Epilepsy—general description

Epilepsy is the most serious common neurological disorder. The lifetime incidence is 2–5%. Epilepsy refers to a group of conditions that have seizures as a common symptom. An epileptic seizure is a transient, abnormal electrical discharge from the neurons in the brain. The region involved will shape the behavioural manifestation of the attack. Seizures may involve motor, sensory, psychic, or autonomic disturbances— alone or in combination. Epileptic seizures are stereotyped. They have a sudden onset but a brief duration (lasting minutes). Seizure occurrence is generally unpredictable. Table 32.1 lists some UK sources of information and/or support for those with epilepsy.

2.1 Classification

Epilepsy is classified according to clinical manifestation and electroencephalographic (EEG) changes (see Table 32.2).

◆ *Partial seizures* begin with epileptic discharges in a localized brain area. Any area of the cortex can be the epileptogenic zone, but the temporal lobes are the most susceptible. Temporal lobe epilepsy constitutes 60–70% of partial epilepsy cases. Following seizures, recovery may be variable. There may be a significant period of drowsiness and malaise (post-ictal phase).

  Seizures may begin partially but then spread to involve the whole brain (secondary generalized seizures).

◆ In *generalized seizures* the epileptogenic activity involves the whole cortex from the outset. Generalized seizures may vary in severity and duration.

  —*Absence seizures* involve a brief arrest of consciousness.

  —*Generalized tonic clonic seizures* are more severe. The patient stiffens and will fall if standing (tonic phase). Jerking limb movements then follow (clonic phase). The patient may be incontinent. The seizure lasts a few minutes and exhaustion and drowsiness may follow.

  —*Atonic* and *tonic seizures* occur suddenly. The individual will fall if standing. Head injuries may often be a sequela. Recovery of consciousness is rapid.

Table 32.1 Sources of information/support in the UK for those with epilepsy and their carers/families

British Epilepsy Association, Anstey House, 40 Hanover Square, Leeds LS3 1BE
Epilepsy Association of Scotland, 48 Govan Road, Glasgow GS1 1JR
Epilepsy Bereaved, PO Box 112, Wantage OX12 8XT
National Society for Epilepsy, The Chalfont Centre, Chalfont St Peter, Bucks SL9 ORJ
Wales Epilepsy Association, Y Pant teg Brynteg, Dolgellau, Gwynedd, Wales LL40 1RP

Table 32.2 The International League against Epilepsy's (1981) classification of epileptic seizures

I Partial seizures (seizures beginning locally)

(a) Simple partial seizures (consciousness not impaired)

With motor symptoms

With somatosensory or special sensory symptoms

With autonomic symptoms

With psychic symptoms

(b) Complex partial seizures (with impairment of consciousness)
Beginning as simple partial seizures and progressing to impairment of consciousness

i with no other features

ii with features as in I(a)

iii with automatisms

With impairment of consciousness at onset

i with no other features

ii with features as in I(a)

iii with automatisms

(c) Partial seizures secondarily generalized

II Generalized seizures (bilaterally symmetrical and without focal onset)

(a) Absence seizures
Atypical absence seizures

(b) Myoclonic seizures

(c) Clonic seizures

(d) Tonic seizures

(e) Tonic clonic seizures

(f) Atonic seizures

III Unclassified epileptic seizures (inadequate or incomplete data)

Most seizures are short-lived and stop spontaneously. *Status epilepticus* refers to serial seizures with inadequate recovery between attacks. It occurs for any seizure type. For tonic clonic seizures, it is a medical emergency. It is more common in children, people with learning difficulties, and in frontal lobe epilepsy. Table 32.3 gives the International League against Epilepsy's classification of epilepsy syndromes.

2.2 Prognosis

Of people with epilepsy, 70–80% become seizure-free. About 50% will be able to discontinue their antiepileptic medication (Sander and Sillanpaa 1998).

Table 32.3 The International League against Epilepsy's (1989) classification of the epilepsy syndromes

I Generalized

(a) Idiopathic generalized epilepsy with age-related onset

    (i)   Benign neo-natal family convulsions

    (ii)   Benign neonatal convulsions

    (iii) Benign myoclonic epilepsy in infancy

    (iv) Childhood absence epilepsy

    (v)   Juvenile absence epilepsy

    (vi) Juvenile myoclonic epilepsy

    (vii) Epilepsy with generalized tonic clonic seizures on awakening

    (viii) Other idiopathic generalized epilepsies

    (ix) Epilepsies with seizures precipitated by specific modes of activation

(b) Cryptogenic or symptomatic

    (i)   West's syndrome

    (ii) Lennox–Gastaut syndrome

    (iii) Epilepsy with myoclonic–astatic seizures

    (iv) Epilepsy with myoclonic absences

(c) Symptomatic generalized epilepsies

    (i)   Epileptic syndromes complicating other disease states

    (ii) Non-specific aetiology

    (iii) Early myoclonic encephalopathy

    (iv) Early infantile encephalopathy with burst suppression

    (v)   Other symptomatic epilepsies not defined above

II Localization-related (focal/local/partial)

(a) Idiopathic with age-related onset

    (i)   Benign epilepsy with centro-temporal spikes

    (ii) Childhood epilepsy with occipital paroxysms

    (iii) Primary reading epilepsy

(b) Symptomatic

    (i)   Temporal lobe epilepsies

    (ii) Frontal lobe epilepsies

    (iii) Parietal lobe epilepsies

    (iv) Occipital lobe epilepsies

    (v)   Epilepsia partialis continua

    (vi) Syndromes characterized by specific modes of precipitation

Table 32.3 (*continued*)

III Epilepsies and syndromes undetermined as to focal or generalized

(a) With both generalized and focal seizures

  (i) Neonatal seizures

  (ii) Severe myoclonic epilepsy in infancy

  (iii) Acquired epileptic aphasia

  (iv) Electrical status epilepticus in slow-wave sleep

(b) Without unequivocal generalized or focal features

2.3 **Causes**

The causes of epilepsy are varied.

- Epilepsy may be genetically determined. Idiopathic generalized epilepsies include childhood absence epilepsy. Of these, 80% remit by adulthood. The mode of inheritance is unclear. It is likely to be multigenetic (Duncan *et al.* 1995). There are a large number of rare inherited disorders with seizures as a common feature. These include tuberous sclerosis and neurofibromatosis, both of which are autosomal dominant. Unverricht Lundborg's disease is autosomal recessive.

- Congenital disturbances of the brain may cause epilepsy. *Cortical dysgenesis* refers to brain abnormalities that have developed during embryogenesis (Sisodiya 2000). The most severe cases involve gyral abnormalities. In *lissencephaly* there is an absence of gyri over the whole brain. Invariably there are severe learning disabilities. Prognosis is poor. There may be more localized areas of dysgenesis, i.e. dysembryoplastic neuroepithelial tumours (DNETs). Disruption of cognitive function may be minimal.

- *Hippocampal sclerosis* is the most common lesion identified in resected tissue following temporal lobectomy. It is strongly associated with a history of a prolonged childhood febrile convulsion(s). Habitual epilepsy may not develop for several years. It remains controversial whether hippocampal sclerosis is the cause or the consequence of febrile convulsions (Gloor 1991).

- The incidence of epilepsy is high following *cerebral infections*. Rates for herpes simplex encephalitis are 25%, for bacterial meningitis 10%, and for human immunodeficiency virus (HIV)-related cerebral toxoplasmosis 25%.

- Epilepsy may develop following a severe head injury. The risk increases when post-traumatic amnesia lasts longer then 24 hours. Intracranial haematoma and open head injuries also increase the risk.

- Seizures can develop *de novo* following *neurosurgery*. The occurrence of seizures will be influenced by the site (increased frontal and temporal), the extent of resection (increased with larger), and the condition for which the craniotomy is performed (e.g. higher for arteriovenous malformations than for intracranial aneurysms).

- *Cerebrovascular disease* may cause epilepsy. It depends on the extent and site of the infarcted area. Lower rates occur for transient ischaemic attacks (TIAs). Higher rates arise for haemorrhagic stroke.
- *Neoplasms* may be an underlying cause of epilepsy. The risk varies with tumour type (oligodenrogliomas 90%; meningiomas and astrocytomas 70%; malignant tumours 35%).
- Dementias and *neurodegenerative conditions* may underlie a seizure disorder. Approximately 25% of Alzheimer's disease cases develop seizures. Response to antiepileptic drug (AED) treatment is reported to be good.
- *Metabolic disorders* are a cause of epilepsy. Changes in blood concentrations of sodium, potassium, calcium, magnesium, and glucose have been documented.
- There are reports of epilepsy following the ingestion of a variety of medications. Drugs implicated include antibiotic, antimalarial, antidepressant, and antipsychotic agents. Epilepsy has been reported following illicit drug use and heavy consumption of alcohol. Drug withdrawal may precipitate seizures.

3 Investigations for epilepsy

3.1 Electroencephalography (EEG)

A diagnosis of epilepsy is commonly made on the basis of a behavioural description. This is generally provided by the family. Rarely do physicians witness an attack. EEG recording is a major diagnostic tool. An EEG trace represents the summation of synchronized excitatory or inhibitory postsynaptic potentials. In about 30% of cases, epileptic abnormalities are seen in routine recordings (20–30 minutes duration). EEGs made during seizures (ictal recordings) show abnormalities in about 95% of cases.

- Generalized spike-and-wave discharges typically occur during absence seizures.
- Evolving temporal slow-wave activity may be seen in temporal lobe epilepsy.

The chances of recording a seizure are low.

More prolonged EEG recordings increase the chances of seizure detection. Small portable EEG machines (ambulatory monitors) allow longer recording periods. The patient may wear these until attacks occur. During videotelemetry, the EEG is combined with synchronized video recording. This allows for the correlation of clinical and electrographical events. Videotelemetry recordings take place in hospital. Drugs can be reduced and/or the patient can be sleep-deprived. Both increase the chances of a seizure occurring.

3.1.1 Intracranial EEG recordings

Intracranial EEG recordings are undertaken on selected surgical candidates. These are usually made when the site of the epileptogenic focus is unclear. Depth electrodes are multicontact wires inserted stereotactically under magnetic resonance imaging (MRI) control. The electrodes can be inserted into brain regions of interest. For temporal lobectomy candidates this may include the hippocampus and other mesial structures.

Subdural grids consist of a large array of electrodes. These are used when the epileptogenic zone is extensive. Intracranial recordings are invasive and there is a significant risk of morbidity.

3.2 Brain scans

Neither MRI nor computerized tomography (CT) scans can be used to diagnose epilepsy. Nevertheless, MRI plays a major role in identifying potential surgical candidates. The MRI scan can reveal subtle structural abnormalities in intractable epilepsy. MRI has been responsible for the rapid growth of surgical treatment (Duncan *et al.* 1995).

3.3 The intracarotid amytal procedure (IAP)

This is a special investigation undertaken on selected surgical candidates. It is used to establish language dominance. It is also used to screen for postoperative amnesia in temporal lobectomy candidates. Each cerebral hemisphere in turn is temporarily anaesthetized. Sodium amobarbital is injected into a single carotid artery via a catheter in the femoral artery. The drug effects last approximately 10 minutes. A transient hemiplegia and EEG changes indicate a lateralized effect. The patient is shown stimuli before and after the injection. Speech arrest and dysphasic difficulties indicate language dominance in the injected hemisphere. Intact memory performance indicates adequate memory in the non-injected hemisphere.

The IAP is an invasive procedure. Its reliability and validity have been questioned. Functional magnetic resonance imaging (fMRI) paradigms are being developed as non-invasive alternatives (Baxendale 2000).

4 Treatment

4.1 Acute management

Convulsive seizures are usually short-lived. No immediate medical treatment is required. Nothing can be done to influence the course of the seizure.

- The patient should be made as comfortable as possible, preferably lying down, or eased to the floor if seated.
- The head should be protected and any tight clothing should be released.
- Clear a space around the person in order to avoid injury.
- Do not attempt to open the mouth and do not force anything between the teeth.
- After the convulsive movements have stopped, roll the person on to his or her side.
- Check that the airway is not obstructed.

- Patients may take a variable time to recover and may wish to sleep or rest.
- Emergency treatment will only be needed if:

—the person sustains an injury;

—the convulsive stage lasts longer than 10 minutes;

—the patient takes a long time to regain consciousness;

—a second convulsive attack follows before full recovery.

Non-convulsive seizures require minimal management.

- Many attacks are very brief and have little impact on behaviour.
- In complex partial seizures the patient may wander and fiddle with items. An attempt should be made to guide the person out of danger if necessary.
- No attempt should be made to restrain. Such attempts can cause agitation and aggression.

4.2 Medication

The majority of people will be treated with antiepileptic drugs (AEDs). The range of drugs available is given in Table 32.4.

Table 32.4 Antiepileptic drugs

Generic name	Brand name	Abbreviation	Dose range (mg)
Carbamazepine	Tegretol	CBZ	600–1800
Clobazam	Frisium	CLB	10–30
Clonazepam	Rivotril	CZP	0.5–3
Ethosuximide	Zarontin	ESM	500–1500
Gabapentin	Neurontin	GBP	900–2400
Lamotrigine	Lamictal	LTG	200–400
Levetiracetam	Kepra	LT	1000–3000
Phenobarbitone	Luminal	PB	60–180
Phenytoin	Epanutin	DPH	200–400
Primidone	Mysoline	PMD	125–500
Sodium valproate	Epilim	VPA	1000–2500
Tiagabine	Gabitril	TGB	30–45
Topiramate	Topimax	TPM	200–400
Vigabatrin	Sabril	GVG	2000–3000

4.3 **Surgical treatment**

The most commonly performed operation is an anterior temporal lobectomy. The most common pathology is hippocampal sclerosis. Two-thirds of cases can be expected to achieve complete seizure control (Polkey 2000*a*). The next most common operation is a frontal resection. A seizure-free outcome is less likely. A hemispherectomy represents the most radical procedure. It involves the deactivation of an entire cerebral hemisphere. Candidates will have prior evidence of major structural abnormalities. The functional capacity of the removed hemisphere is small.

Corpus callosotomy involves disconnecting the callosal fibres between the cerebral hemispheres. The aim is to prevent the spread of epileptic discharges. Most operations involve partial disconnection. A multiple subpial transection may be performed to isolate an epileptic area from the surrounding cortex to prevent seizure spread. Vertical cuts are made in the epileptogenic cortical region. This is undertaken when seizure discharges arise from cognitively important regions such as language areas or motor cortex (Polkey 2000*b*).

Vagal nerve stimulation is a recent development. A stimulator is wrapped around one vagus nerve. It is intermittently stimulated, usually for less than a minute, every 5–10 minutes. An improvement in seizure control has been reported. Complete seizure control is rare. At present, this treatment is confined to patients with severe refractory epilepsy who are not suitable surgical candidates (Schachter and Saper 1998).

4.4 **Psychological treatment**

A number of treatments have been proposed as seizure-reducing techniques (Thompson and Baxendale 1996). From a behavioural viewpoint, a seizure may be viewed as part of a sequence of events. By interrupting the behavioural chain the likelihood of a seizure is reduced. Avoidance has been the most successful treatment in the reflex epilepsies. Individuals with photosensitivity epilepsy can reduce the likelihood of seizures by altering TV viewing habits. Strategies include viewing at a distance, covering one eye, viewing in good ambient lighting, and using polarized glasses. Desensitization, relaxation, bio-feedback, aversive therapy, and positive reinforcement have been employed with variable success.

Cognitive therapy is used more for mood disturbance. It may be helpful where anxiety is an identified seizure trigger. Case studies report success in individual cases with complex partial seizures.

4.5 **Diet and lifestyle changes**

The ketogenic diet is the most established treatment. It is high in fat and low in carbohydrate and protein. It is generally used with children. The diet can be continued for months, or even years. Many children find it unpalatable. This reduces compliance (Duncan *et al*. 1995).

Abstaining from alcohol, regularizing sleep, and improving compliance have been associated with improved seizure control.

5 Neuropsychological deficits in intelligence

Epilepsy has in the past been associated with limited intellectual abilities. This was largely a consequence of biased sampling. Research indicates that people with epilepsy are represented throughout the spectrum of intellectual ability (Thompson and Trimble 1996). However, failed or arrested intellectual development arises in some epilepsy syndromes (Roget 1992).

- Early infantile epileptic encephalopathy has an onset in infancy. The MRI shows abnormalities and atrophy. Many infants die. Survivors have severe and profound learning disabilities. Sensory and motor abnormalities are common.

- Mental retardation is one of a triad of symptoms in West's and Lennox–Gastaut syndromes, the others being frequent seizures and characteristic EEG changes. Developmental delay follows and frequent and severe seizures develop.

- There are a number of conditions where there is comorbidity. Often seizures do not develop until adolescence or adulthood. The estimated risk of seizures in Down's syndrome is 10%; in autism 30%; in cerebral palsy 50%; in tuberous sclerosis 60%; in Angelman's syndrome 80%.

The likelihood of epilepsy increases with the severity of the learning disability. Both the seizures and the cognitive impairment are a consequence of extensive brain damage and immature cerebral development.

There is normal intellectual development in other syndromes. In childhood absence epilepsy the prognosis for cognitive development is good.

5.1 Intellectual deterioration

Follow-up studies show that the intellectual level remains stable unless there is an underlying neurodegenerative disorder (Aldenkamp *et al.* 1990; Holmes *et al.* 1998). Intellectual deterioration may occur when seizures are frequent and severe. Atonic and tonic seizures (drop attacks) carry a poorer prognosis. Episodes of convulsive status epilepticus will result in neuronal death and cognitive decline.

In some rare syndromes, cognitive deterioration is an ongoing feature unless treatment is prompt and successful (Duncan *et al.* 1995).

- *Rasmussen's encephalitis.* The patient presents with constant partial motor seizures. These usually begin in one limb and there is gradual progression to the ipsilateral limb. A hemiplegia may result. Rasmussen's encephalitis is associated with progressive focal atrophy and progressive intellectual decline. In left hemisphere cases there is a decline in verbal intellect. In right hemisphere cases visuospatial abilities decline (assuming typical language dominance).

- *Electrical status epilepticus during slow-wave sleep* (ESES) is characterized by continuous periods of abnormal EEG patterns of generalized spike and wave. Two-thirds of cases have normal development until the onset. Gross intellectual deterioration, attentional, and other significant cognitive difficulties develop. ESES and seizures remit in the majority in adolescence. Intellectual gains thereafter are small.

◆ *Landau–Kleffner syndrome*. ESES, daytime temporoparietal spike wave discharges, and aphasia (see Section 6.2) are the three main features of this syndrome.

◆ *Unverricht Lundborg's syndrome* (*Baltic myoclonous*). The onset is usually between the ages of 5 and 15 years. Early development is normal. Progressive motor and cognitive deterioration occurs.

5.2 Transient cognitive disturbance

Deficits vary in severity and type depending on the duration and site of the epileptic discharge (Thompson and Trimble 1996).

◆ *Transient cognitive impairment* (TCI) is a term used to describe fleeting cognitive lapses that are associated with brief epileptic discharges. TCI may only be apparent during continuous cognitive activity. Where such discharges occur frequently, cognitive disturbance is marked. Localized discharges may have a selective effect. Left temporal discharges may impair verbal but not spatial memory tasks. Epileptic discharges are known to arise from structures deep within the brain. These are not accessible to scalp EEG recordings. Depth electrode studies in patients have shown that runs of epileptic discharges may underlie transient memory disturbance.

◆ Overt seizures may present as more obvious intermittent cognitive disturbances. Word-finding difficulties may be the manifestation of partial seizures arising from dominant lateral temporal regions. Brief episodes of topographical disorientation may reflect seizures in the nondominant temporal lobe. Several cases of ictal amnesia have been documented (Zeman and Hodges 2000).

◆ During *nonconvulsive status epilepticus* individuals may present with severe cognitive impairment (Shorvon 1994). This can mimic dementia. Misdiagnosis is more likely in the elderly and individuals with learning disabilities. EEG recordings can confirm this diagnosis. AED treatment can bring about rapid control. Reversal of the cognitive disturbance follows.

Recovery from seizures can be variable. In the post-ictal phase, disturbed cognition may occur. Cognitive impairment may be selective. Individuals with left temporal lobe seizures may show a selective verbal memory impairment. Such deficits can persist several days following a bout of complex partial seizures.

5.3 Cognitive activity triggering seizures

Reflex epilepsies refer to epileptic disorders for which there is a specific trigger. The most common of the reflex epilepsies is photosensitive epilepsy. The most frequent environmental triggers are watching television and computer use. There are a number of case reports of seizures induced by higher mental processing. Activities implicated include reading, writing, arithmetic, memorizing, and chess and card playing (Matsouka *et al.* 2000).

6 Chronic cognitive disturbance

There is no cognitive deficit or test profile that characterizes epilepsy. The majority of individuals who are well controlled by drug treatment will not experience problems. Accordingly, such patients do not come to the attention of the clinical neuropsychologist. Individuals with intractable epilepsy, however, are at risk of persisting cognitive difficulties. The underlying aetiology is the primary cause. The nature and severity of a deficit will be determined by the location of the brain pathology. Given the increased risk of epilepsy with temporal and frontal pathology, memory and executive deficits are the most frequently encountered in clinical practice.

6.1 Memory

Deficits of new learning have been the subject of most investigations. These are the most common cognitive impairment in temporal lobe epilepsy (Thompson 1997). Memory impairment is most extensive in cases with known bilateral temporal lobe damage. The amnesic syndrome is the most severe scenario. Early reported cases followed bilateral temporal lobectomy. Currently, severe amnesia is most frequently encountered in adult-onset post-encephalitic cases.

Unilateral temporal lobe epilepsy has been associated with material-specific memory disorders. Assuming left hemisphere language dominance, left temporal lobe disturbance is reported to be associated with verbal memory difficulties and right temporal lobe disturbance with spatial memory deficits. Such material-specific memory disorders are more likely to be encountered after temporal lobectomy. In presurgical or nonsurgical unilateral temporal lobe cases, material-specific memory problems are more elusive. They are less likely to be recorded in early-onset epilepsy where the underlying pathology is cortical dysplasia. In such cases, insults early during embryogenesis may result in significant cognitive reorganization as a consequence of cerebral plasticity.

6.2 Language

Most people have language functions lateralized predominantly to the left cerebral hemisphere. Rates are lower for genetic left-handers. Atypical language dominance is more commonly encountered in epilepsy. Language functions are predominantly lateralized to the right hemisphere or bilaterally represented. Predisposing factors include:

- early cerebral insult to the left hemisphere;
- early onset of recurrent seizures;
- left (pathological) handedness;
- weak right handedness.

Language laterality in epilepsy is a clinically relevant variable in surgical cases. It may influence the decision to proceed to surgery, the extent of the resection, and/or the risk of postoperative cognitive deficits. The intracarotid sodium amytal procedure (IAP) is the gold standard for establishing language dominance (Baxendale 2000).

Individuals with epilepsy may experience language problems (Ballaban-Gil 1995; Breier *et al.* 2000). Such difficulties can have a negative impact on academic, occupational, and social functioning. Most at risk are individuals with seizures that emanate from the language dominant hemisphere.

- A seizure focus in the frontotemporal regions may be more likely to interfere with expressive functions.
- More posterior temporal lesions may impair comprehension.
- Parietal lesions may impact on reading and spelling.

Acquired epileptic aphasia (Landau–Kleffner's syndrome) is a rare disorder in which the child presents with language difficulties. The EEG shows severe focal abnormalities. This syndrome usually presents between the ages of 4 and 11 years. Language development prior to onset is unremarkable. The first symptom is usually the experience of receptive language difficulties. The majority of cases go on to develop generalized and partial seizures. Language deterioration occurs over time and total mutism can result. The EEG shows multifocal spike-and-wave. Most often, the abnormalities are in the temporal and parietal occipital regions. Language functions may improve as seizures become less frequent or stop. Many individuals have residual language problems.

6.3 Executive functions

Individuals with frontal lobe epilepsy show a mixed cognitive picture. Research studies have reported impaired programming and coordination of motor sequences, impaired working memory and attention, and reduced response inhibition (Helmstaedter *et al.* 1996; Upton and Thompson 1996). For some, the cognitive burden is very handicapping. Executive function deficits are more evident in individuals with bilateral and/or more widespread frontal damage. Those with late-onset seizures secondary to 'new' pathology (tumours and head injuries) are another at-risk group. Rapid seizure propagation is a characteristic of frontal lobe epilepsy. Neurons in the contralateral frontal lobe and mesial temporal regions are frequently recruited. Consequently, frontal lateralizing cognitive deficits are rarely found. Where seizure activity spreads to temporal regions, memory deficits more characteristic of temporal lobe epilepsy cases may be seen.

7 Neuropsychological impacts of antiepileptic drugs (AEDs) and surgery

7.1 AEDs

There is no evidence that AEDs have any independent cognition-enhancing properties. Improvements in cognition can occur as a consequence of better seizure control.

For individuals with multiple daily absences, effective drug treatment will result in improved attention and information processing. For those at risk of episodes of status epilepticus, effective drug treatment may prevent further neuronal death. This in turn will prevent cognitive deterioration. Where seizures take the form of transient cognitive deficits, effective treatment will eliminate such episodes. Control of seizures does not always result in cognitive improvements. AEDs aim to suppress the symptoms of epilepsy, not the cause. Patients with epilepsy secondary to brain pathology will often experience persisting problems despite good seizure control.

AEDs can be a cause of cognitive impairments (Thompson and Trimble 1996). AEDs should always be considered a possible factor in patients referred due to cognitive complaints. AEDs are given to suppress neuronal overexcitability and they are not selective in their action. Drugs will also affect normally acting neurons. When a single drug controls seizures at small doses, adverse cognitive effects may be negligible. Where seizures are more difficult to control, the risk of adverse cognitive effects is higher. The aim of drug treatment is to achieve maximal seizure control with minimal side-effects. This balance can be difficult to achieve. Any drug can exert a negative effect when serum concentrations are too high. Cognitive disturbance usually presents with other symptoms of drug intoxication, including ataxia and diplopia. Cognitive blunting, however, may be the only sign.

Conflicting results predominate in the research literature. Randomized controlled trials tend to report minimal cognitive side-effects. Such studies may miss adverse drug effects if the response is not uniform across patients. The pharmaceutical industry sponsors most of these studies, which can influence the reporting of the results. Case studies and less rigorously designed investigations report greater negative effects. These designs have their own biases (Meador 1998; Thompson 2001).

The cognitive profile of individual drugs is far from clear. Clinical experience indicates that generalizations are impossible. A drug can cause adverse effects in one patient but not in another. Mental slowness is a common drug effect to which timed tests will be particularly sensitive. Reduced efficiency may be seen on a range of cognitive measures. Specific cognitive deficits are less likely. However, some patients do experience an exacerbation of a pre-existing cognitive problem.

- *Phenobarbitone* is the oldest AED. Adverse cognitive effects have been reported relative to other AEDs.

- *Phenytoin* is a drug with peculiar pharmacokinetics. A small increment in dose may result in a dramatic increase in serum levels. This in turn may produce marked mental slowing. There are reports of reversible dementia.

- Cases of *sodium valproate*-induced dementia have also been documented. This is usually due to raised serum ammonia levels. Marked cognitive slowness does occur when phenobarbitone is co-prescribed.

- *Carbamazepine* has been associated with fewer adverse effects. Some negative cognitive reactions have been reported.

There are few studies of the newer AEDs. Adverse cognitive effects have been reported for *topiramate*. Some patients report experiencing effortful thinking and reduced verbal fluency. Such deficits have been confirmed by neuropsychological testing (Thompson *et al.* 2000). There is some consensus that polypharmacy increases the risk of cognitive deficits. Few AED drug combinations have been adequately studied. Co-therapy with anti-depressants and antipsychotic agents may bring added cognitive risks.

7.2 **Surgery**

7.2.1 Temporal lobectomy

In the 1950s, bilateral temporal lobectomies were undertaken. Profound amnesia was a frequent outcome. Accordingly, such operations were abandoned. Unilateral temporal resections can result in amnesia if contralateral structures are dysfunctional. For this reason, neuropsychological assessment became a vital part of presurgical evaluations. In cases where memory disturbance indicates bilateral temporal pathology, a sodium amytal investigation is needed. In some surgical centres this procedure is performed on all surgical candidates. When the ipsilateral hemisphere is temporarily anaesthetized, normal memory function is expected. When memory is impaired the patient is at risk of postoperative amnesia. Either the patient does not proceed to surgery or has a more limited resection (Baxendale 2000).

Temporal lobe resections give rise to material-specific memory disorders. Verbal memory decline following dominant hemisphere resections is the most common finding. Nonverbal memory impairments arise following nondominant hemisphere resections. Verbal memory decline, however, has been documented by some investigators. Memory deterioration does not always occur. The functional adequacy of the tissue removed is important (Baxendale 1995). Postoperative pathological changes in the remaining structures are also implicated (Baxendale *et al.* 2000). Other risk factors include older age at surgery (>40 years) and above-average preoperative test scores. Impaired processing in the contralateral temporal lobe carries a poor prognosis (Baxendale *et al.* 1998). Some patients show no memory decline postoperatively and some show improvement. Cerebral plasticity earlier in development may underlie these positive outcomes. It is the role of the neuropsychologist to predict the likely cognitive con-sequences. These are shared with the patient. Verbal memory decline has the most impact on everyday functioning. Verbal memory decline can cause problems at work and in social settings.

Language decline can occur after dominant temporal lobe resections. Expressive functions are commonly affected. There is often rapid recovery in the early postoperative weeks. For some cases, naming difficulties persist. Hermann *et al.* (1999) reported that older age at onset and absence of hippocampal sclerosis were predictors of persisting naming problems.

Decrements in intellectual ability following surgery are rare. Some patients show substantial gains. This is more likely in seizure-free patients who have AEDs withdrawn. Low preoperative intellectual level is not a good predictor of outcome. Low IQ should not be used to exclude patients from surgery (Chelune *et al.* 1998).

7.2.2 Frontal lobectomy

The cognitive outcome is variable (Helmstaedter *et al.* 1998). Some cases show exacerbation of existing deficits. Cognitive improvement is most likely with good seizure outcome. Outcome is poorest when seizures continue and in preoperatively cognitively intact cases. Resection involving the pre-motor and sensory motor areas increases risk of impaired response maintenance and inhibition. Marked language disturbance has been reported with dominant hemisphere operations.

7.2.3 Hemispherectomy

This is more often performed in cases where there is evidence of significant hemiatrophy and actual or anticipated cognitive decline is expected if surgery is not performed (e.g. Rasmussen's encephalitis, Sturge–Weber syndrome). Hemispherectomy is usually undertaken in children and the available evidence suggests that the cognitive and behavioural outcomes are good. This is more likely to be so if seizures stop and AED medication can be withdrawn or substantially reduced. Cognitive outcome is better in nondominant cases and with a younger age at operation.

◆ Significant increases in IQ and attentional capacity have been reported.

◆ Some dominant hemispherectomy cases have shown postoperative recovery of language (Bode and Curtiss 2000).

◆ Powers of repetition and language comprehension show the greatest recovery.

◆ Expressive functions may be limited to single words or grammatically simple short sentences.

7.2.4 Corpus callosotomy

Improvements in alertness and general behaviour have been documented. This enables individuals to achieve higher levels of independence (Nordgren 1991). The trend is for greater improvements when seizures, particularly tonic/atonic attacks, are controlled. There is better cognitive outcome when the operation is undertaken at a younger age. Transient deficits such as alien hand syndrome and mutism are rare. These tend to occur in the early postoperative period following total resection.

8 Psychological disorders associated with epilepsy

8.1 Mood disturbance

Professionals need to be aware of possible negative emotional reactions (Lambert and Robertson 1999; Thompson and Grant 2001).

Anxiety and depression are the most commonly encountered mood disorders. Many aspects of epilepsy may contribute.

- Seizures occur unpredictably. There is often the risk of injury, particularly with drop attacks.
- Seizure behaviours can be bizarre and embarrassing.
- Epilepsy is not a benign condition. Mortality rates are elevated. Twenty to forty year olds have an eightfold increased risk of death so that fear of premature death is realistic.
- Patients need to adhere to a restrictive drug regime. Adverse side-effects such as weight gain, facial hair, and cognitive difficulties can undermine confidence. The experience of successive medication failures in intractable epilepsy is stressful.
- The failure of surgical treatment can be more distressing, particularly if this follows years without seizures. Surgical failure occurs in about one-third of cases. Some patients undergo lengthy presurgical assessments, only to be rejected as unsuitable candidates.
- Children may experience teasing and bullying at school and academic expectations may be wrongly lowered.
- Adult employment options are reduced and unemployment rates are high. Employment difficulties may result in restricted finances.
- The anxieties of potential parents with epilepsy may be raised regarding the pregnancy, the birth, and subsequent development of the child.
- Epilepsy still carries a sizeable social stigma and prejudice.

8.2 Psychosis

This may present as a transient ictal phenomenon (Adachi *et al.* 2000). The patient may experience disturbing hallucinations and paranoid thoughts. Episodes may last several hours. AED treatment may be effective. Psychosis can develop between seizures. It is more common when epilepsy is longstanding. It may be a sign of drug intoxication or a drug side-effect. Vigabatrin, topiramate, and ethosuximide have been implicated. Treatment with antipsychotic medication is indicated. Unfortunately, many effective drugs are known to be epileptogenic.

8.3 Aggression

This is less widespread than reported in the past. It is more likely to arise with widespread underlying brain damage. Risk of aggression increases with frontal lobe involvement. Drug treatment may be implicated. Phenobarbitone, benzodiazepines, vigabatrin, and topiramate have been implicated. Aggressive behaviour is a rare ictal phenomenon. It is more common post-ictally, especially if restraint is applied. Ictal aggressive episodes are likely to be stereotyped and to occur in the absence of environmental precipitants. They are not clearly directed toward a specific person or object and do not involve planned or complicated motor actions.

8.4 **Non-epileptic attack disorder (NEAD)**

NEAD is a term used to describe episodic disturbances resembling epilepsy. There are no accompanying epileptic EEG discharges. There is no other physical cause (e.g. hypoglycaemia).

NEAD was previously known as pseudoseizures. The latter term is to be discouraged due to pejorative connotations. It may be a symptom of posttraumatic stress disorder, an anxi-ety disorder, or other psychological conditions (Francis and Baker 1999). There is often a history of past emotional trauma. Physical and/or sexual abuse may feature. Ongoing relationship difficulties may contribute. Occasionally, there is obvi-ous secondary gain. In tertiary referral sites NEAD is diagnosed in up to 25% of epilep-sy cases. The risk of misdiagnosis is high in learning disabilities. Up to 50% of status epilepticus cases at accident and emergency departments have NEADs.

Differentiating between epileptic and non-epileptic seizures is difficult. No clinical phenomena are exclusive to either. Incontinence and injury do not reliably distinguish one from the other. Features suggestive of NEAD include gradual onset, long duration (>5 minutes), and asynchronous limb flailing. Directed actions, especially aggression and react-ivity to external stimulation, may suggest NEAD. Environmental and psy-chological triggers may be readily identifiable.

The presentation of a change of diagnosis needs to be positive. The immediate family should be involved. Precipitating factors need to be ascertained. Functional analysis may be helpful. The circumstances of the first attack may be helpful. Enquiries about sexual trauma should be made. Psychotherapy is often indicated. Response to treat-ment is poorer the longer a history of misdiagnosis (>10 years) and where financial and social support is dependent on epilepsy diagnosis.

9 **Neuropsychological assessment**

9.1 **General**

- Before the assessment, get a seizure description. In partial epilepsy this may provide pointers to the area of cerebral disturbance. If a post-ictal dysphasia is reported this suggests that language areas are implicated. Assessment may need to focus on this area. A seizure description will also enable the prompt recognition of an attack.

- Document drugs taken including dosages and recent changes.

- Measurement of mood is recommended. High rates of anxiety and depression will influence test performance. This in turn will affect the interpretation of the test results.

- Test selection is usually influenced by the referral question (although some centres have a standard battery of tests). Test selection may also be shaped by the results of investigations, e.g. EEG and MRI findings may indicate localized cerebral disturbance.

9.2 A patient complains of memory impairment and/or decline

This is the most common referral for neuropsychological assessment.

- Memory tests should include measures of recall, learning, and recognition of both verbal and nonverbal material. Immediate and delayed retention should be assessed.

- Measures of general intellectual capacity are important. The Wechsler Adult Intelligence Scales WAIS-R or WAIS-III will provide an indication of ability level. This provides the context for interpretation of memory test performance.

- Measures of other skills should be made. Language and executive functions are important. A perceived memory decline may reflect problems in these areas rather than memory deficit *per se.*

- Subjective ratings of memory provide valuable information as to the nature of memory problems encountered in everyday situations.

- Where no cognitive deficits are found a broader and/or more experimental approach may be needed. Measures of remote and autobiographical memory can be included. Memory can be tested at delays longer than 30 minutes.

9.3 Are drugs the cause of cognitive impairments?

It is unlikely that a single assessment will provide the answer. Ideally, testing should be undertaken before and after a drug change. A 2–3 month interval between assessments is recommended. The tests used need to be available in parallel forms or be minimally sensitive to practice effects. Some timed tests should be included. Drugs seem to impact more on speed of processing. Computerized tests enable accurate measurement of information processing speed. Useful tests include digit span, timed cancellation tasks, verbal fluency, and verbal learning.

9.4 Evaluation of candidates for resective surgery

- It is essential to assess for cognitive disturbance concordant with the known lesion and electrophysiological disturbance. With temporal cases the focus will be on memory skills. With frontal cases the clinical focus should be on executive skills.

- A brief assessment of areas of cognition discordant with the known lesion should also be made as a good surgical candidate will function well in these areas.

- The results of the assessment, including any indicators of poor prognosis, should be discussed with the patient. High preoperative functioning, older age at operation, and discordant neuropsychological deficits place individuals at risk of cognitive decline postoperatively. The risks should also be provided in writing.

- For those cases undergoing surgery, postoperative reassessments should be planned. In this way, changes can be monitored.

- Neuropsychological rehabilitation may be necessary in some cases.

10 Neuropsychological rehabilitation

Cognitive problems in epilepsy are varied. Any of the rehabilitation programmes outlined in this volume can be used. Memory complaints are the most frequent reason for referral and memory training is the most widely used therapy. Compensatory strategies are the most commonly applied (Thompson 1997; Hendriks 2001).

People with epilepsy are a good group to work with. Memory problems are less devastating than in some neurological disorders and insight is generally retained. Many people live independently and have no 'carer' to act as a memory support.

Feedback of test results is essential. Individuals may be relieved by the confirmation that a memory difficulty exists. In many cases it may be possible to state that this is not progressive. A young person may be struggling academically to achieve a standard comparable to sibling or parental expectations. Confirmation of a memory deficit may result in reappraisal. Redirection to courses with less reliance on written examinations may be a partial solution. Feedback should also be given in writing. Without this the patient may forget or misremember what is said. Physicians should be informed. Physicians should be encouraged to provide written summaries of clinic visits and proposed drug changes.

Sessions can be offered to focus on memory support strategies.

◆ Clinical experience indicates that external memory aids are the most valuable. Instruction can be given in the use of diaries, box organizers, and wall planners. Computerized diaries and personal organizers are also useful (see Chapter 10, this volume).

◆ Another valuable aid is the drug wallet. This reduces the chances of forgotten tablets and overdose. Drug wallets usually consist of seven small containers—one for each day of the week. Drug wallets are inexpensive and can be obtained from local chemists.

◆ Internal memory aids involving mental strategies have limited use. These are most helpful for small amounts of information.

Neuropharmacological treatment is not widely used and results have been disappointing (Aldenkamp *et al.* 1999).

Selective references

Adachi, N., Onuman, T., Nishiwaki, S., Murauchi, S., Akanuma, N., Ishida, S., and Talei, N. (2000). Interictal and postictal psychosis in frontal lobe epilepsy. A retrospective comparison with psychosis in temporal lobe epilepsy. *Seizure* 9, 328–35.

Aldenkamp, A.P., Alpherts, W.C.J., De Bruine-Sedder, D., and Dekker, J.J.A. (1990). Test retest variability in children with epilepsy. Comparison of WISC-R profiles. *Epilepsy Res.* 7, 165–72.

Aldenkamp, A.P., Hendriks, M., and Vermeulen, J. (1999). Cognitive deficits in epilepsy: is there a treatment? In *Epilepsy: problem solving in clinical practice* (ed. D. Schmidt and S.C. Schachter), pp. 291–301. Martin Dunitz, London.

Ballaban-Gil, K. (1995). Language disorders in epilepsy. In *Recent advances in epilepsy*, no. 6 (ed. T.A. Pedley and B.S. Meldrum), pp. 205–20. Churchill Livingstone, Edinburgh.

Baxendale, S.A. (1995). The hippocampus: functional and structural correlations. *Seizure* 4, 104–17.

Baxendale, S.A. (2000). Carotid amytal testing and other amytal procedures. In *Intractable focal epilepsy: medical and surgical treatment* (ed. J.M. Oxbury, C.E. Polkey, and M. Duchowny), pp. 627–36. W.B. Saunders, London.

Baxendale, S.A., Van Paesschen, W., Thompson, P.J., Harkness, W.H., and Shorvon, S.D. (1998). Hippocampal cell loss and gliosis: relationship to pre-operative and post-operative memory functions. *Neuropsychiatry, Neuropsychol., Behav. Neurol.* 11, 12–21.

Baxendale, S.A., Thompson, P.J., and Kitchen, N.D. (2000). Post-operative hippocampal shrinkage and memory decline. *Neurology* 55, 243–9.

Bode, S. and Curtiss, S. (2000). Language after hemispherectomy. *Brain Cognition* 43, 135–8.

Breier, J.J. Fletcher, J.M., Whiless, J.W., Clark, A., Cass, J., and Constantinou, J.E.C. (2000). Profiles of cognitive performance associated with reading disability in temporal lobe epilepsy. *J. Clin. Exp. Neuropsychol.* 22, 804–16.

Chelune, G.J., Naugle, R.I., Hermann, B.P., Barr, W.B., Trenerry, M.R., Loring, D.W., Perrine, K., Strauss, E., and Westerveld, M. (1998). Does pre-surgical IQ predict seizure outcome after temporal lobectomy? Evidence from the Bozeman Epilepsy Consortium. *Epilepsia* 39, 314–18.

Cull, C. and Goldstein, L.H. (eds.) (1997). *The clinical psychologist's handbook of epilepsy. Assessment and management*. Routledge, London.

Duncan, J.S., Shorvon, S.D., and Fish, D.R. (1995). *Clinical epilepsy*. Churchill Livingstone, New York.

Francis, P. and Baker, G.A. (1999). Non-epileptic attack disorder (NEAD): a comprehensive review. *Seizure* 8, 53–61.

Gloor, P. (1991). Mesial temporal sclerosis: historical background and an overview from a modern perspective. In *Epilepsy surgery* (ed. H. Luders), pp. 689–708. Raven Press, New York.

Helmstaedter, C., Kemper, B., and Elger, C.E. (1996). Neuropsychological aspects of frontal lobe epilepsy. *Neuropsychologia* 34, 399–406.

Helmstaedter, C., Gleibner, U., Zentner, J., and Elger, C.E. (1998). Neuropsychological consequences of epilepsy surgery in frontal lobe epilepsy. *Neuropsychologia* 36, 333–41.

Hendriks, M. (2001). Neuropsychological compensatory strategies for memory deficits in patients with epilepsy. In *Comprehensive care for people with epilepsy* (ed. M. Pfaflin, R.T. Fraser, R. Thorbecke, U. Specht, and P. Wolf), pp. 87–94. John Libbey, London.

Hermann, B., Davies, K., Foley, K., and Bell, B. (1999) Visual confrontation naming outcome after standard left anterior temporal lobectomy with sparing versus resection of the superior temporal gyrus: a randomized prospective clinical trial. *Epilepsia* 40, 1070–6.

Holmes, M.G., Dodrill, C.B., Wilkus, R.S., and Ojermann, G.A. (1998). Is partial epilepsy progressive? Ten year study of EEG and neuropsychological changes in adults with partial seizures. *Epilepsia* 39, 1189–93.

International League against Epilepsy (1981). Proposal for revised clinical and electroencephalographic classification of epileptic seizures. *Epilepsia* 22, 489–501.

International League against Epilepsy (1989). Proposal for revised classification of epilepsies and epileptic syndromes. *Epilepsia* 30, 389–99.

Lambert, M.V. and Robertson, M.M. (1999). Depression in epilepsy: aetiology, phenomenology and treatment. *Epilepsia* 40 (suppl.10), S21–47.

Matsuoka, H., Takahashi, T., Sasaki, M., Matsumoto, K., Yoshida, Y., Saito, H., Ueno, T., and Sato, M. (2000). Neuropsychological EEG activation in patients with epilepsy. *Brain* 123, 318–30.

Meador, K.J. (1998). Cognitive and behavioural assessments in AED trials. In *Antiepileptic drug development* (ed. J. French, I. Leppik, and M.A. Dichter), Advances in Neurology 76, pp. 231–8. Lippincott–Raven Publishers, Philadelphia.

Nordgren, R. (1991). Corpus callosotomy for intractable seizures in the paediatric age group. *Arch. Neurol.* **48**, 364–72.

Polkey, C.E. (2000*a*). Temporal lobe resections. In *Intractable focal epilepsy* (ed. J. Oxburg, C. Polkey, and M. Duchowny), pp. 667–96. W.B. Saunders, London.

Polkey, C.E. (2000*b*). Functional surgery for epilepsy. In *Intractable focal epilepsy* (ed. J. Oxburg, C. Polkey, and M. Duchowny), pp. 735–50. W.B. Saunders, London.

Roget, T. (1992). *Epileptic syndromes in infancy, childhood and adolescence*, 2nd edn. John Libbey, London.

Sander, J.W.A.S. and Sillanpaa, M. (1998). The natural history and prognosis of epilepsy. In *Epilepsy: a comprehensive textbook* (ed. P. Engel and T. Pedley), pp. 69–86. Raven Press, New York.

Schacter, S.C. and Saper, C.B. (1998). Vagus nerve stimulation. *Epilepsia* **39**, 677–86.

Shorvon, S.D. (1994). *Status epilepticus. Its causes and treatment in children and adults.* Cambridge University Press, Cambridge.

Sisodiya, S.M. (2000). Surgery for malformations of cortical development. *Brain* **123**, 1075–91.

Thompson, P.J. (1997). Epilepsy and memory. In *The clinical psychologist's handbook of epilepsy. Assessment and management* (ed. C. Cull and L.A. Goldstein), pp. 35–53. Routledge, London.

Thompson, P.J. (2001). Cognitive and behavioural assessment in clinical trials: when should they be done? *Epilepsy Res.* **45**, 159–61.

Thompson, P.J. and Baxendale, S.A. (1996). Non-pharmacological treatment of epilepsy. In *Treatment of epilepsy* (ed. S.D. Shorvon, F.E. Dreifuss, D.R. Fish, and D.G.T. Thomas), pp. 345–56. Blackwell Science, Oxford.

Thompson, P.J. and Grant L (2001). Epilepsy associated emotional disturbances and the role of coping strategies. In *Comprehensive care for people with epilepsy* (ed. M. Pfafflin, R.T. Fraser, R. Thorbecke, U. Specht, and P Wolf), pp. 59–66. John Libbey and Co, Eastleigh.

Thompson, P.J. and Trimble, M.R. (1996). Neuropsychological aspects of epilepsy. In *Neuropsychological assessment of neuropsychiatric disorders.* 2nd edn (ed. E. Grant and K.M. Adams), pp. 263–87. Oxford University Press, Oxford.

Thompson, P.J., Baxendale, S.A., Duncan, J.S., and Sander, J.W.A.S. (2000). Effects of topiramate on cognitive functions. *J. Neurol., Neurosurg., Psychiatry* **69**, 636–41.

Upton, D. and Thompson, P.J. (1996). Epilepsy within the frontal lobes: neuropsychological characteristics. *J. Epilepsy* **9**, 215–27.

Zeman, A. and Hodges, J.R. (2000). Transient global amnesia and transient epileptic amnesia. In *Memory disorders in psychiatric practice* (ed. G. Berios and J.R. Hodges), pp. 187–203. Cambridge University Press, Cambridge.

Part 7

Neuropsychiatric conditions

Chapter 33

The clinical presentation of neuropsychiatric disorders

Ronan O'Carroll

1 Introduction

Neuropsychology is concerned with the study of brain–behaviour relationships, and has traditionally used the classical lesion-based approach relating focal brain damage to patterns of preserved and impaired cognitive functioning. In the majority of psychiatric disorders, however, focal brain lesions are rare, and the challenge of the new discipline of cognitive neuropsychiatry (Halligan and David 2001) is to understand abnormal behaviour in terms of dysfunctional processing of information. This is more likely to be related to abnormalities of brain systems than to localized brain damage. The determination of brain–cognition relationships is no easy undertaking in psychopathological states.

- Many neuropsychological studies in major psychiatric disorders are conducted on patients who are taking psychotropic medication, and such drugs may well have confounding effects on measures of cognitive functioning.

- It is also important to remember that most psychiatric disorders disturb affective status so that mood and motivation may also critically impact on neuropsychological test performance.

We must also address the issue of diagnosis, i.e. how psychiatric disorders are traditionally grouped. The conventional approach is to adopt the medical model and describe 'illness' states that allegedly share common features. However, many critics have challenged the validity and reliability of standard psychiatric diagnoses, such as schizophrenia, arguing that they represent such heterogeneous groupings that effectively 'apples are being mixed with oranges', and classified as the same fruit (Bentall 1992). In recent years greater attention has been paid to exploring specific syndromes or symptoms rather than 'illnesses'. For example, rather than trying to explain schizophrenia, attempts have been made to explain specific features (e.g. paranoid delusions) in neuropsychological terms.

Clinical neuropsychology also has an important role to play in the assessment of cognitive impairment in clinical practice and in research in psychiatry. Recent advances in knowledge have allowed for more fine-grained cognitive analysis of specific

Table 33.1 Neuropsychiatric disorders considered in this chapter

Amnestic disorder
Anorexia nervosa
Asperger's syndrome
Autism
Bulimia nervosa
Capgras' syndrome
Cotard's syndrome
De Clerambault's syndrome
Dementia
Depression
Frégoli delusion
Ganser's syndrome
Conversion hysteria
Munchhausen's syndrome
Obsessive–compulsive disorder (OCD)
Othello syndrome
Post-traumatic stress disorder (PTSD)
Reduplicative paramnesia
Schizophrenia
Somatoform disorders
Tourette's syndrome

impairments. This in turn can lead to a greater understanding of the neural basis of abnormal behaviour. The development of neuropsychological measures allows for the valid and reliable assessment of treatment efficacy. This is particularly important as 'negative' features (including cognitive impairment) are becoming increasingly recognized as important targets for pharmacological treatment in psychiatry. Furthermore, ecologically valid neuropsychological outcome measures are essential in the rapidly developing field of cognitive rehabilitation.

In the following sections, the clinical presentation and common neuropsychological features of some of the major psychiatric disorders (Table 33.1) will be briefly reviewed.

2 Amnestic disorder

2.1 Clinical presentation

Amnestic disorder is reviewed in Chapter 28, so it will be only briefly covered here. The primary presenting feature of amnestic disorder is a marked inability to lay down new long-term explicit, episodic, or declarative memories, in the presence of spared other cognitive functions, notably intelligence and implicit and short-term memory. There are a variety of possible causes of amnestic disorder (see Section 2.2). The sufferer will often have a clear recollection of episodes in their distant past, but will be unable to recall events that happened 30 minutes ago. In some instances, notably in Korsakoff's syndrome, patients attempt to cover up their memory loss via confabulation, i.e. using their preserved language and intellectual abilities to create elaborate stories in an effort to compensate for the memories they have lost. The memory loss in amnestic syndrome is thought to be largely irreversible.

2.2 Neuropsychological features

The essential features of amnestic syndrome are devastatingly impaired anterograde memory function, with a variable degree of impaired retrograde memory function (usually surrounding the time of the brain insult) in the presence of preserved other cognitive functions. This has often been demonstrated by the use of an intellectual quotient—memory quotient discrepancy. For example, a person who has a Wechsler intelligence quotient (IQ) of 100 with a memory quotient of 70 would have a 30-point discrepancy, which would be consistent with an amnestic profile.

Amnestic disorder can result from a variety of causes of cerebral pathology. Perhaps the most famous case is that of H.M. who was rendered amnesic following bilateral temporal lobectomy for the treatment of his epilepsy (Scoville and Milner 1957). H.M.'s case was influential in clarifying the critical role of temporal lobe structures in episodic memory functioning. Herpes encephalitis resulting in damage to the temporal lobes can also lead to amnestic syndrome (Wilson *et al.* 1995). Korsakoff's syndrome, a consequence of chronic alcoholism and thiamine deficiency, leads to selective atrophy of the mamillary bodies and this can similarly lead to the development of an amnestic syndrome. Many patients with alcohol-induced persisting dementia are misclassified as suffering from amnestic syndrome. However, they often do not have specific and isolated anterograde memory impairment, but rather have widespread cognitive impairments.

A striking feature in amnestic syndrome is preserved implicit memory performance. For example, amnestic patients typically perform normally on implicit tasks such as the pursuit rotor or incomplete figures task, yet will have no explicit memory of having performed these tasks. Such evidence has been important in clarifying the neural substrates that subserve different components of memory function in man.

3 Anorexia nervosa

3.1 Clinical presentation

The essential features of anorexia nervosa are body weight at least 15% below the standard weight (i.e. a body mass index below 17.5) and an intense fear of gaining weight or becoming fat, even though the individual is clearly underweight. There is an associated perceptual disturbance in the way the person's body shape is seen (e.g. in the mirror) and, in women, the presence of amenorrhoea, i.e. the absence of at least three consecutive menstrual cycles. Patients generally eat very little and set themselves restrictive daily calorie limits, e.g. 500 calories per day. Additional strategies to achieve weight loss include laxative abuse, vomiting, and excessive exercise. Anorexia nervosa is 10–20 times more frequent in women than in men and occurs in approximately 1% of young women. Six to 10% of female siblings of patients with anorexia suffer from the condition, compared to 1–2% found in the general population of the same age. This increase may be due to family environment or to genetic influences.

3.2 Neuropsychological features

A variety of biological, psychological, and environmental factors have been implicated in the aetiology of anorexia nervosa.

◆ Hypothalamic dysfunction has been proposed in anorexia as there is a profound disturbance of weight regulation. However, it may be that the endocrine and metabolic abnormalities are a consequence of low weight and disturbed eating habits, rather than the cause.

◆ Brain imaging abnormalities have also been reported, e.g. enlarged ventricles in anorexia nervosa. However, these findings are usually reversed by weight gain, suggesting again that they are also a consequence rather than a cause.

◆ Several studies have reported neuropsychological impairments in anorexia, affecting a variety of cognitive domains (memory, attention, and problem-solving). Cognitive improvements following weight gain suggest again that they are reversible, not primary, and may be related to nutritional status.

4 Asperger's syndrome

4.1 Clinical presentation

Asperger's syndrome is a pervasive developmental disorder, first described by Asperger in 1944. The condition is characterized by marked impairment in social interaction, e.g. avoidance of eye-to-eye gaze and failure to develop relationships and restricted, repetitive, and stereotyped patterns of behaviour, with clinically significant impairment in social functioning. Asperger's syndrome differs from autism because in the former there is no general delay or retardation of cognitive development or language. Nonverbal communication problems and clumsiness are common. Asperger's syndrome is well reviewed by Frith (1991).

4.2 Neuropsychological features

There is relatively little known about neuropsychological functioning in Asperger's syndrome, though theory of mind deficits are commonly observed (see Section 5). It has been suggested that right hemisphere impairments may contribute to the behavioural abnormalities seen in Asperger's syndrome, e.g. face processing problems and poor gaze perception (Ellis and Leafhead 1996). Autism and Asperger's syndrome have been considered to be part of the same spectrum of disorders. Miller and Ozonoff (2000) have recently proposed that Asperger's syndrome may simply reflect high-IQ autism, and that separate categories for the disorders may not be warranted.

5 Autism

5.1 Clinical presentation

Autistic children show deficits in social interaction.

- They fail to show the usual intimate relationship with people close to them, including parents and siblings.
- Many autistic individuals lack a social smile and do not display an anticipatory posture for being picked up, e.g. when a parent approaches, and abnormal eye contact is frequently observed.
- Disturbances of communication and language delay are also common. When autistic individuals do learn to converse, they often lack social competence and their conversations do not exhibit the normal reciprocal responsive interchanges.
- Autistic children often demonstrate abnormalities in play, e.g. engaging in rituals and frequently insisting on 'sameness' and being resistant to change.
- Autistic children may also be over- or underresponsive to sensory stimuli.
- Hyperkinesis is also a common behavioural problem in young autistic children.

5.2 Neuropsychological features

Autism is often associated with developmental conditions that have associated neurological lesions, e.g. rubella, and in untreated or uncontrolled phenylketonuria. Electroencephalographic (EEG) abnormalities are common, although no EEG findings are specific to autism. Approximately 40% of children with infantile autism have IQ scores below 50–55. Some autistic children, however, demonstrate precocious talents, e.g. in cognitive and visuomotor abilities. Examples include 'idiot savants', individuals who have exceptional memory, artistic, musical, or calculating abilities.

A major current theory proposes that autistic children lack a 'theory of mind', i.e. the ability to see the world from the perspective of another. This is commonly assessed using tests such as the 'Sally–Anne problem', where two dolls, Sally and Anne, act out a scene. Sally puts a marble in a basket before leaving the room and Anne then moves it to a box. The question is where will Sally look for it when she returns? Autistic children commonly respond 'in the box' (U. Frith 1991). Happe and Frith (1996) proposed that it is useful to consider three main neuropsychological areas when attempting to understand autism:

- mentalizing impairment;
- executive dysfunction;

◆ weak central coherence (central coherence is a characteristic of normal information-processing—the tendency to draw together diverse information to construct higher-level meaning in context). It is notable that, in autism, weak central coherence can result in performance superior to that of healthy controls on tasks such as the embedded figures test, where one has to try and detect a target hidden in a complex background.

6 **Bulimia nervosa**

6.1 **Clinical presentation**

Bulimia nervosa is characterized by recurrent episodes of binge eating associated with a lack of control over eating during the binge episode. The binge is usually followed by recurrent eliminatory behaviours aimed at preventing weight gain, e.g. vomiting and laxative abuse. The binge eating and eliminatory behaviours occur, on average, at least twice a week for 3 months. As in anorexia nervosa, bulimia is much more common in women than in men. Bingeing tends to precede vomiting by about 1 year in the development of the disorder. Sticking fingers down the throat commonly produces vomiting, though some bulimic patients can vomit at will. Vomiting acts to decrease the abdominal pain and feeling of being bloated. Depressed mood often follows the episode and has been called 'post-binge anguish'.

6.2 **Neuropsychological features**

Attempts have been made in the past to associate cycles of bingeing and purging with various neurotransmitter abnormalities. Treatment with antidepressants, particularly selective serotonin re-uptake inhibitors (SSRIs), has achieved some success, leading to the hypothesis that serotonin is implicated in the aetiology of the disorder. Recent evidence has also suggested the presence of marked impulsivity and problem-solving deficits in patients with bulimia (Ferraro *et al.* 1997).

7 **Capgras' syndrome**

7.1 **Clinical presentation**

Capgras' syndrome involves the belief that impostors have replaced people to whom the sufferer is emotionally close (e.g. loved ones or relatives). It is believed that the impostors have assumed the roles of the persons they impersonate and behave like them. Some patients who suffer from Capgras' syndrome may threaten, harm, or even kill the supposed impostor.

7.2 **Neuropsychological features**

Up to 40% of cases are associated with organic disorders, e.g. head injury and dementia. Right cerebral hemisphere dysfunction has also frequently been reported in patients suffering from Capgras' syndrome.

Ellis and Young (1990) presented a cognitive account of Capgras' syndrome. They proposed two distinct routes to facial recognition:

- a route for the actual identification of the face;
- a route to give it emotional significance.

They proposed that prosopagnosia results from a disruption of the first route, whereas Capgras' syndrome is 'a mirror image' of prosopagnosia. Thus, Ellis and Young (1990) propose that Capgras patients have an intact primary route to face recognition but have a disconnection or damage within the route that gives the face its emotional significance. Ellis *et al.* (1997) demonstrated that people with the Capgras delusion fail to show autonomic discrimination between familiar and unfamiliar faces. Their model proposes that, to the person with Capgras' syndrome, the impostor's face looks identical to that of the familiar person, but the emotional feelings associated with the face are abnormal. Put another way, the patients receive a veridical image of the person they are looking at that stimulates the appropriate semantic data about the person, but the patient lacks another set of confirmatory information that may carry the appropriate affective tone for a loved one. The patient then adopts a rationalization strategy, i.e. the person looks the same but somehow does not feel the same, and therefore the person must be an impostor. The Capgras patient mistakes a change in themselves for a change in others, i.e. 'they must be impostors'. Recent work in his area is reviewed by Ellis and Lewis (2001).

8 **Cotard's syndrome**

8.1 **Clinical presentation**

Cotard's syndrome is essentially the delusion of nihilism. This condition was described by the nineteenth century French psychiatrist, Jules Cotard, who gave an account of several patients who suffered from a syndrome he referred to as 'délirie de négation'. Patients exhibiting this syndrome may complain not only of having lost possessions, status, and strength, but even of having lost internal organs such as the heart and lungs. Patients may not only claim that they are dead, but that corpses have replaced their bodies. They may state that they have no feelings, and it is important to note that many are severely depressed.

8.2 **Neuropsychological features**

Non-specific neurological lesions have been reported in many patients with Cotard's syndrome, e.g. neoplastic, vascular, and encephalopathic lesions. Recent work (Young and Leafhead 1996) proposes a right hemisphere dysfunction, as evidenced by the observation of face-processing impairments in patients with Cotard delusions. In this model, the delusion of being dead is viewed as a misinterpretation of abnormal perceptual experiences in which things seem strange and unfamiliar. There is a lack of emotional responsiveness, together with feelings of emptiness and derealization. The depressed mood of the patient leads him or her to exaggerate the negative effects of the perceptual changes while correctly attributing the changes to oneself. In sum, this model proposes that the Cotard delusion represents a depressed person's attempt to account for abnormal perceptual experience. Berrios and Luque (1995) have suggested that it is useful to distinguish between patients presenting with Cotard's syndrome in the presence or absence of clinical depression, arguing that the former may be best understood in terms of affective disorder, the latter in terms of delusional disorder.

9 De Clerambault's syndrome

9.1 Clinical presentation

De Clerambault's syndrome is one of erotomania. It is currently classified in the *Diagnostic and statistical manual of mental disorders*, 4th edn (DSM-IV; American Psychiatric Association 1994) as a delusional disorder of the erotomanic type. It is exceedingly rare and more commonly a disorder of women. The subject, usually a single woman, believes that a 'higher status' person is in love with her. The target is usually inaccessible as he may be married, or be a famous personality or public figure. The sufferer is convinced that the object of her affection cannot be a happy or complete person without her. People suffering from this syndrome can become extremely difficult for the target of the affection to deal with, and in many cases, police and court involvement may be required in order to protect the target from the sufferer. A proportion of 'stalkers' who threaten celebrities suffer from delusional erotomania (Kamphuis and Emmelkamp 2000). Many patients suffering from De Clerambault's syndrome also suffer from paranoid schizophrenia, and it has been suggested that the syndrome may not exist as a separate nosological entity, but rather is a variant of schizophrenia or affective disorder (Ellis and Mellsop 1985).

9.2 Neuropsychological features

Little is known about neurological or neuropsychological abnormalities in this condition, although the emergence of erotomania has been reported following brain injury (Gelder, 1996). As stated above, the syndrome often presents in the context of schizophrenia, with associated impairments in memory and executive functioning. Kopelman *et al.* (1995) used the case-study approach, and tested the hypothesis that executive dysfunction may underlie delusional memories in erotomania. However, they found executive functioning to be intact, but reported an impairment in retrograde memory for the period around the onset of the patient's psychosis. Kopelman *et al.* (1995) propose that delusional memories may result from slippage in the relationship between memory schemata, leading to a predisposition to interpret the world in particular ways, contingent upon underlying affective or cognitive factors.

10 Dementia

10.1 Clinical presentation

The dementias are reviewed in detail in Chapter 28 and so will be only briefly covered here. The main forms of dementia are Alzheimer's disease (AD) and multi-infarct dementia (MID). Both involve a gradual deterioration in mental capacities to the point where social and occupational functions become impaired. Memory disturbance is the most prominent feature of dementia but, importantly, other cognitive abilities are also compromised, e.g. visuospatial, praxis, and language abilities. The prevalence of dementia rises sharply with age, from about 2% in people aged 65–70 to 20% in those aged over 80 years. Given increasing life expectancies, the burden of care over the next century could be enormous. AD generally has a steady progressive deterioration, whereas in MID the deterioration occurs in abrupt, step-like stages, caused by a series of cerebral infarcts. Acute episodes of deterioration in MID can sometimes be followed by improvements for a time. However, in both conditions, death usually occurs some 2–8 years after onset.

10.2 Neuropsychological features

In dementia the key neuropsychological features are gradual deterioration of memory and other cognitive functions. These are caused by changes in brain structure, notably widespread cortical atrophy and ventricular enlargement. It can be difficult to distinguish between MID and AD. However, MID is usually associated with a step-wise deterioration and a fluctuating course, whereas AD has a more steady progression. In AD, plaques (remnants of lost neurons and β amyloid) are scattered throughout the cortex and neurofibrillary tangles also accumulate within the cell bodies of neurons. Functional brain scanning techniques typically show reduced metabolic activity in the temporoparietal area. In MID the cerebral deterioration is attributable to a series of small infarcts that occur throughout the brain. In AD the cholinergic system is thought to become particularly affected and treatment trials of enhancing the cholinergic neurotransmitter system via acetyl-cholinesterase inhibitors are showing some therapeutic promise.

11 Depression

11.1 Clinical presentation

Depression has been recorded since ancient times. Episodes of major depression are characterized by a period of at least 2 weeks that represents a change from previous functioning associated with either depressed mood or loss of interest or pleasure.

DSM-IV criteria (American Psychiatric Association 1994) for a major depressive episode require five of the following nine features:

1 depressed mood most of the day, nearly every day;
2 markedly diminished interest or pleasure in activities;
3 significant weight loss or weight gain;
4 insomnia or hypersomnia nearly every day;
5 psychomotor agitation and retardation nearly every day;
6 fatigue or loss of energy nearly every day;
7 feelings of worthlessness or excessive or inappropriate guilt;

8   diminished ability to think or concentrate or indecisiveness nearly every day;

9   recurrent thoughts of death.

Unipolar depression (i.e. depression with no episodes of mania) is among the most common psychiatric disorders of adults. In many countries surveyed, at any given moment one person in 20 is significantly depressed, with a lifetime prevalence rate of approximately 15% (twice as prevalent in women as in men). There appears to be a genetic loading for depression in that children of severely depressed patients have a morbid risk of 20% for mood disorder as against about 7% in the relatives of controls. Major depression can be a fatal disorder. Approximately two-thirds of depressed patients contemplate suicide and 10–15% go on to commit suicide.

11.2 Neuropsychological features

Noradrenaline (norepinephrine) and serotonin abnormalities are implicated in the pathophysiology of depression. In addition, abnormalities of the limbic hypothalamic–pituitary–adrenal axis have been the most consistently reported neuroendocrine abnormalities.

◆   The dexamethasone suppression test (DST) has been extensively researched in depression. Dexamethasone is a steroid that suppresses the blood level of cortisol and the DST is abnormal in approximately half the depressed patients. However, the DST has been shown not to be specific for depression and may be abnormal in patients with other disorders such as obsessive–compulsive disorder, eating disorders, etc.

◆   Brain imaging studies have used computerized tomography (CT), magnetic resonance imaging (MRI), and positron emission tomography (PET) to investigate possible brain abnormalities in major depression. The results of these studies have not been consistent. However, several have reported decreased blood flow and metabolism in the dorsolateral prefrontal cortex, the cingulate cortex, and, in some cases, the basal ganglia.

◆   Neuropsychological studies have consistently found psychomotor slowing and impairments in memory and executive functioning (Veiel 1997). Studies using affectively toned stimuli reveal that depressed patients have a memory bias towards negative material, which it is thought may help maintain or exacerbate the depressed mood.

11.2.1 Bipolar disorder

In bipolar disorder (episodes of depression and mania), recent evidence suggests that, while neuropsychological functioning is clearly impaired during illness episodes, some residual impairments can be observed in the euthymic state (Ferrier *et al.* 1999). In addition, a more severe course of illness and a greater number of illness episodes are often associated with more impaired neuropsychological functioning, suggesting that repeated manic episodes may be neurotoxic. The pathophysiological mechanisms are not fully understood, though hypercortisolaemia may be implicated and may result in impaired neuropsychological functioning (McAllister-Williams *et al.* 1998).

Relatively few neuropsychological studies have been conducted on manic patients. Preliminary work suggests that both manic and depressed patients are impaired on tests of memory and planning, but differences have been noted in attentional shifting, with manic patients having difficulty with inhibition of behavioural response and attentional focus and with depressed patients impaired in their ability to shift the focus of their attentional bias (Murphy *et al.* 1999). The same authors confirmed the affective bias for negative material in depression, but also demonstrated the opposite affective bias for positive stimuli in mania.

12 Frégoli delusion

12.1 Clinical presentation

The essence of the Frégoli delusion is that the patient believes that other people are able to disguise themselves to look like anyone they wish in order to achieve some influence—usually a sinister one. The patient will identify a familiar person (usually someone who is believed to be his or her persecutor) and insist that this person takes the form of a variety of others whom he or she comes into contact with. The patient will maintain that, although there is no physical resemblance between the familiar person and the others, nevertheless they are the same person. The syndrome is often associated with schizophrenia.

12.2 Neuropsychological features

Neurological abnormalities are common in Frégoli delusion, e.g. brain atrophy is often reported (Joseph and O'Leary 1987). However, transient forms of the delusion have also been described, e.g. following toxic psychoses induced by cannabis. Ellis and Young (1990) offered a cognitive neuropsychiatric explanation for the Frégoli delusion. They employed an information-processing model of face recognition that deconstructs into three essential stages:

1   an initial structural encoding;

2   the excitation of units sensitive to the unique characteristic of each known phase;

3   the link to other multimodal nodes that access biographical/episodic information about people.

Ellis and Young (1990) propose that it is a malfunction in stage 3 that results in the Frégoli delusion.

13 Ganser's syndrome

13.1 Clinical presentation

This syndrome was first reported by Ganser in 1898, when he observed that three prisoners showed an unusual clinical picture. The condition has four main features:

- giving approximate answers;
- psychogenic physical symptoms;
- hallucinations;
- apparent clouding of consciousness.

The meaning of the 'approximate answers' feature is that, although the answer is plainly wrong, it is clearly related to the correct answer in a way that suggests that the correct response is known. e.g. when asked to multiply four times four, the patient answers 'seventeen'. A distinction has been made between the Ganser symptom (approximate answers) and Ganser's syndrome—the symptom is common and the syndrome extremely rare.

Ganser's syndrome has variously been regarded as akin to hysterical conversion reactions, malingering, organic confusion, and psychotic thought disorder. Ganser's syndrome is often thought to represent the voluntary production of psychiatric symptoms, e.g. in an attempt to avoid imprisonment, and, in fact, has been termed 'prison psychosis'. It may be difficult to distinguish whether the condition is genuine or whether the patient is malingering. However, it should be noted that a number of cases have been reported following head injury. Indeed, of Ganser's original three cases, two had suffered head injury and the third was recovering from typhus fever. The syndrome may also occur in people with other disorders such as schizophrenia and depression.

13.2 Neuropsychological features

Ganser's syndrome is a poorly understood phenomenon. Originally, Ganser proposed that the condition represented an unusual hysterical confusional state. There are no clear and consistent neuropsychological features that provide an adequate explanation for this disorder. As Lishman (1998, p. 480) concluded, exactly 100 years after the syndrome was first described, 'Uncertainty surrounds its nosological status and the mechanisms behind its appearance.'

14 Conversion hysteria

14.1 Clinical presentation

Hysteria was described by the ancient Greeks in order to account for a condition where physical and mental symptoms occurred in the absence of the organic pathology that was thought to cause the clinical features (Halligan and David 1999; Halligan *et al.* 2000). Hysteria has been largely replaced by the terms 'conversion' and 'dissociative' disorders, which distinguish conditions with physical and mental symptoms, respectively. Freud proposed that hysteria was caused by emotionally charged ideas that have become lodged in the unconscious of the patient. Classic examples include paralysis of the arm or 'glove anaesthesia' in the absence of organic pathology to account for the paralysis or anaesthesia. Diagnostic features include:

+ symptoms that suggest a neurological or medical condition;
+ psychological features that are judged to be associated with the symptom;
+ the symptom is not intentionally produced or feigned;
+ the symptom or deficit cannot be fully explained by a medical condition;
+ the symptom or deficit causes clinically significant distress or impairment;
+ the symptom is not limited to pain or sexual dysfunction.

Classically, these disorders are said to produce secondary gain, e.g. arm paralysis leading to the sufferer not having to go to work. In addition, patients are said to display 'la belle indifference', i.e. the patients show less distress than would be expected of someone with these symptoms. It is often difficult to distinguish between hysteria and malingering (see Halligan *et al.* 2001; Halligan, Bass, Oakley, 2003).

14.2 Neuropsychological features

It is important to note that diagnostic criteria for conversion disorder state that the symptom or deficit, after appropriate investigation, cannot be fully explained by a general medical condition. However, in a significant study, Slater and Glithero (1965) followed up a series of patients who had been referred to a neurological hospital after having been diagnosed as having hysteria. Approximately one-third of those patients developed a definite organic illness within 10 years of the original diagnosis and a further third developed depression or schizophrenia. This study has proved very influential, leading to the fear that the diagnosis of hysteria was a fertile source of clinical error, with significant neurological or psychiatric disease often being missed. However, Crimlisk *et al.* (1998) recently followed up 64 patients who had medically unexplained motor symptoms for 6 years. Only three patients were subsequently diagnosed with a neurological disorder that could explain their initial presentation, leading to the conclusion that following up-to-date thorough evaluation, the chance of a missing a neurological condition that could account for the initial complaint is small.

It has also been proposed that conversion disorders have a neuropsychological basis in that it is possible that excess cortical arousal results in inhibition of afferent sensory motor impulses, thus diminishing the awareness of bodily sensations. In some conversion disorders this could explain the observed sensory deficits, e.g. glove anaesthesia. Inhibition of motor impulses in hysterical paralysis has been demonstrated by Marshall *et al.* (1997). Spence (1999) has suggested an interesting avenue to pursue in the study of hysterical paralysis. He proposes using functional neuroimaging to test the extent to which the pathophysiology of hysteria resembles either: (1) the normal functional anatomy of willed action (exercising an intent to deceive) or (2) a failure of the will (through a demonstrable dysfunction of 'higher' centres). We await the conclusions of such experiments. Recent work exploring anatomical/neuropsychological mechanisms in hysteria is presented by Marshall *et al.* (1997) and Halligan *et al.* (2001).

15 **Munchhausen's syndrome**

15.1 **Clinical presentation**

Munchhausen's syndrome is a factitious disorder, i.e. a condition characterized by physical or psychological symptoms that are intentionally produced or feigned. Physical or mental illness is simulated with the objective of assuming the 'sick' role of a patient. Essential features include:

- ◆ intentional production of symptoms;
- ◆ the motivation for the behaviour to assume a sick role;
- ◆ external incentives for the behaviour such as financial gain.

Munchhausen patients are often admitted to hospital with an apparently serious and acute illness that is often supported by a plausible or dramatic history. However, the history is not true and the patient is often found to have attended hospital and deceived doctors on many previous occasions. Discharge often occurs after hospital staff confront the patient with evidence regarding similar fraudulent presentations. The condition is most often seen in young men. Patients are often resistant to make contact with psychologists or psychiatrists and treatment is often refused. Munchhausen syndrome by proxy describes a condition in which parents give a false history to explain their child's signs and symptoms (e.g. history suggestive of appendicitis when, in reality, the parent has been poisoning the child). This is clearly child abuse.

15.2 **Neuropsychological features**

Munchhausen's syndrome is a poorly understood phenomenon, with no consistent neuropsychological features or widely accepted explanatory neuropsychological models.

16 **Obsessive–compulsive disorder (OCD)**

16.1 **Clinical presentation**

Obsessive–compulsive disorder (OCD) is characterized by the presence of obsessions or compulsions.

- ◆ Obsessions are persistent and recurrent thoughts and impulses that cause anxiety and distress, which the person tries to suppress, neutralize, or ignore and which the person recognizes as being the product of his or her own mind.
- ◆ Compulsions are repetitive behaviours or mental acts that the person feels driven to perform, and the behaviour or mental acts are aimed at preventing or reducing distress, or preventing a dreaded event or situation. Common examples include obsessional cleaning and checking. However, the compulsive behaviours or acts are not connected in a realistic way with that which they are designed to neutralize or prevent (e.g. removing all hairs from clothing and carpets in the house in order to prevent a loved one dying in an road traffic accident).

The obsessions or compulsions are recognized by the individual as being unreasonable and frequently cause marked distress. While OCD is classified as an anxiety disorder, obsessional patients are often depressed.

16.2 Neuropsychological features

Brain imaging findings have suggested that abnormalities in the orbitofrontal cortex and caudate nucleus may be common in OCD (Insel and Winslow 1992). Cognitive abnormalities often include executive, nonverbal, and praxic deficits in OCD, consistent with theories of frontostriatal functioning that may represent the cognitive substrate of doubt-related phenomena such as checking (Tallis *et al.* 1999).

17 The Othello syndrome

17.1 Clinical presentation

The Othello syndrome is one of delusional jealousy where the person is convinced (without due cause) that his or her spouse or partner is unfaithful. Pathological jealousy is not an uncommon presentation in psychiatric practice, and is more common in men than in women and, in some cases, the individual may be highly dangerous. The syndrome often is associated with, or may be part of, other conditions such as paranoid schizophrenia, depression, or alcoholism.

17.2 Neuropsychological features

Organic disorders (e.g. head injury) have been suggested as being present in up to 20% of such cases, often involving right hemisphere damage. In addition, drug abuse (e.g. amphetamine and cocaine) can often precipitate delusional jealousy, as can a wide range of brain disorders, including metabolic and endocrine disorders; degenerative conditions, e.g. dementia; infections; and neoplasms. We await convincing and testable neuropsychological models of delusional jealousy.

18 Post-traumatic stress disorder (PTSD)

18.1 Clinical presentation

PTSD is a condition in which exposure to an intense, frightening emotional experience leads to lasting changes in behaviour, affect, and cognition.

- Typically, after a life-threatening incident (e.g. a violent assault, rape, or wartime experience), the individual displays re-experiencing of the event(s), e.g. via intrusive, distressing thoughts, images, 'flashbacks', or nightmares.
- The individual may exhibit phobic avoidance and/or physiological reactivity to reminders of the trauma.
- Increased arousal in terms of sleep disturbance, irritability, and exaggerated startle response are common.

◆ In addition, the individual may exhibit a restricted range of affect, sense of a fore-shortened future, and may lose interest in previously rewarding hobbies or activities.

18.2 Neuropsychological features

As stated above, PTSD is characterized by intrusive distressing memories of the traumatic event. Paradoxically, it is also often associated with marked impairments in learning and memory for new material. Patients often complain that they remember what they do not want to, yet cannot remember what they now wish to. Heightened arousal at the time of encoding may result in modulation (strengthening) of the memory trace, possibly via noradrenaline release in the amygdala (Cahill 2000). Subsequent anterograde memory impairment may be due to the deleterious effects of stress hormones (e.g. long-term hypercortisolaemia) on the hippocampal formation. Several MRI studies have now shown that PTSD is associated with reduction in volume of the hippocampus, a brain area critically involved in new learning and memory (Bremner 1999).

Brewin *et al.* (1996) have recently developed a dual representation theory of PTSD. They propose that two memory systems are implicated in the disorder—one that is verbally accessible and one that is automatically accessed via situational cues. They also propose that clinical features may correspond to chronic or premature inhibition of emotional processing of trauma.

19 Reduplicative paramnesia

19.1 Clinical presentation

Reduplicative paramnesia is a clinical condition in which a patient states that there are two or more places with almost identical attributes, although only one exists in reality. Luzzatti and Verga (1996) describe the clinical presentations of several patients presenting with reduplicative paramnesia. For example, a man who suffered a head injury stated that he was in Grimsby when, in fact, he was in hospital outside Edinburgh. He accounted for this state of affairs by stating 'I call it Grimsby; you call it Scotland.'

19.2 Neuropsychological features

The majority of cases described in the literature suffer from a bilateral frontal lesion associated with lesions in other brain areas. The condition has been proposed as being an orientation problem, a memory problem, a perceptual problem, or a mixture of all three. Luzzatti and Verga (1996) proposed that the disorder might be considered as an adaptive rather than a reduplicative phenomenon. In particular, they suggest a difficulty in integrating the actual perceived reality with one's own internal belief. They propose that this is an exaggeration of normal experience, e.g. when waking up in a strange room the internal belief is compared to the information acquired sensorially from the external world and thus the internal belief adapts to the perceived reality. This integration may be reduced or lost in patients with reduplicative paramnesia and the incapacity to shift from a believed to the perceived reality might be considered a set-shifting or perseverative behaviour. Moser *et al.* (1998) suggest that reduplicative paramnesia is secondary to temporal–limbic–frontal dysfunction giving rise to a distorted sense of familiarity and impaired ability to resolve the delusion via logical reasoning. In some cases events may be reduplicated (Marshall *et al.* 1995).

20 Schizophrenia

20.1 Clinical presentation

Schizophrenia has been described as perhaps the most devastating illness known to man, because it appears in early adolescence and can drastically impair the subsequent life of the sufferer and his or her family. A variety of diagnostic systems have been used over the past 100 years, leading to much confusion. Currently, the DSM-IV system (American Psychiatric Association 1994) requires two or more of the following features:

- delusions;
- hallucinations;
- disorganized speech;
- disorganized or catatonic behaviour;
- negative symptoms.

These must be accompanied by:

- social/occupational dysfunction;
- continuous signs of disturbance that persist for at least 6 months;
- other disorders must have been excluded.

The life-time risk of developing schizophrenia is about 1%, a figure that varies very little around the world. There appears to be a strong genetic component to schizophrenia. For example, if there is a 1% prevalence of schizophrenia in the general population, the probability of developing schizophrenia in a monozygotic twin of a schizophrenic patient is 47% versus 12% in a dizygotic twin of a schizophrenic patient. Many of the syndromes reviewed in this chapter (De Clerambault's, Capgras', Othello, etc.) are considered by many to fall within the broad spectrum of schizophrenia.

20.2 Neuropsychological features

A critical finding in schizophrenia research was the report by Eve Johnstone and colleagues in 1976 that confirmed ventricular enlargement in CT scans in patients with schizophrenia versus controls. In the 1960s, there was a widespread view that schizophrenia was a socially created disorder and family dynamics and, in particular, the 'schizophrenogenic mother' were often blamed. The finding of CT abnormalities shifted the balance back to viewing schizophrenia as a brain/neuropsychological disorder. While several studies have found ventricular enlargement in schizophrenia, only about 30% of patients have an increase of one standard deviation greater than the healthy control mean. Furthermore, MRI studies have also confirmed reductions in temporal lobe volume (Nelson *et al.* 1998). Functional brain imaging studies using PET and fMRI have tended to report a decrease in frontal lobe blood flow (hypofrontality). This is most readily demonstrated during cognitive challenge tasks where patients have to perform a task, such as the Wisconsin Card Sort Test. Patients typically fail to show the same level of frontal lobe metabolic activity as healthy controls. However, it should be borne in mind that the patients often have difficulty in performing the cognitive task, so the finding may tell us more about the neural substrate of the cognitive task performance rather than schizophrenia.

The dopamine hypothesis has been central in attempting to explain schizophrenia and is mainly supported by the fact that virtually all effective antipsychotic drugs are dopamine receptor antagonists, particularly D2 receptors. There are at least two problems with the dopamine hypothesis.

♦ Dopamine antagonists are effective in treating virtually all psychotic and agitated patients *regardless of diagnosis*, i.e. response is not unique to schizophrenia.

♦ There is evidence that dopaminergic neurons may, in fact, *increase* their firing rate in response to chronic exposure to antipsychotic drugs, rather than reduce them.

Furthermore, many patients who have been resistant to treatment with dopamine antagonists have responded to the recently developed atypical antipsychotics such as clozapine and resperidone that target other neurotransmitter systems.

There is a huge neuropsychological literature on schizophrenia. However, as stated in the introduction, this may not have been a particularly fruitful research endeavour given that it may be more profitable from a neuropsychological perspective to try and explain particular signs or symptoms, e.g. auditory hallucinations or passivity.

Neuropsychological abnormalities are, however, consistently reported in patients diagnosed with schizophrenia. The most consistent findings are of impairments in learning, memory, and executive functioning (Heinrichs and Zakzanis 1998). Importantly, these abnormalities can be observed in patients who are drug-free. Recent evidence has also confirmed that low intelligence and poor educational achievement precede early-onset schizophrenic psychosis (Jones *et al.* 1994). Furthermore, young adult relatives of schizophrenics who are at high genetic risk of developing schizophrenia exhibit memory and executive impairments (Byrne *et al.* 1999) together with reductions in hippocampal/amygdala complex volume (Lawrie *et al.* 1999). Taken together, these findings add support to the view of schizophrenia as a neurodevelopmental disorder.

Attempts to explain schizophrenia *per se* in neuropsychological terms have had limited success, possibly because of the hetreogeneity of the disorder. However, certain features, e.g. specific delusions, have been explained via recent testable neuropsychological models (e.g. see Sections 7, 8, and 12). Frith (1992) has been particularly influential in this area, developing a model in which internal stimuli (e.g. thoughts or intentions) are thought to be misclassified and misattributed to an external source. For example,

Frith (1992) has proposed that auditory hallucinations in schizophrenia arise from a failure in the self-monitoring of speech processing. In this model, hallucinations are experienced as a result of a failure of the internal registration of the intention to generate inner speech, i.e. the hallucinating person's inner speech is perceived as alien— attributable to an external source. Frith has extended his model to account for a variety of features of schizophrenia including thought broadcasting, insertion, and withdrawal. A key feature of Frith's theory is that some key features of schizophrenia are due to an inability to monitor the beliefs and intentions of others. This is similar to the theory of mind deficit in autism, with one key difference, 'The autistic person has never known that other people have minds. The schizophrenic knows that other people have minds, but has lost the ability to infer the contents of these minds: their beliefs and intentions. Schizophrenics may even lose the ability to reflect on the contents of their own minds. However, they will still have available ritual and behavioural routines for interacting with people, which do not require inferences about mental states.' (Frith 1992, p. 121).

21 Somatoform disorders

21.1 Clinical presentation

Somatoform disorders share the common feature of the presence of a physical symptom that suggests an underlying general medical condition, but that is not fully explained by a general medical condition. These symptoms cause clinically significant distress or impairment. Unlike those in factitious disorders and malingering, the physical symptoms are *not* thought to be intentional. Gelder (1996) points out that there are several problems with the whole concept of somatoform disorder.

+ There is a lack of clear operational definitions for the overall category and unsatisfactory description of subcategories.

+ Some of the disorders, e.g. hypochondriasis, are so enduring that they could be classified as personality disorders rather than mental disorders.

+ Many patients have clinical features that fit the criteria for more than one diagnostic category.

Somatoform disorders include somatization disorder (historically referred to as hysteria or Briquette's syndrome), undifferentiated somatoform disorder, conversion disorder, pain disorder, hypochondriasis, body dysmorphic disorder, or somatoform disorder not otherwise specified. It is important to note that patients with chronic somatoform disorder can become grossly disabled, e.g. wheelchair-bound (Bass *et al.* 2001).

21.1 Neuropsychological features

There is little consistent evidence regarding neuropsychological abnormalities in the somatoform disorders and, in fact, as indicated above, this may reflect the lack of clear operational definitions for the overall category and the unsatisfactory descriptions of some of the subcategories (see Section 14 on conversion hysteria).

22 Tourette's syndrome

22.1 Clinical presentation

Tourette's syndrome involves multiple motor and one or more vocal tics, e.g. shouting profanities, and was first described by Gilles de la Tourette in 1885. The tics can occur many times a day and the disturbance causes marked distress or significant impairment in social occupational functioning. The onset is before age 18 and the condition is not due to drugs or a general medical condition such as Huntington's disease. The prevalence of Tourette's syndrome is approximately 1 per 2000 and the condition has a high genetic loading with a concordance rate of approximately 50% in monozygotic twins versus 8% in dizygotic twins. Obsessive–compulsive symptoms occur frequently in patients with Tourette's syndrome.

22.2 Neuropsychological features

Visuomotor difficulties are common in Tourette's disorder and abnormal, non-specific EEG findings are also common (Robertson 1989). CT brain scan studies suggest that approximately 10% of those with Tourette's syndrome have a non-specific abnormality, with the cingulate gyrus and basal ganglia often suggested as possible candidate sites for the disorder. The central dopaminergic system is thought to malfunction in Tourette's syndrome as dopaminergic stimulants exacerbate the disorder and dopamine blockers such as chlorpromazine often improve the condition. Attentional dysfunction may be central to the disorder as attention difficulties and poor frustration tolerance often predate the tics. Indeed, approximately 25% of people with Tourette's syndrome have been prescribed stimulants for a diagnosis of attention deficit hyperactivity disorder (ADHD) *before* receiving a diagnosis of Tourette's disorder. Recent work has suggested the presence of executive dysfunction, particularly problems with inhibitory control in patients with Tourette's syndrome.

23 Conclusion

The neuropsychological study of psychiatric disorders is still in its infancy. As C.D. Frith (1991, p. 28) stated in a commentary on a paper on a neuropsychological model of schizophrenia, 'A few years ago articles of this sort would have been unthinkable. For most psychologists, schizophrenia either did not exist or was a social disorder of no interest to hard -headed experimental psychologists. Today, schizophrenia is unquestionably a disorder of the brain (however caused) and, as such, it provides one of the most exciting challenges for linking brain and cognition.' Exciting novel attempts to explain abnormal behaviour in terms of dysfunctional information processing are rapidly being developed. However, it is critical that such models are explicitly amenable to experimental testing and refutation. Only then will significant advances be made in our scientific understanding of abnormal experience. We must be wary of replacing neurotransmitter- or structural lesion-based explanations of psychopathology with seductive, glossy PET or fMRI illustrations, or 'black-box' cognitive models. Demonstrating that a particular patient or patient group has abnormal regional brain metabolism, or a specific cognitive deficit is of interest, but it does not provide a causal explanation of abnormal behaviour or experience. In most instances we still await truly convincing neuropsychological explanations of psychopathological states.

Selective references

American Psychiatric Association (1994). *Diagnostic and statistical manual of mental disorders*, 4th edn. American Psychiatric Association, Washington, DC.

Bass, C., Peveler, R., and House, A. (2001). Somatoform disorders: severe psychiatric illnesses neglected by psychiatrists. *Br. J. Psychiatry* 179, 11–14.

Bentall, R.P. (1992). The classification of schizophrenia. In *Schizophrenia: an overview and practical handbook* (ed. D.J. Kavanagh), pp. 23–44. Chapman Hall, London.

Berrios, G.E. and Luque, R. (1995). Cotard's delusion or syndrome? A conceptual history. *Comprehens. Psychiatry* 36, 218–23.

Bremner, J.D. (1999). Alterations in brain structure and function associated with post-traumatic stress disorder. *Sem. Clin. Neuropsychiatry* 4, 249–55.

Brewin, C.R., Dalgleish, T., and Joseph, S. (1996). A dual representation theory of posttraumatic stress disorder. *Psychol. Rev.* 103, 670–86.

Byrne, M., Hodges, A., Grant, E., Owens, D.C., and Johnstone, E.C. (1999). Neuropsychological assessment of young people at high genetic risk for developing schizophrenia compared to controls: preliminary findings of the Edinburgh High Risk Study (EHRS). *Psychol. Med.* 29, 1161–73.

Cahill, L. (2000). Modulation of long-term memory storage in humans by emotional arousal: adrenergic activation and the amygdala. In *The amygdala: neurobiological aspects of emotion, memory and mental dysfunction* (ed. J. Aggleton), pp. 425–44. Wiley, New York.

Crimlisk, H. L., Bhatia, K., Cope, H., David, A., Marsden, C.D., and Ron, M.A. (1998). Slater revisited: 6 year follow up study of patients with medically unexplained motor symptoms. *Br. Med. J.* 316, 582–6.

Ellis, H.D. and Leafhead, K.M. (1996). Raymond: a study of an adult with Asperger syndrome. In *Method in madness: case studies in cognitive neuropsychiatry* (ed. P.W. Halligan and J.C. Marshall), pp. 79–92. Erlbaum, Hove, East Sussex.

Ellis, H.D. and Lewis, M.B. (2001). Capgras delusion: a window on face recognition. *Trends Cogn. Sci.* 5, 149–56.

Ellis, H.D. and Young, A.W. (1990). Accounting for delusional misidentifications. *Br. J. Psychiatry* 157, 239–48.

Ellis, H.D., Young, A.W., Quayle, A.H., and De Pauw, K.W. (1997). Reduced autonomic responses to faces and Capgras delusion. *Proc. R. Soc.: Biol. Sci. B* 264, 1085–92.

Ellis, P. and Mellsop, G. (1985). De Clerambault's syndrome—a nosological entity? *Br. J. Psychiatry* 146, 90–3.

Ferraro, F.R., Wonderlich, S., and Jocic, Z. (1997). Performance variability as a new theoretical mechanism regarding eating disorders and cognitive processing. *J. Clin. Psychol.* 53, 117–21.

Ferrier, I.N., Stanton, B.R., Kelly, T.P., and Scott, J. (1999). Neuropsychological function in euthymic patients with bipolar disorder. *Br. J. Psychiatry* 175, 246–51.

Frith, C.D. (1991). In what context is latent inhibition relevant to the symptoms of schizophrenia? *Behav. Brain Sci.* 14, 28–9.

Frith, C.D. (1992). *The cognitive neuropsychology of schizophrenia.* Lawrence Erlbaum Associates, Hove, East Sussex.

Frith, U. (1991). *Autism and Asperger's syndrome.* Cambridge University Press, Cambridge.

Gelder, M. (ed.) (1996). *Oxford textbook of psychiatry.* Oxford University Press, Oxford.

Halligan, P.W. and David, A.S. (1999). Conversion hysteria: towards a cognitive neuropsychological account. *Cogn. Neuropsychiatry* 4 (3), 161–3.

Halligan, P.W. and David, A.S. (2001). Cognitive neuropsychiatry: towards a scientific psychopathology. *Nature Neurosci.* 2, 209–15.

Halligan, P.W., Bass, C., and Wade, D.T. (2000). New approaches to conversion hysteria. *Br. Med. J.* 7248, 1488–9.

Halligan, P.W., Bass, C., and Marshall, J.C. (eds.) (2001). *Contemporary approach to the study of hysteria: clinical and theoretical perspectives.* Oxford University Press, Oxford.

Halligan, P.W., Bass, C., Oakley, D. (2003). *Malingering and illness deception.* Oxford University Press, Oxford.

Happe, F. and Frith, U. (1996). The neuropsychology of autism. *Brain* 119, 1377–400.

Heinrichs, R.W. and Zakzanis, K.K. (1998). Neurocognitive deficit in schizophrenia: a quantitative review of the evidence. *Neuropsychology* 12, 426–45.

Insel, T.R. and Winslow, J.T. (1992). Neurobiology of obsessive compulsive disorder. *Psychiatric Clin. N. Am.* 15, 813–24.

Johnstone, E.C., Crow, T.J., Frith, C.D., Husband, J., and Kreel, L. (1976). Cerebral ventricular size and cognitive impairment in chronic schizophrenia. *Lancet* 2, 924–6.

Jones, P., Rodgers, B., Murray, R., and Marmot, M. (1994). Child development risk factors for adult schizophrenia in the British 1946 birth cohort. *Lancet* 344, 1398–402.

Joseph, A.B. and O'Leary, D.H. (1987). Anterior cortical atrophy in Fregoli's syndrome. *J. Clin. Psychiatry* 48, 409–11.

Kamphuis, J.H. and Emmelkamp, P.M. (2000). Stalking—a contemporary challenge for forensic and clinical psychiatry. *Br. J. Psychiatry* 176, 206–9.

Kopelman, M., Guinan, E.M., and Lewis, P.D.R. (1995). Delusional memory, confabulation, and frontal lobe dysfunction: a case in de Clerambault's syndrome. *Neurocase* 1, 71–7.

Lawrie, S.M., Whalley, H., Kestelman, J.N., *et al.* (1999). Magnetic resonance imaging of brain in people at high risk of developing schizophrenia. *Lancet* 353, 30–3.

Lishman, W.A. (1998). *Organic psychiatry. The psychological consequences of cerebral disorder*, 3rd edn. Blackwell Scientific Publications, Oxford.

Luzzatti, C. and Verga, R. (1996). Reduplicative paramnesia for places with preserved memory. In *Method in madness: case studies in cognitive neuropsychiatry* (ed. P.W. Halligan and J.C. Marshall), pp. 187–207. Erlbaum, Hove, East Sussex.

Marshall, J.C., Halligan, P.W., and Wade, D.T. (1995). Reduplication of an event after head injury? A cautionary case report. *Cortex* 31 (1), 183–90.

Marshall, J.C., Halligan, P.W., Fink, G.R., Wade, D.T., and Frackowiak, R.S.J. (1997). The functional anatomy of a hysterical paralysis. *Cognition* 64, B1–B8.

McAllister-Williams, R.H., Ferrier, I.N., and Young, A.H. (1998). Mood and neuropsychological function in depression: the role of corticosteroids and serotonin. *Psychol. Med.* 28, 573–84.

Miller, J.N. and Ozonoff, S. (2000). The external validity of Asperger's disorder: lack of evidence from the domain of neuropsychology. *J. Abnorm. Psychol.* 109, 227–38.

Moser, D.J., Cohen, R.A., Malloy, P.F., Stone, W.M., and Rogg, J.M. (1998). Reduplicative paramnesia: longitudinal neurobehavioural and neuroimaging analysis. *J. Geriatr. Psychiatry Neurol.* 11, 174–80.

Murphy, F.C., Sahakian, B.J., Rubinsztein, J.S., *et al.* (1999). Emotional bias and inhibitory control processes in mania and depression. *Psychol. Med.* **29**, 1307–21.

Nelson, M.D., Saykin, A.J., Flashman, L.A., and Riordan, H.J. (1998). Hippocampal volume reduction in schizophrenia as assessed by magnetic resonance imaging—a meta-analytic study. *Arch. Gen. Psychiatry* **55**, 433–40.

Robertson, M.M. (1989). The Gilles de la Tourette syndrome: the current status. *Br. J. Psychiatry* **154**, 147–69.

Scoville, W.B. and Milner, B. (1957). Loss of recent memory after bilateral hippocampal lesions. *J. Neurol., Neurosurg., Psychiatry* **20**, 150–76.

Slater, E.T. and Glithero, E. (1965). A follow-up of patients diagnosed as suffering from 'hysteria'. *J. Psychosom. Res.* **9**, 9–13.

Spence, S.A. (1999). Hysterical paralyses as disorders of action. *Cogn. Neuropsychiatry* **4**, 203–26.

Tallis, F., Pratt, P., and Jamani, N. (1999). Obsessive compulsive disorder, checking and non-verbal memory: a neuropsychological investigation. *Behav. Res. Ther.* **37**, 161–6.

Veiel, H.O. (1997). A preliminary profile of neuropsychological deficits associated with major depression. *J. Clin. Exp. Neuropsychol.* **19**, 587–603.

Wilson, B.A., Baddeley, A.D., and Kapur, N. (1995). Dense amnesia in a professional musician following herpes simplex virus encephalitis. *J. Clin. Exp. Neuropsychol.* **17**, 668–81.

Young, A.W. and Leafhead, K.M. (1996). Betwixt life and death: case studies of the Cotard delusion. In *Method in madness: case studies in cognitive neuropsychiatry* (ed. P.W. Halligan and J.C. Marshall), pp. 147–71. Erlbaum, Hove, East Sussex.

Chapter 34

The clinical assessment of neuropsychiatric disorders

Meryl Dahlitz, Eli Jaldow, and
Michael D. Kopelman

1 Introduction

The primary objective of the neuropsychiatric clinical assessment is to make a comprehensive and accurate diagnosis and, on that basis, to set up a plan of management or care. It may be necessary to identify what additional information, if any, is required to substantiate the diagnosis (see Chapter 33). This unambiguous objective is nevertheless difficult to achieve and misdiagnoses are common, e.g. between a degenerative dementia and depressive pseudodementia in the elderly (e.g. Garcia *et al.* 1981; Ron *et al.* 1979). In general in neuropsychiatry, the greater the care taken in the clinical assessment, the greater the probability of obtaining the correct diagnosis. On the other hand, over-investigation is expensive, time-consuming, and stressful for the patient. This chapter will discuss the principles of what a neuropsychiatrist attempts to do, and also the particular contributions of the neuropsychologist in assessment and management of neuropsychiatric conditions (see Chapter 33).

2 The clinical interview

The skilful neuropsychiatrist should be self-aware and realize that his or her own general appearance, body language, eye contact, and posture will elicit a reaction from the patient and may critically affect the patient's responses. He or she should know how to listen, to be generally perceptive, to take notes and think simultaneously, to deal inconspicuously with interruptions, and to give the impression that there is no hurry even when time may be very limited. At the very least, the patient will receive respect and begin to build a therapeutic relationship. It is usually necessary to have at least one follow up appointment, to review the results of tests and investigations and/or to assess progress after the initial therapeutic intervention. Findings should be reviewed if follow-up appointments are not attended.

Many patients who are referred to a neuropsychiatrist have complex medical histories. Specialist neuropsychiatric clinics are usually secondary or tertiary referral centres, where neuropsychiatrists and neuropsychologists need to take the time to do the thorough assessment that a GP is unable to do in a 5-minute surgery consultation. It is essential that the neuropsychiatrist reads and, if necessary, rereads the referral letter very carefully, as well as any other information that has been sent before the initial interview. Referral letters often contain essential information. The neuropsychiatrist is severely disadvantaged in the assessment if he or she is not absolutely clear about all the information that is presented in the referral. It is sometimes helpful, particularly in complex cases, to begin by reviewing the referral letter with the patient and identifying variations, if there are any, between the referrer's appraisal at the time of writing and the patient's current version of his problems. In this context, the referrer may be functioning as a collateral historian (see Section 2.1) and, in some cases, this will be the only collateral history available and so has an important status. A review of the reason for referral at the beginning of the clinical interview will focus the neuropsychiatrist and the patient on the objectives of the consultation and identify the major topics to be covered in the interview.

Neurologists and neuropsychiatrists deal with different aspects of both acute and chronic organic reactions. Ideally, their approaches are complementary and neurological input may be useful during the neuropsychiatric assessment. Generally, the neurologist is primarily concerned with the diagnosis and treatment of specific lesions and diseases. The neuropsychiatrist is concerned with the psychiatric manifestations and complications of known neurological disorders, as well as with the diagnosis and management of disorders evidenced by psychological/psychiatric signs and symptoms. These include delirium and dementia, the management of secondary disorders (e.g. depression after head injury or stroke, psychosis in epilepsy or dementia), the prevention of secondary complications, and support for relatives and carers. He/she has responsibility for the coordination of care in the hospital and transfer of care at the time of discharge. Sometimes the neuropsychiatrist will assess an organic contribution to functional disorders, consider detention under the Mental Health Act, or assess issues of compensation or competence. Effective communication skills and the exercise of tact are demanded by the work.

In many branches of medicine it is considered good practice to strive to make a single diagnosis that best accounts for all the symptoms (Occam's razor). Except in geriatrics, the conventional wisdom is to seek the single underlying diagnosis that would account for multiple symptoms. However, in neuropsychiatry (as in geriatrics) it is much more common that there are several concomitant problems (e.g. head trauma resulting in impaired cognition, depression, and posttraumatic stress disorder (PTSD)) that tend to occur together in familiar patterns. This has an impact on the scope of the neuropsychiatric assessment and will be considered further in Section 6.

The patient's complaints should be asked about early in the interview and should be considered very thoroughly and in every detail. Among all the aspects of the history, these initial complaints are most likely to be relevant to diagnosis. Throughout the clinical interview, the neuropsychiatrist will be collecting information that will either support or reject certain possible diagnoses. He/she will systematically ask questions to help confirm or eliminate the differential diagnoses. Table 34.1 shows the common causes of dementia that a neuropsychiatrist may consider. Patients presenting with amnesia are most likely to have Wernicke–Korsakoff syndrome, but herpes encephalitis, vascular episode(s), anoxia, head injury, subarachnoid haemorrhage, space-occupying lesion, pituitary excision and radiotherapy, and transient global amnesia are also possible diagnoses. Mild/moderate memory impairment is frequently the result of a vascular episode, epilepsy, alcohol, hypoxia, or head injury, whilst non-progressive generalized cognitive impairment is most often due to anoxia or head injury (Kopelman and Crawford 1996). Tables 34.2 and 34.3 give some examples of aspects of the presenting

Table 34.1 Prevalence of different causes of dementia in adults referred for evaluation of progressive intellectual deterioration*

Cause	Prevalence (%)
Alzheimer's disease (presumed)	39
Multi-infarct dementia	13
Dementia associated with psychiatric disorder (pseudodementia)	9
Alcoholic	8
Metabolic disorders	4
Hydrocephalus	4
Cerebral neoplasms	3
Huntington's disease	2
Not demented	2
Miscellaneous	15

* Data based on 708 patients from eight world-wide series (Marsden 1985). Note that Lewy body dementia has subsequently been shown to account for up to 20% of patients with dementia at autopsy. AIDS dementia is not included in this series.

Table 34.2 The initial complaint and its diagnostic significance

	Examples and comments
Description	Diagnostically this is the most useful aspect of the history and great care should be taken to obtain detailed and precise information about each complaint or symptom

Mode of onset
   Sudden
   Progressive
   Stepwise
	
	Vascular episode, psychiatric disorder
	Alzheimer's disease, psychiatric disorder
	Multi-infarct dementia, multiple sclerosis

Circumstances of onset	Injury/accident (Did the illness cause the accident? Compensation?)
Course	An episodic course is characteristic of epilepsy, Kleine–Levin syndrome, and mental illness

Table 34.3 The past psychiatric history and its diagnostic significance

Type of history	Examples and comments
Family history	Genetic predisposition?
Personal history	
Childhood	Brain damage, febrile convulsions, and head injuries all increase the risk of epilepsy
Occupations	Educational attainment and peak occupational level are better indicators of premorbid IQ than end-of-bed evaluations. Periods of unemployment may identify past episodes of illness
Habits	The impact of alcohol and other drugs is related to doses consumed and precise daily intake should be determined if possible. Have there been epileptic seizures, amnesic episodes, and/or withdrawal phenomena? Drug injection exposes the body to infections, emboli, and thromboses
Forensic	There may be genetic predisposition to criminal behaviour, e.g. XYY syndrome, Tourette's syndrome
Psychosexual	Unusual behaviour may be diagnostically helpful, e.g. increased libido and sexual disinhibition in mania and Kleine–Levin syndrome. Having multiple partners increases the risk of sexually transmitted diseases. Pregnancy and breastfeeding may effect some investigations and treatments
Sleep	The timing of insomnia may help distinguish between the type and severity of mood disorder. Insomnia is also a feature of delirium. Excessive daytime sleepiness may be primary or secondary (e.g. drugs/toxins, head injury, sleep apnoea)
Past psychiatric history	Previous symptoms, diagnoses, course of illness, and responses to previous treatments are characteristic of some illnesses and this information is often helpful diagnostically. Old brain scans may be very useful for identifying new pathology
Past medical history	Neurological (e.g. head injuries, epilepsy, meningitis/encephalitis, stroke) and endocrinological (e.g. diabetes, thyroid disease) histories are most often relevant
Personality and social history	A collateral history is important if a personality change is suspected

complaint and the past psychiatric history that may be diagnostically helpful and should be enquired about. If there are a number of complaints or symptoms, it is useful to list them numerically at the outset, and then investigate them one by one.

2.1 Collaborative (collateral) clinical history

A careful history from close relatives or friends is required to establish the mode of onset of the disorder, the nature and duration of symptoms, and their subsequent course. The patient's own account may be distorted by confusion, memory lapses, denial, or lack of insight. The collateral history may be taken by a second interviewer in a separate room.

2.2 Mental state examination

The mental state examination begins with appearance and general behaviour.

- Pallor, weight loss, disorders of facial expression, posture, and movement, and standards of self-care draw attention to the possibility of an organic disorder (although some of the features may also be seen in severe depression).

- Are there slow, hesitant responses or evidence of poor comprehension?

- Is the patient impulsive, disinhibited, or insensitive?

- Nursing observations may reveal indifference to events, bewilderment, a perplexed expression, aimless wandering, restlessness, stereotypies, loss of way, memory lapses, losses of consciousness, aggressive, suspicious, or paranoid behaviour, feeding or dressing difficulties, binge eating, or incontinence.

- Speech may be incoherent or perseverative. The patient may wander off the point and deny any difficulties, evade questions, or rationalize his/her failures. Speech may reveal a poverty of content, restriction of theme, concrete thinking, or impaired reasoning ability.

- The delirious patient's mood may shift between periods of mild disinhibition or euphoria and hostile agitation. In early dementia, a quiet perplexity or emotional lability characteristically prevails. An empty, shallow quality to emotional expression is quite common.

- Another sign is the catastrophic reaction, in which failure at a previously accomplished task elicits an intense emotional reaction with crying, negativity, withdrawal, and hostility.

Intelligence has a major modifying effect on the presentation of thought content. A highly intelligent patient may appear less severely impaired by virtue of cognitive compensations for his or her deficits. Doctors should avoid making a glib assessment of intelligence quotient (IQ) based on a conversation—this is a common trap that the medical profession falls into! It is quite possible to have a 'normal' conversation with a person who has considerable intellectual impairment. Far more information can be derived from a few 'bedside' clinical screening tests (Kopelman 1986, 1994; Hodges 1994). In those of low or borderline IQ (adult learning disorder), the experience of unfamiliar abstract phenomena in simple, concrete terms may be due to an inability to appreciate the different modalities of perception and/or a lack of the vocabulary required to accurately describe them, e.g. in the reporting of hallucinations. Ideas of reference and delusions of persecution are common, but often poorly elaborated, vague, shallow, transient, or inconsistently related. Anxious, depressive, or hypochondriacal ideas may co-occur with perceptual distortions, illusions, and hallucinations.

2.3 Assessment of cognitive state

The neuropsychiatrist's assessment of cognitive state is essentially a screening procedure. If abnormalities are found they, combined with the clinical history, should help to focus the referral for neuropsychiatric assessment by a psychologist (see Section 4).

◆ In acute psychotic or neurotic patients without apparent organic pathology, it is sufficient to assess orientation in time, place, and person and either knowledge of three recent news events or immediate and delayed recall of a name and address.

◆ In patients with suspected organic disorders, a brief assessment of orientation, attention/concentration, memory (including general information, remote and recent personal memories and current learning), language (including naming, comprehension, expression, repetition, reading and writing, disorders of form and content), mental calculation, drawing and copying, other agnosic or apraxic deficits, and frontal function is likely to provide relevant insights and direct further assessments.

The scope of this type of assessment is described in Kopelman (1994).

3 Physical examination

A thorough physical examination is required. Of admissions to psychiatric hospitals for mental disorder, 12% have physical signs of an illness that is likely to be contributing directly to the psychiatric disorder (Lishman 1998). The elderly are particularly vulnerable, with about one-third having medical disorders complicating dementia (Lipowski 1990).

◆ The neuropsychiatrist looks carefully at the patient's face to gain an impression of his state of mind, in particular, mood state or an appearance of perplexity and confusion: 'there's no art to find the mind's construction in the face'. Is there a suspicion that the patient is experiencing hallucinations? This may be obvious or quite subtle, and beware not to overinterpret. There may be signs of liver disease: spider naevi, jaundice, and parotid enlargement in an alcoholic.

◆ The head should be examined for signs: scars, unusual head shape, size or asymmetry, hair distribution, and texture.

◆ The eyes, windows of the mind, should be examined particularly carefully. Abnormal pupil size may be affected by drugs. Pupillary accommodation and reaction to a light must be checked if there is a suspicion of syphilis; the Argyll–Robinson 'prostitute's pupil' accommodates but does not react.

◆ The hands may also reveal useful information about the patient's health and lifestyle. Is there a tremor, palmar erythema and leuconychia, nicotine staining, clubbing, or calluses? Are the nails long, broken, bitten, or unclean?

◆ The blood pressure must always be measured and the pulse should be taken. Is there an arrhythmia? Is the pulse fast because the patient is anxious or for some other reason (e.g. thyroid disease)?

The traditional neurological examination is often normal in patients with brain disease. If abnormalities are present they may only be witnessed as 'subtle signs', e.g. clumsiness, motor impersistence, minor parkinsonism, or gait abnormalities.

4 Neuropsychological assessment

Within the context of a neuropsychiatric clinic, neuropsychological assessment has three main purposes.

- The first is to help with diagnosis in the context of other observations and findings from the background history, clinical and mental state examination, and the results of physical investigations. Where all the indices point in the same direction, the assessment is easy. Where they differ, it is more challenging, but particularly important to find an explanation for the discrepancy. A patient may be found, on formal testing, to be either more or less severely impaired than expected. If more severely impaired, it could be that the clinician had underestimated the degree of decrement or that the patient is exaggerating or simulating his/her handicap.

- The second main purpose is to identify and quantify the pattern and severity of cognitive impairments. The details of how this is done are discussed elsewhere in this volume.

- The third main purpose of assessment is to plan strategies of cognitive rehabilitation and/or cognitive behaviour therapy—mood disorders and post traumatic stress disorder being common correlates of cognitive deficits (Kopelman and Crawford 1996). Cognitive rehabilitation is carried out according to principles developed elsewhere (Wilson 1999; Stuss *et al.* 1999).

The actual tests employed in neuropsychiatric settings vary somewhat from clinic to clinic, but do not differ in essence from those considered in relation to specific disorders elsewhere in this volume. Within our own clinic, we commonly employ as initial procedures the National Adult Reading Test-revised (NART-R) for estimating premorbid IQ (Nelson and Willison 1991), the Wechsler Abbreviated Scale of Intelligence (WASI) as a brief assessment of current intelligence, and the Wechsler Adult Intelligence Scale-III (WAIS-III; Wechsler 2001*a*) or Wechsler Adult Intelligence Scale-revised (WAIS-R; Wechsler 1981) for more detailed assessment. Alternative measures of anterograde memory, employed in accordance with clinical need and time availability, include the Wechsler Memory Scale-III (WMS-III; Wechsler 2001*b*), Wechsler Memory Scale-revised (WMS-R; Wechsler 1987), the Doors and People test (Baddeley *et al.* 1994), the Recognition Memory Test (Warrington 1984), and the Kendrick Object Learning test (Kendrick 1985). For naming, we commonly employ the Graded Naming test (McKenna and Warrington 1983) and, for executive function, such tests as verbal fluency (Benton 1968), Modified Card Sorting (Nelson 1976), cognitive estimates (Shallice and Evans 1978), Trailmaking (Reitan 1958), and the Brixton–Hayling tests (Burgess and Shallice 1996). Autobiographical memory is assessed using the Autobiographical Memory Interview (Kopelman *et al.* 1990). All patients are given the Beck depression scale (Beck 1987) and subjective evaluations of memory are also used occasionally (Sunderland *et al.* 1983).

5 Physical investigations

Investigations are primarily directed towards excluding or establishing and quantifying organic pathology.

5.1 Blood tests

A biochemical screen is justified in all cases because, even if the diagnosis is known, electrolyte imbalances may complicate and exacerbate other conditions. Unsuspected physical illness is identified by routine blood screening in many psychotic patients (Hall *et al.* 1980). Biochemical tests are essential to confirm many suspected diagnoses, e.g. thyroid disease, parathyroid disease, Cushing's disease, diabetes, uraemia, liver failure, and syphilis.

5.2 Electroencephalogram (EEG) (see Chapter 42)

The EEG is widely used when organic disorders are suspected, confirming abnormalities of brain structure and function in about 60% of cases. In normal subjects the EEG is symmetrical and classified into four characteristic waveforms depending on frequency: delta, theta, alpha, and beta.

Focal abnormalities are most consistent with localized disorders, such as tumours, abscesses, subdural haematomas, and cerebral infarctions. Diffuse slowing occurs in toxic and metabolic disorders and in advanced degenerative diseases. The EEG is a sensitive indicator of cerebral metabolism. The degree of bilateral diffuse slowing correlates positively with the degree of cognitive impairment in delirium and thus serial EEGs are useful for monitoring its progress.

Triphasic waves occur in liver failure, high-amplitude sharp waves in herpes simplex encephalitis, low-voltage activity with posterior slowing in uraemia, acceleration of alpha in hyperthyroidism, and low-voltage activity in hypothyroidism. In delirium tremens, the EEG may show fast activity rather than slowing. In toxic delirium associated with drugs, the EEG may show drug-specific patterns of fast-wave activity (antidepressants, benzodiazepines) or slowing (phenothiazines). Localized spike and sharp wave complexes usually suggest an intracranial cause for delirium.

In very early Alzheimer's disease the EEG is usually normal, but as the disease advances there is progressive slowing, particularly posteriorly and in the medial temporal regions. Multi-infarct dementia is characterized by an asymmetric trace with focal slowing in over two-thirds of patients. Pronounced flattening of the EEG suggests Huntington's disease. The EEG in typical Creutzfeld–Jakob disease may be floridly abnormal in a patient with only minor cognitive impairments and minimal changes on structural imaging (computerized tomography or magnetic resonance imaging).

Characteristically, repetitive spike discharges with triphasic sharp-wave complexes are present: it can clinch the diagnosis in this disorder. The EEG is often normal in pseudodementia and in 20% of patients with tumours and subdural haematomas.

The EEG is especially useful in the diagnosis of the various forms of epilepsy and of pseudoseizures. Monitoring continuously over several days and with simultaneous video monitoring may be required.

5.3 Computerized tomography (CT) (see Chapter 42)

CT detects most cortical lesions, vascular infarctions, demyelination and white matter change (leukodystrophy), and hydrocephalus. Cerebral atrophy (widened ventricles and enlarged sulci) is often reported in dementia, with the abnormalities increasing as the disease progresses. Problems exist with the interpretation of CT scan findings of cerebral atrophy in dementia in that some degree of atrophy occurs in the ageing process of many healthy ('normal') subjects and it may be absent in early dementia. It is not specific to any particular disorder, being seen in alcohol abuse or following severe head injury or hypoxia, as well as in degenerative dementias.

No feature of the CT scan is diagnostic of Alzheimer's disease, but an increase in ventricular size over 1 year is highly suggestive, in the absence of other known pathologies. Automated volumetric indices of brain atrophy may discriminate between normal ageing and Alzheimer's disease, even in its mild stages. A frontal temporal distribution of brain atrophy may suggest Pick's disease, and caudate atrophy may suggest Huntington's disease or neuroacanthocytosis. Some degree of atrophy may occur in psychiatric disorders, including schizophrenia and affective disorders. Detailed views of the temporal lobes may reveal subtle pathology and improve the discriminating ability of the scan in dementia. It should be noted that CT scan appearances can only be interpreted within the context of the total clinical presentation.

5.4 Magnetic resonance imaging (MRI), single-photon emission computerized tomography (SPECT), and positron emission tomography (PET)

See Chapter 42 for descriptions of MRI, SPECT, and PET.

6 Concluding the neuropsychiatric assessment

Ideally, the clinical history and examination as well as the psychometric testing and the investigations all point to the same diagnosis. However, they often do not and in those cases all the information should be reappraised carefully.

◆ Was part of the history missed?

◆ Is there any reason to suspect that the patient may be faking or embellishing symptoms?

◆ Is the patient depressed or suffering from excessive daytime sleepiness (pseudodementia)? Abnormalities in cognitive testing with a normal MRI support a diagnosis of pseudodementia.

A neuropsychiatrist, having made one probable diagnosis, should then consider other disorders that sometimes co-occur with that diagnosis.

◆ Head injury may result in neurological signs, cognitive deficits, and/or emotional problems such as depression and PTSD.

◆ Alcohol causes a range of problems including withdrawal syndromes, acute hallucinosis or paranoia, hepatic encephalopathy, the Wernicke–Korsakoff syndrome, or more global cognitive deficits as well as a range of physical disorders.

Identification of any one problem increases the likelihood of a related disorder, and the assessment needs to take account of the full range of possibilities.

Having established the diagnosis or diagnoses, it is, of course, essential to establish the impact of these upon daily living. Interviewing family members, carers, and other informants is critical here. The care plans evolved may require the involvement of community nurses, occupational therapists, and social workers as well as clinical psychologists working in different settings. One issue that may need to be discussed will be the heritability of disorders known to have a genetic basis, e.g. Huntington's or Alzheimer dementia. Another issue to discuss is prognosis. This is inevitably gloomy, although variable, in the degenerative dementias but, in other forms of brain injury, there is often greater scope for improvement than the medical (and sometimes the neuropsychological) textbooks imply (Victor *et al.* 1971; Wilson 1991; Stanhope and Kopelman 2000).

Selective references

Baddeley, A.D., Emslie, H., and Nimmo-Smith, I. (1994). *Doors and People: a test of visual and verbal recall and recognition.* Thames Valley Test Company, Bury St Edmunds.

Beck, A.T. (1987). *Beck Depression Inventory.* Psychological Corporation, San Antonio, Texas.

Benton, A.L. (1968). Differential behavioural effects in frontal lobe disease. *Neuropsychologia* 6, 53–60.

Burgess, P.W. and Shallice, T. (1996). Response suppression, initiation and strategy use following frontal lobe lesions. *Neuropsychologia* 34, 263–72.

Fogel, B.S., Schiffer, R.B., and Rao, S.M. (eds.) (1996). *Neuropsychiatry.* Williams and Wilkins, Baltimore.

Garcia, C.A., Reding, M.J., and Blass, J.P. (1981). Overdiagnosis of dementia. *J. Am. Geriatr. Soc.* 29, 407–10.

Gelder, M.G., Lopez-Ibor, J.J., and Andreason, N. (eds.) (2000). *New Oxford Textbook of Psychiatry,* Vols 1 and 2. Oxford University Press, Oxford.

Hall, R.C.W., Gardner, E.R., Stickney, S.K., Le Cann, A.F., and Popkin, M.K. (1980). Physical illness manifesting as psychiatric disease. *Arch. Gen. Psychiatry* 37, 989–95.

Hodges, J. (1994). *Cognitive assessment for clinicians.* Oxford University Press, Oxford.

Jacobson, R. and Kopelman, M.D. (1998). Organic psychiatric disorders. In *General adult psychiatry*, Vol. 2. Royal College of Psychiatrists College Seminar Series (ed. G. Stein and G. Wilkinson), pp. 954–1026. Gaskell.

Kendrick, D. (1985). *Cognitive tests for the elderly*. NFER-Nelson, Windsor.

Kopelman, M.D. (1986). Clinical tests of memory. *Br. J. Psychiatry* **148**, 517–25.

Kopelman, M.D. (1994). Structured psychiatric interview: assessment of the cognitive state. *Br. J. Hosp. Med.* **52** (6), 277–81.

Kopelman, M.D. and Crawford, S. (1996). Not all memory clinics are dementia clinics. *Neuropsychol. Rehabil.* **6** (3), 187–202.

Kopelman, M.D., Wilson, B.A., and Baddeley A.D. (1990). *The Autobiographical Memory Interview*. Thames Valley Test Company, Bury St Edmunds.

Lipowski, Z.J. (1990). *Delirium: acute brain failure in man*. Charles C. Thomas, Springfield, Illinois.

Lishman, W.A. (1998). *Organic psychiatry: the psychological consequences of cerebral disorder*, 3rd edn. Blackwell Scientific Publications, Oxford.

Marsden, C.D. (1985). Assessment of dementia. In *Handbook of clinical neurology*, Vol. 2: *Neurobehavioural disorders* (ed. J.A.M. Fredericks), pp. 221–32. Elsevier Science, Oxford.

McKenna, P. and Warrington, E.K. (1983). *The Graded Naming Tests*. NFER-Nelson, Windsor.

Morris, R.G. and Kopelman, M. (1992). The neuropsychological assessment of dementia. In *Handbook of neuropsychological assessment* (ed. J.R. Crawford, D.M. Parker, and W.W. McKinlay), pp. 295–321. Lawrence Erlbaum Associates, Hove, East Sussex.

Nelson, H.E. (1976). A modified card sorting test. *Cortex* **12**, 313–24.

Nelson, H.E. and Willison, J.R. (1991). *The National Adult Reading test—Revised*. NFER-Nelson, Windsor.

Reitan, R.M. (1958). Validity of the Trail Making test as an indicator of organic brain damage. *Percept. Motor Skills* **8**, 271–6.

Ron, M.A., Toone, B.K., Garralda, M.E., and Lishman W.A. (1979). Diagnostic accuracy in presenile dementia. *Br. J. Psychiatry* **134**, 161–8.

Shallice, T. and Evans, M.E. (1978). The involvement of the frontal lobes in cognitive estimates. *Cortex* **14**, 294–303.

Stanhope, N. and Kopelman, M.D. (2000). Art and memory: a 7 year follow-up of herpes encephalitis in a professional artist. *Neurocase* **6**, 99–110.

Stuss, D.T., Winocur, G., and Robertson, I.H. (eds.) (1999). *Cognitive rehabilitation*. Cambridge University Press, Cambridge.

Sunderland, A., Harris, J.E., and Baddeley, A.D. (1983). Do laboratory tests predict everyday memory? A neuropsychological study. *J. Verbal Learning Verbal Behav.* **22**, 341–56.

Victor, M., Adams, R.D., and Collins, G.H. (1971). *The Wernicke–Korsakoff syndrome*. F.A. Davis, Philadelphia.

Warrington, E.K. (1984). *The Recognition Memory Test*. NFER-Nelson, Windsor.

Wechsler, D. (1981). *The Wechsler Adult Intelligence Scale—Revised*. Psychological Corporation, San Antonio, Texas.

Wechsler, D. (1987). *Wechsler Memory Scale—Revised*. Psychological Corporation, San Antonio, Texas.

Wechsler, D. (2001*a*). *Wechsler Adult Intelligence Scale—III*. Psychological Corporation, San Antonio, Texas.

Wechsler, D. (2001*b*). *The Wechsler Memory Scale—III.* Psychological Corporation, San Antonio, Texas.

Wilson, B.A. (1991). Long-term prognosis of patients with severe memory disorders. *Neuropsychol. Rehabil.* 1, 117–34.

Wilson, B.A. (1999). *Case studies in neuropsychological rehabilitation.* Oxford University Press, Oxford.

Chapter 35

Neuropsychological rehabilitation of schizophrenia

Bjørn Rishovd Rund

1 Introduction

Schizophrenia is a disturbance, or a spectrum of disorders, that is diagnostically defined (*Diagnostic and statistical manual of mental disorders*, 4th edn (DSM-IV); American Psychiatric Association 1994) by a duration of at least 6 months, with at least 1 month of an active psychotic phase. Two or more of the following symptoms should be present during the active phase:

◆ delusions;

◆ hallucinations;

◆ disorganized speech;

◆ grossly disorganized or catatonic behaviour;

◆ negative symptoms (i.e. affective flattening, alogia, or avolition).

Even though modern antipsychotics and psychosocial treatment programmes are effective in moderating symptoms and reducing the rate of relapses, most patients with schizophrenia do not function well outside structured, routine settings, such as hospital wards. Outcomes other than symptom improvement and relapse prevention have not been well documented (Lehman *et al.* 1995; Hogarty and Flesher 1999). A majority of patients with schizophrenia interact in ordinary social settings in a conspicuous way and also do not manage an ordinary work or school situation very well. On average, only 10–30% of patients with schizophrenia are employed at any time, and few of these are able to maintain their vocational gains (Attkisson *et al.* 1992; Hogarty and Flesher 1999). What is the reason for this?

1.1 Cognitive dysfunction and outcome in schizophrenia

Many clinicians now claim that the reason is the serious cognitive disturbances of these patients. Several prominent researchers and clinicians have pointed out that cognitive dysfunction is the enduring core feature of schizophrenia. Some have called schizophrenia a thought disorder. Evidence from neuropsychological, neuropathological, and neuroimaging studies has documented schizophrenia as a neuropsychiatric disease. Most cognitive dysfunctions seem to some degree to remain impaired even when symptoms improve. Andreasen (1999) argues that the definition of schizophrenia should be based on basic cognitive disturbances rather than on phenomenology.

The fundamental importance of cognitive deficits in schizophrenia is also substantiated by the fact that cognitive functions have proven to be of much greater significance in the prediction of prognosis and outcome than the symptoms of the illness. Patients with the most serious cognitive dysfunctions appear to have the poorest outcome. Different dysfunctions seem to relate to different functional outcomes.

- Verbal memory is related to all types of functional outcomes.
- Vigilance predicts social problem-solving and the acquisition of social skills.
- Executive functioning predicts the ability to function in the community (Sharma 1999).
- Impairment in cognitive processing seems to mediate the acquisition of behavioural competencies in schizophrenia.

We still have limited knowledge, however, about the underlying mechanisms through which cognitive dysfunctions operate on behaviour and social functions.

1.2 The importance of cognitive prodromal symptoms for early diagnosis

What Hogarty and Flesher (1999) term social cognition, i.e. the ability to act wisely in social interactions, is an important determinant of social and vocational recovery. Klosterkötter and Schultze-Lutter (2000) have shown that cognitive prodromal symptoms are the only ones with a high diagnostic efficiency. These symptoms have high specificity and positive predictive powers as well as satisfactory percentages of false-positive predictions and a good classification rate. Klosterkötter and Schultze-Lutter (2000) claim that, because of the high predictive value of these cognitive symptoms, a diagnosis in the initial schizophrenic prodrome seems possible. They conclude that in the future an early intervention related thereto might enable prevention of early psychotic episodes.

1.3 Cognitive dysfunction as a target for treatment and rehabilitation

The fact that deviance in cognitive functions is a core deficit in schizophrenia makes them an appropriate target for treatment and rehabilitation. The obvious area to address is the one that is most impaired and most damaging for the person's psychosocial functioning. However, the targeting of cognitive and neuropsychological deficits in schizophrenia for therapeutic interventions has so far been greatly neglected. Attempts at cognitive remediation have been relatively sparse. Effective techniques for normalizing or neutralizing cognitive impairments would be a decisive addition to the treatment armamentarium for patients with a psychotic illness in general and patients with schizophrenia in particular. Neuropsychologists have contributed strongly to the development of the few cognitive remediation programmes for patients with schizo-phrenia that exist today, primarily the process-oriented approach (see Section 3). This treatment strategy originated in the areas of experimental psychopathology and the neuropsychology of schizophrenia. In this approach, specific cognitive impairments detected in the laboratory are targeted for change, first in the laboratory and later in increasingly realistic situations (Spaulding *et al.* 1999). As such, this treatment approach has much in common with the models for rehabilitation of head traumas.

There are two distinctly different approaches in cognitive therapy with schizophrenic patients. One focuses on cognitive content, while the other is process-oriented, emphas-izing the correction of basic cognitive deficits.

2 The content-oriented approach to therapy

This is carried out according to the principles of cognitive therapy, e.g. as described by Beck *et al.* (1979) for the treatment of depression and other emotional disorders. However, some modifications that are necessary for severely disturbed patients are included. Outstanding advocates for this approach in schizophrenia treatment are Perris (1989), Fowler and Morley (1989), Bentall and collaborators (1994), and Kingdon and Turkington (1994).

- ◆ Perris's metacognitive approach has been developed in small, community-based and family-style treatment centres in Sweden. Most of the treatment takes place in small groups.

- ◆ Bentall *et al.* (1994) have developed a more behaviourally oriented treatment package that directly targets persistent auditory hallucinations. Their therapeutic programme consists of procedures for fostering attribution of hallucinations to the self rather than to external sources, and for diminishing distress provoked by hearing voices.

- ◆ Kingdon and Turkington (1994) contend that people with schizophrenia are not inherently irrational, but instead suffer from a circumscribed set of irrational beliefs. Their therapeutic approach attempts to help patients to alleviate the impact of these beliefs.

- ◆ The treatment programme of Fowler and colleagues (Garety *et al.* 1994) focuses on techniques aimed at modifying psychotic thoughts.

3 The process-oriented approach to cognitive therapy

This approach focuses on remediation of deficits in cognitive processes rather than changing distorted thoughts, attitudes, beliefs, or hallucinations (Adams *et al.* 1981). This chapter will be limited to this approach and the empirical studies examining the effects of such therapeutic programmes.

There were a few clinical studies in the late 1960s and 1970s reporting encouraging results. After this promising beginning, research lay dormant for more than a decade. Interest in cognitive training programmes based on empirical research was to some extent rekindled in the 1990s. Some few comprehensive training programmes have been developed, and the effects of certain of these have been examined (Fowler 1992; Brenner *et al.* 1995; Spaulding *et al.* 1999). In addition to these well-founded treatment programmes, there have also been several attempts to remediate more specific elementary attentional and conceptual functions.

3.1 The integrated psychological therapy (IPT) programme

Brenner *et al.* (1992, 1995) developed the most complete therapeutic programme, the so-called Integrated Psychological Therapy (IPT). This is a multi-element hierarchical programme in which there is an attempt to enhance basic cognitive capacities before problem-solving and motor skills training is implemented. IPT is a step-by-step procedure devised for groups of 5–7 patients. It is comprised of five subprogrammes:

- cognitive differentiation;
- social perception;
- communication skills;
- interpersonal problem-solving;
- social skills training.

The rationale behind the IPT is that remediation of cognitive deficits will facilitate acquisition and maintenance of more complex skills. A series of studies of IPT has demonstrated significant treatment effects on cognitive functions and reduction of symptomatology (Hodel and Brenner 1994). However, it has not been documented that remediation of cognitive functions has a pervasive effect on social behaviour.

In the USA Will Spaulding has adapted and elaborated Brenner's IPT programme. Spaulding *et al.* (1999) published the results from a study in which 90 subjects with severe and disabling psychiatric conditions, predominantly schizophrenia, participated in a controlled-outcome trial. Patients receiving the cognitive training programme, consisting of the three cognitive modules in Brenner's IPT, were compared to control subjects who received supportive group therapy. Patients receiving cognitive training showed incrementally greater gains compared with controls on the primary outcome measures. There was equivocal evidence for greater improvement in the cognitive training group on a disorganization factor for psychiatric symptoms (the Brief Psychiatric Rating Scale), and strong evidence for greater improvement on a laboratory measure of attention processing. Significant improvement was also found on two measures of attention, memory, and executive functioning.

3.2 A trial of individual neurocognitive therapy

Wykes *et al.* (1998) reported the preliminary results of a controlled trial of individual neurocognitive therapy. The effects of cognitive remediation were compared to those of a control therapy that consisted of intensive occupational therapy to control for non-specific effects of treatment. In a randomized control trial of 33 patients with schizophrenia, results suggested a differential effect in favour of cognitive rehabilitation for tests in the cognitive flexibility and memory subgroups, as well as for self-esteem, but not on symptoms or social functioning. However, generalized improvements in cognitive flexibility were related to improvements in social functioning.

3.3 Remediation of conceptual and attentional skills and memory

The attempts to remediate more specific cognitive dysfunction have mainly concentrated on two areas: conceptual skills and attentional skills.

3.3.1 Remediation of conceptual skills

Conceptual skills have been trained primarily by means of the Wisconsin Card Sorting Test (WCST). These studies all show some positive effects of training. The greatest gains have been attained by providing positive reinforcement for correct solutions. It has not been possible to demonstrate any evidence of generalization for improved executive functions. Bellack and co-workers (1996) showed that schizophrenic patients trained on one of two problem-solving tasks similar to the WCST exhibited a marked improvement on the trained task. However, subjects trained on one test performed no better on the other instrument than subjects who received practice only.

3.3.2 Remediation of attentional skills

Regarding attentional skills (for reviews, see Silverstein *et al.* 2001; Suslow *et al.* 2001), two of the most common measures are the Continuous Performance Test (CPT) and the Span Task. Benedict and associates (1994) used six training tasks that all required sustained vigilance and a high degree of mental effort. Results showed improved performance on the training tasks for the experimental group. However, no significant changes on the outcome measures were observed. Benedict and associates (1994) therefore conclude that the rather substantial practice effect demonstrated did not denote an improved fundamental cognitive skill.

The conclusion of Benedict and associates (1994) is in accordance with the view of Bellack *et al.* (1996). They are sceptical as to whether cognitive rehabilitation of schizophrenic patients is an achievable goal. They admit that practice on tasks can improve performance on that specific task, but state that there is little evidence for the generalizability of such training. Thus, they claim that the task for schizophrenia researchers is to develop real-world training programmes.

Several more positive attempts to train attentional deficits in patients with schizophrenia have been carried out recently.

♦ Kern and associates (1995) compared four groups of schizophrenic patients in regard to improved performance on a Span task. The findings revealed that the combination of monetary reinforcement and instructional cues was superior to other interventions. In the Oslo Cognitive Training Programme that will be outlined in Section 4, we have included an intensive Span training with reinforcement, similar to that used by Kern and associates.

◆ Hermanutz and Gestrich (1991) showed that it was possible to reduce the distraction of schizophrenic patients on reaction-time tasks.

◆ Olbrich *et al.* (1993) found clearly positive effects of a training module that addresses a combination of attentional, mnemonic, and conceptual skills.

◆ Van der Gaag (1992) employed a clinical rehabilitation programme and showed that, although the training programme was effective in some processing domains, it did not affect tasks that rely on fast processing of information.

◆ Medalia *et al.* (1998) assessed the impact of attention training with chronic schizophrenia patients. They found that it is feasible to use practice and behavioural learning to remediate core attention deficits in this patient group.

3.3.3 Remediation of memory

In addition several attempts have also been made to improve memory in schizophrenic patients. For instance, Koh *et al.* (1976) showed that patients were able to increase recall on a memory task to levels close to that of normal control subjects when their encoding was aided by rating stimuli (words) in terms of pleasantness.

3.4 Other views on cognitive remediation in schizophrenia

In a recent issue of *Schizophrenia Bulletin* (no. 1, 1999), the theme was interventions for neurocognitive deficits in schizophrenia. Here several outstanding therapists and researchers ask pertinent questions about the results and designs of cognitive remediation research. Bellack *et al.* (1999) point out that the critical question in selecting neurocognitive targets is one of generalizability. They question how far-reaching the effects of training in any basic information-processing domain are. Bellack and collaborators propose an alternative to the cognitive rehabilitation programmes mentioned above. They claim that a compensatory model is much more appropriate. Their emphasis is not on eliminating impairment so much as on minimizing the resulting disability. Bellack and associates are critical of the belief that the neurodevelopmental nature of impairments defies simple solution. Further, they don't find that rehabilitation strategies depending primarily on repeated practice of neuropsychological tasks yield much improvement in the underlying cognitive operations, or have much benefit for community functioning.

Green and Nuechterlein (1999) point out another important issue. Some neurocognitive deficits in schizophrenia are rather stable over time and thus it would be unreasonable to expect longstanding deficits to improve permanently after a short-term treatment. They also point out that the key question is whether changes in neurocognition translate into changes in functional outcome.

Studies using the process-oriented approach are summarized in Table 35.1.

Table 35.1 The process-oriented approach. Characteristics of outcome studies

Study*	Outcome of cognitive training
Koh et al. 1976	Increased recall on memory task
Hermanutz and Gastrich 1991	Reduced distraction
Van der Gaag 1992	No sign of improvement
Benedict et al. 1994	Improvement on attention task
Hodel and Brenner 1994	Reduction of symptoms
Kern et al. 1995	Improved span of apprehension
Bellack et al. 1996	Marked improvement on WCST
Medalia et al. 1998[†]	Positive effect on attention
Spaulding et al. 1999[‡]	Improvement on cognitive function
Wykes et al. 1999	Improvement in cognitive flexibility/memory

* The groups studied are schizophrenic patients unless otherwise indicated.

[†] This was a study comprising chronic schizophrenic patients.

[‡] This was a study comprising chronic psychotic patients.

4 The Oslo Cognitive Training Programme

The cognitive training programme developed at the Sogn Centre for Child and Adolescent Psychiatry (SCCAP) in Oslo aims to improve cognitive functioning and to develop and strengthen cognitive skills. It takes into account the specific psychopathological characteristics of schizophrenia. The development of the Oslo Cognitive Training Programme is based on research demonstrating that the most significant dysfunctions in schizophrenia can be related to the areas of attention, memory, and executive functions. Using the 'Oslo approach', we have attempted to develop a programme that covers all these areas of dysfunction.

The treatment programme is, however, also based on the presumption that cognitive impairment is a key characteristic in other psychotic disorders. A broad spectrum of psychotic patients is thus included in the study (Rund and Borg 1999).

The controlled treatment study at SCCAP aims to investigate to what extent this cognitive training programme can be a positive clinical supplement to a previously documented psychoeducational training programme that has proven quite effective (Rund et al. 1994). The psychoeducational programme was carried out at SCCAP in the late 1980s and early 1990s. The outcome of this programme was compared with that of a standard reference treatment. Clinical outcome was assessed by relapses during the 2-year treatment period and by changes in psychosocial functioning as measured by the Global Assessment Scale (GAS). The results indicated that the most effective programme as measured by relapse was also the cheapest—namely, the psychoeducational programme. Psychosocial functioning improved more, close to significance, in the psychoeducational group. Patients with poor premorbid psychosocial functioning benefit most from this treatment.

In the controlled treatment study now taking place at SCCAP, the question of whether a cognitive training programme can add anything to the effects of a psychoeducational programme alone, will be assessed by comparing two groups at baseline, post-treatment, and at a 1 year follow-up.

- Group A receives a psycho-educational programme alone.
- Group B receives the same psychoeducational treatment package as group A plus the cognitive training programme.

We have chosen a battery of outcome measures for evaluating treatment effects on cognition as well as psychiatric symptoms (Brief Psychiatric Rating Scale (BPRS)) and psychosocial functioning (GAS).

4.1 The training programme

The programme is arranged in four modules: cognitive differentiation; attention; memory; and social perception.

- The *cognitive differentiation module* is based on the supposition of a generalized impairment in verbal intelligence, abstraction–flexibility, and auditory processing that is congruent with a left-hemispheric dysfunction hypothesis. Much of Brenner *et al.*'s (1995) original methodology is adapted for these tasks.
- The *attention module* considers impairment of attention as a central feature of schizophrenia. With the assumption that deficits in attention are part of an underlying mechanism of other cognitive dysfunctions, tasks aim to strengthen sustained attention over time, as well as train selective attention and scanning abilities.
- The *memory module* is based on studies involving both verbal and visual memory. Tasks that primarily involve short-term recall aim to improve the patient's ability to recall an increasing number of items.
- The *social perception module* involves the cognitive processes that allow the patient to respond and adapt appropriately to his or her environment.

Training in verbal communication, attention, memory, and social perception is conducted by administering systematic training procedures.

- During the cognitive differentiation module patients learn to discriminate among stimulus categories by participating in a card-sorting task. After demonstrating competence on this task, patients are introduced to a concept formation task in which they are instructed to match antonyms and synonyms, distinguish concepts with different definitions, and establish a hierarchy of related concepts (Brenner *et al.* 1992).
- Attention and memory modules are presented simultaneously with the concept formation task.

+ Following these modules, patients participate in the social perception module where they are trained to encode social stimuli by viewing a series of slides showing actors in different social activities and demonstrating emotions of varied intensity.

In the social perception module the focus is on improving the patient's ability to attend to the statements of others and to understand accurately what was said, as well as to encourage association between the patients' thoughts and the statements of those with whom they interact. This training attempts to address the lack of integration between strategies that target information processing and social learning dysfunction.

4.2 Programme structure

The four modules are systematically introduced to the patient over a period of 8–10 weeks. The training consists of 30–35 hours of individual training with 15-minute work sessions. The programme is designed so that the patient begins with elementary tasks and progresses to more difficult ones. The rate of progression is determined by the individual's functioning, though a standard protocol provides the structure for progression.

In addition to the cognitive training programme outlined in Section 4.1, all patients in Group B participate in an intensive span of apprehension training. Patients are administered the same computerized version of the Span of Apprehension task (Asarnow and Nuechterlein, version 1987) in six different sessions:

+ session 1, baseline;
+ sessions 2–4, 3 consecutive days of intervention;
+ session 5, immediate post-test;
+ session 6, at the 10-day follow-up.

The Span task is run on an IBM computer. There are 128 test trials, consisting of 3- and 12-letter arrays. Patients are instructed to identify which of two target letters (T or F) appear on the screen by pressing one of two buttons (marked T or F, respectively) on a control pad as quickly as possible. During interventions 2, 3, and 4, patients receive both monetary reinforcement and enhanced instructions. The reward (50 øre) is given immediately following a correct response by dropping the coin into a metal container placed to the patient's right.

4.3 Initiation of the programme

Following completion of baseline measures of the patient's current level of functioning, he/she is given a standard introduction to the training programme and develops a training schedule together with the therapist. We have chosen to implement our programme individually instead of in a group.

+ Early on in the development of the training, it became clear that the patients themselves preferred individual sessions.

◆ In addition, these allow the therapist to take into consideration patients' tremendous variation in cognitive functioning, and thus progress at an appropriate rate while adhering to the standard protocol.

The cognitive training for the most part takes place in the school at the clinic. A teacher is responsible for this part of the programme. A few tasks, such as the visual scanning task 'Where is Willy', take place in the ward.

4.4 Some preliminary results from the Oslo study

The primary question asked in the present study is whether the Cognitive Training Programme adds anything to the psychosocial (psychoeducative) programme. We have examined two central WCST measures at baseline, at post-test (after 5 months of treatment), and at follow-up 1 year later. The results show an improvement in both groups' performance, but no difference in degree of performance between those who have received cognitive training and those who have not. The same pattern is evident for the Backward Masking task as well as the CPT. (Backward masking is a measure of early information processing.) The conclusion that can be drawn from these preliminary results is that the treatment (or the natural course of the illness) contributes to an improvement in patients' cognitive functioning. However, it is uncertain whether the cognitive training programme contributes specifically to the improvement.

The second question that can be asked at the present stage of the study is, 'Is it possible to improve patients' attentional performance (concentration) by intensive training over a week, and with monetary reinforcement and enhanced instructions added to the intervention?' Results indicate that span of apprehension can be improved by cognitive training (Ueland *et al.* 2003).

5 Conclusions

Considering the results from the studies of Hans Brenner, Will Spaulding, and Til Wykes, as well as the preliminary findings in our project, the following answers to the questions asked in this study emerge.

1 Can basic cognitive functions be remediated?
Yes, cognitive remediation works in the sense that it is possible to remediate cognitive dysfunctions in psychotic patients. What works is uncertain, however. Our preliminary results provide no basis for assuming that the cognitive training programme is more effective than the psychoeducational programme alone. This stands in a certain contrast to the findings of Will Spaulding and Til Wykes. It might be, however, that our psychoeducational therapy includes elements that are more effective in improving cognitive skills than the treatment given to the comparison groups in the two other studies. It is also possible that the number of training hours in The Oslo Cognitive Training Programme is not sufficient and needs to be increased in order to obtain significant results.

2   Is it possible to generalize training effects to other functions, and register this by use of appropriate (cognitive and clinical) follow-up instruments?

There is little evidence in the studies mentioned above for a generalizability of cognitive training.

3   Is it possible to improve attentional skills by intensive Span training?

Yes, more intensive training sessions, combined with reinforcement, are effective in improving concentration (continuous focusing of attention). This has been shown in the present study, as well as in several previous studies (Koh *et al.* 1976; Hermanutz and Gestrich 1991; Kern *et al.* 1995). The challenge is to determine how to obtain lasting results which have an impact on the patient's daily functioning.

We have learned that it is difficult to carry out a systematic and consistent cognitive training programme in a clinical setting.

◆   It is difficult to be totally sure that the treatment provided to the two patient groups is in accordance with the therapy manuals.

◆   It is also very difficult to determine the effects of neuroleptics. It would be impossible, for ethical reasons, either to withdraw all patients from antipsychotic medication or to give all patients a standard dosage of medicines.

◆   Further, the researcher cannot require that all patients be on the same drug and the same dosage over a treatment period that lasts for at least 18 months.

Should the 'experiment' of cognitive remediation of psychotic patients continue? In my opinion, the answer is yes. We have sufficient positive results to support this conclusion. We have not received any reports of negative results or negative consequences of cognitive training. More data and new analyses of which variables are related to each other might throw light on which factors are influencing cognitive functions. Most probably, the improvement found in our study cannot be attributed to the inherent process of the illness alone (spontaneous remission), independent of the treatment received. We have sufficient empirical evidence that the typical course of schizophrenia is one with many relapses, in which the level of patients' social and cognitive functioning goes up and down. With a longitudinal design such as ours, with patient assessment at intervals of 5 and 18 months, there is reason to assume that no improvement would have been found on the average for the group if no treatment factors had been influencing cognitive functioning.

It is important to remediate cognitive dysfunctions in patients with schizophrenia. Treatment programmes that do not take cognitive functions into consideration are of limited interest and value. From this point of view, there are no alternatives to cognitive training programmes at the present time. Therefore, it is necessary to further develop useful therapeutic interventions. The only way to do this is to gather empirical evidence for what works in this connection and what does not work. From a clinical perspective, it is warranted to individualize the cognitive training programmes for each patient according to the deficits disclosed through baseline assessments. A related challenge is to find out which patients benefit from cognitive training and which do not.

In order to answer these and related questions it may be necessary to undertake case studies. However, research based on individualized therapeutic interventions continues to be problematic. Thus, a first step in creating evidence-based therapy for patients with schizophrenia—to assess what works and what does not work—seems to be controlled-effect studies in which the effects of therapeutic programmes/manuals are studied at a group level.

Selective references

American Psychiatric Association. (1994). *Diagnostic and statistical manual of mental disorders,* 4th edn. American Psychiatric Association, Washington, DC.

Adams, H.E., Malatesta, W., Brandley, P.J., *et al.* (1981). Modification of cognitive procesesses: a case study of schizophrenia. *J. Consult. Clin. Psychol.* 49, 460–4.

Andreasen, N.C. (1999). A unitary model of schizophrenia. Bleuler's 'Fragmented Phrene' as schizencephaly. *Arch. Gen. Psychiatry* 56, 781–6.

Attkisson, C., Crook, J., Karno, M., *et al.* (1992). Clinical services, research. *Schiz. Bull.* 18, 561–626.

Beck, A.T., Rush, A.J., Shaw, B.J., *et al.* (1979). *Cognitive therapy of depression.* Wiley, Chichester.

Bellack, A.S, Blanchard, J.J., Murphy, P., *et al.* (1996). Generalization effects of training on the Wisconsin Card Sorting Test for schizophrenia patients. *Schizophren. Res.* 19, 189–94.

Bellack, A.S., Gold, J.M., and Buchanan, R.W. (1999). Cognitive rehabilitation for schizophrenia: problems, prospects, and strategies. *Schizophren. Bull.* 25, 257–74.

Benedict, R.H.B., Harris, A.E., Markow, T., *et al.* (1994). The effects of attention training on information processing in schizophrenia. *Schizophren. Bull.* 20, 537–46.

Bentall, R.P., Haddock, G., and Slade, P.D. (1994). Cognitive behaviour therapy for persistent auditory hallucinations: from theory to therapy. *Behav. Ther.* 25, 51–66.

Brenner, H.D., Hodel, B., Roder, V., *et al.* (1992). Treatment of cognitive dysfunctions and behavioural deficits. *Schizophren. Bull.* 18, 21–6.

Brenner, H., Roder, W., Hodel, B., *et al.* (1995). *Integrated psychological therapy for schizophrenic patients.* Hogrefe and Huber, Bern.

Fowler, D. (1992). Cognitive behaviour therapy in management of patients with schizophrenia. Preliminary studies. In *Psychotherapy of schizophrenia: facilitating an abstractive factor* (ed. A. Verbart *et al.*), pp. 145–53. Scandinavian University Press, Oslo.

Fowler, D. and Morley, S. (1989). The cognitive behavioural treatment of hallucinations and delusions: a preliminary study. *Behav. Psychother.* 17, 267–82.

Garety, P.A., Kuipers, L., Fowler, D., *et al.* (1994). Cognitive behavioural therapy for drug resistant psychosis. *Br. J. Med. Psychol.* 67, 259–71.

Green, M.F. (1998). *Schizophrenia from a neurocognitive perspective.* Probing the impenetrable darkness. Allyn and Bacon, Boston.

Green, M.F. and Nuechterlein, K. (1999). Should schizophrenia be treated as a neurocognitive disorder? *Schizophren. Bull.* 25, 309–19.

Hermanutz, M. and Gestrich, J. (1991). Computer-assisted attention training in schizophrenics. A comparative study. *Eur. Arch. Psychiatry Clin. Neurosci.* 240, 282–7.

Hodel, B. and Brenner, H.D. (1994). Cognitive therapy with schizophrenic patients: conceptual basis, present state, future directions. *Acta Psychiatrica Scand.* **90** (suppl. 384), 108–15.

Hogarty, G.E. and Flesher, S. (1999). Developmental theory for a cognitive enhancement therapy of schizophrenia. *Schizophren. Bull.* **25**, 677–92.

Kern, R.S., Green, M.F., and Goldstein, M.F. (1995). Modification of performance on the span of apprehension, a putative marker of vulnerability to schizophrenia. *J. Abnorm. Psychol.* **104**, 385–409.

Kingdon, D.G. and Turkington, D. (1994). *Cognitive–behavioural therapy of schizophrenia.* Guilford Press, Hillside, New Jersey.

Klosterkøtter, J. and Schultze-Lutter, F. (2000). Diagnosing schizophrenia in the initial prodomal phase [abstract]. *Schiz. Res.* **41**, 10.

Koh, S.D., Kayton, L., and Peterson, R.A. (1976). Affective encoding and consequent remembering in schizophrenic young adults. *J. Abnorm. Psychol.* **85**, 56–166.

Lehman, A.F., Carpenter, W.T., Goldman, H.H., *et al.* (1995). Treatment outcomes in schizophrenia: implication for practice, policy and research. *Schizophren. Bull.* **21**, 669–74.

Medalia, A., Aluma, M., Tryon, W., *et al.* (1998). Effectiveness of attention training in schizophrenia. *Schizophren. Bull.* **24**, 147–52.

Olbrich, R., Voss, E., Mussgay, L., *et al.* (1993). A weighted time budget approach for the assessment of cognitive and social activities. *Soc. Psychiatric Epidemiol.* **28**, 184–8.

Perris, C. (1989). *Cognitive therapy for patients with schizophrenia.* Cassel, New York.

Rund, B.R. and Borg, N.C. (1999). Cognitive deficits and cognitive training in schizophrenic patients: a review. *Acta Psychiatrica Scand.* **99**, 1–12.

Rund, B.R., Moe, L., Sollien, T., *et al.* (1994). The Psychosis Project: outcome and cost-effectiveness of a psychoeducational treatment programme for schizophrenic adolescents. *Acta Psychiatrica Scand.* **89**, 211–18.

Sharma, T. (1999). Cognitive effects of conventional and atypical antipychotics in schizophrenia. *Br. J. Psychiatry* **174** (suppl. 38), 44–51.

Silverstein, S.M., Menditto, A.A., and Stuve, P. (2001). Shaping attention span: an operant conditioning procedure to improve neurocognition and functioning in schizophrenia. *Schizophren. Bull.* **27**, 247–57.

Spaulding, W.D., Reed, D., Sullivan, M., *et al.* (1999). Effects of cognitive treatment in psychiatric rehabiliation. *Schizophren. Bull.* **25**, 657–76.

Suslow, T., Schonauer, K., and Arolt, V. (2001). Attention training in the cognitive rehabilitation of schizophrenic patients: a review of efficacy studies. *Acta Psychiatrica Scand.* **103**, 15–23.

Ueland, T., Rund, B.R., Borg, N.E., *et al.* (2003). Modification of performance on the span of apprehension task in a group of young people with early onset psychosis. *Scand. J. Psychol.*, in press.

Van der Gaag, M. (1992). *The results of cognitive training in schizophrenic patients.* Eburon Publishers, Delft.

Wykes, T., Reeder, C., Corner, J., *et al.* (1999).The effects of neurocognitive remediation on executive processing in patients with schizophrenia. *Schizophren. Bull.* **25**, 291–307.

Chapter 36

Treatment and rehabilitation of neuropsychiatric disorders

Laura H. Goldstein

1 Introduction

This chapter will consider some issues and provide a number of guidelines that should be borne in mind when considering the psychological treatments of neuropsychiatric disorders. Neuropsychiatry itself has been defined in a number of ways (Seli and Shapiro 1997) but for present purposes is best conceptualized as 'an aspect of psychiatry that seeks to advance the understanding of clinical problems through increased knowledge of brain function and structure' (Lishman 1992) and, as indicated by Lishman (1992), neuropsychiatry has greater applicability to some forms of mental illness than others. In practice, neuropsychiatry services tend to see three broad categories of patients:

- those whose psychiatric disorders result from clearly identifiable brain dysfunction;
- patients with psychiatric problems with neurological comorbidity;
- patients who present with neurological symptoms in the absence of underlying neurological disease (Lishman 1992).

It is towards the third of these groups of patients that psychological interventions are most likely to be targeted and therefore most attention will be given to these conditions within this chapter. However, since neurological and psychiatric disorders are clearly not mutually exclusive, issues relevant to the treatment of one class of disorders may be applicable to the other.

2 Assessment

Chapters 33 and 34 has described some of the neuropsychiatric conditions and investigations necessary to enable the clinician to arrive at a neuropsychiatric diagnosis. However, when commencing treatment, further assessment by the clinical psychologist will inevitably be necessary in order to document the nature of the thought pattern that may be problematic (e.g. in depression, where the patient will be required, in a cognitive behavioural therapy framework, to record negative automatic thoughts as well as activity schedules), the patient's psychophysiological disturbance, or the frequency or pattern of occurrence of the behaviour that is to be changed (e.g. challenging behaviour after head injury or tics in Tourette's syndrome). Even pharmacological treatments of disorders will require good baseline recording of the behaviour or thought pattern to be changed so that clinical psychologists' skills in this area can also contribute to the careful evaluation of treatment efficacy.

2.1 The antecedents–behaviour–consequences (A–B–C) model

In terms of behavioural assessments, the classical approaches to functional analysis remain of considerable value (see Goldstein 1993). The simplest of these is the A–B–C model, which assesses the antecedents and setting events of the behaviour, the behaviour itself, and the consequences of the behaviour. This can be applied to challenging behaviour (e.g. aggression following closed head injury) or brief dissociative events such as non-epileptic seizures (see Section 4.2.4), although it would be less commonly applied to the assessment of psychiatric symptoms such as might be present in delusional disorders. However, the A–B link might be worthy of consideration in attempting to examine any potential relationship between psychotic phenomena (the 'behaviour' in this example) and the occurrence of epileptic activity (the 'antecendent' in this example) in individuals being investigated with respect to the possible diagnosis of a post-ictal psychosis.

2.2 Other models of functional analysis

- Other models of functional analysis (e.g. Gardner 1971) extend the area of enquiry to the *interrelationship between problem behaviours*, and the therapist will need to become aware of the broader environment in which the patient exists and identify the resources available to the person to assist in treatment as well as the factors that might exert aversive control over them and their behaviour.

- *Motivational analysis* can also be used to increase the likelihood of treatment success (Kanfer and Saslow 1969), and to identify behavioural strengths as well as weaknesses that can help maximize the opportunities for facilitating progress in therapy (Yule 1987).

- The therapist should also consider *developmental factors* (relevant biological, sociological, and behavioural changes that have occurred in the person's life) since these may also impact on therapy and its likely outcome, as may the interrelationship between the social, cultural, and physical aspects of the person's life.

- More recently, it has become common to consider the *predisposing, precipitating,* and *perpetuating factors* that account for a patient's problems (e.g. Mayou *et al.* 1995; Sharpe *et al.* 1995*a*).

- Further insight into the nature of the behaviour and the pattern of its occurrence can be gained through the use of *analogue conditions* where the possible A–B–C relationships can be manipulated (e.g. Iwata *et al.* 1982).

- During treatment using cognitive behaviour therapy, the use of *behavioural experiments*, where the validity of patients' automatic thoughts can be challenged, can be used to test out the content of their beliefs and then disconfirm them.

How behaviour is measured will to some extent depend on the behaviour itself and the resources available. For thought patterns, self-report is necessary. However, for overt behaviours a variety of techniques exists, each with their advantages and disadvantages (Murphy 1987). In each case the clinician should, wherever possible, use measures with proven validity and reliability so that the extent of change can be estimated accurately.

3 Applying psychological interventions to neuropsychiatric disorders

3.1 The importance of awareness and insight

As discussed by Manchester and Wood (2000), cognitive behaviour therapy has been applied to a range of psychiatric disorders in which the awareness of, or insight into, the inappropriate behaviour or thoughts might be sufficient to facilitate change in the person's thoughts and behaviour, via therapy. With respect to psychiatric disorders, insight might be conceived as awareness by the person that they are suffering from a mental disturbance that may constitute an illness and acceptance of the resulting medical implications and of the need for treatment (Surguladze and David 1999). As Surguladze and David (1999) indicate insight is not considered as an 'all-or-none' phenomenon but rather a dimensional one, with individuals having varying levels of awareness of their condition.

As Manchester and Wood (2000) note, impaired awareness is an important characteristic of many neuropsychiatric disorders, and as such has implications for the access to and continued contact with services, relapse rates, and morbidity (Kent and Yellowlees 1994; Kemp and David 1995). Husted (1999), defining insight in terms of awareness of having an illness, attributing one's symptoms to the illness, and acknowledging the need for treatment, observes that one of the difficulties in delivering continuous voluntary treatment for people with severe mental illnesses is that these disorders reflect disrupted brain function and in turn affect the person's reasoning ability so that they often do not believe that they are ill or that their illness will respond to pharmacological (or other) treatments.

Impaired insight is frequently found in schizophrenia (Husted 1999) and is also of importance in bipolar disorder (Husted 1999). It is worth noting that insight in bipolar disorder has been shown to be more severely affected than has insight in affective disorders (Michalakeas *et al.* 1994; Ghaemi *et al.* 1995). Importantly, insight may not recover with treatment (Peralta and Cuesta 1998). As suggested by Surguladze and David (1999), the clinician should be aware that insight may be impaired in other neuropsychiatric disorders such as obsessive–compulsive disorder (Eisen *et al.* 1994) and anorexia nervosa (Feighner *et al.* 1972) and thus the concept is relevant to those undertaking therapy with a wide range of patients.

The clinician should recognize that insight, or lack of it, cannot be simply related to neuropsychological test performance, as the results from a number of studies across different disorders are contradictory (Surguladze and David 1999). However cognitive abilities, whether one is focusing on executive function or more general abilities, may nonetheless be related to measures of insight and to specific activities that require the person to undertake cognitively demanding introspection into particular aspects of their own mental life (Surguladze and David 1999). As noted by Surguladze and David (1999), a number of approaches to the assessment of insight in psychiatric disorders have been developed (e.g. McEvoy *et al.* 1989; Amador and Strauss 1990; David 1990; Markova and Berrios 1992; Birchwood *et al.* 1994; Kemp and David 1997).

It is widely accepted that lack of awareness or insight is a common feature of people who have sustained brain damage, whether of a traumatic or of a neurodegenerative nature (Migliorelli *et al.* 1995; Zanetti *et al.* 1999). The integrity of insight or awareness has been shown to relate to the success of neurorehabilitation (Ben-Yishay and Gold 1990; Prigatano 1991) although some inconsistencies have been noted, possibly relating to differences in measuring or defining insight and outcome (Malia 1997). Of clinical relevance also are recent observations that individuals may be unaware of some deficits but not others (Dalla Barba *et al.* 1999). Manchester and Wood (2000) suggest that, whilst most therapeutic interventions can be modified to accommodate poor memory, attention, and concentration, it is the need to overcome poor awareness, and also poor motivation, that may often be the crucial factor in bringing about treatment success. Issues relating to motivation will be considered next.

3.2 Motivation to change

Manchester and Wood (2000) have suggested a pivotal role for the establishment of a good therapeutic relationship as a means of increasing both the awareness of people with brain damage concerning their problems and their motivation to change. They stress the importance of therapist variables such as warmth, support, empathy, non-judgemental attitude, and the expectation that change will occur (Leber and Jenkins 1996). They also emphasize the need for therapists to understand their patients' thinking patterns and to engage in a collaborative rather than confrontational approach to therapy. Although there is no supportive empirical evidence to date, they favour the use of motivational interviewing as a means of raising questions about the viability of the person's thinking and behaviour. They also note that it may be useful, in line with Miller and Rolnick (1991), to consider motivation for change in people with brain damage as something that fluctuates over time and across situations. The potential use of a motivational approach for people with cognitive impairment has also obtained some support from its, albeit limited, application in the field of learning disabilities (Rose and Walker 2000).

3.2.1 A six-stage model of change

Manchester and Wood (2000) outline and recommend the use of Prochaska and DiClemente's (1982) six-stage model of change in providing a useful guide to therapy, both from the point of developing awareness of problems, and increasing motivation to change. These stages are:

- the *pre-contemplation stage* where others are aware that there is a problems but the patient has not yet considered the possibility of changing;
- the *contemplation stage* where the patient is aware of the need to change but may feel ambivalence over this;
- the *determination stage* where the patient decides to take action;
- the *action stage* where the patient undertakes activities to achieve change;
- the *maintenance stage* where additional skills are learned to prevent relapse;
- the *relapse stage* where the patient learns to cope with relapse.

Manchester and Wood (2000) illustrate the use of this model with two patients with very different behavioural problems following acquired brain injury.

With respect to one of these cases, the individual had sustained severe cognitive impairment and therapy was designed to increase his motivation to stop absconding from the treatment unit in response to negative feedback from staff about his sexually inappropriate behaviour.

- The *pre-contemplation* and *contemplation* stages involved first asking the patient why he absconded and what the consequences (positive and negative) of this were, with respect both to the short and longer term. Where negative consequences could not be identified explicitly, the patient was asked to describe how the events following his absconding made him feel.

- The *determination* and *action* stages of treatment involved facilitating the generation of longer-term goals by the patient and his commitment to attempt alternative behaviour in order to achieve these. In this case the longer-term goal was to achieve discharge from the unit and alternative behaviours included more appropriate ways of responding to criticism by unit staff. The process was then reviewed by the therapist and by the patient; the patient was asked to state the behavioural trigger, the old response and its negative consequences, and the new response and its positive consequences. The patient's commitment to change was praised, the difficulty involved in changing behaviour was acknowledged, and the need for practice to achieve the consistent establishment of the new responses was emphasized.

- The *maintenance* stage involved the development of a verbal script for the patient to employ and role-play exercises.

- Finally instances of *relapse* were used to identify difficulties the patient experienced in applying the new behaviours and these were incorporated into role-play exercises.

Other approaches to increasing awareness do exist, however (see Malia 1997 for a recent account of techniques), and formal evaluation of such approaches will ultimately guide the therapist's choice of techniques. It may also be necessary to bear in mind that it is sometimes difficult to distinguish between the lack of awareness of deficits due to clear evidence of brain damage and the use of denial as a defence mechanism (Malia 1997; Manchester and Wood 2000). Both Malia (1997) and Manchester and Wood (2000) highlight the need for clinicians to consider that both psychological factors and the direct impact of brain damage may interact to produce the level of awareness that is apparent in an individual patient.

4 The application of cognitive behavioural therapy to neuropsychiatric disorders

4.1 Disorders with an identifiable organic basis

Relatively little attention has been paid to the application of cognitive behavioural techniques to neuropsychiatric disorders in which the resulting cognitive impairment might itself necessitate modification of the techniques in use. Manchester and Wood (2000) suggest that, where there is cognitive impairment:

◆ The clinician may need to make therapy sessions more highly structured;

◆ The sessions may need to occur with greater frequency.

◆ The sessions might need to deal with more specific behaviours, possibly in a more concrete way.

In addition:

◆ It may be necessary to adapt therapy techniques and materials to overcome a person's memory or reading impairments (e.g. Newsom-Davis *et al.* 1998), and here note must be taken of findings from neuropsychological assessments that have been undertaken.

◆ Where an assessment of cognitive functions has not been done, such an assessment may be of value in order for therapy to be targeted at the appropriate level.

However, in general, there is little to guide the clinician as to when cognitive and neurological signs might predict poor response to treatment. For example a recent study found that neuropsychological abnormalities and neurological soft signs in adults with obsessive–compulsive disorder did not predict a poor response to behavioural treatment (Bolton *et al.* 2000). Similarly, no data yet exist to indicate whether cerebral activation abnormalities recently detected in a patient with conversion disorder (Marshall *et al.* 1997) might have any implications for treatment.

In the field of adult mental health, cognitive behaviour therapy (CBT) has been widely applied to people with depression and various anxiety disorders (e.g. Hawton *et al.* 1989) and is also now being applied to disorders such as schizophrenia and bipolar disorder where insight or awareness of difficulties may be an issue (e.g. Kuipers *et al.* 1998; Lam *et al.* 2000).

◆ Kuipers *et al.* (1998) reported that 9 months of CBT, directed at medication-resistant symptoms of *psychosis*, led to a reduction in the distress caused by delusions and in the frequency of hallucinations, with the improvement persisting at an 18-month follow-up. They reported clinical improvements in 65% of the CBT group and in only 17% of the standard care group.

- With respect to *bipolar disorder*, preliminary evidence (Lam *et al.* 2000) suggests that, in comparison to standard care, people undergoing CBT (incorporating a psychoeducational model, using CBT skills to enable people to cope with prodromes, emphasizing the importance of routine and sleep and dealing with long-term vulnerabilities and difficulties resulting from the illness, and undertaken during 12–20 sessions over 6 months) experienced fewer hypomanic and total bipolar episodes, demonstrated better medical compliance, and had higher social functioning and better coping strategies for bipolar prodromes.

However, there are few formal evaluations of the use of CBT to treat affective disorders in patient groups where there is clear evidence of acquired organic pathology such as might be present in disorders more typically presenting with neurological sequelae.

- Larcombe and Wilson (1984) demonstrated the effectiveness of brief, group-based, weekly CBT sessions in reducing depression in a sample of patients with multiple sclerosis for whom depression was the major problem, and at least of moderate severity.

- Davis *et al.* (1984) similarly applied CBT in a group format to a small number of patients with epilepsy, who showed a subsequent reduction in depression scores on various measures.

In neither study was it reported that the CBT required modification in response to any cognitive difficulties of the participants.

More recently, Lincoln *et al.* (1997) reported a number of A–B single-case designs employing CBT with depressed stroke patients, comparing the results of no more than 10 sessions of treatment within a 3-month period, with baseline. Of the 19 patients treated, only eight were noted to show definite although modest improvement. Lincoln *et al.*'s (1997) findings would appear to indicate that:

- stroke patients with intercurrent illness and further stroke might not benefit from treatment;

- patients with impaired memory and reasoning abilities might be less able to understand the concepts underpinning the treatment and therefore might have difficulty applying them independently.

Thus clinicians should bear these difficulties in mind when planning the use of effective CBT for stroke patients. However, clinicians should remember the benefits of facilitating increased leisure activities in improving psychological well-being after stroke if formal CBT proves difficult to implement (Drummond and Walker 1996).

4.2 Medically unexplained disorders

4.2.1 The nature of the problem

Neuropsychiatry services may deal with a range of patients presenting with physical or cognitive disorders for which no medical basis can ultimately be detected, or that are in excess of what is known about the person's medical disorder. These medically unexplained disorders would not include recognized psychiatric symptoms such as delusions and hallucinations.

Within *Diagnostic and statistical manual of mental disorders*, 4th edition (DSM-IV; American Psychiatric Association 1994) such disorders come within the classifications of somatoform disorders (e.g. somatization disorder, conversion disorder, hypochondriasis), factitious disorders, and dissociative disorders. The clinician should be aware that there is ongoing debate about the extent to which such classifications are adequate (Rief and Hiller 1999). In addition, the terminology itself has been questioned (Sharpe *et al.* 1995*b*). Within ICD-10 (World Health Organisation 1992) disorders of interest here, such as dissociative non-epileptic seizures, are classified within the category of dissociative (conversion) disorders.

It is well recognized that medically unexplained disorders pose a sizeable problem for medical services (e.g. Mayou *et al.* 1995; Bass *et al.* 2001; Nimnuan *et al.* 2001). It is worth remembering that patients referred to specialist tertiary services with somatoform or conversion disorders may experience very severe levels of disability in the absence of any underlying organic disorder (Davison *et al.* 1999) or present with symptoms, only some of which will have a clear medical explanation. Here treatment can be useful in enabling the patient to distinguish between those symptoms that are disease-based and those that have a psychological basis (Sharpe *et al.* 1992). However, it is likely that specialist services will see only a fraction of patients with such presentations (Mayou *et al.* 1995).

4.2.2 Approaches to treatment

There is increasing evidence that a cognitive behavioural approach may be of considerable value in treating a number of such disorders (Kroenke and Swindle 2000), although there has been relatively little systematic evaluation of the benefits of psychodynamic psychotherapy (Sharpe *et al.* 1995*a*). Nonetheless, Guthrie (1995) has outlined treatment considerations of relevance to psychodynamic psychotherapists working with patients with functional somatic disorders. Other therapeutic approaches for somatization disorder have included behaviour therapy, exploratory psychotherapy, and group psychotherapy (see review by Wilkinson and Mynors-Wallis 1994). With respect to conversion disorders, where patients present with symptoms that appear to be neurological in nature (e.g. weakness, paralysis, dysphonia, sensory impairment, or memory deficits) the treatment emphasis, within relatively limited studies, appears to be predominantly behavioural (Silver 1996), and the consideration of psychosocial factors would also seem crucial. It is likely, however, that cognitive behavioural therapy will also be applicable to this group of patients (Halligan *et al.* 2000).

Sharpe *et al.* (1992) have described the psychological treatment of what they call functional somatic symptoms, and Speckens *et al.* (1995) have described the additional and successful use of CBT in treating what has more recently been termed 'medically unexplained symptoms', which would appear to include somatization disorder.

Cognitive behavioural treatments for these different disorders vary somewhat, but also share common features. It is likely therefore that the aims considered by the clinician will be:

♦ reducing the patient's stress and disability;

♦ decreasing the patient's symptoms;

♦ limiting inappropriate use of medical and other care (Sharpe *et al.* 1992).

4.2.3 Issues to consider when implementing treatment

Prior to treatment by a clinical psychologist or other psychotherapist such patients are likely to have undergone medical investigations for their symptoms. Bass and Benjamin (1993) have suggested that maintenance of symptoms for longer than 6 months would justify describing the person's disorder as chronic and, given the time that many medical investigations may take to organize, clinicians may well find that they are indeed being asked to treat patients whose symptoms would appear to fall in this category.

The task facing the clinician embarking on psychological interventions with such patients will depend in part on the prior medical approach the patient has experienced. Bass and Benjamin (1993) suggest that such patients require unambiguous information about the results of their medical investigations, and that there should have been a limit set for the range of investigations that might be appropriate, if possible negotiated and agreed between doctor and patient. They highlight the difficulty of doctors worrying about failing to find a treatable medical disorder but not about missing a treatable psychological problem.

♦ Patients should come for psychological treatment having been told clearly what illness(es) they do and do not have, and the symptoms and disability that will and will not be attributable to any such illnesses.

♦ They should come for treatment already knowing that they are to see someone who will be treating their disorder from a psychological perspective, and not from a medical one (Bass and Benjamin 1993).

♦ This should be preceded by a clear account to the patient that all necessary investigations have been undertaken. It would be unwise to embark upon a psychological intervention whilst medical investigations are continuing, as it is important that a certainty about diagnosis can be reached, and that the patient can be given an unambiguous account of the aetiology of their disorder, prior to the commencement of treatment.

Despite these recommendations, it is often unclear to the clinician undertaking the psychological intervention exactly what patients have previously been told about the medical basis or otherwise of their condition. Indeed, some patients will perceive that they have been incorrectly referred for psychological treatment, believing that their problems continue to have a physical basis (Salkovskis 1989). They may also be concerned about the stigma attached to having a psychiatric or psychological as opposed to medical diagnosis (House 1995).

- The clinician should seek early clarification from the referring doctor as to what the patient was told prior to referral. It will be important for the treating clinician to understand the basis on which the patient's diagnosis was made so that a consistent explanation can be given to the patient during therapy and any persisting erroneous beliefs can be corrected (Sharpe *et al.* 1995*a*).

- It may be appropriate for one person to coordinate all the different aspects of the patient's care (medical and psychological) (Sharpe *et al.* 1992; Bass and Benjamin 1993) so that throughout the patient receives consistent explanations about their disorder as well as consistent approaches to treatment. This may be particularly relevant for patients with multiple somatic symptoms (e.g. Smith 1995).

- In addition, there ultimately needs to be a clear communication to the patient's general practitioner about the diagnosis and management (Davison *et al.* 1999) so that treatment is not undermined at this level of care provision.

In all cases, the close liaison between the treating and referring teams is extremely important.

Where possible other, parallel treatments for the same symptoms should be terminated or at the very least suspended while the psychological intervention is underway (Sharpe *et al.* 1992). Withdrawal of medication, which in some instances may actually be having a detrimental effect on the person's condition, should be undertaken in consultation with the prescribing doctor (Salkovskis 1989). However, a role remains for antidepressant medication (Bass and Benjamin 1993).

In terms of treatment success, Bass and Benjamin (1993) review evidence that suggests that sociodemographic factors, pain-related factors, and psychological factors can predict treatment success. Thus age, employment, pain-related financial compensation, pain nature and history, and the extent of dysfunctional illness beliefs and beliefs about illness aetiology as well as mode of referral may all be relevant. However, it is also of considerable importance that the patient:

- engages in treatment;
- accepts that psychological/psychosocial factors are important in maintaining the problem;
- is willing and able to negotiate treatment goals.

4.2.4 The use of CBT with somatoform, factitious, and dissociative conversion disorders

A CBT approach to the treatment of these disorders will essentially be a collaborative one but, depending on the disorder, may require differing numbers of sessions. The essence will be to formulate the person's problems in psychological terms even when their occurrence is complicated by the presence of an existing medical condition (Salkovskis 1989). The clinician needs to remember that the patient may have been used to a more passive role, undergoing medical tests and taking medication (Sharpe *et al.* 1992), and thus may need time to adjust to playing a more active role in their own treatment. As with any psychotherapeutic intervention it will be important for the clinician to establish a good working relationship with the patient, provide a plausible treatment rationale, offer hope for improvement (as a cure may not be a realistic goal; Salkovskis 1989), and be sympathetic to the patient's worries (Sharpe *et al.* 1992).

In the case of dissociative, somatization, or conversion disorder, it will be important to:

- reassure the patient that they are not thought to be 'putting it on' but that their symptoms are real, especially if previous contacts with services have been characterized as dismissive of the patient's symptoms;

- determine whether the patient is misinterpreting bodily signs or symptoms as evidence of illness or whether they have misunderstood or misinterpreted what they have been told by doctors or others so that they perceive slight deviations from the norm as representing serious impairment (Salkovskis 1989).

In the case of factitious disorder, where there is deliberate production or feigning of physical or psychological symptoms, this being motivated by the adoption of the sick role, then therapy needs to assist patients to understand why they are acting in that way, in a non-judgemental manner (Kinsella 2001).

An important aspect of treatment will be for the clinician to involve the family members/carers, and to provide them with the same treatment rationale. This will allow for the involvement of a co-therapist, who can facilitate generalization of treatment strategies beyond the treatment session.

Somatization disorders   The application of a CBT approach to the treatment of somatic symptoms has largely involved the identification and modification of dysfunctional automatic thoughts and the use of behavioural experiments to break the vicious cycle of the symptoms and their consequences (Speckens *et al.* 1995), with this treatment often taking place in specialist services. Such an approach is often more sophisticated in terms of its components than the previously described, more limited therapeutic approaches designed for use in primary care settings, involving reattribution and problem-solving (Goldberg *et al.* 1989; Wilkinson and Mynors-Wallis 1994). This latter treatment approach seemed to be most beneficial for those people:

- whose somatization had lasted for less than a year;

- who acknowledged prior to treatment that they had psychosocial problems;

- who suffered from anxiety disorders.

In the case of a more traditional CBT approach, clinicians might expect that patients with a high level of illness behaviour might have a relatively poor prognosis (Speckens *et al.* 1997).

Hypochondriasis   Whereas the clinician treating somatization disorders may be faced with the patient who needs to be reassured that the results of their medical investigations have proved negative, the effective use of CBT with a patient with hypochondriasis will need to enable the patient to identify clear evidence that their problem was health anxiety itself (Warwick *et al.* 1996). This may be important in preventing patients from becoming preoccupied with a new disease once they have successfully overcome their fears about the original illness (Warwick *et al.* 1996).

Factitious disorder Little guidance is available for the treatment of factitious disorder (used also to describe patients with what has also been termed 'pseudologia fantastica': e.g. Newmark *et al.* 1999, and Munchausen's syndrome, e.g. Fink and Jensen 1989). Certainly it is important to remember that factitious disorder can occur in the context of organic brain damage (e.g. Lawrie *et al.* 1993).

Within DSM-IV, factitious disorder is defined as involving the intentional production or feigning of physical or psychological signs or symptoms, the motivation for which is the assumption of the sick role and there are no external incentives (such as financial gain, avoiding legal responsibility, or improving physical well-being). This is in contrast to *malingering*, where the person again deliberately produces false or exaggerated physical or psychological symptoms but where the motivation is financial (including compensation for injury), evading legal responsibility, avoiding military duty or other forms of work, or obtaining drugs.

A cognitive–behavioural perspective on factitious disorder has recently been outlined. In such patients the clinician may find the coexistence of symptoms of somatization, factitious disorder, and even malingering (Kinsella 2001). Kinsella (2001) discusses the use of nonpunitive confrontation in cases of factitious disorder. However, nonconfrontational, possibly 'face-saving' approaches may also be of use but require very consistent application by a multidisciplinary team. The clinician should be aware that confrontation may meet with different responses from patients, and Kinsella provides most guidance on the use of CBT with those factitious disorder patients who recognize that they need to stop their pattern of behaviour, are able to admit their need to stop this pattern, and seek help. He suggests that therapy should:

- help the person understand their behaviour;
- address face-saving issues and the benefits and disadvantages of revealing the true picture to family and other professionals;
- identify triggers for the behaviour;
- stress the disadvantages of repeated, often dangerous medical investigations.

In addition, Kinsella recommends that activity scheduling should be used to provide the person with a more pleasurable way of meeting their needs, and the patient's unhelpful cognitive schemas should be addressed. However, as yet there is no formal evaluation of such treatment to guide the clinician as to its effectiveness.

Dissociative conversion disorders In terms of the treatment of dissociative conversion disorders some preliminary evidence, drawn from an open trial of CBT in patients with dissociative non-epileptic seizures (Mitchell-O'Malley *et al.* 2001) exists. Approaches similar to those described above for somatization disorders may be effective in reducing the occurrence of events that superficially resemble epileptic seizures but that do not have an epileptic basis. For a more detailed account see Halligan, Bass, and Marshall 2001). These patients too can be difficult to engage, having probably had multiple prior contacts with medical services.

- They will require a clear message that their attacks do not have an epileptic basis.

- It is essential, however, that these patients are not made to feel that they have been fabricating their seizures but that they are real events, in that they are significant episodes of disturbed behaviour that are disruptive to the person's life and represent the expression of psychological distress.

- The treatment of this group of patients is collaborative in nature and will benefit from the involvement of other key people in the person's life to facilitate appropriate changes to behaviour outside of the treatment session, and to assist with exposure to situations and activities that the person had avoided through fear of having a seizure.

- Specific techniques may be used to distract the person from symptoms warning them that they might be about to experience a seizure and to encourage relaxation, thereby reducing symptoms of anxiety that might precede a seizure.

- Treatment would also involve the use of problem-solving techniques and the challenging of negative automatic thoughts.

- Additional problems that might lead to low mood or act as seizure triggers require attention.

- As with all the other disorders discussed here the therapist needs to consider strategies to enable the patient to prevent relapse of their symptoms.

4.2.5 Treatment of somatic symptoms in older adults

Specific attention has also been paid to the treatment of somatic symptoms in older adults (Pearce and Morris 1995). In this area of work clinicians will need to consider the many age-related changes that may influence symptoms found in the elderly. Thus, in an older age group, in particular, somatic symptoms may be wholly organic in origin, partially explained by disease, or completely functionally determined. In practice, it is more likely for older adults to present with a mixture of organically and functionally based symptoms than younger adults (Pearce and Morris 1995). Thus there will be an emphasis on determining whether the physical condition is a sufficient explanation for the level of disability experienced. In addition, it will be necessary to remember that physical failings can give rise to emotional distress, and early dementias can be accompanied by mood change and concerns over health. Pearce and Morris (1995) suggest that many of the treatment approaches used for somatoform disorders in younger adults may be appropriately modified for use with older adults.

5 Conclusions

Whether treating psychological disorders that have a purely organic basis, that are determined by organic and psychological factors, or that are purely psychological in their aetiology, the clinical psychologist working with a neuropsychiatric population has a number of treatment approaches to employ that require similarly good skills of problem assessment and formulation as well as engagement of what can be very difficult to treat patients. However, the refinement of treatment approaches will be ongoing and the clinician is advised to keep abreast of the accumulating literature relating to developments that continue to occur in this challenging area of clinical work.

Acknowledgements

I am grateful to Dr John Mellers for helpful comments on an earlier version of this chapter.

Selective references

Amador, X.F. and Strauss, D.H. (1990). *The Scale to Assess Unawareness of Mental Disorders* (*SUMD*). Columbia University and New York State Psychiatric Institute, New York.

American Psychiatric Association (1994). *Diagnostic and statistical manual of mental disorders*, 4th edn. American Psychiatric Association, Washington, DC.

Bass, C. and Benjamin, S. (1993). The management of chronic somatisation. *Br. J. Psychiatry* **162**, 472–80.

Bass, C., Peveler, R., and House, A. (2001). Somatoform disorders: severe psychiatric illnesses neglected by psychiatrists. *Br. J. Psychiatry* **179**, 11–14.

Ben-Yishay, Y. and Gold, J. (1990). Therapeutic milieu approach to neuropsychological rehabilitation. In *Neurobehavioural sequelae of traumatic brain injury* (ed. R.L. Wood), pp. 194–215. Taylor and Francis Ltd, New York.

Birchwood, M., Smith, J., Drury, V., Healy, J., Macmillan, F., and Slade, M. (1994). A self-report Insight Scale for psychosis: reliability, validity and sensitivity to change. *Acta Psychiatrica Scand.* **89**, 62–7.

Bolton, D., Raven, P., Madronal-Luque, R., and Marks, I.M. (2000). Neurological and neuropsychological signs in obsessive compulsive disorder: interaction with behavioural treatment. *Behav. Res. Ther.* **38**, 695–708.

David, A.S. (1990). Insight and psychosis. *Br. J. Psychiatry* **156**, 798–809.

Davis, G.R., Armstrong, H.E., Donovan, D.M., and Temkin, N.R. (1984). Cognitive–behavioural treatment of depressed affect among epileptics: preliminary findings. *J. Clin. Psychol.* **40**, 930–5.

Davison, P., Sharpe, M., Wade, D., and Bass, C. (1999). 'Wheelchair' patients with non-organic disease: a psychological inquiry. *J. Psychosom. Res.* **47**, 93–103.

Dalla Barba, G., Bartolomeo, P., Ergis, A.-M., Boissé, M.-F., and Bachoud-Lévi, A.-C. (1999). Awareness of anosognosia following head trauma. *Neurocase* **5**, 59–67.

Drummond, A. and Walker, M. (1996). Generalisation of the effects of leisure rehabilitation for stroke patients. *Br. J. Occup. Ther.* **59**, 330–4.

Eisen, S.V., Dill, D.L., and Grob. M.C. (1994). Reliability and validity of a brief patient-report instrument for psychiatric outcome evaluation. *Hosp. Community Psychiatry* **45**, 242–7.

Feighner, J.P., Robins E., Guze, S.B., Woodruff, R.A. Jr, Winokur, G., and Munoz, R. (1972). Diagnostic criteria for use in psychiatric research. *Arch. Gen. Psychiatry* **26**, 57–63.

Fink, P. and Jensen, J. (1989). Clinical characteristics of the Munchausen syndrome. A review and 3 new case histories. *Psychother. Psychosom.* **52**, 164–71.

Gardner, W.I. (1971). *Behaviour modification in mental retardation*. University of London Press, London.

Ghaemi, S.N., Stoll, A.L., and Pope, H. (1995). Lack of insight in bipolar disorder—the acute manic episode. *J. Nerv. Ment. Dis.* **183**, 464–7.

Goldberg, D., Gask, L., and O'Dowd, T. (1989). The treatment of somatization: teaching techniques of reattribution. *J. Psychosom. Res.* **33**, 689–95.

Goldstein, L.H. (1993). Behaviour problems. In *Neurological rehabilitation* (ed. R. Greenwood, M. Barnes, T. McMillan, and C. Ward), pp. 389–401. Churchill Livingstone, London.

Guthrie, E. (1995). Treatment of functional somatic symptoms: psychodynamic treatment. In *Treatment of functional somatic symptoms* (ed. R. Mayou, C. Bass, and M. Sharpe), pp. 144–60. Oxford University Press, Oxford.

Halligan, P.W., Bass, C., and Wade, D.T. (2000). New approaches to conversion hysteria. *Br. Med. J.* **320**, 1488–9.

Halligan, P.W., Bass, C., and Oakley, D. (2001). *Contemporary Approaches to the Study of Hysteria.* Oxford University Press, Oxford.

Hawton, K., Salkovskis, P.M., Kirk, J., and Clark, D.M. (eds.) (1989). *Cognitive behaviour therapy for psychiatric problems.* Oxford University Press, Oxford.

House, A. (1995). The patient with medically unexplained symptoms: making the initial psychiatric contact. In *Treatment of functional somatic symptoms* (ed. R. Mayou, C. Bass, and M. Sharpe), pp. 89–102. Oxford University Press, Oxford.

Husted, J.R. (1999). Insight in severe mental illness: implications for treatment decisions. *J. Am. Acad. Psychiatry Law* **27**, 33–49.

Iwata, B.A., Dorsey, M.F., and Slifer, K.J. (1982). Towards a functional analysis of self injury. *Anal. Intervent. Devel. Disabil.* **2**, 3–20.

Kanfer, F.M. and Saslow, G. (1969). Behavioural diagnosis. In *Behaviour therapy: appraisal and status* (ed. C.M. Franks), pp. 417–44. McGraw Hill, New York.

Kemp, R. and David, A. (1995). Psychosis: insight and compliance. *Curr. Opin. Psychiatry* **8**, 357–61.

Kemp, R. and David, A. (1997). Insight and compliance. In *Treatment compliance and the treatment alliance in serious mental illness* (ed. B. Blackwell), pp. 61–86, Harwood Academic, The Netherlands.

Kent, S. and Yellowlees, P. (1994). Psychiatric and social reasons for frequent rehospitalisation. *Hosp. Community Psychiatry* **45**, 347–50.

Kinsella, P. (2001). Factitious disorder: a cognitive behavioural perspective. *Behav. Cogn. Psychother.* **29**, 195–202.

Kroenke, K. and Swindle, R. (2000). Cognitive–behavioural therapy for somatisation and symptom syndromes: a critical review of controlled clinical trials. *Psychother. Psychosom.* **69**, 205–15.

Kuipers, E., Fowler, D., Garety, P., Chisholm, D., Freeman, D., Dunn, G., Bebbington, P., and Hadley, C. (1998). London East Anglia randomised control trial of cognitive–behavioural therapy for psychosis. III: Follow-up and economic evaluation at 18 months. *Br. J. Psychiatry* **173**, 61–8.

Lam, D., Bright, J., Jones, S., Hayward, P., Schuck, N., Chisholm, D., and Sham, P. (2000). Cognitive therapy for bipolar illness—a pilot study of relapse prevention. *Cogn. Ther. Res.* **24**, 503–20.

Larcombe, N.A. and Wilson, P.H. (1984). An evaluation of cognitive–behaviour therapy for depression in patients with multiple sclerosis. *Br. J. Psychiatry* **145**, 366–71.

Lawrie, S.M., Goodwin, G., and Masterton, G. (1993). Munchausen's syndrome and organic brain disorder. *Br. J. Psychiatry* **162**, 545–9.

Leber, W. and Jenkins, M.R. (1996). Psychotherapy with clients who have brain injuries and their families. In *Neuropsychology for clinical practice* (ed. R.L. Adams, O.A. Parsons, J.L. Cuthbertson, and S.J. Nixon), pp. 489–506. American Psychological Association, Washington, DC.

Lincoln, N.B., Flannaghan, T., Sutcliffe, L., and Rother, L. (1997). Evaluation of cognitive behavioural treatment for depression after stroke: a pilot study. *Clin. Rehabil.* 11, 114–22.

Lishman, W.A. (1992). What is neuropsychiatry? *J. Neurol. Neurosurg. Psychiatry* 55, 983–5.

Malia, K. (1997). Insight after brain injury: what does it mean? *J. Cogn. Rehabil.* May/June, 10–16.

Manchester, D. and Wood, R.L. (2000). Applying cognitive therapy to neurobehavioural rehabilitation. In *Neurobehavioural disability and social handicap following traumatic brain injury* (ed. R.L. Wood and T.M. McMillan), pp. 157–74. Psychology Press, Hove, East Sussex.

Markova, I.S. and Berrios, G.E. (1992). The assessment of insight in clinical psychiatry: a new scale. *Acta Psychiatrica Scand.* 86, 159–64.

Marshall, J.C., Halligan, P.W., Fink, G.R., Wade, D.T., and Frackowiak, R.S.J. (1997). The functional anatomy of a hysterical paralysis. *Cognition* 64, B1–B8.

Mayou, R., Bass, C., and Sharpe, M. (1995). Overview of epidemiology, classification and aetiology. In *Treatment of functional somatic symptoms* (ed. R. Mayou, C. Bass, and M. Sharpe), pp. 42–65. Oxford University Press, Oxford.

McEvoy, J.P., Apperson, L.J., Appelbaum, P.S., Ortlip, P., Brecosky, J., Hammill, K., Geller, J.L., and Roth, L. (1989). Insight in schizophrenia: its relationship to acute psychopathology. *J. Nerv. Ment. Dis.* 177, 43–7.

Michalakeas, A., Skoutas, C., Charalambous, A., Peristeris, A., Marinos, V., Keramari, E., and Theologou, A. (1994). Insight in schizophrenia and mood disorders and its relation to psychopathology. *Acta Psychiatrica Scand.* 90, 46–9.

Migliorelli, R., Tesón, A., Sabe, L., Petracca, G., Petracchi, M., Leiguarda, R., and Starkstein, S.E. (1995). Anosognosia in Alzheimer's disease: a study of associated factors. *J. Neuropsychiatry Clin. Neurosci.* 7, 338–44.

Miller, W. and Rolnick, S. (1991). *Motivational interviewing.* Guilford Press, New York.

Mitchell-O'Malley, S., Deale, A., Goldstein, L.H., Toone, B., and Mellers, J.D.C. (2001) The cognitive behavioural treatment of non-epileptic seizures: a 6 month follow-up report. *Epilepsia* 42 (Suppl 2) 53.

Murphy, G. (1987). Direct observation as an assessment tool in functional analysis and treatment. In *Assessment in mental handicap. A guide to assessment practice, tools and checklists* (ed. J. Hogg and N.V. Raynes), pp. 190–238. Croom Helm, London.

Newmark, N., Adityanjee, and Kay, J. (1999). Pseudologica fantastica and factitious disorder: review of the literature and a case report. *Comprehens. Psychiatry* 40, 89–95.

Newsom-Davis, I., Goldstein, L.H., and Fitzpatrick, D. (1998). Fear of seizures: an investigation and treatment. *Seizure* 7, 101–6.

Nimnuan, C., Hotopf, M., and Wessely, S. (2001). Medically unexplained symptoms. An epidemiological study in seven specialities. *J. Psychosom. Res.* 51, 361–7.

Pearce, J. and Morris, C. (1995). The treatment of somatic symptoms in the elderly. In *Treatment of functional somatic symptoms* (ed. R. Mayou, C. Bass, and M. Sharpe), pp. 371–87. Oxford University Press, Oxford.

Peralta, V. and Cuesta, M.J. (1998). Lack of insight in mood disorders. *J. Affect. Disord.* 49, 55–8.

Prigatano, G.P. (1991). Disturbances of self awareness of deficit after traumatic brain injury. In *Awareness of deficit after brain injury: clinical and theoretical issues* (ed. G.P. Prigatano and D.L. Schacter), pp. 111–26. Oxford University Press, New York.

Prochaska, J.O. and DiClemente, C.C. (1982). Transtheoretical therapy: towards a more integrative model of change. *Psychother.: Theory, Res., Practice* 19, 276–88.

Rief, W. and Hiller, W. (1999). Toward empirically based criteria for the classification of somatoform disorders. *J. Psychosom. Res.* 46, 507–18.

Rose, J. and Walker, S. (2000). Working with a man who has Prader–Willi syndrome and his support staff using motivational principles. *Behav. Cogn. Psychother.* **28**, 293–302.

Salkovskis, P.M. (1989). Somatic problems. In *Cognitive behaviour therapy for psychiatric problems* (ed. K. Hawton, P.M. Salkovskis, J. Kirk, and D.M. Clark), pp. 235–76. Oxford University Press, Oxford.

Seli, T. and Shapiro, C.M. (1997). Neuropsychiatry—the mind embrained? *J. Psychosom. Res.* **43**, 329–33.

Sharpe, M., Peveler, R., and Mayou, R. (1992). The psychological treatment of patients with functional somatic symptoms: a practical guide. *J. Psychosom. Res.* **36**, 515–29.

Sharpe, M., Bass, C., and Mayou, R. (1995a). An overview of the treatment of functional somatic symptoms. In *Treatment of functional somatic symptoms* (ed. R. Mayou, C. Bass, and M. Sharpe), pp. 66–85. Oxford University Press, Oxford.

Sharpe, M., Mayou, R., and Bass, C. (1995b). Concepts, theories and terminology. In *Treatment of functional somatic symptoms* (ed. R. Mayou, C. Bass, and M. Sharpe), pp. 3–16. Oxford University Press, Oxford.

Silver, F.W. (1996). Management of conversion disorder. *Am. J. Phys. Med. Rehabil.* **75**, 134–40.

Smith, G.R. Jr. (1995). Treatment of patients with multiple symptoms. In *Treatment of functional somatic symptoms* (ed. R. Mayou, C. Bass, and M. Sharpe), pp. 175–87. Oxford University Press, Oxford.

Speckens, A.E.M., van Hemert, A.M., Spinhoven, P., Hawton, K.E., Bolk, J.H., and Rooijmans, H.G.M. (1995). Cognitive behavioural therapy for medically unexplained physical symptoms: a randomised controlled trial. *Br. Med. J.* **311**, 1328–32.

Speckens, A.E.M., Spinhoven, P., van Hemert, A.M., and Bolk, J.H. (1997). Cognitive behavioural therapy for unexplained physical symptoms: process and prognostic factors. *Behav. Cogn. Psychother.* **25**, 291–4.

Surguladze, S. and David, A. (1999). Insight and major mental illness: an update for clinicians. *Advan. Psychiatric Treat.* **5**, 163–70.

Warwick, H., Clark, D.M., Cobb, A.M., and Salkovskis, P.M. (1996). A controlled trial of cognitive–behavioural treatment of hypochondriasis. *Br. J. Psychiatry* **169**, 189–95.

Wilkinson, P. and Mynors-Wallis, L. (1994). Problem-solving therapy in the treatment of unexplained physical symptoms in primary care: a preliminary study. *J. Psychosom. Res.* **38**, 591–8.

World Health Organisation. (1992). *The ICD-10 classification of mental and behavioural disorders. Clinical descriptions and diagnostic guidelines.* World Health Organisation, Geneva.

Yule, W. (1987). Identifying problems: functional analysis and observation and recording techniques. In *Behaviour modification for people with mental handicaps*, 2nd edn (ed. W. Yule and J. Carr), pp. 8–27. Croom Helm, London.

Zanetti, O., Vallotti, B., Frisoni, G.B., Geroldi, C., Bianchetti, A., Pasqualetti, P., and Trabucchi, M. (1999). Insight in dementia: when does it occur? Evidence for a nonlinear relationship between insight and cognitive status. *J. Gerontol.: Psychol. Sci.* **54B**, 100–6.

Part 8

Forensic neuropsychology

Chapter 37

Forensic issues in neuropsychology

William W. McKinlay and Michaela McGowan

1 Introduction

A neuropsychologist may be called on to assist in civil cases, e.g. in personal injury claims after traumatic brain injury (TBI) and other brain injury including medical negligence (e.g. anaesthetic accident). A neuropsychologist may also assist in criminal cases, where issues of competency (including fitness to plead and present evidence) and disposal (sentencing) arise in relation to individuals who are neuropsychologically impaired.

2 Civil cases

2.1 Why is a neuropsychologist's opinion required?

Serious brain injury typically results in:

- physical/sensory sequelae;
- cognitive sequelae;
- emotional/behavioural sequelae.

Psychological factors (cognitive and emotional/behavioural sequelae) are the most important determinants of disability—including reduced ability to work and need for care/supervision. The sequelae of brain injury, especially emotional/behavioural changes, cause stress on family members and sometimes family breakdown, making issues of care more pressing (See McKinlay and Watkiss 1999 for a fuller, referenced account). Loss of earnings and costs of care are often the two main drivers of the amount of damages in these cases. The neuropsychological assessment is often the key assessment identifying the factors that may impede return to work and give rise to the need for care and supervision.

2.2 What information do the lawyers and the court need?

In order to decide what, if any, compensation is due, the court must decide on two broad areas:

- *liability*: did the defending party cause loss injury and damage to the plaintiff (England) or pursuer (Scotland) or claimant/petitioner (some other jurisdictions)?
- the *quantum (amount) of damages*, which depends on the extent and implications of the loss injury and damage suffered.

In cases brought before the courts in the UK damages will be awarded under two broad headings. (In America, punitive damages may also arise, and in other jurisdictions the basis of calculation may differ.)

- There is a sum for *general damages* (England) or *solatium* (Scotland). The extent of pain and suffering is relevant here, as is the extent of the injured person's awareness: the more the injured person is aware of his/her predicament, the greater this element of the damages, other things being equal.

- There is a sum for *special damages*, often by far the larger part of the damages awarded in cases of serious injury. Key factors in calculating the quantum of special damages include extent of loss of earnings and extra costs arising from disability.

It follows that key information lawyers seek to take from neuropsychologists' reports (and, in their respective fields, from other clinicians) is:

- the nature and extent of any impairment, disorder, or other effect of injury;
- the causality: did the injury cause or substantially contribute to the difficulties suffered?
- the prognosis (with and without treatment), including timescale;
- the functional implications, especially for work and care needs.

The neuropsychologist should therefore consider the following:

- What is the nature/extent of neuropsychological impairment and emotional–behavioural change? What abilities remain intact? It is important to look for intact as well as impaired abilities as these are relevant to rehabilitation and work prospects, and prognosis.

- Are the impairments/disorders/etc. more likely to be due to the injury than to any other cause? Failing this, has the injury made a significant contribution to these impairments/disorders/etc.?

- Is further treatment/rehabilitation indicated (and, if so, what kind with what aims)? What is the prognosis? Is it too soon to estimate long-term outcome (as the likely long-term prognosis will seldom be clear until at the very least 2–3 years after serious brain injury?

- What implications—in broad terms—do the impairments and other changes have for functional outcome, including ability to work and lead a social life, and need for care/supervision?

Civil cases are decided on the *balance of probability*. The question is, for example, is it more likely than not that the trauma (rather than some other factor) caused—or materially contributed to—the problems found? It is also important to remember that the court will nearly always make a once-for-all decision, based on the best evidence available at the time. Damages in the UK and many other countries are not punitive: the sum of money awarded is intended to put the injured person in the same position as he/she would have been but for injury. In the UK, an exception to this general rule, sadly, is the damages awarded to the victims of criminal assault via the Criminal Injuries Compensation Authority (CICA). In recent years, the usual rules for calculating civil damages have been replaced for CICA cases by a tariff system for general damages/solatium, and, moreover, the total award for damages is capped at a very much lower level than the sums that are often awarded in the civil courts. The current maximum total damages for any CICA case in 2001 is UK £0.5 million, this being in effect the total of general damages or solatium plus special damages.

2.3 How should the assessment be conducted?

2.3.1 Stage 1: Before the examination

Before accepting instructions, ensure that you can do what is asked, i.e. can you comment on all of the questions raised? Amongst the questions there may be some—such as life expectancy and risk of epilepsy—that are matters for other experts. You should point this out at the outset. There may be strict time requirements—especially in England under Lord Woolf's Civil Procedure Rules (CPR). You should only accept if you can meet these. If you cannot, there may be room for negotiation but you should do this at the outset. There is no harm in agreeing at the outset, at least broadly, the level of fee and when it will be paid.

Lawyers will often seek a report from a professional who is *not* the treating doctor, to avoid any conflict of interest, and obtain a view from someone not committed to the treating unit. If you are involved in the case already, you should consider if there would be any conflict before accepting instructions.

It is good practice to have all the records you need prior to assessment, so that you are properly briefed, and also so that issues arising can be clarified with patient/relative. Lack of records is often a key reason for assessments being plain wrong. The following records are often useful.

◆ *GP medical records* should make evident any significant pre-injury disorders or handicaps and other factors or conditions (e.g. poorly controlled diabetes, alcohol/drug abuse, previous injuries, etc.) that may impact significantly on neuropsychological function.

◆ *Educational records* (especially for younger people recently in education) or *employment records* (where available) may help confirm test-based estimates of premorbid ability. Sometimes, due to young age at injury or acquired language deficits, the usual methods for assessing premorbid ability (e.g. National Adult Reading Test) cannot be used, and these records will be even more important.

◆ *Early hospital records* relating to the admission after injury should be reviewed to confirm that there was indeed a significant injury. Information on Glasgow Coma Scale, scan results, and any clinical evidence of focal neurological signs is important. Duration of posttraumatic amnesia (PTA) is often not explicitly recorded, but orientation may be. The return of orientation and the ending of PTA cannot be assumed to occur at exactly the same time, but the ending of PTA is seldom long delayed after the return of orientation. Information about orientation is often in the notes—if not in the reports, then in the handwritten clinical notes of the psychologist, speech and language therapist, and other therapists and nurses.

All of these points relate to injury severity, which is a key consideration if seeming deficits are to be reconciled with the injury. If you do not know from a source independent of the patient/relative how severe the injury was, there is a danger of incorrect assessment/diagnosis. In particular, patients with post-concussion symptoms (PCS) following mild–moderate injury (a condition that is considered to be maintained by anxiety) may show similarities to patients with aspects of more severe brain injury. There is also the risk of malingering. It is probably rare but it is not unknown for long coma, long PTA, and great disability to be claimed falsely after mild or moderate injury.

♦ Later hospital/rehabilitation records should also alert the assessor to behavioural problems. These may not emerge in the calm, contained environment of the neuropsychological examination, but may be a problem in day-to-day interactions with others, and must not be overlooked.

2.3.2 Stage 2: The examination

It should go without saying that the broad approach to assessment should be neutral in the sense of not seeking to favour either side in the litigation, but simply conducting a careful and thorough assessment. It is very hard to do a satisfactory assessment without also speaking to a relative or close friend, given that the patient may very well have memory gaps and limited insight. In practice, it is very rare indeed for patient/relative not to agree to separate interviews (if the need is well explained). It is, however, not unknown for follow-ups (usually nonpsychological) to be based on a cursory interview with the patient alone, and therefore to be potentially misleading.

Joint interview Since the patient may well have retrograde amnesia and posttraumatic amnesia, information about events around the time of injury is often best collected with a relative also present. Further information that may best be collected with both present—in case of memory or communication problems—is social and health background.

Separate interviews Due to the problem of lack of insight on the part of the injured person, there is a danger of underreporting. It is useful to think of insight using the four stages suggested by Fleming *et al.* (1996):

♦ lack of awareness (or admission) of deficit;

♦ awareness of deficit;

♦ awareness of functional implications of deficit;

♦ ability to set realistic goals.

These stages typically are worked through first in relation to physical limitations, and then cognitive limitations, and lastly emotional/behavioural limitations. However, by no means every injured person completes the process.

It is therefore essential for an interview with a relative or 'significant other' to be carried out, if at all possible, separately. While the relative's view cannot be assumed to be the 'gold standard', there is evidence that suggests it is more likely to be accurate. Sunderland *et al.* (1983*a*) found relatives' accounts had greater validity as regards memory failure then those of patients. The separate interviews with patient and relative should *each* cover the main possible sequelae of injury. Deficits of functional significance may arise in the following areas.

- The physical/sensory changes (including epilepsy) are, of course, primarily matters for others, but nevertheless a broad view of them should be kept in mind in considering the psychological picture.

- There may be symptoms such as headaches, dizziness, poor balance, intolerance of noise, tiredness, changes in sleep/wake pattern, loss of libido. Some of these, especially tiredness, are very common and can be very disabling. Tiredness can exacerbate behavioural disturbances, and can 'bring out' otherwise silent residual deficits. It can also impact upon an individual's ability to participate in rehabilitation.

- The cognitive changes should be reviewed, and an attempt made to identify how they affect daily life.

- The emotional/behavioural changes should likewise be reviewed. Some patients will deny all such problems while other evidence (relative's account, records) suggests otherwise.

- Progress in returning to education or employment should, of course, be considered. Careful questions about how they spend their time ('an average day') should be asked. Family and social life and maintenance of friendships, should be explored. Social isolation is the major long-term danger for many patients and their families (Morton and Wehman 1995).

The above list is not exhaustive and, as in other settings, questions about other life events and about such factors as alcohol/drug abuse are relevant. Distinctions that are relevant to good clinical practice in any event are even more important in medicolegal reporting, and it is important to be clear about the following points:

- the distinction between *spontaneous* and *elicited* complaints;

- the *source* of information should be clear (patient, relative, test scores, or records?);

- the distinction between what is *reported* and *observed* and *inferred* should be made clear.

Neuropsychological examination   There are several areas that it is important to assess. It is probably not productive in a chapter such as this to debate the merits and demerits of particular tests. Perfectly sound neuropsychological examinations may be based on varying selections of tests, so long as the tests are suitable for the purpose and the proper range of abilities is sampled. The key areas that should be covered are described and referenced in McKinlay and Watkiss (1999). In brief, they are as follows;

◆ A language screen should include consideration of spontaneous speech and brief tests of repetition, naming, word-finding, obeying commands, reading, writing, as Lezak (1995) has described.

◆ Intellectual level—premorbid and current. A caution should be entered against using an 'overall' intelligence quotient (IQ) score in this context. Scores that average subtests vulnerable to the effects of brain injury with subtests that are not vulnerable will mask the nature and extent of impairment. Separate consideration of subtests or indices is therefore better in this context than IQ scores.

◆ Both verbal and visuospatial memory should be assessed. It is worth bearing in mind that verbal memory (especially as assessed by Logical Memory from the Wechsler scale) is one of the tests best related to 'everyday' memory failures (Sunderland *et al.* 1983*b*) and failure to return to work (see McKinlay and Watkiss 1999).

◆ Another key area to consider is attention/concentration. Difficulties in 'divided attention' are especially common.

◆ Impairments of executive functions, which are associated with frontal lobe damage, are also common and can be very disabling even where other aspects of cognitive function are not grossly impaired.

◆ 'Focal' problems (e.g. dyspraxia, agnosia, etc.) should not be overlooked, although they are not especially common in marked form after TBI.

◆ Some clinicians include questionnaire measures of emotional adjustment. However, it should be borne in mind that—in a medicolegal context—these are often essentially a series of leading questions. The manuals of many such measures caution against their use in a medicolegal context. They need to be interpreted with great care.

A caution should be entered against what Lezak has called 'neuropsychology by the numbers'. Test scores must be interpreted in the context of information from interviews, records, and qualitative observations—how the patient tackles tasks as well as the final scores.

2.3.3 Stage 3: Reporting and giving evidence

The next stage is to write the neuropsychological report. As the great majority of cases are settled before reaching an actual court hearing, the report will often be the only means by which the neuropsychologist's opinion will be communicated to the court.

What should be included in a medicolegal neuropsychological report?   The report (like other medicolegal reports) should set out the instructions given, state where and when the patient and relative were assessed/interviewed, and describe the documentation studied. The nature and severity of injury should be considered, drawing on patient/relative interview and evidence from the records. As always, the social and health background should be described. The information from patient/relative interviews and from the neuropsychological examination should be presented. Neuropsychologists differ in whether they include scores, centiles, etc. in the report or use terms such as 'moderate' or 'very severe' impairment. Some argue that actual scores may be misinterpreted by nonpsychologists, but without scores one is left only with vague and non-operational terms such as 'severe impairment'. One solution for those unwilling to include actual scores in the body of the report is to provide a technical summary as an appendix in which scores, test versions used, etc are listed. This facilitates later assessment by other neuropsychologists.

The report should set out conclusions on the key areas of relevance to the court, as set out more fully above, i.e. nature/extent of impairment and change, cause and effect, treatment and prognosis, and functional implications.

What areas should be addressed with caution?   There are also areas that it is not appropriate to cover as they are primarily a matter for related reports. To stray into these areas may confuse the issues and give rise to unnecessary contradictions in the evidence. It may be quite appropriate for a neuropsychologist to say that someone has such severe deficits that they are likely to be incapable of open-market employment, or would be capable only of restricted/simple work. However, to speculate as to what jobs may be available in more detail may be unwise. Normally, such questions are for an employment expert with knowledge of availability of employment in the appropriate travel-to-work area, knowledge of factors that might militate against employment in the relevant field, knowledge of competition for such jobs, and so on.

There will often also be a report on future needs (a 'needs report' or 'rehabilitation cost consultant's report' or related term). This will cover various areas, attaching costs. It is unhelpful for clinicians to be too specific on care needs. The details are a matter for a care specialist who knows the practicalities of care provision, and can seek to match what is practicable with the patient's needs. It would, however, be appropriate and helpful in a neuropsychological report to offer a view as to the broad level of care/supervision needed.

However, a particular aspect of future needs—rehabilitation—may well merit fuller discussion. After brain injury, many patients, at least in the UK, will not receive an adequate (or indeed any) programme of specialized rehabilitation. One cannot consider prognosis without considering what services may be available, and it will often be appropriate to make recommendations for rehabilitation, which may require funding. It is important to remember the following.

- You should not hold out to patient/family the definite prospect of rehabilitation or other treatment until and unless funding is in place.
- If there is a case for such rehabilitation, you should do no more than discuss it with patient/family as a possibility, to gauge their receptiveness, then raise the matter with your instructing lawyers.
- The lawyers acting for the injured person may be able to obtain funding for this purpose, either by means of an interim award of damages, or through negotiation with the defenders. However, that is a matter for them to pursue where possible and the clinician's role is to provide them with any evidence that such rehabilitation may be of benefit.

- The lawyers acting for the defenders may also be able to arrange funding for this purpose, and the idea of doing so may be attractive to defenders on the grounds that such an investment now may reduce disability (and therefore damages) later. Again, the clinician's role is to explain any grounds to believe that such rehabilitation may be of benefit.

- It will often be possible for any privately funded rehabilitation/treatment to be provided by a service with which you (the person who recommended it) have no connection. If the service may be provided by a unit with which you do have a connection, it is wise to declare a possible conflict of interest. Suggesting the lawyers get a review of your recommendations by a disinterested clinician would be a way to defuse concern about conflict of interest.

If called to present evidence in court, it is well worth reading some relevant material about the court in advance, or seeking to speak to a colleague with court experience. Carson (1990), a lawyer who describes the methods barristers or advocates use to 'test' witnesses, provides a view from the 'other side' that is very helpful for prospective witnesses. There are several publications by psychologists that provide useful advice (Cooke 1990; Beaumont 1994; McKinlay 1992). Other useful UK publications are *Psychologists as expert witnesses in Scotland* and *Psychologists and the new rules in civil procedure* published by the British Psychological Society.

2.4 Further issues

2.4.1 Malingering

The possibility of malingering is something to be borne in mind (see Halligan *et al.* 2003). Malingering is the 'intentional production of false or grossly exaggerated [symptoms or deficits] motivated by external incentives' (*Diagnostic and statistical manual of mental disorders*, 4th edn (DSM-IV); American Psychiatric Association 1994). Although probably rare in brain injury cases (McKinlay *et al.* 1983), it obviously should be borne in mind when financial or other external incentives are present. (See Rogers 1997)

In some studies, subjects, including psychology students, have been asked to simulate ('fake') deficits. Such 'fakers' tend do badly across the board—as if reluctant to do well even on easy items. TBI patients usually still find some tasks quite easy. Typically (although not invariably), they show:

- little deficit on measures of personal information, basic language function, verbal IQ, and forwards digit span;

- a degree of difficulty on measures of performance IQ;

- major difficulty on tests of memory and attention/concentration (the latter including backwards digit span, Digit Symbol, and Paced Auditory Serial Addition Task (PASAT)).

Some also have great difficulty with 'frontal' (executive function) tests.

A 'flat' profile—doing badly across the board—is suspicious. Various methods can be used. One is to derive a score or profile from a test in common use, such as calculating a Simulation Index from Raven's Standard Progressive Matrices (Gudjonsson and Shackleton 1986) which is based on this principle. Another approach that may help with this issue is to use a 'floor effect' test—one so easy that TBI patients can do it, but that appears difficult. Rey's 15-item 'memory' test is an example (see Lezak 1995), although it probably only appears difficult to the less able. Forced-choice testing is another approach that may help. Such testing is in multiple-choice format, and those who score below chance are thought to be deliberately performing poorly. However, there can be exceptions. For example, on certain tasks, Broca's aphasics are routinely misled by aspects of sentence structure, performing below chance (Grodzinsky 1995).

There is also a more general caveat that surprising and hard-to-understand behaviour should not too readily be taken to suggest malingering, as there may be an underpinning organic explanation. For example, the first author has come across a case of 'foreign accent syndrome' in which the subject spoke (after a mild stroke allegedly due to medical negligence) with a 'mid-European' sounding accent, despite no connection with that part of the world. The question of malingering had been raised. However, although rare, this condition has been reported to arise sometimes with and sometimes without aphasia and to be related to anterior left (dominant) hemisphere lesions, generally of the frontal and precentral gyri (e.g. Kurowski *et al.* 1996; Moonis *et al.* 1996; Takayama *et al.* 1993), as was the case with the subject.

However, there is no doubt that some compensation claimants seek to invent or exaggerate deficits, and that neuropsychological examination has an important part to play in detecting them. There are two scenarios.

1   Forced-choice tasks are occasionally used in neuropsychological examination and, where the patient performs significantly worse than chance, obviously the question of malingering arises as a very strong possibility. Indeed, Binder has said that, where forced-choice answers are worse than chance, 'the probability of an explanation other than malingering is nil' (see Adams and Rankin 1996). Presumably, he excepts the Broca's aphasia cases noted above, although that is a very small and specific exception. While this is a strong statement, it is hard to escape the conclusion that Binder is nearly always right. However, a hysterical reaction should also be considered although, as Lishman (1997) has noted, that need not exclude some element of conscious malingering.

2   A more common scenario is where the patient produces responses that are implausibly poor. For example, he/she may do badly across the board, rather than producing the selective deficits found after brain insult, or the deficits may be severe despite the injury being mild or moderate. Other examples are very poor performance on memory tests despite detailed recall of symptoms and grievances about the

case, or evidence of non-organic 'deficit' from special tests, e.g. André Rey's 15-item 'memory' test (see Lezak 1995) or the Rate of Decay index for the Standard Progressive Matrices (Gudjonsson and Shackleton 1986). Where the performance is implausibly poor, not consistent with any brain injury sustained, again malingering should be strongly suspected. Obviously, severe depression or anxiety should be considered as alternative explanations. However, in order to produce 'deficits', an individual who is not actually impaired must persist, during what is usually quite a lengthy examination, in performing less well than he/she can perform despite the guidance and encouragement of the neuro-psychologist. Unlike, say, an orthopaedic examination, there is no fear of pain to 'excuse' less than full cooperation.

Overall, key areas to look for are:

- atypical test performance, with seemingly great difficulty on simple tests;
- marked inconsistencies in what is expected from the nature of injury and the patient's presentation and self-reports.

It is also worth bearing the following in mind.

- Did the claimant consult a lawyer before seeking full clinical assessment and/or help with 'post-injury' problems?
- Have symptoms shown typical progression over time?
- Is the claimant's account at interview consistent with the records?

2.4.2 Premature ageing

An increased risk of 'premature ageing' (or even 'premature dementia') has been suggested by some. The idea that the injured brain may be less able to resist the effects of ageing and/or dementia has some plausibility. Bell (1992) is sometimes quoted in support of such a view. Lawyers, naturally, may raise the issue. If it were the case that accelerated ageing did occur, it would have implications for long-term care and therefore costs, and it would only be right that the diligent lawyer pursue the issue. There is now a fairly large literature on this topic. There are many retrospective studies reporting an association between previous head injury and onset of Alzheimer's disease but these are of little interest as the relatives (whose accounts have generally been the basis of these studies) may be making an effort to 'explain' the dementia. There remains a debate about whether there is a link between brain injury and increased risk of premature decline in later years, as well as a lack of specification of what that would mean. There is some evidence to the contrary albeit from a different injury type, e.g. the war veterans with missile wounds of the brain reported in Newcombe's (1969) classic research had remarkably good late outcomes, although one has to bear in mind that these were focal rather than diffuse injuries. Nevertheless, the developing research and debate in this area are highly relevant in a medicolegal context.

2.5 **The impartiality of the expert witness**

Excellent advice on presenting expert evidence was provided in Deutsch and Parker's (1995) brief publication for rehabilitation professionals, which applies just as well to neuropsychologists. The need to maintain a consistency of approach from case to case and to maintain intellectual honesty is paramount. It is perhaps easier to do this by always keeping in mind that you are involved in the legal process as an educator—to give the court the benefit of your knowledge and experience. You are not there as an advocate. It is the lawyers' not the expert's job to advance arguments for one side or the other.

In England and Wales, Lord Woolf's Civil Procedure Rules (CPR) now emphasize that the overriding duty of the expert witness is to the Court, to help the Court on matters within the expert's field of expertise, and that this duty overrides any obligation to the instructing party. CPR has also made the process more transparent. Experts must state the instructions received (both written and oral) and must summarize the range of opinion (views expressed by another neuropsychologist involved in the case) stating, where it arises, why they disagree. It is explicitly unacceptable—as it always was for the honest expert—for any 'negative comments' to be confined to a covering letter, as sometimes lawyers used to request. There is an increasing tendency for the Court to require the appointment of a Single Joint Expert, reporting jointly to both sides simultaneously. This places even greater responsibility on the expert witness, as there is not in these cases the check, in effect, of an experienced colleague also doing an assessment. The requirements of experts (in England and Wales) under CPR are to be found on the Lord Chancellor's website (www.lcd.gov.uk). Part 35 of the rules, and the Practice Directions that are a supplement to that part ('Practice direction—experts and assessors'), are relevant. Various organizations offer courses for expert witnesses and on being a Single Joint Expert.

Although the CPR seek to limit the range of experts called to those 'proportionate' to the case (i.e. not allowing an army of experts), the admissibility of neuropsychological evidence has not presented problems in the authors' experience. Common sense would suggest that there is no issue. In ordinary clinical practice, it is neuropsychologists who possess the sharpest instruments for assessing the outcome and implications of brain injury, and it is to neuropsychologists that the clinical team turns to make these assessments.

An exception is in defining 'patients' for Court of Protection purposes, i.e. deciding who is unable to manage his/her own affairs. Here the advice of medical practitioners is required, although in day-to-day clinical practice the clinical team will often seek guidance from the neuropsychologist. It is nevertheless relevant to tell the instructing solicitor if there are concerns arising from the neuropsychological examination about the ability of the person assessed to manage his or her affairs. Such concerns may arise due to lack of insight, inability to comprehend the concepts involved, extreme memory impairment, etc. It is, however, important to make clear that, as things stand at present, they would need a certificate from a medical practitioner under the present law.

The law in Scotland is changing at the time of writing in relation to consideration of such matters: instead of an all-or-none position whereby an individual is deemed to have full capacity or no capacity, there is a staged introduction under the (Scottish) Adults with Incapacity Act of provisions to allow for the vulnerable individual to have help with selected aspects of their affairs, while they retain control over other aspects. A similar approach, to allow increased flexibility, is under consideration for England and Wales. (The websites of the Public Guardians for England and Wales, and for Scotland, provide further information.)

3 Criminal cases

The evidence of a neuropsychologist (as opposed to a forensic psychologist) is less often required in criminal than in civil cases. However, there are certain circumstances in which neuropsychological issues bear on issues arising in criminal proceedings, and it may well be that in the future the range of neuropsychological issues arising in this setting will increase.

3.1 Peritraumatic loss of memory in TBI

Possible loss of memory at the time of an accident or assault is a particular issue that sometimes involves neuropsychologists in criminal cases. A period of retrograde amnesia (RA) and PTA is the signature of a significant concussional head injury. The individual recalls nothing from sometime before injury until sometime after it. This obviously may lead to difficulty in criminal cases. The victim of an assault may well be unable to recall events just prior to assault due to RA, or the immediate aftermath due to PTA, and this can lead to problems in bringing the perpetrators to justice. Another instance is after road traffic accidents when the injured person may have been the victim or may have been a driver suspected of an offence. RA/PTA may mean the injured person has no recall of the event. In all cases where RA/PTA is an issue, study of the contemporaneous records is a key step in trying to clarify how extensive RA/PTA are likely to have been, as the injured person may have a motive for claiming to remember or forget what happened.

It is worth bearing in mind that although RA and PTA are always found with significant *concussional* head injury, not all assaults are of this sort. In assaults, depressed fractures or penetrating wounds are not uncommon. Where concussion is not the main mechanism of brain injury, the injured person may recall the actual incident, and may have succumbed to unconsciousness later.

It should be borne in mind that many people who commit murder/violent acts claim to have no memory of the act. It is thought that this commonly occurs as a result of emotional shock/psychological trauma (Kopelman 1987). Obviously, this should not be confused with RA/PTA. It is hard to conceive of a concussed person being able to carry out such an act.

3.2 Neuropsychological deficits

The lasting neuropsychological deficits in cognition and emotional adjustment that may follow TBI or other brain insult/disorder are also of potential relevance. Neuropsychologists may be asked to comment on vulnerabilities that affect the competency of a person with brain injury to stand trial, or give evidence as victim or witness. In the context of the police interview and testifying in court, the term 'psychological vulnerabilities' refers to psychological characteristics or mental states that render a witness prone to providing information that is inaccurate, unreliable, or misleading (Gudjonsson 1999).

3.2.1 Cognitive deficits

As well as RA/PTA, people who have had TBI or other brain insult/disorder may have ongoing memory and other cognitive impairments. The issue may arise as to whether such impairments undermine the ability to follow questions and marshal facts in giving evidence. Obviously, the bar should not be set too high. In ordinary cases, where there is no neuropsychological deficit, some accused or witnesses may be of well below average ability. It would be wrong and arguably would undermine the aims of justice to say that merely because a witness has some loss of sharpness they could not give evidence, because that might well mean that no charges would be brought and justice would be defeated. However, where there are substantial difficulties—e.g. dysexecutive syndrome, word-finding difficulties, or memory problems—there may be very specific difficulties in giving evidence. Some individuals after severe TBI may be at such a disadvantage in the dock or witness box that attempts at examination and cross-examination would be in serious danger of ending in farce. In this context, the fact that some neuropsychologically compromised individuals may be subject to extreme emotion (e.g. 'catastrophic reaction') is also relevant.

There is, however, a lack of hard indicators (such as test cutting scores), and clinical judgement is required. As regards the *defendant*, a trial cannot be fair if the individual is unable to understand the court proceedings, instruct his or her lawyer, and participate in the court proceedings. The exact criteria set down in the law to ensure a fair trial vary to some extent from jurisdiction to jurisdiction.

Where issues of intellectual and related impairment may arise (e.g. due to head injury, neurological disorder, etc.), a neuropsychological assessment is necessary to define the nature and extent of the limitations. However, competency cannot be measured by just evaluating mental capacity and there is a need to assess the functional ability of a defendant matched to the contextual demands of the case (Grisso 1986). Therefore, in addition to standard IQ measures, there is a move towards the use of screening measures specifically designed to assess fitness to stand trial. Two North American measures include the Fitness Interview test (Roesch *et al.* 1998), a semi-structured interview evaluating understanding of proceedings, consequences, and communication with counsel, and the MacArthur Competence Assessment Tool

(Bonnie *et al.* 1996), which assesses ability to participate in a trial, rational thinking, and recognition of relevant information, using case scenarios. These screening tools have no cut-off scores for 'fitness' and it is recommended that clinicians use these tests in conjunction with neuropsychological assessment (Roesch *et al.* 1999). However, they do provide a useful framework to aid assessment.

Such assessment will be a key part of the decision-making process as to whether charges are brought, although the final decision will not be for the psychologist to make. It is important to remember that 'impairment' on neuropsychological measures or, indeed, the presence of a mental disorder (one in e.g. DSM-IV) does not necessarily mean a lack of capacity to participate in a trial, either as accused or as a witness.

As regards *witnesses*, some similar considerations apply. A witness may be unable to give evidence if deemed not to have the intellectual capacity to understand questions, articulate answers, and understand the implications of their answers. However, to date there is little research in this area (Gudjonsson 1999).

3.2.2 Suggestibility

Suggestibility is the tendency to yield to leading questions and submit to interrogative pressure (Gudjonsson 1999). Suggestibility can be assessed by the use of behavioural tests, such as the Gudjonsson Suggestibility Scales, that assess an individual's response to 'leading questions' and 'negative feedback'. Many neuropsychologists will have no experience of such measures and may wish to cross-refer to forensic psychologists. Evidence suggests that low intellectual functioning, memory impairment, anxiety, and low levels of self-esteem affect an individual's cognitive appraisal within an interrogative/interview situation and the coping strategies that they adopt (Gudjonsson 1992). Consequently, they may be misled by some questions, and vulnerable to giving inaccurate testimony when interviewed by police or cross-examined.

3.2.3 Other variables

A neuropsychologist might also be asked to comment on various further (criminal) forensic issues to the extent that neuropsychological impairments interfere, or may interfere, with the ability of the accused, or of a witness, to recall or describe events. The factors that may affect the witness's ability to recall details of a crime at a later date are primarily of interest to forensic psychologists rather than neuropsychologists. These factors include 'estimator variables', which may affect witness's recall (such as witness age, weapon focus, duration of exposure to the crime, effects of stress/arousal), and duration, which occur at the time of the event, and 'system variables' which occur during the investigation process (impact of misleading questions, exposure to 'mug shots'/photographs leading to false memories). Neuropsychological impairments may impact on ability to recall information about crime and perpetrators reliably. However, this is not a mainstream neuropsychological concern and detailed discussion is outside the scope of this chapter. Those interested might consult Loftus (1993) and Cutler and Penrod (1995).

3.3 Recovered memories of childhood abuse

This is a controversial area. Some propose that when a person encounters a traumatic event they may engage in an unconscious process of forcing the traumatic memory from conscious awareness. This 'repressed' memory may be expressed through flash-backs and dreams and 'recovered' under certain conditions (e.g. during psychotherapy). However, there is substantial controversy over the validity of recovered memories, espe-cially when initially 'recovered' during psychotherapy. Critics argue that factors known to distort memory are present within some psychotherapy sessions, and that many indi-viduals who report recovered memories are highly suggestible (Loftus 1993). While advocates of recovered memory argue that adult survivors of sexual abuse can 'forget' traumatic experiences and later access the repressed memory during psychotherapy, the issue remains controversial (Cercy *et al.* 1997). Cases of this nature (where there is a lack of independent evidence) are unlikely to go to court as police, lawyers, and judges are reluctant to accept recovered evidence as being of itself substantial evidence.

3.4 Disposal

An issue that occasionally arises, in the authors' experience, is that of 'disposal', or sen-tencing. A neuropsychologist may be called upon to comment on whether there is treatment or rehabilitation available that may help, which might be taken as an alternat-ive to fines or imprisonment.

Acknowledgements

We are grateful to the following for their helpful comments on specific issues: Robert Swanney, Partner, Digby Brown and Co, Solicitors, Glasgow; Hugh Potter, Partner, Hugh Potter and Co, Serious Injury Solicitors, Manchester; Hugh Jones, Partner, Pannone and Partners, Manchester; Anna Watkiss, Psychologist, Case Management Services Ltd, Edinburgh.

Selective references

Adams, R.L. and Rankin, E.J. (1996). A practical guide to forensic neuropsychological evaluations and testimony. In *Neuropsychology for clinical practice* (ed. R.L. Adams, O.A. Parsons, J.L. Culbertson, and S.J. Nixon), pp. 455–87. American Psychological Association, Washington, DC.

American Psychiatric Association (1994). *Diagnostic and statistical manual of mental disorders*, 4th edn. American Psychiatric Association, Washington, DC.

Beaumont, J.G. (1994). Expert witness. *Psychologist* (Nov.) 511–12.

Bell, D.S. (1992). *Medicolegal assessment of head injury*. Charles C. Thomas, Springfield, Illinois.

Bonnie, R.J., Hodge, S.K., Monohan, J., and Poythres, N. (1996). The MacArthur Adjudicative Competence Study: a comparison of criteria for assessing the competence of criminal defendants. *J. Am. Acad. Psychiatry Law* 25, 249–59.

Carson, D. (1990) *Professionals and the courts: A handbook for expert witnesses*. Birmingham Venture Press.

Cercy, S.P., Schretlen, D.J., and Brandt, J. (1997). Simulated amnesia and the pseudo-memory phenomena. In *Clinical assessment of malingering and deception*, 2nd edn (ed. R. Rodgers), pp. 85–107. Guilford Press, New York.

Cooke, D.J. (1990). Do I feel lucky? Survival in the witness box. *Neuropsychology* 4, 271–85.

Cutler, B.L. and Penrod, S.D. (1995). *Mistaken identification: the eye witness psychology and the law*. Cambridge University Press, Cambridge.

Deutsch, T.M. and Parker, E.C. (1995). *Rehabilitation testimony: maintaining a professional perspective*. Matthew Bender, Albany, New York.

Fleming, J.M., Strong, J., and Ashton, R. (1996). Self-awareness of deficits in adults with traumatic brain injury: how best to measure? *Brain Injury* 10, 1–15.

Grisso, T. (1986). *Evaluating competencies: forensic assessment and instruments*. Plenum Press, New York.

Grodzinsky, Y. (1995) Trace deletion, theta roles, and cognitive strategies. *Brain and Language* 51, 469–97.

Gudjonsson, G.H. (1992). *The psychology of interrogations, confessions and testimony*. John Wiley and Son, New York.

Gudjonsson, G.H. (1999). Testimony from persons with mental disorder. In *Analysing witness testimony: a guide for legal practitioners and other professionals* (ed. A. Heaton-Armstrong, E. Shepherd, and D. Wolchover), pp. 62–75. Blackstone Press, London.

Gudjonsson, G.H. and Shackleton, H. (1986). The pattern of scores on Raven's Matrices during 'faking bad' and 'non-faking' performance. *Br. J. Clin. Psychol.* 25, 35–41.

Halligan, P.W., Bass, C. and Oakley, D. (2003). Malingering and Illness Deception. Oxford University Press, Oxford.

Kopleman, M.D. (1987) Amnesia: organic and psychogenic. *British Journal of Psychiatry.* 150, 428–42.

Kurowski, K.M., Blumstein, S.E., and Alexander, M. (1996). The foreign accent syndrome— a reconsideration. *Brain Language* 54, 1–25.

Lezak, M.D. (1995). *Neuropsychological assessment*, 3rd edn. Oxford University Press, New York.

Lishman, W.A. (1997). *Organic psychiatry*, 3rd edn. Blackwell Science, Oxford.

Loftus, E.F. (1993). Psychologists in the eye witness world. *Am. Psychol.* 48, 550–2.

McKinlay, W.W. (1992). Assessment of the head injured for compensation. In *A handbook of neuropsychological assessment* (ed. J.R. Crawford, D.M. Parker, and W.W. McKinlay), pp. 381–92. Lawrence Erlbaum, Hove, East Sussex.

McKinlay, W.W. and Watkiss. A. (1999). Cognitive and behavioural effects of brain injury. In *Rehabilitation of the adult and child with traumatic brain injury*, 3rd edn (ed. M. Rosenthal *et al.*), pp. 74–86 F.A. Davis Co, Philadelphia.

McKinlay, W.W., Brooks, D.N., and Bond, M.R. (1983). Post-concussional symptoms, financial compensation and outcome of severe blunt head injury. *J. Neurol. Neurosurg. Psychiatry* 46, 1084–91.

Moonis, M., Swearer, J.M., Blumstein, S.E., Kurowski, K.M., Licho, R., Kramer, P., Mitchell, A., Osgood, D.L., and Drachman, D.A. (1996). Foreign accent syndrome following a closed head injury—perfusion deficit on single-photon emission tomography with normal magnetic-resonance imaging. *Neuropsychiatry, Neuropsychol. Behav. Neurol.* 9, 272–9.

Morton, M.V. and Wehman, P. (1995). Psychosocial and emotional sequelae of individuals with traumatic brain injury: a literature review and recommendations. *Brain Injury* 9, 81–92.

Newcombe, F. (1969). *Missile wounds of the brain*. Oxford University Press, London.

Roesch, R., Zapf, P.A., Eaves, D., and Webster, C.D. (1998). *Fitness Interview Test.* Mental Health, Law, and Policy Institute, Simon Fraser University, Vancouver.

Roesch, R., Zapf, P.A., Golding, S.L., and Skeen, J.L. (1999). Defining and assessing competency to stand trial. In *The Handbook of forensic psychology* (ed. A.K. Hess and I.B. Weiner), pp. 327–50. Wiley and Sons, New York.

Rogers, R. (1997). *Clinical assessment of malingering and deception.* The Guilford Press, New York.

Sunderland, A., Harris, J.E., and Baddeley, A.D. (1983*a*). Assessing everyday memory after severe head injury. In *Everyday memory, actions and absentmindedness* (ed. J.E. Harris and D.E. Morris), pp.191–206. Academic Press, London.

Sunderland, A., Harris, J.E., and Baddeley A.D. (1983*b*). Do laboratory tests predict everyday memory? A neuropsychological study. *J. Verbal Learn. Verbal Behav.* 22, 341–57.

Takayama, Y., Sugishita, M., Kido, T., Ogawa, M., and Akigushi, I. (1993). A case of foreign accent syndrome without aphasia caused by a lesion of the left precentral gyrus. *Neurology* 43, 1361–3.

Part 9

Functional neuroanatomy

Chapter 38

Functional neuroanatomy of spatial perception, spatial processes, and attention

Gabriella Bottini and Eraldo Paulesu

1 Introduction

Functional neuroimaging measures haemodynamic changes—blood flow in the case of positron emission tomography (PET; Raichle 1987) and blood oxygenation in the case of functional magnetic resonance imaging (fMRI; Turner 1997; Ogawa *et al.* 1998; Logothetis 2001). These indices are used as indirect measures of synaptic activity and neural firing. PET and fMRI have rapidly become the major sources of neurophysiological information in humans. Since their early inception, they have been extensively used to characterize the neural bases of spatial cognition. The amount of available empirical information is now sufficiently large to allow for the formulation of a summary that may prove useful for the experimental and clinical neuropsychologist.

The empirical data of experimental psychology, neurophysiology in the primate, and neuropsychological observations in patients remain the primary source of experimental hypotheses for functional neuroimaging experiments in spatial neurocognition:

◆ the way in which space is mapped from early sensory codes (e.g. retinotopic maps, somatotopic maps) through the transformation in higher-order coordinates;

◆ the multicomponent nature of space representation and the existence of several spatial frames (e.g. far as opposed to near space);

◆ the distinction between object- and space-based visual cognition;

◆ the relationship between space and motion cognition;

◆ the modulation of spatial representation and perception through attentional mechanisms.

In this review we will discuss the above areas of enquiry. These themes will be introduced by a brief summary of the relevant comparative information drawn from primate physiology literature and neuropsychology. As the reader will notice, there is no complete agreement between lesion data and functional imaging data of spatial processing and attention: this we regard as a source of major interest for further research.

2 Building spatial neural representation from earlier sensory codes

2.1 The higher-order nature of spatial representation

Space, perceived as unitary, is in fact mapped by several systems all of which provide a representation relevant for a given set of actions and for different parts of space itself, including the body (Fig. 38.1) (Anderson *et al.* 1997; Colby and Goldberg 1999; Rizzolatti *et al.* 2000). Evidence for a dissociation between spatial representations and individual sensory codes in perception and directional coding of movement is provided by the cases of brain-damaged patients:

♦ with relatively spared elementary perceptual (e.g. visual, tactile) or motor skills and an impaired ability to report, respond to, or orient towards stimuli presented in different portions of space (spatial unilateral neglect: see review in Bisiach and Vallar 2000);

♦ with altered visuomotor integration in reaching tasks (see reviews in Jeannerod 1997).

Studies in spatial neglect have allowed us to dissociate elementary somatotopic and retinotopic codes from body-centred coordinate frames (see reviews in Bisiach

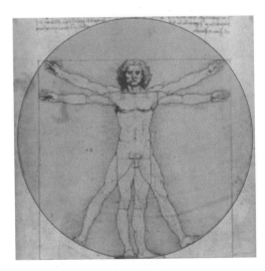

Fig. 38.1 Classification of spatial frames. The body; the space within reaching distance; and far space. Neuropsychology and neurophysiology provide evidence that the brain has separate representations for these different spatial frames. Personal space is somatosensory space mapped as a body schema independently from visual space. Extrapersonal space involves also visual space. This can be based on egocentric coordinates (within reaching distance) in that visual space is organized with reference to head, trunk, and limbs. Extrapersonal space can be mapped in allocentric (object-based) coordinates. (See also 'Plates' section.)

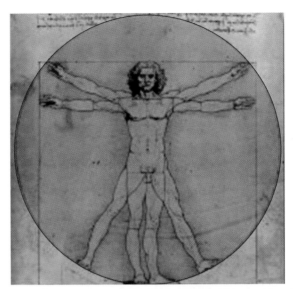

Plate 1 Classification of spatial frames. The body; the space within reaching distance; and far space. Neuropsychology and neurophysiology provide evidence that the brain has separate representations for these different spatial frames. Personal space is somatosensory space mapped as a body schema independently from visual space. Extrapersonal space involves also visual space. This can be based on egocentric coordinates (within reaching distance) in that visual space is organized with reference to head, trunk, and limbs. Extrapersonal space can be mapped in allocentric (object-based) coordinates.

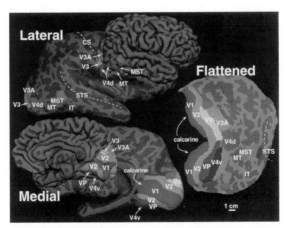

Plate 2 Visual areas with well characterized retinotopic organization identified by fMRI. The brain regions are superimposed on lateral and mesial views of the human cerebral hemispheres and on flattened visual cortex. CS, central sulcus; STS, superior temporal sulcus; MT, motion temporal area; MST, medial superior temporal; IT, inferior temporal; VP, ventral posterior. (Courtesy of Martin Sereno; © 2001, Lippincott, Williams and Wilkins; Sereno *et al.* 1995; Bear *et al.* 2001).

Three imaging studies on line bisection

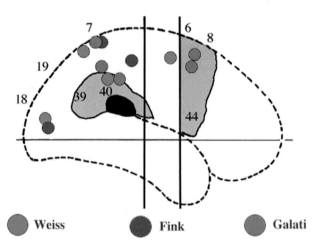

Plate 3 Brain areas associated with spatial neglect (shaded areas) and meta-analysis of three functional neuroimaging experiments using line bisection. Circles represent the location of activation peaks expressed in stereotactic space from three different imaging studies (Weiss *et al.* 2000; Fink *et al.* 2000a; Galati *et al.* 2000). Only the activations on the lateral surface of the right hemisphere are reported. The horizontal line represents the plane passing through the two commissures. The two vertical lines represent the coronal planes passing through each of the two commissures. Mesial ventral occipital activations are not shown.

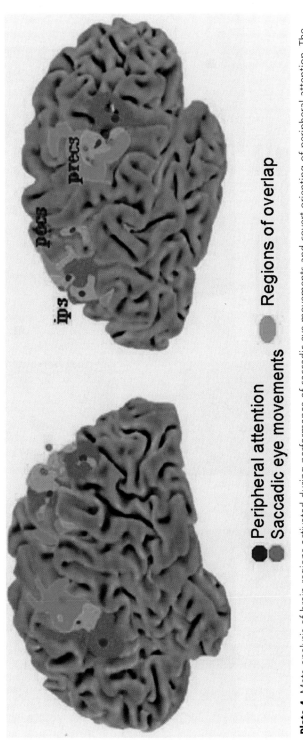

Plate 4 Meta-analysis of brain regions activated during performance of saccadic eye movements and covert orienting of peripheral attention. The picture shows areas for performance of saccadic eye movements, for covert orienting of peripheral attention, and areas shared, at the macroscopic anatomical level, by the two processes. ips, Intraparietal sulcus; pocs, postcentral sulcus; precs, precentral sulcus. (Source: Corbetta 1998: Courtesy of Maurizio Corbetta; © 1998, National Academy of Sciences, USA.)

● Peripheral attention
● Saccadic eye movements
● Regions of overlap

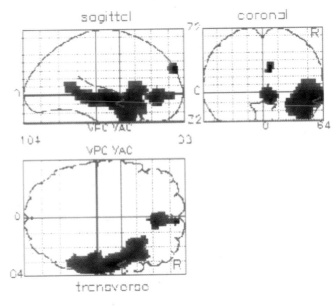

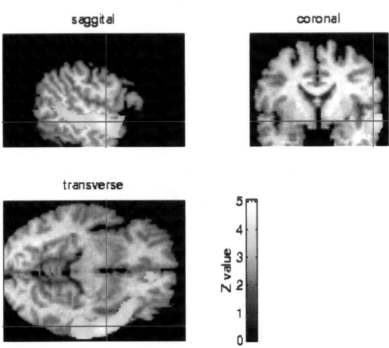

SPM analysis – date: 28–Sep–95 user: grl

Plate 5 Positron emission tomographic (PET) results, showing activated brain regions of an individual, imaging episodes of his past.

and Vallar 2000; Vallar 1998). A third source of evidence for the role of sensory afferents in the building of spatial representations comes from the effects of lateralized or direction-specific stimulations of peripheral sensory systems, such as caloric vestibular stimulation (CVS), posterior neck muscle mechanical vibration (NV) and optokinetic stimulation (OKS) (review in Vallar *et al.* 1997). In normal subjects these stimulations can induce a distortion of egocentric coordinates, causing, e.g. a deviation of the subjective straight ahead (an index of spatial representation) in pointing tasks (relevant literature quoted in Bottini *et al.* 2001). Therefore, the internal representation of space may involve the integration of different sensory inputs—visual, somatosensory–proprioceptive, vestibular, auditory—yielding reference frames that are not based on individual peripheral sensory codes, organized, as they are, in egocentric (e.g. head, trunk, arm) and object- or environment-centred coordinates (Andersen *et al.* 1997; Rizzolatti *et al.* 2000; Graziano and Gross 1994). To illustrate the integrative nature of the neural representation of space, we first need to consider, briefly, the individual sensory modalities. We have constrained our review to visual and somatosensory space. We will then discuss how these individual modalities are combined into multimodal representations and to what extent functional imaging has contributed to describing the anatomical bases of these representations in humans.

2.2 **Visual space**

Visual space is mapped primarily by the geniculostriate pathway where magnocellular, parvocellular, and koniocellular information arrives segregated to different layers of primary visual cortex (area V1) (Livingstone and Hubel 1988; Zeki 1993; Hendry and Reid 2000). Area V1 information is then conveyed to extrastriate visual cortex through divergent pathways, usually referred to as the ventral (object-centred or 'what') stream and the dorsal (space-related or 'where') stream (Mishkin *et al.* 1983). Neurons of the visual cortices have receptive fields (RFs) of increasing complexity and size from area V1 to extrastriate visual cortex. The farther from V1, the more complex the receptive fields of the neurons, with neurons having an RF nearly as big as the whole visual field. Cortical visual areas may show a retinotopic organization in that a single neuron responds to visual events arising from the same part of the retina. The part of the visual world mapped by these neurons varies with the position of the eyes in the orbit. There is now clear evidence that the brain makes extensive use of both retinotopic and non-retinotopic representations of visual space (reviews in Rizzolatti *et al.* 2000; Graziano and Gross 1994; Andersen 1994; Galletti and Fattori 2002). Even from an intuitive point of view, this appears to be an efficient computational strategy to enable stable phenomenological perception in situations, e.g. when the eyes move, the perceived world remains stable despite the movements of the retinal images. Actions such as reaching and grasping benefit from visual descriptions centred on moving body segments (peripersonal space) or centred on objects in space (allocentric space).

2.2.1 Where are the visual cells with increasingly complex RF properties located?

In the primary visual cortex (area V1), visual space is mapped in purely retinotopic space. Each neuron has a receptive field, a sort of small window, that captures a portion of the visual field. Suppose we observe a basket full of red apples and fixate on one of the apples. A given single visual cell in V1 will provide the same information when the eyes are fixating on the closest apple at the left end or the farthest apple at the right end of the basket. That is to say, single neurons in V1 do not discriminate between spatial locations.

A first departure from a purely retinotopic mapping of the visual field is observed in the so-called gaze-dependent cells (Andersen 1994). In these cells the firing frequency depends not only on what strikes their receptive field but also on the position of the eyes in the orbit or the dynamic component of gaze. Initially found in the posterior parietal cortex (PPC), particularly in area 7a, and in the lateral intraparietal sulcus (LIP), they have been found in extrastriate visual areas V3, V3A, V5/MT, MST, and V6 (see Figs 38.2 and 38.3) (Galletti and Fattori 2002; Galletti et al. 1993). These neurons have retinotopically organized RFs and therefore do not yet encode visual space in a manner that is independent of the eye position.

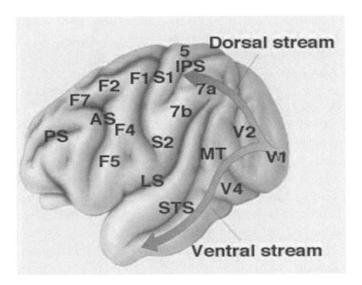

Fig. 38.2 Left cerebral hemisphere of the macaque brain. IPS, intraparietal sulcus; MT, motion temporal area (V5); S1, primary somatosensory area; S2, second somatosensory area; CS, central sulcus; LS, lateral sulcus; STS, superior temporal sulcus; AS, arcuate sulcus; PS, principal sulcus. The nomenclature of motor areas follows Matelli et al. (1985, 1991). Some of the visual areas (V3, V6) cannot be seen on the lateral surface of the brain.

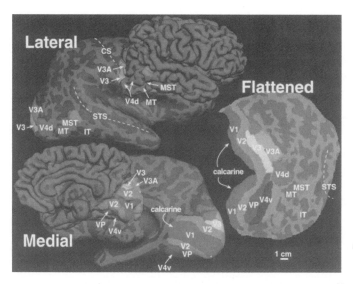

Fig. 38.3 Visual areas with well characterized retinotopic organization identified by fMRI. The brain regions are superimposed on lateral and mesial views of the human cerebral hemispheres and on flattened visual cortex. CS, central sulcus; STS, superior temporal sulcus; MT, motion temporal area; MST, medial superior temporal; IT, inferior temporal; VP, ventral posterior. (Courtesy of Martin Sereno; © 2001, Lippincott, Williams and Wilkins; Sereno *et al.* 1995; Bear *et al.* 2001). (See also 'Plates' section.)

2.2.2 How does the brain build an eye-position-independent coding of visual space?

There are two competitive hypotheses on this issue.

♦ One maintains that this further level of visual space representation may arise by the temporal integration of an extensive system of gaze-dependent visual cells (Andersen *et al.* 1997).

♦ A second theory postulates the existence of real-position cells, in which visual stimuli given to the same part of space cause similar neuronal responses in spite of the actual direction of gaze and position of the eyes in the orbits. Cells of this kind have been described in the PPC (area V6a or PO; Galletti *et al.* 1993), in the ventral intraparietal cortex (Duhamel *et al.* 1992), and in the premotor cortex (area F4) (Graziano and Gross 1994; Fogassi *et al.* 1996). Their property may arise from convergent input from a set of gaze-dependent cells. The space coded by such cells can be called extrapersonal space. Evidence from patients with unilateral neglect and neurophysiological evidence in the monkey show that extrapersonal space can be further divided into peripersonal space (the space within reaching distance) and far space (review in Rizzolatti *et al.* 2000).

2.3 **Somatosensory and personal space**

Cortical somatosensory representation of the body surface, joints, and muscles includes areas of the postcentral gyrus (areas of the S1 complex, Brodmann areas (BAs) 3, 1, 2), areas of the dorsal posterior parietal region (BA 5 of the monkey and human BAs 5 and 7), the secondary somatosensory area (area S2, BA 43). which is located in the ventral bank of the parietal operculum, the granular insula, the retroinsular cortex. and the more rostral part of the inferior parietal lobule (area 7b of the monkey and human area 40 (reviews in Kaas 1990; Paulesu *et al.*1997). Much as for the visual areas, the RFs of individual neurons of the various somatosensory areas and the overall grain of the resulting maps change from area S1 to area S2, granular insula, retroinsular cortex, and supramarginal gyrus.

♦ S1 has the finest grained somatotopy with strictly contralateral receptive fields and limited callosal connections.

♦ S2 has a large proportion of neurons with bilateral or even with ipsilateral receptive fields.

The same applies to the other somatosensory cortices (for a synopsis of the properties of the somatosensory cortices, see Paulesu *et al.* 1997)

♦ Input to these cortices remains purely somatosensory only in area S1 proper (area 3b) and in area 1.

♦ The retroinsular cortex, part of area 3a, area S2, the cortex at the tip of the intraparietal sulcus, and area 7b receive vestibular input as well.

♦ Area 7b has about 20% of neurons responding to visual stimuli.

♦ Signals from the neck muscles reach the retroinsular cortex, the insula, and area S2 (Guldin and Grüsser 1998).

♦ In keeping with the functional properties of these cortices, the afferent thalamic inputs to these areas are strictly from the specific ventroposterior somatosensory nucleus for area 3b and 1 and from multiple thalamic nuclei for the remaining areas.

Polymodal neurons with tactile and visual properties have also been found in the lateral premotor cortex (review in Rizzolatti *et al.* 2000), which also receives vestibular signals (Guldin and Grüsser 1998).

The integrative nature of body schema representation goes well beyond a body map of the skin such as that represented in area 3b. The body schema is probably based on a number of body-centred spatial frames, including knowledge about the spatial relationship of body segments. The midsagittal plane of the body appears a robust neural/mental construct: its representation is easily tested with tasks involving the appreciation of the straight ahead coordinate in pointing or visual detection tasks and may arise from the neural operations of the brain regions receiving joint input from tactile, muscle/joint receptors and from the vestibular receptors. Orientation of the midsagittal plane can be pathologically rotated towards the side of the brain damage in patients with spatial neglect or physiologically rotated in normal subjects by asymmetric input from the vestibular or from the neck-muscle receptors (Karnath 1994; Karnath *et al.* 1994). The space coded by this neural system is called personal space.

2.4 Merging visual, somatosensory, and motoric spatial representations

Recently, the important discovery was made of a class of bimodal neurons responding to visual stimuli and to tactile stimuli. These bimodal neurons have been found in:

- the premotor cortex (area 6 or F4);
- the inferior parietal cortex (area 7b);
- the putamen (Graziano and Gross 1994).

In these regions, a hand bimodal neuron responds to both tactile stimuli delivered to the hand while the animal's eyes are closed and to a visual stimulus delivered in the space surrounding the hand (about 20 to 100 cm away). Interestingly, the visual field of these bimodal neurons moves with the position of the limb and is independent of the position of the eyes. The space coded by these neurons is indeed peripersonal space.

The aforementioned evidence of the existence of visual neurons in premotor area 6 contributes to the now overwhelming demonstration that space (visual, somatosensory, and even auditory) is not just represented in posterior sensory regions but also in frontal-lobe regions, including the agranular and dysgranular premotor cortex, which has motor-like functions (review in Rizzolatti *et al.* 2000). The premotor cortex (areas 6 and 8) has neurons that enter in the descending motor tracts or are connected to primary motor cortex. In addition, in the same regions, there are visual neurons with clear visual or visuomotor properties and a recognizeable visual receptive field. In the frontal eye-fields (FEFs), the region that triggers saccadic eye movements to reach spatial location with gaze, there are visual and visuomotor neurons whose firing is enhanced by visual stimuli when the stimulus represents a target for an ocular movement (Goldberg and Bushnell 1981). The visual receptive field of these neurons is based on retinotopic coordinates. On the other hand, as mentioned above, in the ventral premotor cortex (particularly in area F4), along with the motoric neurons involved in reaching and grasping, there are also visual neurons, or bimodal visuotactile neurons, whose visual receptive field is anchored to body segments and moves with them. The response of these neurons does not depend on retinotopic coordinates. It rather contributes to egocentric/peripersonal space representation. These premotor cortices are electively and orderly connected with posterior parietal regions of the inferior parietal lobule, of the intraparietal sulcus, and of the superior parietal lobule, sharing some functional properties related to the space mapped. Area F4 is functionally related to area the inferior parietal lobule (BA 7b) and to the anterior intraparietal area—they both predominantly encode peripersonal space within reaching distance. The FEFs are functionally connected with the lateral intraparietal cortex and with the posterior part of the inferior parietal lobule (BA 7a). They have to do with eye movements and visual space coded in retinotopic and craniocentric coordinates.

Another interesting description of neuronal properties of the premotor and parietal network is based on a task-dependent classification of motor behaviour within space at reaching distance (Jeannerod *et al.* 1995; Wise *et al.* 1997). The dorsal stream is proposed as a modular visuomotor transformation network.

- There is now abundant evidence that the most dorsal part of the parietofrontal network (superior parietal cortex and dorsal premotor cortex) is primarily concerned with reaching tasks and contributes to compute distance between target and limb and spatial location of targets.

- The more ventral premotor and parietal network is more concerned with grasping and the relevant dynamic hand-shaping processes.

Objects are therefore represented at multiple levels.

- In the ventral stream objects are represented in allocentric coordinates related to object semantics, i.e. features such as shape, texture, colour.

- In the dorsal stream objects are coded for their spatial position in an egocentric/peripersonal spatial frame used for generations of reaching and grasping behaviour.

Dissociation of these spatial frames is supported by human neuropsychological evidence: object discrimination can be severely impaired by ventral visual-cortex lesions, while accurate reaching and grasping may still be possible. The opposite anatomo-behavioural dissociation is also on record (Goodale and Milner 1992).

3 Space representation in humans: evidence from lesion studies

A major source of evidence comes from studies on unilateral neglect and from studies on patients with reaching disorders not associated with neglect. The evidence is somewhat limited by the nature of the acquired brain lesions, which are by default vast and not constrained to discrete cytoarchitectural areas. Acquired lesions also usually involve subcortical white matter, making interpretation of the anatomoclinical associations not simple.

3.1 Anatomical basis of spatial neglect (see Chapter 5)

Reviews on the anatomical basis of spatial neglect can be found in Bisiach and Vallar (2000), Mesulam (1990), and Heilman *et al.* (1994). The distribution of cortical lesions observed in neglect, according to Vallar (1998), is presented in Fig. 38.4 (shaded areas). In short, unilateral neglect, which is characterized by the inability of representing and exploring the side of space contralateral to the brain lesion, is usually observed after damage to the inferior parietal lobule: lesions are centred on the supramarginal gyrus,

Three imaging studies on line bisection

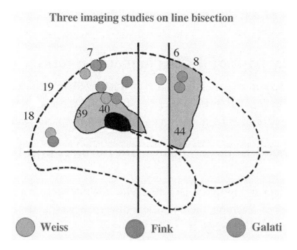

Fig. 38.4 Brain areas associated with spatial neglect (shaded areas) and meta-analysis of three functional neuroimaging experiments using line bisection. Circles represent the location of activation peaks expressed in stereotactic space from three different imaging studies (Weiss *et al.* 2000; Fink *et al.* 2000a; Galati *et al.* 2000). Only the activations on the lateral surface of the right hemisphere are reported. The horizontal line represents the plane passing through the two commissures. The two vertical lines represent the coronal planes passing through each of the two commissures. Mesial ventral occipital activations are not shown. (See also 'Plates' section.)

with involvement of the neighbouring inferior parietal and superior temporal areas. Lesion of the premotor cortices (BA 6, 44) can bring about neglect dominated by motor symptoms rather than by perceptual symptoms. Yet, this dichotomy does not seem to be always a valid one (Mattingley *et al.* 1998).

Neglect has also been observed after thalamic lesions or subcortical white matter lesions. It is much more frequent for right- rather than left-hemisphere lesions. It has recently been suggested that parietal neglect may be confounded by visual field deficits. It has been proposed that lesion of the superior temporal cortex might be a purer anatomical correlate of space exploration deficit (Karnath *et al.* 2001; Samuelsson *et al.* 1997). On the other hand, damage restricted to primary motor or sensory areas does not bring about neglect. This supports the higher-level nature of the spatial disorder observed in patients with spatial neglect.

Taken together, the anatomy of spatial neglect suggests a distributed neural architecture for spatial representation with a functional specialization of the right hemisphere.

One area in which lesion data have not been informative as yet is that of the dissociation of symptoms within the neglect syndrome. Patients may present neglect symptoms only in one spatial frame (e.g. near space but not far space; Halligan and Marshall 1991) or in the same peripersonal space, in one task (e.g. line bisection) but not in another (target cancellation tasks; Halligan and Marshall 1992). These dissociations are not corroborated as yet by clear anatomical differences of lesion location (review in Vallar 2001).

3.2 Anatomical basis of deficits in reaching tasks

The other major acquired spatial disorder is characterized by deficits in reaching tasks. Lesions are usually located in the superior parietal lobule and the disorder usually involves the contralateral limb in reaching in both sides of space (Jeannerod 1997).

3.3 Discrepancies between data from humans and those from monkeys

How do human data and monkey data fit together? While there is a substantial agreement for disorders of reaching, there is a clear discrepancy as far as the location of the key lesion that brings about neglect.

- In the monkey, neglect is more severe for ventral premotor cortical lesions or for lesions in the superior temporal sulcus.
- In humans, the manifestations of neglect are more severe in the case of parietal lesions (for reviews, see Rizzolatti et al. 2000 and Bisiach and Vallar 2000).

Another important discrepancy is the hemispheric asymmetry observed in humans and not in primates.

4 Functional anatomical studies of space perception

4.1 Visual and somatosensory space

Functional imaging has the advantage of allowing one to explore the organization of the normal, as well as, the diseased human brain *in vivo*. Yet, it should be kept in mind that the temporal and spatial resolution of imaging is not that of invasive electrophysiology in the primate brain. To give an example of an area where imaging may be difficult to compare with electrophysiology, the progressive making of spatial representation from early sensory visual codes may prove difficult to demonstrate. With the current techniques it has not been possible to isolate signals of neuronal populations of cells with gaze-dependent visual response, nor to isolate responses that can be plausibly interpreted as real-position like. There are obvious reasons why this may remain difficult with imaging. Such cells are present in small areas that contain simpler cells as well. Even in the primate brain, real-position cells coexist in the same area with gaze-dependent cells.

In spite of the above limitations, a substantial part of the detailed information derived from the primate brain is reproducible using functional imaging in humans. A large number of retinotopically organized areas have been now identified outside area V1 and area V2. Historically, the existence of separate extrastriate areas specialized in colour and motion perception, respectively, was first shown. These are likely homologues of the monkey areas V4 and V5 (Zeki et al. 1991). An even more detailed cartography of retinotopically organized extrastriate areas has now been described through the use of fMRI (see Fig. 38.3) (Sereno et al. 1995).

The receptive fields of the neurons within these areas are increasingly complex, with neurons mapping also the ipsilateral visual field starting from area V3a and area MT/V5 (Tootell *et al.* 1998). Together with the increasing complexity of the visual receptive field, an increasing complexity of processing is observed, e.g. in the ventral stream, while posterior regions are preferentially activated by object attributes such as colours or scrambled objects, more anterior regions of the temporal lobe are activated by intact objects or faces (review in Kastner and Ungerleider 2000).

The neural representation of somatosensory space has been explored using a variety of approaches. Simple experiments in which somatosensory stimuli were delivered to the hands or feet have broadly confirmed the well-established notion of a somototopic organization of area S1. A possible somatotopic organization of area S2 has also been reported (Ruben *et al.* 2001). In keeping with primate data, receptive fields in S1 appear to be strictly unilateral, while bilateral activation of area S2 is observed for stimuli delivered to either side of the body, suggesting the presence in the human S2 of cells with at least bilateral, if not ipsilateral RFs (review in Paulesu *et al.* 1997).

4.2 The different frames of space as assessed by functional imaging

Coming to higher-order spatial representations, one area of enquiry that was approached as soon as functional imaging became available, was the demonstration of the broad dichotomy between the two visual streams (the 'what' and 'where' pathways). This has proved a relatively easy task. Haxby *et al.* (1991) were the first to compare a face-matching task (a ventral 'what' stream task) and a dot location task (a spatial 'where' task). A sensorimotor task with no relevant visual stimuli served as a control task. Compared to baseline, both experimental tasks showed activation of the lateral occipital cortex. Face discrimination alone activated a region of the occipitotemporal cortex, whereas the spatial location alone activated a region of the lateral superior parietal cortex.

This dichotomy has been demonstrated and further characterized several times (Haxby *et al.* 1994), particularly with reference to visual working memory. In keeping with electrophysiological data in the monkey (Goldman-Rakic 1996), when visual processing involves active maintenance of the spatial location of visual stimuli and delayed response, a dorsolateral prefrontal cortex activation is also observed (Courtney *et al.* 1998). Consistent again with primate data (Wilson *et al.* 1993; Chelazzi *et al.* 1993), active maintenance of object-oriented visual information involves the more ventral part of lateral prefrontal cortex together with the ventral visual cortex (Courtney *et al.* 1996). Therefore, the what (ventral) and where (dorsal) dichotomy is also present in frontal cortex (for a review of human functional imaging data of various forms of visual working memory, see Ungerleider *et al.* 1998).

The experiment of Haxby *et al.* (1991) involved extrapersonal spatial coordinates. The systematic exploration of other spatial frames has become the focus of research in several laboratories.

4.2.1 Object-centred (allocentric) space

Interestingly, a number of tasks have been used in which patients with spatial neglect may fail, showing either an overall impairment or a specific and dissociated impairment, depending on the nature of the task and the spatial frame explored by it. Object-centred (allocentric) spatial judgements have been studied in at least three experiments (Weiss *et al.* 2000; Fink *et al.* 2000*a*; Galati *et al.* 2000). The stimuli used were computerized variations of Milner's landmark task in which stimuli are pre-bisected segments. The subjects had to judge whether the vertical bar that bisects a longer horizontal segment is placed in the middle of the segment or not. A meta-analysis of the main activations detected in the right hemisphere in these experiments is presented in Fig. 38.4. Baseline tasks were designed to subtract components other than spatial awareness. Activation foci are superimposed on a standard stereotactic view of the right hemisphere. The shaded areas represent the brain regions usually damaged in unilateral neglect (Vallar 1998). A common involvement of the lateral extrastriate cortex, of the most dorsal part of area 40 in the inferior parietal lobule, and the intraparietal sulcus, the superior parietal lobule, and dorsal premotor cortex is clearly evident. This network closely resembles the visuomotor transformation network involved in reaching tasks in the monkey and in humans (Jeannerod 1997).

In the same experiment described above, Galati and co-workers (2000) devised an additional task in which subjects had to judge whether the vertical bar was located to the left or to the right of the subjective (egocentric) midsagittal plane of their body. In comparison with the same baseline, a similar, yet larger, bilateral pattern of activation emerged in the superior posterior parietal cortex (mesial and lateral), in the dorsal premotor cortex (bilaterally), and in the left temporoparietal cortex. The premotor cortex, the medial dorsalparietal cortex, and the right intraparietal cortex were more active when compared with the 'allocentric' task. In turn, there was a larger activation in the medial ventral extrastriate cortex when the allocentric task was compared with the egocentric one (not shown in Fig. 38.4). This seems a reproducible result. A similar finding was made by Fink *et al.* (2000*b*) when comparing a bisection judgement performed on a one-dimensional object (a segment) or a two-dimensional object (a square).

Larger activation of the ventral occipital cortex was also observed by Weiss *et al.* (2000), when comparing pointing tasks (including bisection) in far space as opposed to near space. On the other hand, they found that the left hemispheric parietal cortex, the dorsal occipital cortex, and the premotor cortex were more active when comparing activations for near space as opposed to far space.

4.2.2 Egocentric (personal) space

Representations for egocentric (personal) space have been also explored recently using a different approach by Bottini *et al.* (2001). As discussed in Section 1, one possible mechanism by which spatial representations could be achieved is through integration through convergence of different afferent inputs. Within this level of spatial body-centred description, tactile, vestibular, and proprioceptive stimuli, including those conveyed by the muscle spindles of the neck, play an important role. In the monkey, a perisylvian network of cortices including the parietoinsular and retroinsular cortex, the ventral premotor cortex, and the tip of the intraparietal sulcus, all receive inputs from the vestibule, from the body surface, and from muscle spindles, including those of the neck muscles. Using this rationale, Bottini *et al.* (2001) have mapped the cortical areas that are activated by either vestibular signals or by the neck muscle spindles, as appropriate stimulations of these systems can induce spatial bias towards the stimulated side in normal controls and reduce spatial disorder of unilateral neglect. As for the monkey, the perisylvian somatosensory cortex (retroinsular cortex, area S2, supramarginal gyrus) appears to be a site of convergence of these inputs, suggesting that these brain regions contribute to egocentric space representation (Bottini *et al.* 2001).

4.2.3 Is there dissociation between allocentric and egocentric frames of reference?

The picture that emerges from the above experiments is not yet fully coherent in showing a clear-cut dissociation of allocentric and egocentric frames of references. This may be due to a not complete equivalence between experimental and baseline tasks used in the various experiments and to the assumption of lack of spatial demands made when choosing such baselines. In addition, subjects responded to the stimuli in different ways, in each of the experiments. There was button pressing in three experiments, pointing with a laser light in one, and no response in another.

However, taken together, the results of Fink *et al.* (2000*a*), Galati *et al.* (2000), and Weiss *et al.* (2000) seem to indicate a weak dissociation in a distributed and partially overlapping system for spatial representation of peripersonal and extrapersonal space.

- ◆ The visuomotor transformation network implied in the reaching behaviour is activated, with greater emphasis on the dorsal parietal and premotor cortex, when the experimental task implies attending spatial locations that are within reaching distance.

- ◆ Ventral retinotopically organized and object-based visual cortices are more active when the comparisons of blood flow maps isolate the processing of spatial locations that are either outside reaching distance (far space) or when reaching is (relatively) de-emphasized.

The difference in results between the 'egocentric task of Galati *et al.* (2000) and the experiment of Bottini *et al.* (2001), an experiment that, no doubt, tackles the convergent afferents that contribute to the representation of egocentric space, remains particularly striking. It is likely that the task in hand, and the reference baseline adopted, dominate the picture of the activations that can be observed with imaging. These factors alone may somewhat explain the discrepancies. Alternatively, one may speculate on the existence of multiple levels of neural/cognitive representations for the same spatial frame. If this were the case, behavioural dissociations based on lesion data would be needed to make this a more concrete possibility.

The consistency of each of the above observations with lesion data of neglect will be discussed in Section 6.

5 Spatial attention

The space surrounding us has far too many items for the brain to be able to process them all efficiently and consciously at the same time. The mental ability that permits to deal explicitly with a subset of behaviourally relevant stimuli is usually referred to as attention. In the definition made by the psychologist William James (1890/1950), 'Attention is . . . the taking possession by the mind . . . of one out of what seem several simultaneously possible objects or trains of thought. . . . It implies withdrawal from some things in order to deal effectively with others.' This definition emphasizes attention as a process of selection.

The advantage of attention in perceptual/motor tasks can be appreciated even introspectively. We know that we are more efficient in responding to environmental stimuli when we attend to them. In addition to introspection, there are quantitative behavioural techniques to measure the advantage of attention. Various indices can be used: reaction times are faster for responses to visual stimuli that fall in attended parts of visual field; discrimination of stimuli is enhanced (for an extensive review of behavioural phenomena measured during spatial attention experiments, see Umiltà 2000).

If we consider visual space, the process of orienting attention usually implies fast saccadic eye movements, which are made to bring into foveal space the visual stimuli. Yet there is definitive evidence that spatial attention can be oriented without eye movements—covert (endogenous) orienting.

- Endogenous orienting of attention is frequently referred to as a top–down or controlled process that is effortful and depends on will. The classic paradigm devised by Posner (1980) taps this form of attention (Umiltà 2000; Posner 1980). This paradigm, with small *ad hoc* adaptations, has been used in a number of functional imaging experiments and is illustrated in Fig. 38.5.

- Spatial attention can also be attracted automatically by the sudden appearance of a stimulus in the visual field or by the perceptual salience of a stimulus among others (e.g. a vertical bar among other bars all tilted 30° to the right). These other phenomena are called bottom–up or exogenous processes (Fig. 38.6).

Once attention has been oriented towards a stimulus, it may become necessary to re-orient attention to a different spatial location which implies disengagement from the former stimulus to re-orient towards a different one.

5.1 Does spatial attention have a dedicated neural system in the human brain?

The research agenda into spatial attentional processes using functional neuroimaging (see also the box, p. 712.) includes:

- identification of brain regions involved in spatial attention and assessment of the degree of overlap between attentional, perceptual, and premotor networks, particularly with reference to the neural system for eye movement;

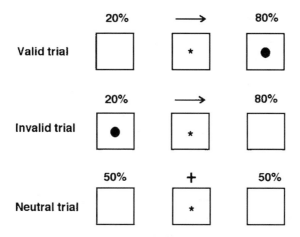

	20%	→	80%
Valid trial		⋆	●

	20%	→	80%
Invalid trial	●	⋆	

	50%	+	50%
Neutral trial		⋆	

Fig. 38.5 Posner's attentional paradigm. In Posner's paradigm, subjects are instructed by a symbolic central cue (an arrow) that a target stimulus (a filled circle) will occur with 80% of chance in a given spatial location. Subjects are instructed to fixate a central mark, not to move their eyes, and to press a key as fast as possible when the filled circle appears. Covert attention is measured as the reaction time benefit in responding to target that appears in the attended location (valid trials) as opposed to response for targets appearing in unattended locations (invalid trials) or to neutral trials, when another symbol (+) indicates that the filled circle has a 50% chance of appearing in either box (Posner 1980).

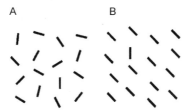

A   B

Fig. 38.6 Difference between controlled and automatic attentional processes. In display A, detection of a vertical segment is a demanding attention-seeking (top–down) process that can be oriented endogenously or through verbal instructions. Detection of a vertical segment in display B is stimulus driven and automatic (redrawn from Kastner and Ungerleider 2000).

- ◆ characterization of top–down processes (like those involved in covert, or endogenous, orienting) as opposed to attentional phenomena based on perceptual salience (bottom–up processes; exogenous orienting);
- ◆ assessment of orienting versus disengaging attention;
- ◆ space- versus object-based attention;
- ◆ global (diffuse) and local attentional processes.

Some of these issues have been illuminated by functional imging.

Attention from the neurophysiologist's perspective

While psychologists characterize attentional effects in the form of reaction time benefits or costs, the neurophysiologist records the neuronal firing rate associated with presentation of a stimulus or with the execution of a motoric response. Which kind of response is then interpreted as attentional in nature by the neurophysiologist? The most robust and established effects are 'enhancement effects', increases of baseline activity, and suppressions of unwanted information.

◆ *Enhancement effects.* Goldberg and Wurtz (1972) made the important observation that the firing rate of a visual neuron of the superior colliculus can be enhanced when a stimulus is delivered to the receptive field of that neuron if the animal is covertly paying attention to that spatial location. The enhancement effects in the superior colliculus are present only when the animal is about to generate a saccadic eye movement towards the stimulus. Similar neurons can be found in cortical structures involved in eye-movement control, such as the frontal eye-fields (Goldberg and Bushnell 1981). Importantly, in a given neuron the 'enhancement effect' is not present if the saccadic eye movement is performed towards a spatial location outside the receptive field of the neuron. Enhancement effects are not necessarily associated with the generation of saccadic eye movements. Such 'purer' enhanced responses have been seen in the pulvinar, but also in parietal cortex (Colby *et al.* 1996) and temporal cortex (Chelazzi *et al.* 1993). In the cortex of the parietal lobe the enhancement is related to spatial location of the stimulus. In the temporal lobe enhancement effects are related to stimulus attributes rather than to its spatial location.

◆ *Increase of baseline activity.* While the enhancement effect occurs at the time that the stimulus is presented, increase of baseline activity has been observed in neurons of area V2 or area V4 even before the presentation of a stimulus, providing the experimental animal is paying attention to the spatial location that corresponds to the receptive field of the neuron (Luck *et al.* 1997).

◆ *Filtering of unwanted information.* When two objects are present in the receptive field of the same neuron of the temporal lobe (e.g. an object that activates the neuron and an object that activates it less strongly), a mutual suppression of neural response is observed so that the neural firing is roughly the average of the firing rates induced by each object at the time. This suppression can be modulated by attention towards one of the two objects so that the response is similar to that for that object presented in isolation (Reynolds *et al.* 1999).

All of these general effects have been seen in humans using functional imaging.

Enhancement effects have been seen in subjects who were paying attention to certain visual features of a display in comparison to when they were passively viewing the same display.

Attention from the neurophysiologist's perspective *(continued)*

♦ Attention to colour was associated with enhanced response in modality-specific visual cortices such as area V4.

♦ Attention to shape was associated with enhanced response in area V3.

♦ Enhancement for speed and motion was associated with area V5/MT (Corbetta *et al.* 1991).

A shift in baseline activity in specific cortical areas has been described using fMRI. Even in the absence of any actual change in the visual stimulus, the baseline activities of the visual motion area V5/MT or of colour area V4 are enhanced if subjects are expecting to detect a change of motion or in colour in a visual display (Chawla *et al.* 1999). Conversely, if subjects are distracted by a highly demanding language task while observing a display of moving dots, activation of area V5/MT disappears, contrary to what happens in the same conditions when the distracting task is an easy one (Rees *et al.* 1997*b*).

fMRI data that are compatible with the filtering of unwanted visual information by visual cortex have recently been reported (Kastner *et al.* 1998).

The contribution of functional imaging to these fundamental issues has been crucial to progress. In fact, lesion data are not conclusive for the same reason that some disorders of spatial exploration and representation, such as spatial neglect, are not universally interpreted as due to an attentional deficit (for a review of competing interpretations of spatial neglect, see Bisiach and Vallar 2000). Event-related potentials are able to reveal changes of brain response but they cannot tell in which part of the brain these effects are generated. In a very influential paper, Posner and Petersen (1990) summarized the then available evidence, including very early functional imaging data, on the existence of attentional networks. They proposed the following three tenets.

♦ The attentional system is anatomically separate from the data-processing system and, in this sense, it is like other sensory and motor systems.

♦ The attentional system involves a distributed network:

—a posterior attentional system;

—an anterior attentional system;

—an ascending attentional system.

♦ Within the network different components have different specializations that can be described in cognitive terms.

The cognitive operations involved are:

♦ orienting to sensory events;

♦ detecting signals for focal processing;

♦ maintaining vigilance.

In this account of spatial attention, each component has its neural machinery.

- Orienting to sensory events usually implies the foveation of a stimulus (overt orienting). The brain regions involved are: the posterior parietal cortex (Goldberg and Bruce 1985); the pulvinar nucleus of the thalamus (LaBerge and Buchsbaum 1990); and the superior colliculus (Goldberg and Wurtz 1972). These regions represent the posterior attentional system. Based on observation made in patients with parietal lesions (Posner *et al.* 1984), Posner and Petersen (1990) maintain that:

  —the posterior parietal cortex is involved in disengagement from an attentional focus towards a target located in the opposite direction of the side of brain lesion;

  —the superior colliculus would also be involved in shifting attention, whether or not attention was already focused elsewhere;

  —the pulvinar nucleus is thought to contribute to engagement with the new target location of the attentional focus.

- Posner and Petersen (1990) also proposed that the anterior (frontal and cingulate) cortical regions might represent an amodal system that primes the posterior system to detect signals for focal processing. The anterior system is postulated to mediate selective attention and cognitive control. Early PET experiments on divided attention and on control of response for conflictual stimuli (like those of the Stroop task) support this assumption (Pardo *et al.* 1990; Corbetta *et al.* 1991).

- Finally, Posner and Petersen (1990) proposed that alerting is a function of the right hemisphere and of the ascending noradrenergic system (see also Heilman *et al.* 1993).

This cognitive–anatomical model for attention is not unanimously accepted. For example, it sharply contrasts with a competing model that postulates that the attentional networks are embedded with the same networks involved in perception and action. One such model, in fact, postulates that spatial attention is the consequence of the activation, even in the absence of overt motor response, of the neural system that mediates sensory motor transformation (Rizzolatti *et al.* 1994).

We will next discuss the extent to which assumptions proposed by Petersen and Posner have been confirmed by the recent imaging literature, together with a short review of other relevant experiments on spatial attention.

5.2 The physiology of eye movements and spatial attention

A crucial test of Posner and Petersen's (1990) model is the assessment of the degree of independence of areas activated by covert orienting of visual attention (as in Posner's paradigm illustrated in Fig. 38.5) and actual performance of saccadic eye movements. Behavioural evidence would suggest that the two systems are somewhat embedded (for reviews see Umiltà 2000 and Corbetta 1998). On this particular issue there are a number of specific functional imaging experiments (Corbetta *et al.* 1998; Nobre *et al.* 2000) and detailed meta-analyses (Corbetta 1998; Nobre *et al.* 1997).

In short, both covert orienting attention (as in Posner's paradigm; see Fig. 38.5) and generation of saccades share neural resources in:

- the parietal regions of the intraparietal sulcus and superior parietal lobule;
- the dorsal lateral premotor cortex (human homologue of frontal eye fields);
- the mesial dorsal premotor cortex (human supplementary frontal eye-fields) (Fig. 38.7).

Therefore, one can reject complete independence of regions involved in covert orienting and saccadic eye movements. However, in the meta-analysis of Corbetta *et al.* (1998), the overlap between the two systems, while considerable, is clearly not perfect.

- Eye movements are associated with more extensive involvement of regions near primary motor and somatosensory cortices.
- Covert orienting shows a larger involvement of prefrontal regions and, posteriorly, of the lateral occipitoparietal junctions.

The additional areas seen in the saccadic eye movements, can be readily explained by the fact that subjects are actually moving the eyes. The additional areas seen in covert orienting may represent the more cognitive neural counterpart of the task. Indeed, the discrepancy between the motor task (saccadic eye movements) and the more controlled orienting task is reminiscent of the difference seen in tasks of different nature in which one task involves more controlled and cognitive demanding factors. For instance, in the case of articulation of a stereotyped string of digits as opposed to random generation of digits, the latter task also involves more anterior prefrontal regions (Petrides *et al.* 1993). A meta-analysis performed by Kastner and Ungerleider (2000) also shows that the distribution of the activation during covert orienting of visual

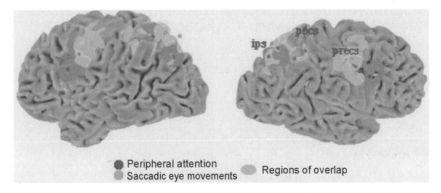

Fig. 38.7 Meta-analysis of brain regions activated during performance of saccadic eye movements and covert orienting of peripheral attention. The picture shows areas for performance of saccadic eye movements, for covert orienting of peripheral attention, and areas shared, at the macroscopic anatomical level, by the two processes. ips, Intraparietal sulcus; pocs, postcentral sulcus; precs, precentral sulcus. (Source: Corbetta 1998: Courtesy of Maurizio Corbetta; © 1998, National Academy of Sciences, USA.) (See also 'Plates' section.)

attention, while maintaining central fixation, is independent of the specific require-ments of the visuospatial task, i.e. detecting a stimulus and discriminating or tracking its movement. Interestingly, the pattern of activation looks very similar to that identi-fied in the meta-analysis presented in Fig. 38.4.

What is the impact of eye movements on the firing rate of the brain regions outside those directly implicated in the motor commands? There is evidence of a substantial inhi-bition of occipital visual areas during saccades. This has been seen for reflexive saccades induced by vestibular stimuli where the lateralization of deactivation (on the opposite side of the areas of major activation by vestibular stimuli) suggests that a specific neurobiolog-ical mechanism is involved. It is also interesting that deactivations include, amongst oth-ers, the visual motion perception area MT/V5. The modulatory effect of eye movements on visual areas has also been described by Paus *et al.* (1996). Volunteers lay in the dark and moved their eyes at different rates during a series of scans. Activity in the frontal eye fields was positively correlated with the rate of eye movements. However, in visual cortex and visual association areas, activity was negatively correlated with rate of eye movements.

Fink and colleagues (1997) have explored another important issue, the interaction of eye movements in object- as opposed to space-based attention. They found that brain activation during attention is modulated by eye movements, particularly for object-based attention. Greater parietal activations were seen when foveation was not allowed, as if object-based attention, in these conditions, becomes 'more spatial' in nature. The stimuli used by Fink and colleagues were devoid of any semantic information (simple lines with a square), nor were graspable objects or body segments used. Further studies are needed to address the same issue using ecologically relevant objects in two- and three-dimensional presentations.

5.3 Top–down and bottom–up processes in spatial attention: where is 'the top' and where is 'the bottom'?

Whichever model of attention one considers, it is necessary to consider whether con-trolled processes can be distinguished anatomically from automatic orienting of atten-tion. While there is a general consensus that enhancement effects observed in extrastriate visual cortex (see the box) may represent the effect of top–down modula-tions from areas outside visual cortex, the source of the modulation remains elusive.

Kastner and Ungerleider (2000) propose that the source of top–down modulation may be located in the brain areas involved in covert orienting of attention. The obvious way to test this assumption would be to compare Posner's task with another task in which spatial attention is driven exogenously. This was tried by Nobre and collabor-ators (1997). They compared a task in which a peripheral visual cue indicated that a subsequent stimulus was 80% likely to occur in the same location with the situation in which the same cue meant that a subsequent stimulus was 80% likely to occur in the opposite part of the visual field. The latter task is more tightly associated to a con-trolled attentional process, while the former tackles almost fully an exogenous process. However, the two tasks did not show a clear-cut dichotomy either when compared with a reference task or when the two tasks were compared directly to each other. Both tasks were associated with a system compatible with that described in Fig. 38.7.

Rees *et al.* (1997*a*) approached the same problem in an experiment in which top–down factors were assessed by trying to distinguish tonic biasing mechanisms from stimulus-dependent mechanisms. This is not easy to achieve given the temporal resolution of imaging techniques (Rees *et al.* 1997*a*). However, by changing the rate of the visual stimuli requiring attention, they were able to show that the inferior temporal cortex had rate-dependent changes of attention-induced activity, while activity in the right dorsal premotor cortex (BA8) was independent of the stimulus presentation rate. This data is compatible with the idea that the inferior temporal cortex is a site of modulation while the right premotor region is a source of top–down modulatory effects on the visual cortices.

Kastner *et al.* (1999) used fMRI to investigate patterns of activation in the presence and absence of visual stimuli. Sustained activity was observed, even in the absence of actual stimulation, in the dorsal parietal regions and premotor regions usually involved in covert orienting of attention. This sustained activity was of the same magnitude as the activity observed during stimulus presentation. On the other hand, in ventral extrastriate visual areas, activity in the absence of visual stimuli was comparatively smaller. This evidence supports the proposal that the dorsal brain areas involved in orienting attention are the source of modulatory signals towards ventral extrastriate visual areas. The role of the superior parietal cortex in orienting attention, rather than stimulus detection, has been recently demonstrated by Corbetta *et al.* (2000).

Is the source of these modulatory effects unique? We believe that this is unlikely. Although direct imaging evidence is still scanty, there is behavioural evidence that shows that biasing effects in visual stimuli detection can be induced in tasks that are very different from Posner's covert orienting paradigm or from the other tasks used so far in imaging experiments. For instance, preparing a given grasping response facilitates visual detection of objects with a shape compatible to that grip (Craighero *et al.* 1999). Grasping and observation of grasping depend on different and more ventral sets of premotor and parietal cortices than those involved in eye movements (Rizzolatti *et al.* 2000). As a consequence, it can be speculated that the source of the biasing effects will move according to the nature of the task in hand. This conjecture is supported by recent fMRI evidence. Sustained attention to and observation of finger movements modulate ventral premotor and rostral superior parietal regions, both involved in the actual performance of the same movements and their observation. These are regions, particularly the ventral premotor cortex, well outside the network for eye movements, suggesting a modular organization of the neural systems for attention (Iacoboni *et al.* 1999).

6 A discrepancy between imaging data on spatial attention and processing and the anatomy of spatial neglect

As also remarked by others (Kastner and Ungerleider 2000), the evolving picture of the functional anatomy of spatial attention and, as described here, of spatial processing in general, presents a nontrivial discrepancy with the published anatomy of spatial neglect (Vallar 1998, 2001). Consider the distribution of the lesions observed in neglect and summarized by the shaded areas in Fig. 38.4 (Vallar 1998). It is quite clear that the pattern of activation reported for a line bisection task (a sensitive test of spatial neglect; see meta-analysis in Fig. 38.4) involves brain regions of the parietal lobe that are over-all more dorsal. On the other hand, the more ventral regions are systematically seen in experiments on the central projections of the vestibular system, an important finding given the well known ability of vestibular signals to recalibrate spatial misperception and representation in neglect patients (review in Paulesu *et al.* 1997).

The same remark on the topography of parietal and premotor activations applies to the anatomy of covert orienting of attention (see Fig. 38.7) (Corbetta 1998), which appears overall more dorsal than the anatomy of spatial neglect. Indeed, given the lim-ited overlap of the two anatomical patterns, the available data seem to justify the posi-tion that spatial neglect does not merely represent a disorder of attention, as maintained by some influential students of neglect (review in Bisiach and Vallar 2000).

Another source of nontrivial discrepancy with the anatomy of neglect is the lateraliza-tion of brain activations. A predominant activation of the right hemisphere was found in some studies on spatial attention (e.g. Nobre *et al.* 1997) and in studies on sustained attention (Pardo *et al.* 1991). However, meta-analyses of experiments on covert orient-ing attention show substantially bilateral and symmetrical patterns of dorsal premotor and superior parietal and intraparietal activity (Kastner and Ungerleider 2000; Corbetta 1998). The functional predominance of the left hemisphere for near space reported in the PET experiment of Weiss *et al.* (2000) awaits to be tested in brain-damaged patients.

Mismatch between functional imaging and lesion data is nothing new. This has been seen before for episodic memory (Dolan *et al.* 1997). Resolution of these discrepancies in spatial neurocognition may contribute to a better understanding of spatial neglect, of normal human spatial processing and attention, and of the nature of the right hemi-spheric dominance for spatial processing. To achieve this, more studies are needed on the anatomy of neglect and of spatial processing in normal subjects and in patients with acquired lesions. The anatomy of neglect needs to be mapped by recruiting patients using a wider range of tasks and looking for large groups of patients showing dissociations of behavioural deficit. Indeed, so far, the available data have been collected primarily by recruiting patients on the basis of cancellation tasks that cover spatial exploration in peripersonal space alone. If the overall pattern of brain lesion of neglect can be replicated using different tasks, it then becomes very important to characterize the spatial properties of those brain areas in humans, a task that has proved to be not obvious using paradigms taken from clinical practice in spatial neglect.

Selective references

Andersen, R. (1994). Coordinate transformation and motor planning in posterior parietal cortex. In *The cognitive neurosciences* (ed. M. Gazzaniga), pp. 519–33. MIT Press, Boston.

Andersen, R., Snyder, L., Bradley, D., and Xing, J. (1997). Multimodal representation of space in the posterior parietal cortex and its use in planning movements. *Ann. Rev. Neurosci.* **20**, 303–30.

Bear, M., Connors, B., and Paradiso, M. (2001). *Neuroscience. Exploring the brain*. Lippincott, Williams and Wilkins, Baltimore.

Bisiach, E. and Vallar, G. (2000). Unilateral neglect in humans. In *Handbook of neuropsychology*, 2nd edn (ed. F. Boller, J. Grafman, and G. Rizzolatti), pp. 1–44. Elsevier, Amsterdam.

Bottini, G., Karnath, H.-O., Vallar, G., *et al.* (2001). Cerebral representations for egocentric space: functional–anatomical evidence from caloric vestibular stimulation and neck vibration. *Brain* **124**, 1182–96.

Chawla, D., Rees, G., and Friston, K.J. (1999). The physiological basis of attentional modulation in extrastriate visual areas. *Nature Neurosci.* **2**, 671–6.

Chelazzi, L., Miller, E.K., Duncan, J., and Desimone, R. (1993). A neural basis for visual search in inferior temporal cortex [see comments]. *Nature* **363**, 345–7.

Colby, C.L. and Goldberg, M.E. (1999). Space and attention in parietal cortex. *Ann. Rev. Neurosci.* **22**, 319–49.

Colby, C.L., Duhamel, J.R., and Goldberg, M.E. (1996). Visual, presaccadic, and cognitive activation of single neurons in monkey lateral intraparietal area. *J. Neurophysiol.* **76**, 2841–52.

Corbetta, M. (1998). Frontoparietal cortical networks for directing attention and the eye to visual locations: identical, independent, or overlapping neural systems? *Proc. Natl Acad. Sci., USA* **95**, 831–8.

Corbetta, M., Miezin, F.M., Dobmeyer, S., Shulman, G.L., and Petersen, S.E. (1991). Selective and divided attention during visual discrimination of shape color and speed functional anatomy by positron emission tomography. *J. Neurosci.* **11**, 2383–402.

Corbetta, M., Akbudak, E., Conturo, T.E., *et al.* (1998). A common network of functional areas for attention and eye movements. *Neuron* **21**, 761–73.

Corbetta, M., Kincade, J.M., Ollinger, J.M., McAvoy, M.P., and Shulman, G.L. (2000). Voluntary orienting is dissociated from target detection in human posterior parietal cortex. *Nature Neurosci.* **3**, 292–7.

Courtney, S.M., Ungerleider, L.G., Keil, K., and Haxby, J.V. (1996). Object and spatial visual working memory activate separate neural systems in human cortex. *Cerebral Cortex* **6**, 39–49.

Courtney, S.M., Petit, L., Maisog, J.M., Ungerleider, L.G., and Haxby, J.V. (1998). An area specialized for spatial working memory in human frontal cortex. *Science* **279**, 1347–51.

Craighero, L., Fadiga, L., Rizzolatti, G., and Umiltà, C. (1999). Action for perception: a motor-visual attentional effect. *J. Exp. Psychol.: Hum. Percept. Perform.* **25**, 1673–92.

Dolan, R., Paulesu, E., and Fletcher, P. (1997). Human memory systems. In *Human brain function* (ed. R. Frackowiak), pp. 367–404. Academic Press, San Diego.

Duhamel, J., Colby, C., and Goldberg, M. (1992). The updating of the representation of visual space in parietal cortex by intended eye movements. *Science* **255**, 90–2.

Fink, G.R., Dolan, R.J., Halligan, P.W., Marshall, J.C., and Frith, C.D. (1997). Space-based and object-based visual attention: shared and specific neural domains. *Brain* **120** (pt. 11), 2013–28.

Fink, G., Marshall, J., Shah, N., *et al.* (2000*a*). Line bisection judgements implicate right parietal cortex and cerebellum as assessed by fMRI. *Neurology* **54**, 1324–31.

Fink, G., Marshall, J., Weiss, P., *et al.* (2000*b*). 'Where' depends on 'what': a differential functional anatomy for position discrimination in one- versus two-dimensions. *Neuropsychologia* **38**, 1741–8.

Fogassi, L., Gallese, V., Fadiga, L., Luppino, G., Matelli, M., and Rizzolatti, G. (1996). Coding of peripersonal space in inferior premotor cortex (area F4). *J. Neurophysiol.* **76**, 141–57.

Galati, G., Lobel, E., Vallar, G., Berthoz, A., Pizzamiglio, L., and Bihan, D.L. (2000). The neural basis of egocentric and allocentric coding of space in humans: a functional magnetic resonance study. *Exp. Brain. Res.* **133**, 156–64.

Galletti, C. and Fattori, P. (2002). Posterior parietal networks encoding visual space. In *The cognitive and neural bases of spatial neglect* (ed. H. Karnath, D. Milner, and G. Vallar), pp. 59–69. Oxford University Press, Oxford.

Galletti, C., Battaglini, P.P., and Fattori, P. (1993). Parietal neurons encoding spatial locations in craniotopic coordinates. *Exp. Brain Res.* **96**, 221–9.

Goldberg, M.E. and Bruce, C.J. (1985). Cerebral cortical activity associated with the orientation of visual attention in the rhesus monkey. *Vision Res.* **25**, 471–81.

Goldberg, M.E. and Bushnell, M.C. (1981). Behavioral enhancement of visual responses in monkey cerebral cortex. II. Modulation in frontal eye fields specifically related to saccades. *J. Neurophysiol.* **46**, 773–87.

Goldberg, M.E. and Wurtz, R.H. (1972). Activity of superior colliculus in behaving monkey. II. Effect of attention on neuronal responses. *J. Neurophysiol.* **35**, 560–74.

Goldman-Rakic, P.S. (1996). The prefrontal landscape: implications of functional architecture for understanding human mentation and the central executive. *Phil. Trans. R. Soc., London B: Biol. Sci.* **351**, 1445–53.

Goodale, M. and Milner, A. (1992). Separate visual pathways for perception and for action. *Trends Neurosci.* **15**, 20–5.

Graziano, M. and Gross, C. (1994). The representation of extra-personal space: a possible role for bimodal visual–tactile neurons. In *The cognitive neurosciences* (ed. M. Gazzaniga), pp. 1021–34. MIT Press, Boston.

Guldin, W. and Grüsser, O.-J. (1998). Is there a vestibular cortex. *Trends Neurosci.* **21**, 254–9.

Halligan, P.W. and Marshall, J.C. (1991). Left neglect for near but not far space in man. *Nature* **350**, 498–500.

Halligan, P.W. and Marshall, J.C. (1992). Left visuo-spatial neglect: a meaningless entity? *Cortex* **28**, 525–35.

Haxby, J.V., Grady, C.L., Horwitz, B., *et al.* (1991). Dissociation of object and spatial visual processing pathways in human extrastriate cortex. *Proc. Natl Acad. Sci., USA* **88**, 1621–5.

Haxby, J.V., Horwitz, B., Ungerleider, L.G., Maisog, J.M., Pietrini, P., and Grady, C.L. (1994). The functional organization of human extrastriate cortex: a PET-rCBF study of selective attention to faces and locations. *J. Neurosci.* **14**, 6336–53.

Heilman, K.M., Watson, R.T., and Valenstein, E. (1994). Localization of lesions in neglect and related disorders. In *Localization and neuroimaging in neuropsychology* (ed. A. Kertesz). Academic Press, San Diego.

Hendry, S.H. and Reid, R.C. (2000). The koniocellular pathway in primate vision. *Ann. Rev. Neurosci.* **23**, 127–53.

Humphreys, G., Duncan, J., and Treisman, A. (Eds.) (1998). *Attention, space and action.* Oxford University Press, Oxford.

Iacoboni, M., Woods, R.P., Brass, M., Bekkering, H., Mazziotta, J.C., and Rizzolatti, G. (1999). Cortical mechanisms of human imitation. *Science* **286**, 2526–8.

James, W. (1890/1950). *Principles of psychology.* Dover, New York.

Jeannerod, M. (1997). *The cognitive neuroscience of action.* Blackwell, Oxford.

Jeannerod, M., Arbib, M., Rizzolatti, G., and Sakata, H. (1995). Grasping objects: the cortical mechanisms of visuomotor transformation. *Trends Neurosci.* **18**, 314–20.

Kaas, J.H. (1990). Somatosensory system. In *The human nervous system* (ed. G. Paxinos), pp. 813–44. Academic Press, San Diego.

Karnath, H. (1994). Subjective body orientation in neglect and the interactive contribution of neck muscle proprioception and vestibular stimulation. *Brain* 117, 1001–12.

Karnath, H., Sievering, D., and Fetter, M. (1994). The interactive contribution of neck muscle proprioception and vestibular stimulation to subjective 'straight ahead' orientation in man. *Exp. Brain Res.* 101, 140–6.

Karnath, H., Ferber, S., and Himmelbach, M. (2001). Spatial awareness is a function of the temporal not the posterior parietal lobe. *Nature* 411, 950–3.

Kastner, S. and Ungerleider, L.G. (2000). Mechanisms of visual attention in the human cortex. *Ann. Rev. Neurosci.* 23, 315–41.

Kastner, S., De Weerd, P., Desimone, R., and Ungerleider, L.G. (1998). Mechanisms of directed attention in the human extrastriate cortex as revealed by functional MRI. *Science* 282, 108–11.

Kastner, S., Pinsk, M.A., De Weerd, P., Desimone, R., and Ungerleider, L.G. (1999). Increased activity in human visual cortex during directed attention in the absence of visual stimulation. *Neuron* 22, 751–61.

LaBerge, D. and Buchsbaum, M.S. (1990). Positron emission tomographic measurements of pulvinar activity during an attention task. *J. Neurosci.* 10, 613–19.

Livingstone, M. and Hubel, D. (1988). Segregation of form, color, movement, and depth: anatomy, physiology, and perception. *Science* 240, 740–9.

Logothetis, N. (2001). Neurophysiological investigation of the basis of the fMRI signal. *Nature* 412, 150–7.

Luck, S., Chelazzi, L., and Hillyard, S. (1997). Neural mechanisms of spatial selective attention in areas V1, V2 and V4 of macaque visula cortex. *J. Neurophysiol.* 77, 24–42.

Matelli, M., Luppino, G., and Rizzolatti, G. (1985). Patterns of cytochrome oxidase activity in the frontal agranular cortex of the macaque monkey. *Behav. Brain Res.* 18, 125–36.

Matelli, M., Luppino, G., and Rizzolatti, G. (1991). Architecture of superior and mesial area 6 and the adjacent cingulate cortex in the macaque monkey. *J. Comp. Neurol.* 311, 445–62.

Mattingley, J., Husain, J., Rorden, C., Kennard, C., and Driver, J. (1998). Motor role of human inferior parietal lobe revealed in unilateral neglect patients. *Nature* 392, 179–82.

Mesulam, M. (1990). Large-scale neurocognitive networks and distributed processing for attention, language, and memory. *Ann. Neurol.* 28, 597–613.

Mishkin, M., Ungerleider, L., and Macko, K. (1983). Object vision and spatial vision: two cortical pathways. *Trends Neurosci.* 6, 414–17.

Nobre, A., Sebestyen, G., Gitelman, D., Mesulam, M., Frackowiak, R., and Frith, C. (1997). Functional localization of the system for visuospatial attention using positron emission tomography. *Brain* 120 (pt. 3), 515–33.

Nobre, A.C., Gitelman, D.R., Dias, E.C., and Mesulam, M.M. (2000). Covert visual spatial orienting and saccades: overlapping neural systems. *Neuroimage* 11, 210–16.

Ogawa, S., Menon, R., Kim, S., and Ugurbil, K. (1998). On the characteristics of functional magnetic resonance imaging of the brain. *Ann. Rev. Biophys. Biomol. Struct.* 27, 447–74.

Pardo, J.V., Pardo, J.P., Janer, K.W., and Raichle, M.E. (1990). The anterior cingulate cortex mediates processing selection in the Stroop attentional conflict paradigm. *Proc. Natl Acad. Sci., USA* 87, 256–9.

Pardo, J.V., Fox, P.T., and Raichle, M.E. (1991). Localization of a human system for sustained attention by positron emission tomography. *Nature* 349, 61–4.

Paulesu, E., Frackowiak, R., and Bottini, G. (1997). Maps of somatosensory systems. In *Human brain function* (ed. R. Frackowiak), pp. 183–242. Academic Press, San Diego.

Paus, T., Marrett, S., Evans, A.C., and Worsley, K. (1996). Imaging motor-to-sensory discharges in the human brain: an experimental tool for the assessment of functional connectivity. *Neuroimage* 4, 78–86.

Petrides, M., Alivisatos, B., Meyer, E., and Evans, A.C. (1993). Functional activation of the human frontal cortex during the performance of verbal working memory tasks. *Proc. Natl Acad. Sci., USA* 90, 878–82.

Posner, M.I. (1980). Orienting of attention. *Quart. J. Exp. Psychol.* 32, 3–25.

Posner, M.I. and Petersen, S.E. (1990). The attention system of the human brain. *Ann. Rev. Neurosci.* 13, 25–42.

Posner, M.I., Walker, J.A., Friedrich, F.J., and Rafal, R.D. (1984). Effects of parietal injury on covert orienting of attention. *J. Neurosci.* 4, 1863–74.

Raichle, M.E. (1987). Circulatory and metabolic correlates of brain function in normal humans. In *Handbook of physiology. The nervous system. Higher functions of the brain* (ed. V.B. Mountcastle, F. Plum, and S.R. Geiger), pp. 643–74. American Physiological Society, Bethesda, Maryland.

Rees, G., Frackowiak, R., and Frith, C. (1997a). Two modulatory effects of attention that mediate object categorization in human cortex. *Science* 275, 835–8.

Rees, G., Frith, C.D., and Lavie, N. (1997b). Modulating irrelevant motion perception by varying attentional load in an unrelated task. *Science* 278, 1616–19.

Reynolds, J., Chelazzi, L., and Desimone, R. (1999). Competitive mechanisms subserve attention in macaque areas V2 and V4. *J. Neurosci.* 19, 1736–53.

Rizzolatti, G., Riggio, L., and Shaliga, B. (1994). Space and selective attention. In *Attention and performance*, Vol. 15 (ed. C. Umiltà and M. Moscovitch), pp. 231–65. MIT Press, Cambridge, Massachusetts.

Rizzolatti, G., Berti, A., and Gallese, V. (2000). Spatial neglect: neurophysiological bases, cortical circuits and theories. In *Handbook of neuropsychology*, 2nd edn (ed. F. Boller, J. Grafman, and G. Rizzolatti), pp. 303–37. Elsevier, Amsterdam.

Ruben, J., Schwiemann, J., Deuchert, M., *et al.* (2001). Somatotopic organization of human secondary somatosensory cortex. *Cerebral Cortex* 11, 463–73.

Samuelsson, H., Jensen, C., Ekholm, S., Naver, H., and Blomstrand, C. (1997). Anatomical and neurological correlates of acute and chronic visuospatial neglect following right hemisphere stroke. *Cortex* 33, 271–85.

Sereno, M.I., Dale, A.M., Reppas, J.B., *et al.* (1995). Borders of multiple visual areas in humans revealed by functional magnetic resonance imaging. *Science* 268, 889–93.

Tootell, R.B., Mendola, J.D., Hadjikhani, N.K., Liu, A.K., and Dale, A.M. (1998). The representation of the ipsilateral visual field in human cerebral cortex. *Proc. Natl Acad. Sci., USA* 95, 818–24.

Turner, R. (1997). Signal sources in bold contrast fMRI. *Adv. Exp. Med. Biol.* 413, 19–25.

Umiltà, C. (2000). Visuospatial attention. In *Handbook of neuropsychology*, 2nd edn (ed. F. Boller, J. Grafman, and G. Rizzolatti), pp. 394–425. Elsevier, Amsterdam.

Ungerleider, L.G., Courtney, S.M., and Haxby, J.V. (1998). A neural system for human visual working memory. *Proc. Natl Acad. Sci., USA* 95, 883–90.

Vallar, G. (1998). Spatial hemineglect in humans. *Trends Cogn. Sci.* 2, 87–97.

Vallar, G. (2001). Extrapersonal visual unilateral neglect and its neuroanatomy. *NeuroImage* 14, S52–8.

Vallar, G., Guariglia, C., and Rusconi, M. (1997). Modulation of the neglect syndrome by sensory stimulation. In *Parietal lobe contributions to orientation in 3D space* (ed. P. Thier and H.-O. Karnath), pp. 555–78. Springer-Verlag, Heidelberg.

Weiss, P., Marshall, J., Wunderlich, G., *et al.* (2000). Neural consequences of acting in near versus far space: a physiological basis for a clinical dissociation. *Brain* 123, 2531–41.

Wilson, F., O'Schalaide, S., and Goldman-Rakic, P. (1993). Dissociation of object and spatial processing domains in primate prefrontal cortex. *Science* 260, 1955–60.

Wise, S.P., Boussaoud, D., Johnson, P.B., and Caminiti, R. (1997). Premotor and parietal cortex: corticocortical connectivity and combinatorial computations. *Ann. Rev. Neurosci.* 20, 25–42.

Zeki, S. (1993). *A vision of the brain.* Blackwell, Oxford.

Zeki, S., Watson, J., Lueck, C., Friston, K., Kennard, C., and Frackowiak, R. (1991). A direct demonstration of functional specialization in human visual cortex. *J. Neurosci.* 11, 641–9.

Chapter 39

Functional neuroanatomy of learning and memory

Hans J. Markowitsch

1 Introduction

This chapter will state what kinds of learning and memory are relevant for clinical practice and how they are defined and delineated (see Chapters 9 and 10). Basically, two main lines will be followed—one that divides information processing with respect to *time*, and another that divides it with respect to *contents*. Then information will be given on how information is transmitted to the brain ('encoded'), stored or represented in it, and how information is retrieved. The anatomical circuits and networks engaged in these processes will be described and reference will be made to the brain's biochemistry (transmitters, hormones), as far as relevant for learning and memory or its disorders.

2 Learning and memory—the behavioural view

Learning and memory constitute those intellectual processes of a human being that differentiate him or her most clearly from other animals and that allowed the evolution of tradition, culture, and foresight. Both human society as a whole and each individual are strongly dependent on remembering their experiences and comparing present or planned situations with previous ones. Hering in 1870 formulated the importance of memory by stating: 'Memory connects innumerable single phenomena into a whole, and just as the body would be scattered like dust in countless atoms if the attraction of matter did not hold it together so consciousness—without the connecting power of memory—would fall apart in as many fragments as it contains moments.' (transl. in Hering 1895)

Learning is a universal attribute of the animal kingdom and is consequently diversified from most simple forms of adaptation to the environment to sophisticated inferential ones. Table 39.1 gives a crude overview and definition of various forms of learning. Generally speaking, learning and memory can be defined as follows.

- *Learning* is a relatively permanent change in a behavioural tendency that occurs as a result of reinforced practice (Kimble 1961).

- *Memory* is the learning-dependent storage of ontogenetically acquired information. This information integrates into phylogenetic neuronal structures selectively

Table 39.1 Taxonomy of learning (after Gagné 1965)

1 *Signal learning or classical conditioning*

This form of learning became most well known as Pavlovian conditioning. The dog, who after a few pairings of a bell with a piece of meat soon salivates already to the sound, is an example. In classical conditioning the unconditioned stimulus occurs independently of the subject's behaviour

2 *Stimulus–response learning or instrumental conditioning*

Instrumental conditioning is dependent on the subject's behaviour. The subject learns the association between a stimulus and a response

3 *Chaining (including verbal association)*

Chaining refers to several consecutive responses where each response determines the next (e.g. only several responses that build upon each other may lead to a reward)

4 *Multiple discrimination*

Learning to differentiate between stimuli that have one or more attributes in common

5 *Concept learning*

Learning to respond in the same way to a variety of objects or attributes of objects that have something in common

6 *Principle learning*

Acquiring knowledge on how to master a set of problems that have common attributes

7 *Problem-solving*

Making proper use of learned principles and having insight (being able to draw inferences)

* Gagné saw this sequence as hierarchical or as proceeding from simple to complex forms of learning.

and with respect to the given species so that it can be retrieved at all times. This means that it can be provided for situation-dependent behaviour. Generally formulated, memory is based on conditioned changes of the transfer properties in neuronal nets so that under specific circumstances those system modifications (engrams) that correspond to neuromotoric signals and behavioural tendencies become reproducible in full or partly (Sinz 1979).

Memory can be subdivided with respect to both time and content. In terms of duration memory can be subdivided into:

- *sensory* (*'iconic', 'echoic'*) *memory*: the retaining of information along the sensory channels (duration ~50–500 milliseconds);
- *short-term memory* (online processing of information): storage of memory for a period ranging from seconds to a few minutes (7 ± 2 bits of information);
- *long-term memory*: principally lifelong retention of information.

(See Fig. 39.1 for a comparison of short- and long-term memory.) The processing of information in memory over time can also be subdivided into stages:

- *registration*: initial perception and transfer to cortical routes;
- *encoding*: further initial processing of information (binding, associating);

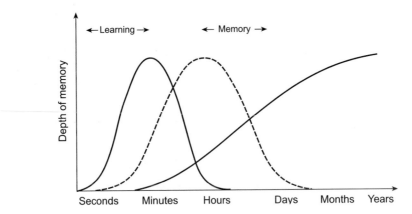

Fig. 39.1 Sketch of the relations between memory strength and duration for the two principal time-related memory systems, short-term and long-term memory (solid lines), and an intermediate, rarely cited, memory system (broken line).

♦ *consolidation*: deep encoding and embedding of information (engram formation);
♦ *storage*: stable representation of information in the nervous system;
♦ *retrieval*: reproduction of information (recall).

In terms of content, memory can be subdivided into:

♦ *episodic memory* (memory for episodes): context-embedded autobiographical memory allowing mental time-travelling;
♦ *declarative memory* (memory for facts; knowledge system): storage of context-free information;
♦ *procedural memory*: memory for skills, rules, sequences;
♦ *priming*: higher likelihood of re-identifying previously perceived stimuli;
♦ other forms of memory: lower forms of memory such as classical conditioning or sensitization.

See Fig. 39.2 for examples of these subtypes of memory.

The term *anterograde amnesia* is used when the long-term acquisition ('new learning') of information is lost and *retrograde amnesia* is used when a patient is unable to retrieve stored (already long-term acquired) information (Fig. 39.3). It is no longer common to use the term 'global amnesic syndrome', as recent research has shown that patients usually have different memory systems affected and that they have to be termed 'demented' if they indeed have major deficits along all memory systems. The hypothetical memory trace is called the *engram* and, recently, an already old expression, 'ecphory', has regained attention. *Ecphory* refers to the process wherein retrieval cues interact with stored information so that an image or a representation of the desired information becomes activated.

The concept of ecphory implies that there are different ways in which information can be retrieved.

Memory

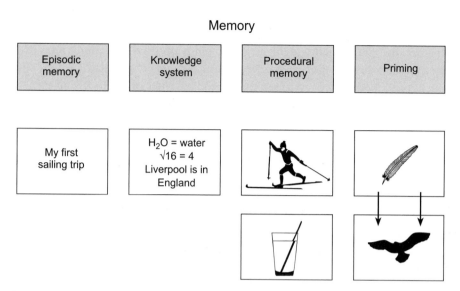

Fig. 39.2 The four principal memory systems important for human information processing. The episodic memory system is context-specific with respect to time and place. It allows mental time travel. Examples are episodes such as the last holiday or the previous night's dinner. Declarative memory is context-free and refers to general facts. It is termed semantic memory or the knowledge system. Procedural memory is largely motor-based, but includes also sensory and cognitive skills ('routines'). Priming refers to a higher likelihood of re-identifying previously perceived stimuli.

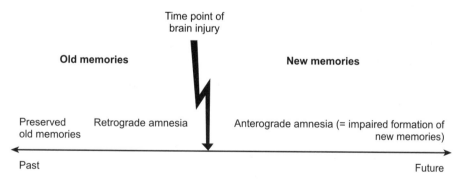

Fig. 39.3 Possible consequences of brain injury on old and new memories.

- The most demanding form is 'free recall', the voluntary recall of learned information without external help or cueing.
- 'Cued recall' is recall with the help of cues.
- Finally, the easiest and least demanding way of retrieving information is recognition by simply selecting a previously presented stimulus out of a larger number of stimuli.

3 Disorders of learning and memory

Memory disorders are among the most frequently observed symptoms after brain damage. They can also occur as a consequence of a number of psychiatric illnesses. The kind of memory disorder and its severity depend of course on the locus and extent of affected brain tissue. In this regard it has to be assumed that in patients with psychiatric diseases memory disorders are due to temporary alterations in the nervous system—most probably due to changes in neurotransmitter availability and distribution or in changes in hormones on the brain level. Indeed, recent neuroimaging data have shown that memory disorders evoked by psychic trauma can lead to lasting changes in brain tissue metabolism (Markowitsch *et al.* 2000), and there may be considerable similarities between changed neural metabolisms in amnesias occurring after organic brain damage

Table 39.2 Overview of patient groups who usually demonstrate memory disorders

Aetiology	Common lesion sites
Intracranial tumours	Medial and anterior thalamus, medial temporal lobe, posterior cingulate cortex
Cerebral infarcts, ruptured aneurysms	Medial temporal lobe, limbic nuclei of the thalamus (posterior cerebral artery), orbitofrontal cortex, basal forebrain (anterior communicating artery)
Closed head injury	Temporal pole, orbitofrontal and prefrontal cortex
Viral infections (e.g. herpes simplex encephalitis)	Hippocampal region, limbic and paralimbic cortex
Avitaminoses (e.g. B_1 deficiency)	Limbic thalamus, mammillary bodies (e.g. Korsakoff's disease)
Neurotoxin exposure	Hippocampal formation
Temporal lobe epilepsy	Hippocampus and medial temporal lobe
Anoxia or hypoxia (e.g. after heart attack or drowning)	Hippocampus (CA1 sector)
Degenerative diseases of the CNS (e.g. Alzheimer's or Pick's diseases)	Temporal and other association cortices
Drugs (e.g. anticholinergics, benzodiazepines)	Limbic system
Electroconvulsive therapy	Probably limbic system
Transient global amnesia	Probably medial temporal lobe and/or medial thalamus (when an aetiology is found)
Paraneoplastic limbic encephalitis	Limbic structures in medial temporal lobe
Mnestic block syndrome	Massive glucocorticoid release leading to a disruption in the memory-processing pathways of the medial temporal lobe
Dissociative disorders	Amnesia possibly due to hormonal changes in the brain

and in those occurring after psychiatric illnesses (Markowitsch 1999a,b). Table 39.2 gives an overview of patient groups who usually show memory disturbances.

4 Anatomical bases of learning and memory

Much of our current understanding of basic memory-related neuronal changes and modifications stems from the pioneering research of Eric Kandel and his co-workers (Martin *et al.* 2000; Kandel 1998) who largely used an invertebrate, the marine mollusc *Aplysia* for their studies. *Aplysia* contains only limited number of neurons, many of which are individually identified and labelled. Initially, these authors investigated simple memory mechanisms such as sensitization and habituation and found that there are both short- and long-term forms of these. They found that the physiological correlates of the short-term forms are facilitated neuronal responses (increases in the magnitude of the excitatory postsynaptic potentials formed between sensory and motor neurons). The long-term forms (repeated stimulus applications) required new ribonucleic acid (RNA) and protein synthesis, involving the growth of new synaptic connections between sensory and motor neurons. Later, Kandel and co-workers extended their work to gene expression and transcription factors that provided the genetic switch for memory consolidation and storage. Other workers from both the invertebrate and vertebrate side demonstrated, for example, that adenylyl cyclase is an important enzyme for short-term memory (Zars *et al.* 2000) and long-term potentiation (LTP) as well as long-term depression (LTD)—all important mechanisms for memory consolidation (Lynch 2000). Still others, however, questioned the necessity of such mechanisms for memory formation. Zamanillo and co-workers (1999), for example, provided evidence against LTP as an essential prerequisite for memory formation.

On the vertebrate and especially the mammalian level, the important questions are less how information is processed, but where it is processed. The brain is, of course, involved from the initial stages of information registration. However, both the time and content dimensions of memory interact in the neural processing of information. This complicates the description of the neural pathways, circuits, and networks implicated in information processing. I will first describe the neural bases of the simpler forms of memory and then those of declarative and episodic memory.

4.1 The neural bases of simpler forms of memory

Classical conditioning and other simple forms of memory largely occur within the spinal cord and brainstem. Certain subtypes may, however, engage structures in various other loci of the brain.

♦ Fear conditioning, for example, involves the amygdala.

♦ Priming, a non-reflected, unconscious transmission of information, activates cortical areas—largely, though probably not exclusively, within the particular modality of the stimulus ('unimodal' primary and association cortex).

♦ Procedural memory engages the basal ganglia in particular. It may also involve portions of the cerebellum, though the evidence is mixed here.

4.2 The neural bases of declarative and episodic memory

The most complex routes are followed for processing declarative and episodic memory (Tulving and Markowitsch 1998). For these forms it is necessary to differentiate between the stages of information transfer as given in Section 2.

Information for the declarative and episodic memory systems enters the brain via the sensory channels, and is then stored online or short-term in cortical association areas, particularly those of the lateral parietal cortex (Markowitsch 2000). From there it is transmitted to the limbic system, to use the classical term. Here, within the various structures and fibre networks of this system, the processes of selecting, binding, associating, and assigning are located. While the hippocampal formation can be regarded as the core of the limbic system, there are several other important components. Table 39.3 lists the most relevant ones.

Most of the patients who in former times were declared to be globally amnesic had bilateral damage to either the medial temporal lobe or medial diencephalic regions. The most well-known example is patient H.M., who in 1953 received a bilateral resection of the medial temporal lobes due to otherwise intractable epileptic attacks (Fig. 39.4) (Scoville and Milner 1957). While the attacks were largely reduced, H.M. became grossly anterogradely amnesic and still remains so. Consequently, bilateral resections of the hippocampal region are usually avoided.

While infarcts usually do not affect the hippocampal region bilaterally, such bilateral damage is not uncommon after medial diencephalic infarcts (Fig. 39.5). The consequences with respect to amnesia are largely the same as seen after bilateral medial temporal lesions, though they may be more severe with respect to the patient's ability for conscious reflection (Markowitsch 2000). While H.M. stated that, for him, 'Every day is alone, whatever enjoyment I've had, and whatever sorrow I've had', a patient with bilateral diencephalic damage was unable to acknowledge his severe amnesia and instead considered his memory to be 'normal' (Markowitsch *et al.* 1993).

These two examples stand for the two principal groups of patients with major and lasting anterograde amnesia for the episodic and declarative domains—the medial diencephalic and the medial temporal group. While the contributions of individual nuclear or areal portions within these regions for memory are still under discussion (cf. Table 39.2), there is rarely damage confined to single structure. An exception is the hippocampus or individual hippocampal sectors after hypoxic or toxic states. The high vulnerability of the so-called 'Sommer's sectors' to epilepsy or hypoxia was noted as long ago as 1880 (Sommer 1880).

The basal forebrain most probably constitutes a third region relevant to memory. Reasons for this may include its intimate connection with the other two networks, the

Table 39.3 Structures of the limbic system and their principal functional implications

Structure	Functional involvement(s)
Diencephalon	
Anterior nuclear complex	(Anterograde) memory, emotion, attention
Mediodorsal nucleus	(Anterograde) memory, consciousness, sleep, emotion
Non-specific thalamic nuclei	Consciousness (?), (anterograde) memory (?)
Mammillary bodies	(Anterograde) memory, emotion (?)
Telencephalon (subcortical)	
Basal forebrain	Emotional evaluation, (anterograde) memory
Amygdaloid body	Emotional evaluation of information, motivations, olfaction
Telencephalon (cortical)	
Hippocampal formation	(Anterograde) memory, spatial–temporal integration
Entorhinal region	(Anterograde) memory
Cingulate gyrus	Attention, drive, pain perception
Associated regions	
Medial and orbitofrontal cortex	Emotional evaluation, social behaviour, initiative (initiation of retrieval of information)
Insula	Sensory–motivational integration (?)
Temporal pole	Memory-related sensory integration, initiation of retrieval, recruitment of engrams
Fibre systems	
Fornix	(Anterograde) memory (?)
Medial internal lamina	(Anterograde) memory (?)
Mammillothalamic tract	(Anterograde) memory (?)
Uncinate fascicle	Retrograde memory (?)

fornix being an example. Under the term basal forebrain, a number of components of divergent evolutionary origin, connections, and biochemistry are subsumed:

- the cholinergic systems (basal nucleus of Meynert, septal nuclei, diagonal band of Broca);
- the nucleus accumbens;
- other parts of the ventral striatum.

The cholinergic system has long been implicated in the highest cognitive functions—memory and consciousness (Perry *et al.* 1999).

5 Brain circuits

5.1 Brain circuits for encoding and consolidating

A common view of information processing assumes that information enters the brain via the sensory organs and then is stored for a short term—most probably

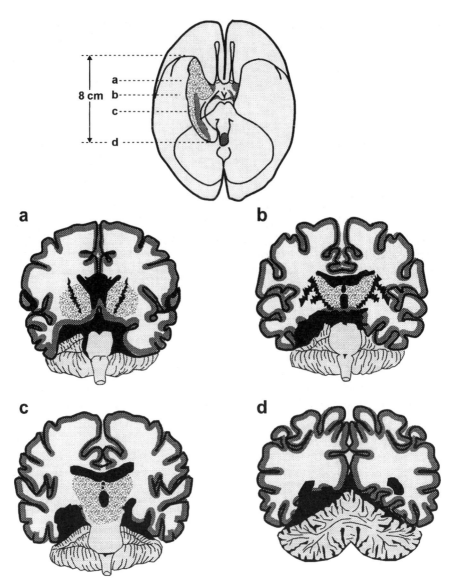

Fig. 39.4 Drawings of the extent of the principal surgical removal within H.M.'s temporal lobe. The top diagram shows a basal view of his brain with the locations of four levels a–d indicated. The lower section of the diagram shows four coronal sections at the levels a–d, respectively. The extent of the surgical resection is blackened on the left side of the brain only, although the removal was bilateral and symmetrical. (After fig. 2 of Scoville and Milner 1957.)

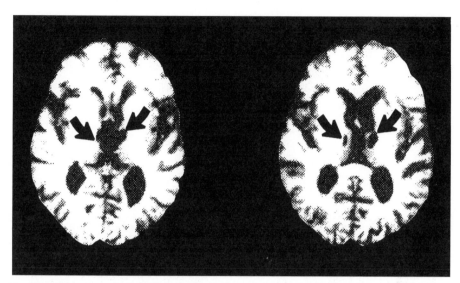

Fig. 39.5 The extent of bilateral diencephalic damage in a patient with preserved intelligence, but severe and persistent anterograde amnesia. (After fig. 2 of Markowitsch *et al.* 1993.)

in portions of the parietal and possibly also the prefrontal cortex. Information then is transmitted into the limbic system, a phylogenetically old system of structures and fibre connections that originally was associated with olfaction, then (more generally) with emotions, and presently is seen as relevant for the processing of emotional as well as of cognitive forms of information. In particular, it is assumed that the limbic system is responsible for evaluating incoming (and short-term stored) information and for assigning this information to the final storage networks, which, for episodic and declarative memories, can be found distributed in cortical networks.

There are several structures within the limbic system that have a closer affinity to the emotional-affective side (e.g. the amygdala and the septum) and others (e.g. the hippocampal formation) that have a closer relation to the cognitive side. It is possible to speak of two circuits for information selection, binding, and transfer (Fig. 39.6). One is named the medial (or Papez) circuit and the other the basolateral limbic circuit.

◆ The basolateral limbic circuit is composed of three structures and their interconnecting fibres:

—the amygdala;

—the mediodorsal thalamus;

—the subcallosal area within the basal forebrain.

The unidirectional ventral amygdalofugal pathway leads from the amygdala to the mediodorsal thalamus. From there fibres reach the subcallosal area and then

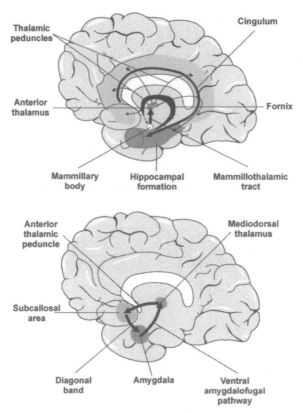

Fig. 39.6 The medial (or Papez) circuit and the basolateral limbic circuit. The medial circuit is probably more relevant for the cognitive acts of memory processing, the basolateral one for the affective evaluation of information. Both circuits interact with each other. The Papez circuit interconnects the hippocampal formation via the (postcommissural) fornix to the mammillary bodies and connects these via the mammillothalamic tract (or tractus Vicq d'Azyr) to the anterior thalamus. The anterior thalamus with its cortical projection targets reaches the cingulate gyrus and the subicular part of the hippocampal formation and the cingulum fibres in addition project back from the cingulate gyrus into the hippocampal formation. (The precommissural fornix in addition provides a bidirectional connection between the hippocampal formation and the basal forebrain.) The basolateral limbic circuit links the amygdala, mediodorsal thalamic nucleus, and area subcallosa with each other by distinct fibre projections, namely the ventral amygdalofugal pathway, the inferior thalamic peduncle, and the bandeletta diagonalis.

project via the bandeletta diagonalis back into the amygdaloid body. This circuit evaluates the affective side of incoming information and interacts with the second, the medial circuit.

♦ The medial circuit traditionally includes four structures:

—the mammillary bodies;

—the anterior thalamus;

—the cingulate cortex;

—the hippocampal formation.

Of these, the cingulate cortex can be omitted—both because of its functional engagement and because of the existence of direct projections between the anterior thalamus and parts of the hippocampal formation. The interconnecting fibres are given in Fig. 39.6. The medial (or Papez) circuit is regarded as the traditionally relevant circuit for evaluating, binding, and assigning information for long-term storage.

It is evident that the medial temporal lobe and the medial diencephalic system are embedded in these circuits. It has also to be noted that there are more structures of relevance than those immediately belonging to the two circuits. Even for the limbic system, there is an ongoing discussion of what to include in it and in what directions to expand it. Structures within the basal forebrain are just one example. Another one can be found within the medial temporal lobe system containing hierarchically organized allocortical structures that converge to subdivisions of the hippocampus (Fig. 39.7).

It needs also to be noted that, after encoding and transfer to the cortex for long-term storage, the engram is not yet fixed. Instead, memories are further consolidated by

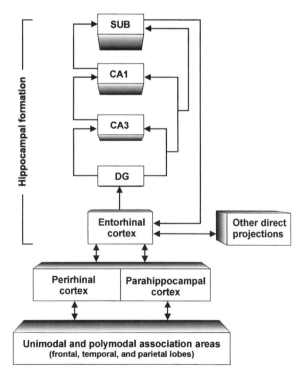

Fig. 39.7 The hierarchical organization within the medial temporal lobe. (After Squire and Knowlton 2000.) Abbreviations: CA1, CA3: sectors of the hippocampus (cornu ammonis), DG: dentate gyrus, SUB: subicular complex.

matching the recently encoded information with that already in existence and by further assimilating, assigning, and embedding the recently encoded information within the wealth of already stored engrams. The mind tends (and apparently intends) to form a congruent or consistent Gestalt of its memory repertoire.

5.2 Brain circuits for storage

In general, information is assumed to be stored in widespread networks. For episodic and declarative information these networks are principally situated within neocortical structures ('association' or 'polysensory cortex'), but may recruit additional allocortical and subcortical regions. In particular, episodic information, which is usually emotionally coloured, most probably requires (emotion-charging) input from the amygdala and/or the septal region. As episodic information per definition is consciously reflected, it is further dependent on a respective network activation from the brainstem reticular formation to the neocortex (Markowitsch 2003).

5.3 Brain circuits for retrieval

As stated initially, retrieved biographical information, especially more complex information, is usually not identical with the originally encoded information. The combined action of cues and mood states present at the time of retrieval interacts with the engrams and forms an actual representation (this process is termed 'ecphory'). Functional neuroimaging data have shown that portions of the (right) prefrontal and the anterior temporal cortex are necessary for ecphorizing *old* autobiographic episodes (G.R. Fink *et al.* 1996). The retrieval of recently learned information may primarily engage prefrontal regions. It can be assumed that the prefrontal cortex provides the impetus or trigger signal to retrieve memories that are largely laid in networks of the posterior association cortices and that the regions within the (anterior) temporal lobe are especially active with respect to the affective side of the ecphorized episodes and with respect to a possible re-encoding (which then engages the hippocampal formation as well). Figure 39.8 provides an example of the activated brain regions of an individual imaging episodes of his past.

5.3.1 Prospective memory, meta-memory, source memory

In recent years, memory experts have stressed the existence of so-called higher forms of memory—meta-memory, source memory, and prospective memory. These are forms of memory that need a reflection on its contents. It is necessary to know where information comes from or what one intends to do with information in the future. Aspects of effortful generation of information and of time—sometimes including sequential ordering and recency discriminations—are especially important for these forms of memory. 'Future intention', 'temporary storage of intended acts', and 'timely performance of planned actions' are phrases for prospective memory.

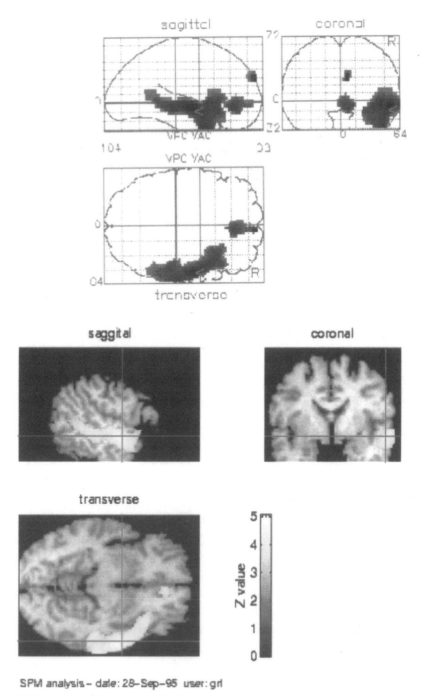

Fig. 39.8 Positron emission tomographic (PET) results, showing activated brain regions of an individual, imaging episodes of his past. (See also 'Plates' section.)

Usually seen as part of the episodic memory system, these forms seem to depend in particular on frontal lobe structures (in addition to their dependence on structures of the limbic system; Shimamura 1995) and it has been found that, in particular, patients with dementia show an early deterioration of these memory functions (Maylor 1995).

6 The brain's biochemistry and the mnestic block syndrome

It has long been known that information processing can be impaired not only after a neural morphology, but that psychiatric illnesses may also lead to a damaged memory. The effects of drugs and hormonal (G. Fink *et al.* 1996) and neurotransmitter alterations have been the subjects of numerous studies employing animals and, more recently, of several using human subjects. The process of memory consolidation especially can be influenced by a wide range of pharmacological substances (Lynch 1998).

For psychiatric illnesses, changes in the brain's biochemistry can be assumed to lead to memory impairments. These changes sometimes are obvious, e.g. the lack of dopamine in Parkinson's disease resulting in procedural memory detriments. There is also substantial evidence for an involvement of acetylcholine in memory processing (Hasselmo 1999; Perry *et al.* 1999) and for the view that cholinergic dysfunction may lead to both neurological (Babic 1999) and psychiatric diseases (Sarter and Bruno 1999). Other transmitters such as gamma-aminobutyric acid (GABA; Kalueff and Nutt 1996), and glutamate, serotonin, and noradrenaline (norepinephrine) have numerous interactive effects especially in the memory-relevant hippocampal region (Vizi and Kiss 1998). Even histamines have been found to enhance memory processing (Passani *et al.* 2000). Vizi and Kiss (1998) suggested that even transmitter release without synaptic contact plays an important role in the fine tuning of communication between neurons within a given circuit.

Kaufer *et al.* (1998) pointed to stress-related changes in cholinergic gene expression, and Markowitsch *et al.* (1999, 2000) hypothesized that the acute or chronic release of glucocorticoids (stress hormones) on the brain level may lead to what they termed 'mnestic block syndrome'. The mnestic block syndrome is considered to be a psychic reaction towards stress or trauma situations leading to an inability to retrieve old and/or to acquire new information on a long-term basis. The syndrome may be transient (if properly treated; see Markowitsch *et al.* 2000), but frequently will show little improvement over time. It is an example of the manifold ways in which the environment may feed back on the brain's ability to code and re-code signals.

7 Conclusions

The nervous system has evolved to allow the individual flexible responses and adaptations to the environment, thereby strengthening the possibility of long-term survival. The individual learned to distinguish between edible and poisonous food and learned to remember smells in order to distinguish between dangerous and sexually arousing members of its species. Such emotionally coloured messages were initially largely processed by the limbic system and made this a primary centre for memory control and, during evolution, for the highest form of information representation—episodic or autobiographical conscious memory. Other, principally reactive forms of memory were used for routines and to increase the adaptability to the environment (procedural memory, priming). All forms together provide an optimal basis for survival in an increasingly complex and demanding environment.

Selective references

Babic, T. (1999). The cholinergic hypothesis of Alzheimer's disease: a review of progress. *J. Neurol., Neurosurg. Psychiatry* 67, 558.

Fink, G., Sumner, B.E., Rosie, R., Grace, O., and Quinn, J.P. (1996). Estrogen control of central neurotransmission: effect on mood, mental state, and memory. *Cell. Mol. Neurobiol.* 16, 325–44.

Fink, G.R., Markowitsch, H.J., Reinkemeier, M., Bruckbauer, T., Kessler, J., and Heiss, W.-D. (1996). Cerebral representation of one's own past: neural networks involved in autobiographical memory. *J. Neurosci.* 16, 4275–82.

Gagné, R.M. (1965). *The conditions of learning*. Holt, Rinehart and Winston, New York.

Hasselmo, M.E. (1999). Neuromodulation: acetylcholine and memory consolidation. *Trends Cogn. Sci.* 3, 351–9.

Hering, E. (1895). *Memory as a general function of organized matter*. Open Court, Chicago.

Kalueff, A. and Nutt, D.J. (1996). Role of GABA in memory and anxiety. *Depress. Anxiety* 4, 100–10.

Kandel, E.R. (1998). A new intellectual framework for psychiatry. *Am. J. Psychiatry* 155, 457–69.

Kaufer, D., Friedman, A., Seldman, S., and Soreq, H. (1998). Acute stress facilitates long-lasting changes in cholinergic gene expression. *Nature* 393, 373–7.

Kimble, G.A. (1961). *Hilgard and Marquis' conditioning and learning*. Appleton Century-Crofts, New York.

Lynch, G. (1998). Memory and the brain: unexpected chemistries and a new pharmacology. *Neurobiol. Learning Memory* 70, 82–100.

Lynch, G. (2000). Memory consolidation and long-term potentiation. In *The new cognitive neurosciences*, 2nd edn (ed. M.S. Gazzaniga), pp. 139–58. MIT Press, Cambridge, Massachusetts.

Markowitsch, H.J. (1999a). Functional neuroimaging correlates of functional amnesia. *Memory* 7, 561–83.

Markowitsch, H.J. (1999b). Neuroimaging and mechanisms of brain function in psychiatric disorders. *Curr. Opin. Psychiatry* 12, 331–7.

Markowitsch, H.J. (2000). Memory and amnesia. In *Principles of cognitive and behavioral neurology* (ed. M.-M. Mesulam), pp. 257–93. Oxford University Press, New York.

Markowitsch, H.J. (2003). Autonoetic consciousness. In *The self and schizophrenia: a neuropsychological perspective* (ed. A.S. David and T. Kircher), in press. Cambridge University Press, Cambridge.

Markowitsch, H.J., von Cramon, D.Y., and Schuri, U. (1993). Mnestic performance profile of a bilateral diencephalic infarct patient with preserved intelligence and severe amnesic disturbances. *J. Clin. Exp. Neuropsychol.* 15, 627–52.

Markowitsch, H.J., Kessler, J., Russ, M.O., Frölich, L., Schneider, B., and Maurer, K. (1999). Mnestic block syndrome. *Cortex* 35, 219–30.

Markowitsch, H.J., Kessler, J., Weber-Luxenburger, G., Van der Ven, C., and Heiss, W.-D. (2000). Neuroimaging and behavioral correlates of recovery from 'mnestic block syndrome' and other cognitive deteriorations. *Neuropsychiatry, Neuropsychol., Behav. Neurol.* **13**, 60–6.

Martin, K.C., Bartsch, D., Bailey, C.H., and Kandel, E.R. (2000). Molecular mechanisms underlying learning-related long-lasting synaptic plasticity. In *The new cognitive neurosciences* (ed. M.S. Gazzaniga), pp. 121–37. MIT Press, Cambridge, Massachusetts.

Maylor, E.A. (1995). Prospective memory in normal ageing and dementia. *Neurocase* **1**, 285–9.

Passani, M.B., Bacciottini, L., Mannaioni, P.F., and Blandina, P. (2000). Central histaminergic system and cognition. *Neurosci. Biobehav. Rev.* **24**, 107–13.

Perry, E., Walker, M., Grace, J., and Perry, R. (1999). Acetylcholine in mind: a neurotransmitter correlate of consciousness? *Trends Neurosci.* **22**, 273–80.

Sarter, M. and Bruno, J. P. (1999). Abnormal regulation of corticopetal cholinergic neurons and impaired information processing in neuropsychiatric disorders. *Trends Neurosci.* **22**, 67–74.

Scoville, W.B. and Milner, B. (1957). Loss of recent memory after bilateral hippocampal lesions. *J. Neurol., Neurosurg., Psychiatry* **20**, 11–21.

Shimamura, A.P. (1995). Memory and frontal lobe function. In *The new cognitive neurosciences* (ed. M.S. Gazzaniga), pp. 803–13. MIT Press, Cambridge, Massachusetts.

Sinz, R. (1979). *Neurobiologie und Gedächtnis*. Gustav Fischer, Stuttgart.

Sommer, W. (1880). Erkrankung des Ammonshorns als aetiologisches Moment der Epilepsie. *Arch. Psychiatrie* **10**, 631–75.

Squire, L.R. and Knowlton, B.J. (2000). The medial temporal lobe, the hippocampus, and the memory system of the brain. In *The new cognitive neurosciences*, 2nd edn (ed. M.S. Gazzaniga), pp. 765–79. MIT Press, Cambridge, Massachusetts.

Tulving, E. and Markowitsch, H. J. (1998). Episodic and declarative memory: role of the hippocampus. *Hippocampus* **8**, 198–204.

Vizi, E.S. and Kiss, J.P. (1998). Neurochemistry and pharmacology of the major hippocampal transmitter systems: synaptic and nonsynaptic interactions. *Hippocampus* **6**, 566–607.

Zamanillo, D., Sprengel, R., Hvalby, O., Jensen, V., Burnashev, N., Rozov, A., Kaiser, K.M., Koster, H.J., Borchardt, T., Worley, P., Lubke, J., Frotscher, M., Kelly, P.H., Sommer, B., Andersen, P., Seeburg, P.H., and Sakmann, B. (1999). Importance of AMPA receptors for hippocampal synaptic plasticity but not for spatial learning. *Science* **284**, 1805–11.

Zars, T., Fischer, M., Schulz, R., and Heisenberg, M. (2000). Localization of a short-term memory in Drosophila. *Science* **288**, 672–5.

Chapter 40

Functional neuroanatomy of language disorders

Claudius Bartels and Claus-W. Wallesch

1 Introduction

This chapter will attempt a synopsis of the representation of language functions in the brain with a focus upon disorders based upon three sources of information:

- lesion studies, i.e. what is known from the effects of pathology upon language behaviour in patients (see Chapter 14);
- the anatomical interpretation of normal function based upon physiological measurements during language operations in normal subjects;
- a combination of the two, namely, physiological measurements recorded during language processing in aphasic patients.

Computer-generated three-dimensional brain images into which imaging software places coloured regions of increased or decreased 'function' have great appeal and are well suited for title pages of scientific and other journals. However, the underlying methodology is highly complex and prone to artefacts and misinterpretations. Therefore, we shall include a brief discussion of functional imaging methodology.

2 Basic anatomy

The hemispheric surface is divided into the frontal, temporal, parietal, and occipital lobes (Fig. 40.1). The depth of the sylvian fissure, which separates the temporal from the parietal and frontal lobes, harbours a hidden part of cerebral cortex, the insula, which is covered by lips (the opercula) of the adjacent lobes.

The forebrain is walnut-shaped with one strong (the corpus callosum) and two minor (commissura anterior and posterior) interconnections between the hemispheres. The core of the medial surface of the hemispheres does not continue the lobar structure. One single large gyrus, the cingulum, surrounds the corpus callosum.

Cortical processing interacts with the function of subcortical neuronal structures, the basal ganglia and the thalamus, by reciprocal connections with specific nuclei of the latter, and loop systems that include both the basal ganglia and the specific thalamic nuclei (Alexander *et al.* 1986). A similar action upon cortex has been proposed by Schmahmann and Pandya (1997) for the cerebellum. The basal ganglia consist of the

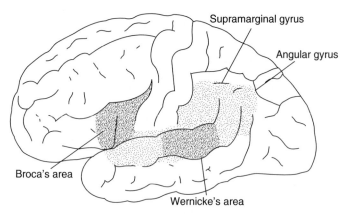

Fig. 40.1 The surface of the left hemisphere. Of special interest for language representations are the following structures of the left hemisphere: the insular cortex and a number of cortical areas that are close to the sylvian fissure, namely, Broca's area in the foot of the second and third frontal convolution, Wernicke's area in the posterior third of the first temporal convolution, and, surrounding the posterior end of the sylvian fissure, the supramarginal and angular gyrus (see the text for a discussion of lateralization of language representations).

putamen and caudate nucleus, the pallidum, the subthalamic nucleus, and a number of minor nuclei that need not be considered here. The thalamus contains more than 30 nuclei that subserve different relay functions: in cortico–subcortico–cortical loops; in ascending sensory and cerebellar projections; and in non-specific ascending pathways that subserve, e.g. cortical activation and the awake state (Fig. 40.2).

In most subjects, almost all right-handers and a majority of left-handers, the left hemisphere dominates language processing, although the degree of cerebral dominance differs interindividually. Anatomically, the planum temporale, which corresponds to the core of Wernicke's area, is larger on the left in about 75 % of normal people (Steinmetz 1996). This asymmetry seems genetically predetermined and can be found in fetuses (Chi *et al.* 1977). Nevertheless, whether or not the planum temporale is an area that is inherently specialized for language function is currently being debated both on neurobiological and on neurolinguistic grounds (Marshall 2000).

The temporal lobe association cortex, of which Wernicke's area is a part, integrates auditory, visual, and even somatosensory information. It is closely interconnected with the temporal limbic cortex and the amygdalohippocampal system that subserve both memory and emotional functions. Broca's area is part of the precentral association cortex, which is located between the cortical motor strip and the prefrontal cortex. The precentral cortex is involved in movement preparation, but the exact function of Broca's area is still under debate. Another frontal lobe cortical area, the left supplementary motor area at the medial aspect of the frontal lobe, is involved in language production, especially in the initiation of speech acts. Functionally, this area is part of the anterior cingulum. (See the box on p. 743 for a discussion of localization of functions in the brain.)

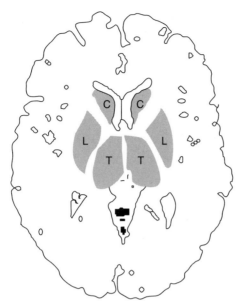

C = (head of) caudate nucleus
L = lentiform nucleus
T = thalamus

Fig. 40.2 The subcortical nuclei of the cerebral hemispheres.

Localization of functions within the brain

The extent to which functions can be localized in the brain is variable. The primary sensory and motor areas are quite circumscribed. The more cognitive a function is, the less well it can be assigned to defined cortical areas. Cerebral maps even of primary areas are not fixed representations but may vary in response to functional demand (Merzenich *et al.* 1983). It has been proposed that neuronal networks are a general feature of cerebral organization with quite distributed networks for cognitive functions (McClelland and Rumelhart 1986; Harley 1996). The extent of such networks has been demonstrated by functional magnetic resonance imaging (fMRI; Carpenter and Just 1999).

3 The anatomical foundation of aphasia

The most common cause of aphasia is stroke in the area of supply of the middle cerebral artery. Stroke results in circumscribed lesions, the anatomical analysis of which is rather unambiguous. Damage to some regions is more likely to cause lasting aphasia than damage to others, and there is some interaction between lesion configuration and chronic aphasia syndromes. Poeck *et al.* (1984) found core lesions for Broca's aphasia in the anterior insula, frontal operculum, and the underlying white matter; for Wernicke's aphasia in the posterior superior temporal lobe (Wernicke's area); and for global aphasia in the middle and posterior insula and a much larger white matter lesion including the deep white matter. Naeser *et al.* (1987) confirmed the association between Wernicke's area lesion and Wernicke's aphasia, and stressed the role of deep white matter pathways for the pathogenesis of global aphasia (Naeser *et al.* 1989). Whether or not the deep lesion in global aphasia signifies involvement of white matter pathways or rather a lesion of the basal ganglia that combines detrimentally with a cortical lesion is under debate (Wallesch 1997). A recent investigation based on magnetic resonance (MR)-documented lesions came to the following conclusions (Kreisler *et al.* 2000).

◆ Nonfluent aphasia depends on the presence of frontal or putaminal lesions.

◆ Repetition disorder depends on insular or external capsule lesions.

◆ Comprehension disorder depends on posterior lesions of the temporal gyri.

◆ Verbal paraphasia depends on temporal or caudate lesions.

We will not discuss in detail the anatomy of lesions that may lead to transient aphasia. It may suffice that almost any lesion in the area of supply of the left middle cerebral artery, but also of the left anterior cerebral artery, and lesions of the left thalamus may cause transient speech or language disturbances. Lesions of the left supplementary motor area (SMA) transiently lead to mutism that progresses to transcortical motor aphasia and finally to normal language production with some nonfluency. With bilateral lesions, mustim may persist. There is some agreement that the cingular region, of which the SMA is part, is not involved in linguistic processes, but rather in the initiation of speech (von Stockert 1975).

Kertesz and Wallesch (1993) summarized why the functional neuroanatomy must be different between acute and chronic aphasia: 'The early deficit that may be related to edema, cellular dysfunction, transient ischemia, etc., is followed by a great deal of early spontaneous recovery in trauma or stroke. The chronic deficit is related not only to a loss of function, but to compensatory changes by functionally connected structures such as homologous contralateral areas or neighbouring areas during subsequent stages of recovery'.

Of interest for the issue of lateralization and more widespread, bilateral representations of language functions are cases of aphasia in right-handers with right hemisphere lesions (crossed aphasia). In some well analysed cases an anomalous pattern of lateralization was found, with some linguistic functions lateralized to the right, although for most functions the left hemisphere was dominant (Alexander and Annett 1996). The occurrence of such individual lateralization patterns may explain why the aphasic symptomatology cannot be predicted from imaging data.

There are some language functions that suffer greater impairment from right than from left hemisphere damage (for a review, see Joanette and Goulet 1993):

◆ the identification of emotional words and sentences (Borod *et al.* 1992);

◆ the production of effective prosody in a tonal (Thai) language (Gandour *et al.* 1995).

When analysing the clinical imaging data of large numbers of aphasic patients it becomes apparent that some linguistic functions (e.g. grammaticalization) seem to be focally represented in the left periinsular cortex, whereas others, e.g. the processes that underlie naming and word finding, are more broadly distributed in the brain. It is often argued that the clinical symptomatology should not be attributed to the damaged region but to other undamaged structures that subserve the respective functions after the lesion occurred. This view is based on a localization assumption, namely, that brain regions subserve a function and, if they are destroyed, other brain areas, which originally subserved another function, have to compensate, or that there is redundancy in the system. In recent years, another theory has gained ground, namely, that cognitive functions have a distributed representation in neural networks, which have compensatory facilities of their own. The properties of the network may explain the symptomatology (Plaut 1995).

The role of the basal ganglia and the thalamus in the pathogenesis of aphasic symptoms is still controversial. A central reason is that exact lesion anatomy is difficult to define because of common vascular supply to various structures and anatomical variability. Physiologically, a role for the loop systems, which run from cortex via basal ganglia and thalamus back to executive cortex and which execute an output gating is plausible and can explain the symptoms of so-called subcortical aphasia (Wallesch 1997).

4 The functional neuroanatomy of normal language processing

Literally hundreds of positron emission tomography (PET) and fMRI studies have been published since the landmark investigation of Petersen *et al.* (1988) that described the activation of brain areas in normal subjects during language tasks. With respect to many assumed representations of language functions, the data are conflicting. The studies can be replicated only if the experimental setting is exactly reproduced (for a discussion of methodology, see Section 6). However, certain aspects of language-related activations converge between studies, and some of these are briefly outlined in the box on p. 747. Furthermore, PET (Absher *et al.* 2000) and fMRI activations have been found to correlate with electrophysiological event-related potentials, which indicates their validity. In general, fMRI seems more sensitive than PET due to its superior signal-to-noise ratio (Sadato *et al.* 1998). In this review, we shall not separate PET from fMRI studies.

Electrophysiologically, some language processes, especially those that can be analysed by the comparison of two stimuli with identical structure over time and a discrete event that separates them, can be analysed by the method of averaged event-related potentials (ERPs). Of special interest for psycholinguistic analysis is the N400 wave, with which subjects react to semantic or syntactic incompatibility. These phenomena are highly interesting for the physiology of language processing, but give little evidence for its underlying anatomy, even when the method of brain mapping is employed (for further details, see Rugg and Coles 1995).

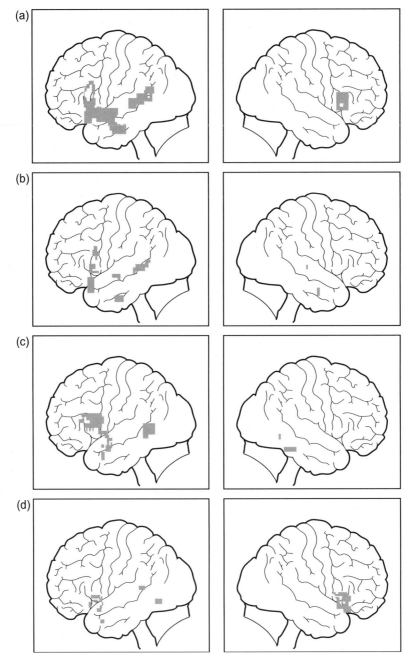

Fig. 40.3 Activation of cortical regions by reading words of different class and concreteness versus pseudowords in a lexical decision task: a) activation by words compared to pseudowords; b) commonalities of activation by all words; c) verbs compared to nouns; d) abstract words compared to concrete words. (Taken with permission from Perani et al. 1999a, fig. 1.)

Some language-related activations of brain areas

PET studies using language comprehension (story listening) and production (covert verb generation to a semantically related noun) paradigms and analysing their covariance in comparison to a resting state were able to identify three areas involved in language processing, roughly the regions of Broca's and Wernicke's area, and the anterior part of the left inferior temporal gyrus (Papathanassiou *et al.* 2000).

Activation of Broca'a area has been found with receptive syntactic processing (Caplan *et al.* 2000). Broca's area was not activated by word repetition, but rather the left anterior insula and lateral premotor cortex were activated (Wise *et al.* 1999).

Lexical–semantic processing of words activates an extensive, mainly left hemisphere network of brain structures (Perani *et al.* 1999*a*, see Fig. 40.3), with a larger left frontal activation for verbs than nouns. A number of studies have found a left fusiform gyrus (a parahippocampal structure of the temporal lobe) activation with semantic access (Murtha *et al;* 1999, Kuperberg *et al.* 2000). With respect to semantic category judgements, Perani *et al.* (1999*b*) found a left fusiform gyrus activation with the processing of living things, and of the left middle temporal gyrus for tools. It can be expected that abundant information on the cerebral basis of semantics will be available from fMRI studies in the near future. It can also be expected that future studies will reveal a great degree of interindividual variability, as subgroups of normal subjects show bilateral temporal activation with semantic retrieval (Warburton *et al.* 1999).

5 The functional neuroanatomy of language processing in aphasics

The lesions underlying aphasia interfere with task-related activation of the affected brain structures. However, functional imaging demonstrated changes in the functional organization of language processing in aphasics. Depending on the language task, aphasic patients seem to activate ipsi- and contralesional cortical areas in addition to spared structures (Ohyama *et al.* 1996). The superior repetition performance in transcortical aphasia seems to be based on right hemisphere mechanisms (Berthier *et al.* 1991). Alterations in language processing in aphasic patients can also be demonstrated by neurophysiological analysis. ERP and MEG (magnetoencephalography) studies have the advantage of superior temporal resolution over fMRI and PET (but inferior spatial resolution). Friederici *et al.* (1998) were able to show that ERP-correlates of the automatic analysis of syntactic structures were absent in Broca's aphasia.

Recovery from aphasia seems to depend mainly upon three functional anatomical mechanisms:

♦ recruitment of perilesional left cortical areas for language processing (Warburton *et al.* 1999);

- an activation of the left supplementary motor area;
- an activation of contralesional homologues in the right hemisphere.

Some studies suggest that early recovery is related to left and long-term improvement to right hemisphere activation (Karbe *et al.* 1998). Patients who were able to recruit dominant language structures exhibited better recovery (Heiss *et al.* 1999). It has been proposed that speech therapy may aid in the activation of the dominant hemisphere and that right hemisphere activation may be dysfunctional (Belin *et al.* 1996). On the other hand, improvement with intensive comprehension training in Wernicke's aphasia was shown to correlate with task-dependent activation in the posterior part of the right superior temporal gyrus (Musso *et al.* 1999).

Pizzamiglio *et al.* (2001) pointed out that the function-related changes in cerebral activation patterns after lesion may have different meanings.

- In some cases, spared neuronal populations involved in a given function may undergo reorganization providing the basis for functional recovery.
- In other cases, different regions of the brain, which process information in a completely different way, are recruited after a lesion to compensate for a functional loss.

6 Methodological problems of functional imaging

Functional images represent spatially and temporally integrated measures of regional cerebral blood flow during the performance of a task in contrast to flow distribution during another task (or a resting state). A detailed discussion of the methodological aspects of functional language studies is given by Grabowski and Damasio (2000). These authors' summary of items to be included in processing the complex data includes:

- modelling and removal of artefacts;
- spatial transformation to a standard anatomical space (usually based upon Talairach and Tournoux 1988);
- spatial filtering to improve signal-to-noise ratio, to overcome anatomical variability, and to meet parametric assumptions of statistical analysis (see end of this section);
- statistical analysis;
- construction of a statistical parametric map;
- significance thresholding of the test statistic images;
- inference;
- representations of the results (Grabowski and Damasio 2000, pp. 430–2).

The method is based on a number of assumptions that are difficult to control.

- It supposes that the experimental task states differ only with respect to the tasks (problems, e.g. effort, demand on working memory, subjective reaction).
- Brains differ anatomically and cannot completely be mapped upon a standard anatomical space (Rajkowska and Goldman-Rakic 1995).

- It is assumed that the experimental tasks isolate a single cognitive function.
- It is assumed that task-related activation is insensitive to practice effects.

In fact, practice changes activation patterns. Furthermore, the sheer rate of presentation of stimuli affects activation (Raichle *et al.* 1994).

In many experiments, the crucial experimental task differed in a number of aspects (e.g. difficulty, propositionality, size, and number of activated semantic fields) from those it was compared with. Generally, the so-called subtraction method assumes that cognitive variables that affect different stages of processing are simply added and can be revealed by the subtraction of two states, one that includes the process in question from a similar other that does not. This approach was very fruitful in the analysis of reaction times. The use of this method with language tasks poses many problems, among which the following cause the greatest concern.

- Automatic activation of language processing even when subjects are instructed not to pay attention to linguistic content.
- Changes in activation may be a characteristic of the control task.
- The assumption of addition of a processing state may be inherently false (Friston *et al.* 1996).

Parametric designs are able to overcome some of these problems. Statistical parametric mapping is based upon spatially extended statistical processes that compare spatially distributed events with a probabilistic distribution. Improbable effects within the map are interpreted as regionally specific effects due to the experimental manipulation. 'The fundamental difference between subtractive and parametric approaches lies in treating a cognitive process not as a categorical invariant but as a dimension or attribute that can be expressed to a greater or a lesser extent' (Friston 1997). An important next step is the introduction of nonparametric statistics ('statistical nonparametric mapping'; Poline *et al.* 1997). Functional connectivity between two regions can be statistically established by factorial designs (Friston *et al.* 1997).

7 Summary

From the above discussion, it becomes obvious that the methodological problems of functional imaging are not settled. Although experiments can be replicated, if the exact situation is restaged, results are still conflicting, depend upon the strategy of analysis, and cannot be generalized yet (Friston *et al.* 1997; Grabowski and Damasio 2000). However, it is also clear that functional imaging, especially fMRI, has a great potential for the analysis of cerebral processes, particularly those that are involved in cognition and emotion. In our opinion, the analysis of interindividual differences will become increasingly important.

Selective references

Absher, J.R., Hart, L.A., Flowers, D.L., Dagenbach, D., and Wood, F.B. (2000). Event-related potentials correlate with task-dependent glucose metabolism. *NeuroImage* 11, 517–31.

Alexander, G., DeLong, M.R., and Strick, P. (1986). Parallel organization of functionally segregated circuits linking basal ganglia and cortex. *Ann. Rev. Neurosci.* **9**, 357–81.

Alexander, M.P. and Annett, M. (1996). Crossed aphasia and related anomalies of cerebral organization: case reports and a genetic hypothesis. *Brain Language* **55**, 213–39.

Belin, P., van Eeckhout, P., Zilbovicius, M., *et al.* (1996). Recovery from nonfluent aphasia after melodic intonation therapy. *Neurology* **47**, 1504–11.

Berthier, M.L., Starkstein, S.E., Leiguarda, R., *et al.* (1991). Transcortical aphasia. Importance of the non-speech dominant hemisphere in language repetition. *Brain* **114**, 1409–27.

Borod, J.C., Andelman, F., Obler, L.K., Tweedy, J.R., and Welkowitz, J. (1992). Right hemisphere specialization for the identification of emotional words and sentences: evidence from stroke patients. *Neuropsychologia* **30**, 827–44.

Caplan, D., Alpert, N., Waters, G., and Olivieri, A. (2000). Activation of Broca's area by syntactic processing under conditions of concurrent articulation. *Hum. Brain Mapping* **9**, 65–71.

Carpenter, P.A. and Just, M.A. (1999). Modeling the mind: very-high field functional magnetic resonance imaging activation during cognition. *Topics MRI* **10**, 16–36.

Chi, J.G., Dooling, E.C., and Gilles, F.H. (1977). Left–right asymmetries of the temporal speech areas of the human fetus. *Arch. Neurol.* **34**, 346–8.

Frackowiak, R.S.J., Friston, K.J., Frith, C.D., Dolan, R.J., and Mazziotta, J.C. (eds.) (1997). *Human Brain Function.* Academic Press, San Diego.

Friederici, A.D., Hahne, A., and von Cramon, D.Y. (1998). First-pass versus second-pass parsing processes in a Wernicke's and a Broca's aphasic: electrophysiological evidence for a double dissociation. *Brain Language* **62**, 311–41.

Friston, K.J. (1997). Analyzing brain images: principles and overview. In *Human brain function* (ed. R.S.J. Frackowiak, K.J. Friston, C.D. Frith, R.J. Dolan, and J.C. Mazziotta), pp. 25–41. Academic Press, San Diego.

Friston, K.J., Price, C.J., Fletcher, P., Moore, C., Frackowiak, R.S.J., and Dolan, R.J. (1996). The trouble with cognitive subtraction. *NeuroImage* **4**, 97–104.

Friston, K.J., Price, C.J., Buechel, C., and Frackowiak, R.S.J. (1997). A taxonomy of study designs. In *Human brain function* (ed. R.S.J. Frackowiak, K.J. Friston, C.D. Frith, R.J. Dolan, and J.C. Mazziotta), pp. 141–59. Academic Press, San Diego.

Gandour, J., Larsen, J., Dechongkiet, S., Ponglorpisit, S., and Khunadorn, F. (1995). Speech prosody in affective contexts in Thai patients with right hemisphere lesions. *Brain Language* **51**, 422–43.

Grabowski, T.J. and Damasio, A.R. (2000). Investigating language with functional neuroimaging. In *Brain mapping: the systems* (ed. A.W. Toga and J.C. Mazziotta), pp. 425–61. Academic Press, San Diego.

Harley, T.A. (1996). Connectionist modelling of the recovery of language functions following brain damage. *Brain Language* **52**, 7–24.

Heiss, W.D., Kessler, J., Thiel, A., Ghaemi, M., and Karbe, H. (1999). Differential capacity of left and right hemispheric areas for compensation of poststroke aphasia. *Ann. Neurol.* **45**, 430–8.

Joanette, Y. and Goulet, P. (1993). Verbal communication deficits after right-hemisphere damage. In *Linguistic disorders and pathologies* (ed. G. Blanken, J. Dittmann, H. Grimm, J.C. Marshall, and C.W. Wallesch), pp. 383–8. De Gruyter, Berlin.

Karbe, H., Thiel, A., Weber-Luxenburger, G., Herholz, K., Kessler, J., and Heiss, W. (1998). Brain plasticity in poststroke aphasia: what is the contribution of the right hemisphere? *Brain Language* **64**, 215–30.

Kertesz, A. and Wallesch, C.W. (1993). Cerebral organization of language. In *Linguistic disorders and pathologies* (ed. G. Blanken, J. Dittmann, H. Grimm, J.C. Marshall, and C.W. Wallesch), pp. 120–37. De Gruyter, Berlin.

Kreisler, A., Godefrey, O., Delmaire, C., *et al.* (2000). The anatomy of aphasia revisited. *Neurology* 54, 1117–23.

Kuperberg, G.R., McGuire, P.K., Bullmore, E.T., *et al.* (2000). Common and distinct neural sustrates for pragmatic, semantic and syntactic processing of spoken sentences: an fMRI study. *J. Cogn. Neurosci.* 12, 321–41.

Marshall, J.C. (2000). Planum of the apes: a case study. *Brain Language* 71, 145–8.

McClelland, J.L. and Rumelhart, D.E. (1986). *Parallel distributed processing: explorations in the microstructure of cognition.* Vol. 2: *Psychological and biological models.* MIT Press, London.

Merzenich, M.M., Kaas, J.H., Wall, J., Nelson, R.J., Sur, M., and Felleman, D. (1983). Topographic reorganisation of somatosensory cortical areas 3b and 1 in adult monkeys following restricted deafferentation. *Neuroscience* 8, 33–55.

Murtha, S., Chertkow, H., Beauregard, M., and Evans, A. (1999). The neural substrate of picture naming. *J. Cogn. Neurosci.* 11, 399–423.

Musso, M., Weiller, C., Kiebel, S., Müller, S.P., Bülau, P., and Rijntjes, M. (1999). Training induced brain plasticity in aphasia. *Brain* 122, 1781–90.

Naeser, M.A., Helm-Estabrooks, N., Haas, G., Auerbach, S., and Scrinivasan, M. (1987). Relationship between lesion extent in Wernicke's area on computed tomographic scan and predicting recovery of comprehension in Wernicke's aphasia. *Arch. Neurol.* 44, 73–82.

Naeser, M.A., Palumbo, C.L., Helm-Estabrooks, N., Stiassny-Eder, D., and Albert, M.L. (1989). Severe nonfluency in aphasia. Role of the medial subcallosal fasciculus and other white matter pathways in recovery of spontaneous speech. *Brain* 112, 1–38.

Ohyama, M., Senda, M., Kitamura, S., Ishii, K., Mishina, M., and Terashi, A. (1996). Role of the nondominant hemisphere and undamaged area during word repetition in poststroke aphasics. A PET activation study. *Stroke* 27, 897–903.

Papathanassiou, D., Etard, O., Mellet, E., Tago, L., Mazoyer, B., and Tzourio-Mazoyer, N. (2000). A common language network for comprehension and production: contribution to the definition of language epicenters with PET. *NeuroImage* 11, 347–57.

Perani, D., Cappa, S.F., Schnur, T., *et al.* (1999*a*). The neural correlates of verb and noun processing. A PET study. *Brain* 122, 2337–44.

Perani, D., Schnur, T., Tettamanti, M., Gorno-Tempini, M., Cappa, S.F., and Fazio, F. (1999*b*). Word and picture matching: a PET study of semantic category effects. *Neuropsychologia* 37, 293–306.

Petersen, S.E., Fox, P.T., Posner, M.I., Mintun, M., and Raichle, M.E. (1988). Positron emission tomographic studies of the cortical anatomy of single word processing. *Nature* 331, 585–9.

Pizzamiglio, L., Galati, G., and Committeri, G. (2001). The contribution of functional neuroimaging to recovery after brain damage: a review. *Cortex* 37, 11–31.

Plaut, D.C. (1995). Double dissociation without modularity: evidence from connectionist neuropsychology. *J. Clin. Exp. Neuropsychol.* 17, 291–321.

Poeck, K., de Bleser, R., and von Keyserlingk, D.G. (1984). Computed tomography localization of standard aphasia syndromes. *Advan. Neurol.* 42, 71–89.

Poline, J.B., Holmes, A., Worsley, K., and Friston, K.J. (1997). Making statistical inferences. In *Human brain function* (ed. R.S.J. Frackowiak, K.J. Friston, C.D. Frith, R.J. Dolan, and J.C. Mazziotta), pp. 85–106. Academic Press, San Diego.

Raichle, M.E., Fiez, J., Videen, T.O., *et al.* (1994). Practice-related changes in human functional anatomy during nonmotor learning. *Cerebral Cortex* 4, 8–26.

Rajkowska, G. and Goldman-Rakic, P.S. (1995). Cytoarchitectonic definition of prefrontal areas in the normal human cortex: II: Variability in locations of areas 9 and 46 and relationship to the Talairach coordinate system. *Cerebral Cortex* 5, 323–37.

Rugg, M.D. and Coles, M.G.H. (1995). *Electrophysiology of mind. Event-related potentials and cognition.* Oxford University Press, Oxford.

Sadato, N., Yonekura, Y., Yamada, H., Nakamura, S., Waki, A., and Ishii, Y. (1998). Activation patterns of covert word generation detected by fMRI in comparison with 3D PET. *J. Comput. Assisted Tomogr.* **22**, 945–52.

Schmahmann, J.D. and Pandya, D.N. (1997). The cerebrocerebellar system. In 'The cerebellum and cognition' [volume edited by J.D. Schmahmann]. *Int. Rev. Neurobiol.* **41**, 31–60.

Steinmetz, H. (1996). Structure, function and cerebral asymmetry: *in vivo* morphometry of the planum temporale. *Neurosci. Behav. Rev.* **20**, 587–91.

Talairach, J. and Tournoux, P. (1988). *Co-planar stereotaxic atlas of the human brain.* Thieme, New York.

Toga, A.W. and Mazziotta, J.C. (eds.) (2000). *Brain Mapping: the systems.* Academic Press, San Diego.

Von Stockert, T.R. (1975). Aphasia sine aphasia. *Brain Language* **1**, 277–82.

Wallesch, C.W. (1997). Symptomatology of subcortical aphasia. *J. Neurolinguistics* **10**, 267–75.

Warburton, E., Price, C.J., Swinburn, K., and Wise, R.J. (1999) Mechanisms of recovery from aphasia: evidence from positron emission tomography studies. *J. Neurol. Neurosurg. Psychiatry* **66**, 155–61.

Wise, R.J., Greene, J., Büchel, C., and Scott, S.K. (1999). Brain regions involved in articulation. *Lancet* **353**, 1057–61.

Chapter 41

Functional neuroanatomy of executive process

Joaquín M. Fuster

1 Introduction

The cortex of the frontal lobe contains the highest stages of the hierarchy of neural structures dedicated to motor representation and processing. The lowest stage of that hierarchy consists of motor neurons in the anterior horns of the spinal cord. Above, in ascending order, are the motor nuclei of the brainstem, the cerebellum, and the diencephalon, including nuclei of the hypothalamus, the thalamus, and the basal ganglia. The cortex of the convexity of the frontal lobe is itself hierarchically organized and devoted to motor actions. At the bottom of the cortical motor hierarchy lies the primary motor cortex, for the representation and execution of elementary skeletal movements. Above it lies the premotor cortex, for more complex movements, which are defined by goal and trajectory. Some premotor areas are involved in speech organization. At the top is the cortex of association of the frontal lobe, commonly called prefrontal cortex. This cortex, especially in its lateral region, contains neuronal networks that represent broad schemas and plans of sequential action and are crucially involved in their enactment. Thus, the lateral prefrontal cortex (LPC) has been sometimes identified with the 'central executive' and also called 'the executive of the brain'. In this chapter, the executive functions of the LPC are considered (see Chapters 17 and 18). Before dealing with them, the chapter deals with the anatomy, the connectivity, and the neuropsycho-logy of the prefrontal cortex in general.

2 Anatomy and connectivity of the prefrontal cortex

The prefrontal cortex is one of latest regions of the neocortex to develop, phylogenetically as well as ontogenetically. In evolution, it reaches its greatest relative expansion in the brain of the human, where it constitutes almost one-third of the neocortex. Most of that expansion takes place in the lateral convexity of the frontal lobe, that is, in the LPC. In ontogeny, the prefrontal cortex—the LPC in particular—is one of the last regions to reach full myelination of afferent, efferent, and intrinsic fibres. The LPC is also late in reaching maturity by other indices, e.g. number and volume of neurons, and size and number of dendritic spines. In the normal human subject, the prefrontal cortex does not reach full morphological maturation until late adolescence. The late maturation of the LPC is probably related to the late maturation of its cognitive functions.

The prefrontal cortex is profusely connected with other brain structures. It receives afferent fibres from the brainstem, the hypothalamus, the limbic system (especially amygdala and hippocampus), the thalamus, the basal ganglia, and other areas of the neocortex, especially the association cortex behind the sylvian fissure (parietal, temporal, and occipital regions).

- The afferents from the brainstem, the hypothalamus, and limbic formations bring the prefrontal cortex information about the internal milieu.

- The inputs from the hippocampus are probably essential for the formation of motor or executive memory.

- The afferents from posterior association cortex appear to be involved in higher-order sensorimotor integrations.

The prefrontal cortex reciprocates afferent inputs from all those cerebral structures with efferent outputs to them.

Several neurotransmitter systems of brainstem origin converge on various areas of the prefrontal cortex. They mediate interactions at the synaptic level between subcortical structures and that cortex. The most prominent among them are the dopamine systems, which vary in terms of the types of receptors by which they mediate the transmission of information between cells.

- Dopamine plays an important role in orbital prefrontal cortex, where it mediates neural transactions related to rewards and emotional behaviour. Furthermore, dopaminergic prefrontal pathways mediate motor behaviour through the basal ganglia.

- Noradrenaline (norepinephrine) and serotonin, with sparser distributions in the prefrontal cortex, are probably involved in cortical arousal and attention mechanisms.

- A powerful cholinergic system, originating in the basal nucleus of Meynert and widely distributed throughout the neocortex, is most probably also involved in those attention mechanisms and in short-term memory.

- In the prefrontal cortex, as in other parts of the cortex, γ-aminobutyric acid (GABA) is the most abundant inhibitory neurotransmitter. It participates in the filtering or exclusionary mechanisms of attention and working memory.

- Glutaminergic neurotransmitters, such as those operating on *N*-methyl-D-aspartate (NMDA) receptors, most probably play a role in the formation of executive memory in the prefrontal cortex.

Intervening in this process are probably the reciprocal connections between the hippocampus and the LPC, which have been demonstrated in the monkey.

3 Neuropsychology of the prefrontal cortex

For more than a century, the study of the behavioural and cognitive effects of prefrontal damage from disease or trauma has been a major source of knowledge about the functions of the prefrontal cortex. This knowledge is largely inferential, based on the assumption that the deficit from the lesion of a cerebral structure such as the prefrontal cortex results from the interference with the normal function(s) of that structure. This assumption is not always tenable, because the lesion may secondarily and imponderably affect other—neighbouring or connected—structures. Furthermore, the deficit is commonly relative, i.e. only quantitatively different from the dysfunction induced by lesions elsewhere in the brain. In any event, the inferences from clinical lesion are generally confounded by considerable individual variability—in terms of the extent and location of the lesion as well as its effects. Nonetheless, a massive literature is now available on the clinical and psychological manifestations of frontal-lobe injury. This literature allows us to characterize those manifestations with considerable confidence. A particular cluster of symptoms and signs can be reliably observed after damage to each of the three principal regions of the prefrontal cortex (Fig. 41.1):

- medial;
- orbital;
- lateral (LPC).

3.1 Medial/cingulate region

The lesions of the medial region of the prefrontal cortex induce disorders of drive and motivation. Apathy and disinterest are the dominant manifestations of medial prefrontal damage. Related to them is the lack of spontaneity in all domains of action, including speech. The patient is generally hypokinetic. In cases with large lesions of medial prefrontal cortex, hypokinesia turns into akinesia (akinetic mutism when speech is involved). Circumscribed lesions of the anterior cingulate cortex (areas 24 and 32) commonly result in deficits of attention. The patient with such a lesion has difficulty focusing on the performance of tasks that require sizeable effort and attention to detail. Thus the patient appears not only neglectful, but also unable to gather the energy to respond to cognitively challenging situations.

In all probability, the lack of interest, the aspontaneity, and the inattentiveness of patients with medial/anterior-cingulate lesion reflect the disruption of a general adaptive function of goal-directed drive that is indispensable for selective attention. The connectivity of medial prefrontal cortex with limbic structures probably plays a role in that general function. Mesulam (1981) has postulated an 'anterior attentional system', of which the anterior cingulate region would be a crucial part. That system also includes gaze-control areas of parietal and lateral prefrontal cortex.

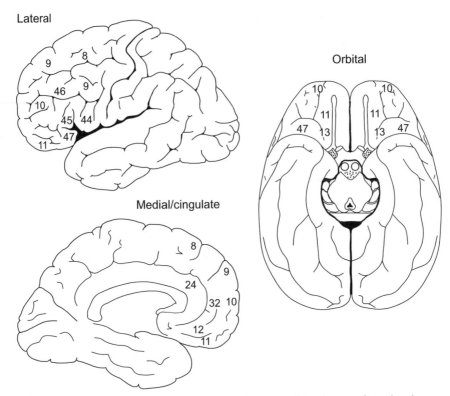

Fig. 41.1 Diagram of the human cerebral cortex. The areas of the three prefrontal regions are numbered in accord with Brodmann's cytoarchitectonic map.

3.2 **Orbital region**

Lesions of ventral (orbital) prefrontal cortex ordinarily induce a relatively uniform syndrome. An attentional disorder is here again in the foreground, but this one is not so much characterized by absence of drive as by failure of the exclusionary aspect of attention. The patient is abnormally distractable, unable to inhibit the interference from external stimuli that are extraneous to the action in progress, whatever that may be. Together with distractability, and probably related to it, is a general tendency to hyperactivity and hyperreactivity. On formal testing, the patient commonly fails to perform correctly the Stroop task, the Wisconsin Card Sorting Test (WCST), and other tests that require the attentional suppression of interference.

Furthermore, the affect of the orbital patient is labile and unpredictable. Together with a sporadic tendency to euphoria, the patient commonly exhibits inappropriate and coarse humour. In addition, he or she is unable to inhibit instinctive drives, and thus inclined to frequent displays of quarrelsomeness, hypersexuality and hyperphagia. The disinhibition of instinct, accompanied by lack of moral judgement, often leads the patient to unruly behaviour and conflict with the law. Sociopathy is almost the hallmark of the orbital syndrome.

In brief, the patient with damage of the orbital prefrontal cortex commonly exhibits a variety of abnormalities of emotional and social behaviour (Damasio *et al.* 1994; Fuster 1997). At the root of these abnormalities, there appears to be a deficit in the inhibitory control functions of this cortex. In normal attentive processing, inhibitory control is probably exerted through efferent connections of orbital cortex upon the thalamus and upon areas of frontal and posterior association cortex. In normal social behaviour, that control is exerted upon the hypothalamus and other limbic structures. Both kinds of control fail in the patient with orbitofrontal damage.

3.3 Lateral region (LPC)

The most characteristic cognitive deficits from frontal-lobe injury are those that result from damage to the associative cortex of the lateral frontal convexity—the LPC. In subjects with a large LPC lesion, the most common disorder is the inability to conceptualize and to carry out plans and goal-directed sequences of actions. It is from this disorder that the notion emerged of a critical role of the LPC in the representation and execution of organized behaviour (Luria 1966; Fuster 1997). The planning deficit, which extends to the representation and construction of language (Luria 1970), is now generally considered a consistent manifestation of large lateral LPC lesion. One aspect of this deficit is a difficulty in mentally representing sequences of speech or behaviour. Another is a difficulty in executing them in orderly fashion. The aggregate of these difficulties constitutes what Baddeley (1986) calls the 'dysexecutive syndrome'. This syndrome, like the medial and orbital syndromes, usually includes a severe attentional disorder, though this disorder differs qualitatively from those that result from medial or orbital lesion. Shallice (1988) characterizes the LPC disorder as the failure of 'supervisory attentional control'. By this he means the inability to summon and sustain selective attention on a series of goal-directed actions. This aspect of attention is essential to executive initiative, decision-making, and the temporal organization of novel and complex behaviour.

Any reasonable analysis of the functions of the LPC must distinguish between its *representational* role and its *operational* role. The former can be inferred from the deleterious effects of LPC lesions on the mental representations of plans and schemata of sequential action. The study of these effects has led to the concept of the LPC as the substrate of executive memory, which includes the schemata or plans of past or future action. Plans can be considered 'memory' inasmuch as they consist of fragmentary representations of previous actions—rearranged for future planning. Executive memory is held in wide arrays of interconnected neuronal networks of the LPC (Fuster 1995).

The operational role of the LPC essentially consists of the orderly activation of those networks in the construction of goal-directed sequences or temporal 'gestalts' of executive action. Temporal integration is the most general function of the LPC.

This operation is served by at least four cognitive functions that this cortex controls in cooperation with subcortical structures and with other regions of the neocortex. Those functions are:

+ attention;
+ working memory;
+ prospective set;
+ response monitoring.

They are closely entwined and cannot be extricated from one another physiologically. None is represented exclusively in any discrete LPC area. Any demonstrable specialization of LPC areas is not so much attributable to the topographical distribution of those cognitive functions as to the kind of executive information they process. Thus some areas are dedicated to motor actions, others to eye movement, and still others to speech. In any given area, all four cognitive functions operate at the service of the temporal integration of the kind of executive information in which the area specializes.

4 Temporal integration and its ancillary executive functions

Temporal integration, i.e. the capacity to integrate information across time, is the essence of temporal order. This applies to behaviour, speech, and logical reasoning. The central role of the LPC in the organization of actions in those three domains is crucially based on its ability to mediate contingencies across time ('if now this, then later that; if earlier that, then now this'). Both the choice and the timing of an act in a goal-directed sequence are contingent on the plan of action, on the goal, and on other acts that have preceded that act or are expected to succeed it (Fig. 41.2). Inasmuch as the LPC is needed for the mediation of cross-temporal contingencies, it is needed for the temporal organization of behavioural, linguistic, and cognitive actions.

The most widely used behavioural paradigms for testing the role of LPC in temporal integration are the so-called 'delay tasks', e.g. delayed response, delayed matching-to-sample. In these tasks, the subject is required to retain a discrete item of information in order to execute, a few seconds later, an action that is contingent on that information. For correct performance, therefore, each trial requires the integration of information across time, i.e. across the delay. It has long been known (Jacobsen 1931) that monkeys that have sustained lesions of LPC are rendered incapable of learning and performing delay tasks, especially when the information is complex and the delay long (>10 seconds).

In the past 30 years, electrophysiology and neuroimaging have established the operational role of the LPC in all four of its temporal integrative functions. Many of the studies contributing the supporting evidence have been carried out in monkeys or humans performing delay tasks.

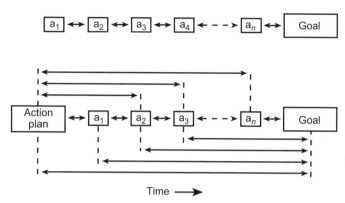

Fig. 41.2 Temporal sequencing of acts ($a_1 \ldots a_n$) toward a goal. (Above) Chain of acts in a routine and well-practised sequence. Contingencies (arrows) are present only between successive acts. (Below) A novel and complex sequence of acts that necessitates the mediation of cross-temporal contingencies, a function of the LPC.

4.1 **Sensory attention**

Attention is the selective allocation of neural resources to behaviour and cognition. It operates at many levels of sensory and motor systems. It is essential in the cerebral cortex for the efficient processing of information in its vast systems of intersecting networks. For a behavioural sequence to attain its goal, continuous selective attention is required on the sensory stimuli that guide it and on the motor actions that constitute it. This is fundamentally a cortical function. Its mechanisms are still poorly understood and they can be assumed to include excitation as well as inhibition. The results of their operation are:

- selective focusing;
- enhanced contrast;
- suppression of extraneous information.

All forms of attention required for the organization of behavioural and cognitive sequences are under executive prefrontal control. As noted in Section 3, medial and cingulate areas contribute to the motivational aspects of attention and orbital areas to the inhibitory control of interference or distraction. Areas of the LPC, on the other hand, contribute to the aspects of attention more directly related to temporal integration. Sensory attention is one of them. Several LPC areas—notably area 8—are involved in visual attention, as they specialize in the control of gaze and eye movements. Lesions of these areas lead to visual neglect and to the inability to shift attention between locations in the visual field. Functional neuroimaging provides further evidence for the role of LPC in selective sensory attention, as it supports a variety of temporal integrative tasks (Duncan and Owen 2000).

Working memory and prospective set, the two LPC functions that are essential to bridge time (see Sections 4.2 and 4.3), can also be considered forms of selective attention. Both constitute attention that is directed to internal representations. Both appear to depend on the selective activation of cortical and subcortical structures under the control of the LPC (Desimone and Duncan 1995; Fuster 1995).

4.2 **Working memory**

Working memory (Baddeley 1986) is the temporary retention of information for the performance of an act that is contingent on that information. All forms of cognitive and behavioural performance requiring the mediation of cross-temporal contingencies depend to some degree on working memory. Working memory is the first cognitive function of the LPC to have been substantiated at the neuronal level by microelectrode methods. In delay tasks, during the retention of a sensory cue for a prospective action, neurons in the dorsolateral prefrontal cortex of the monkey exhibit sustained elevated discharge (Fuster 1973). This discharge, which may last anywhere between a few seconds and 2 or 3 minutes, is correlated with accuracy of performance and can be obliterated or attenuated by distraction. Cells with these characteristics have been called 'memory cells'. During the performance of spatial delayed-response tasks, in which the animal must retain the position of a visual cue, some LPC cells are involved in the retention of spatial information. In other kinds of delay tasks, memory cells have been found for colours, auditory cues, and tactile information. In any case, the participation of LPC cells in working memory seems strictly related to the need to retain information for an action that is contingent on that information.

In the human, the use of functional neuroimaging by positron emission tomography (PET) or magnetic resonance (MR) reveals the activation of the LPC in a number of working memory tasks (Grasby *et al.* 1993; Petrides *et al.* 1993; Smith *et al.* 1996). The activation has a different topography depending on the nature of the memorandum or information that the subject must temporarily retain. It is reasonable to assume that the activation reflects the excitation of large assemblies or networks of memory cells that encode that information in working memory. LPC networks have been thus substantiated for visuospatial, visual–nonspatial, and verbal memoranda.

4.3 **Prospective set**

Prospective or preparatory set is another form of internalized attention under LPC control. Like working memory, it helps the organism to mediate cross-temporal contingencies. Whereas working memory is retrospective memory, prospective set is 'memory of the future'. It is attention focused on the representation of prospective action. Thus, the prospective-set function can be considered a kind of motor, or executive, attention. By this function and mechanisms that are still unknown, the LPC primes executive systems for anticipated action.

A well-known electrical correlate of prospective set is the contingent negative variation (CNV), a slow surface potential that develops over the frontal lobe in the interval between a sensory stimulus and a motor response that depends on it (Brunia *et al.* 1985). Another such correlate is the *Bereitschaftspotential* or 'readiness potential', which develops over motor cortex immediately before the response. In monkeys performing a delay task in which the animal had to remember a colour for a hand movement to the right or to the left, some LPC were found to react specifically to colours and others to direction of manual response (Quintana and Fuster 1999). During the delay or memory period, the cells of the first type (colour-coupled) showed a gradual descent of discharge (Fig. 41.3). Conversely, those of the second type (direction-coupled) showed an acceleration of discharge. Furthermore, the degree of that acceleration varied in proportion to the certainty with which the animal could predict response direction (different colours predicted direction with different degrees of probability).

To sum up, the slow potentials in anticipation of an action, and the presence of cells in LPC that seem to predict the action, indicate that the LPC participates in the preparation of the motor apparatus to act. At lower stages, that apparatus includes structures such as the premotor cortex, the basal ganglia, and the pyramidal system. All may take

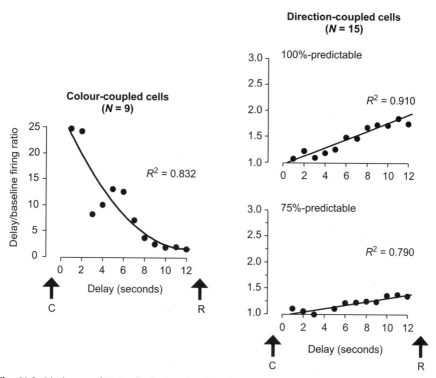

Fig. 41.3 Discharge of LPC cells during the delay between a colour and the manual response associated with it (C, colour; R, response). (Left) Discharge of colour-coupled memory cells. (Right) Discharge of direction-coupled cells. The latter cells anticipate the response with an acceleration of firing that is greatest (top graph) when the animal can predict response direction with certainty.

part in the preparatory modulation of motor systems under LPC control. That kind of preparatory control can also be inferred from the activation of the LPC observed by neuroimaging during planning tasks (Partiot *et al.* 1995; Baker *et al.* 1996).

4.4 **Response monitoring**

Response monitoring is a fourth integrative function of the LPC. This function is based on both internal and external feedback arriving in this cortex during organized action. The internal feedback consists of signals from internal receptors activated by movement. Such signals include inputs from the motor system in the form of so-called 'efferent copies' of muscular movement and inputs from proprioceptors. The aggregate of these internal signals related to movement generates in the LPC what has been termed *corollary discharge* (Teuber 1972). This consists of neural impulses that flow into sensory systems and prepare them for changes resulting from anticipated movement. Corollary discharge would thus stabilize perception despite changes in the relative position of sensory receptors with respect to the environment.

In addition, various kinds of feedback from sensory receptors carry to the LPC information about the changes that actions in a behavioural sequence induce in the environment. Thus, a more or less continuous stream of sensory signals arrive in LPC with information on the consequences of one's successive actions. These signals include indicators of the success or failure of each act with respect to the goal of the sequence. The LPC will integrate that information to prepare the organism for subsequent actions and to induce in them corrective modifications.

Neuroimaging supports the involvement of the LPC in response monitoring (Petrides *et al.* 1993; Fink *et al.* 1999). Further evidence of this involvement comes from electrophysiology in patients with LPC lesions (Gehring and Knight 2000). Both imaging and electrophysiology also indicate a parallel role of the anterior cingulate cortex in the monitoring of response errors.

5 **The perception–action cycle**

All four integrative functions of the LPC just mentioned operate within the broad physiological framework of the perception–action cycle (Fuster 1997). This physiological cycle constitutes the extension into the cerebral cortex—and thus into the cognitive sphere—of a basic physiological principle of sensorimotor adaptation of the organism to its environment. It may be considered to be part of the 'homeostatic' mechanisms of the organism inasmuch as adaptation to the environment protects stability of the internal milieu. The cycle is made of the circular cybernetic flow of information between the environment, sensory structures, and motor structures. Those neural structures are hierarchically organized along the nerve axis, and so are the levels of the cycle that unites them. The LPC and the posterior association cortex are at the summit of the perception–action cycle (Fig. 41.4).

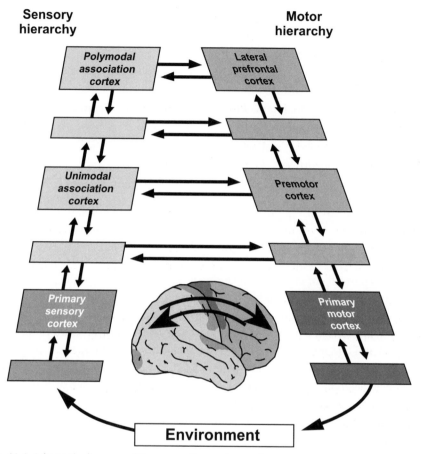

Fig. 41.4 Schematic diagram of the perception–action cycle.

In the course of a goal-directed sequence of behavioural acts, the sensory information that guides the sequence is processed upward in successive stages of the
hierarchy of sensory cortical areas. That processing leads to outputs to motor areas,
where actions are integrated. The actions induce changes in the environment, which
generate new sensory inputs, which lead to new actions, and so on. Automatic and routine behaviours can be integrated at lower stages of sensory and motor hierarchies,
without need for intervention of higher cortices. Novel and complex behaviours,
however, require processing at the highest levels of the perception–action cycle
and thus involve the prefrontal cortex and the cortex of polymodal sensory association.
The LPC intervenes whenever those behaviours necessitate the mediation of cross-
temporal contingencies. Temporal integration, and thus the temporal organization
of those behaviours, are then made possible by the executive functions of the LPC
summarized above.

As can be gleaned from the structure and operations of the perception–action cycle and the position of the LPC in it, the latter performs its executive functions in close cooperation with other cortical regions (Fuster 2001).

◆ The LPC controls the focus of attention by its modulation of sensory association areas of posterior cortex.

◆ Working memory is maintained by reverberation of activity in connective loops that link the LPC with those areas.

◆ Prospective set involves the downflow of priming influences from LPC upon premotor and motor cortices.

◆ Finally, the monitoring of motor responses and their consequences is in large part mediated by signals that arrive in LPC after being processed in hierarchically lower sensory and motor cortices.

6 Conclusions

The neural substrate for executive processing is organized hierarchically. At every level of the hierarchy, neuronal assemblies serve both the representation and the execution of actions. In the upward progression of executive levels, from the spinal cord to the neocortex, the actions represented and executed increase in complexity, as well as in the spatial and temporal remoteness of their goal. The association cortex of the convexity of the frontal lobes, or lateral prefrontal cortex (LPC), constitutes the highest level of that hierarchy. Its primary function is the temporal organization of goal-directed behaviour, speech, and reasoning. The organization of actions in those domains is essentially based on the capacity of the LPC to integrate temporally discontinuous information. In that process of temporal integration, the LPC mediates contingencies across time by cooperating with other cortical structures in the cognitive functions of the perception–action cycle, which include attention, working memory, prospective set, and response monitoring.

Selective references

Baddeley, A. (1986). *Working memory*. Clarendon Press, Oxford.

Baker, S.C., Rogers, R.D., Owen, A.M., Frith, C.D., Dolan, R.J., Frackowiak, R.S.J., and Robbins, T.W. (1996). Neural systems engaged by planning: a PET study of the Tower of London task. *Neuropsychologia* 34, 515–26.

Brunia, C.H.M., Haagh, S.A.V.M., and Scheirs, J.G.M. (1985). Waiting to respond: electrophysiological measurements in man during preparation for a voluntary movement. In *Motor behavior* (ed. H. Heuer, U. Kleinbeck, and K.-H. Schmidt). Springer, New York.

Damasio, H., Grabowski, T., Frank, R., Galaburda, A.M., and Damasio, A.R. (1994). The return of Phineas Gage: clues about the brain from the skull of a famous patient. *Science* 264, 1102–5.

Desimone, R. and Duncan, J. (1995). Neural mechanisms of selective visual attention. *Ann. Rev. Neurosci.* 18, 193–222.

Duncan, J. and Owen, A.M. (2000). Common regions of the human frontal lobe recruited by diverse cognitive demands. *Trends NeuroSci.* 23, 475–83.

Fink, G.R., Marshall, J.C., Halligan, P.W., Frith, C.D., Driver, J., Frackowiak, R.S., and Dolan, R.J. (1999). The neural consequences of conflict between intention and the senses. *Brain* 122, 497–512.

Fuster, J.M. (1973). Unit activity in prefrontal cortex during delayed-response performance: neuronal correlates of transient memory. *J. Neurophysiol.* 36, 61–78.

Fuster, J.M. (1995). *Memory in the cerebral cortex—an empirical approach to neural networks in the human and nonhuman primate.* MIT Press, Cambridge, Massachusetts.

Fuster, J.M. (1997). *The prefrontal cortex—anatomy, physiology, and neuropsychology of the frontal lobe,* 3rd edn. Lippincott-Raven, Philadelphia.

Fuster, J.M. (2001). The prefrontal cortex—an update: time is of the essence. *Neuron* 30, 319–33.

Gehring, W.J. and Knight, R.T. (2000). Prefrontal–cingulate interactions in action monitoring. *Nature Neurosci.* 3, 516–20.

Grasby, P.M., Frith, C.D., Friston, K.J., Bench, C., Frackowiak, R.S.J., and Dolan, R.J. (1993). Functional mapping of brain areas implicated in auditory-verbal memory function. *Brain* 116, 1–20.

Jacobsen, C.F. (1931). A study of cerebral function in learning: the frontal lobes. *J. Comp. Neurol.* 52, 271–340.

Luria, A.R. (1966). *Higher cortical functions in man.* Basic Books, New York.

Luria, A.R. (1970). *Traumatic aphasia.* Mouton, The Hague.

Mesulam, M.-M. (1981). A cortical network for directed attention and unilateral neglect. *Neurology* 10, 309–25.

Partiot, A., Grafman, J., Sadato, N., Wachs, J., and Hallett, M. (1995). Brain activation during the generation of non-emotional and emotional plans. *NeuroReport* 6, 1269–72.

Petrides, M., Alivisatos, B., Evans, A.C., and Meyer, E. (1993). Dissociation of human mid-dorsolateral from posterior dorsolateral frontal cortex in memory processing. *Proc. Natl Acad. Sci., USA* 90, 873–7.

Quintana, J. and Fuster, J.M. (1999). From perception to action: Temporal integrative functions of prefrontal and parietal neurons. *Cerebral Cortex* 9, 213–21.

Shallice, T. (1988). *From neuropsychology to mental structure.* Cambridge University Press, New York.

Smith, E.E., Jonides, J., and Koeppe, R.A. (1996). Dissociating verbal and spatial working memory using PET. *Cerebral Cortex* 6, 11–20.

Teuber, H.L. (1972). Unity and diversity of frontal lobe function. *Acta Neurobiolagiae Experimentalis* 32, 615–56.

Part 10

Clinical context and resources

Chapter 42

Clinical and laboratory examinations relevant to clinical neuropsychology

Udo Kischka

1 Introduction

The methods described in this chapter are used by clinicians to gain insight into the structure and the functions of a patient's nervous system. Computerized tomography (CT) and magnetic resonance imaging (MRI) are the methods of choice to demonstrate the anatomical structure and deviations thereof, such as trauma, stroke, tumour, or inflammation. They help visualize where a lesion is localized. All the other methods mentioned in this chapter are used to examine the extent of functioning of parts of the nervous system. In the context of this handbook, only those methods that deal with the brain rather than the spinal cord and the peripheral nervous system will be considered.

For the neuropsychologist, the outcomes of these examinations are relevant for several different reasons.

◆ The intactness of a patient's sensory and motor functions influences his/her performance in the neuropsychological tests. For instance, a visual field defect renders tests that require reading more difficult, and a weakness (*paresis*) or clumsiness (*ataxia*) in the responding arm will put the patient at a disadvantage in a test demanding motor responses. Thus, the knowledge of a clinical neurological deficit informs the choice of the neuropsychological tests that can be used and can help with the interpretation of their results.

◆ If a patient's cognitive performance fluctuates significantly within a short period of time, he/she might be suffering from *partial complex epileptic seizures*, whereby consciousness is altered for some minutes without being lost completely. In this case, an EEG may provide confirmation of the clinical suspicion of seizures.

◆ The MRI and CT scans make it possible to relate findings of neuropsychological deficits to damaged brain structures.

◆ A patient who displays a slow cognitive decline might suffer from one of a variety of possible neurological conditions, e.g. tumour, recurring strokes, or progressive brain atrophy in Alzheimer's disease. A CT or MRI scan then demonstrates the nature and extent of the pathological brain process.

Some of the methods described in this chapter (MRI, CT, electroencephalography (EEG), and parts of the clinical neurological examination) therefore yield results that can be related to neuropsychological findings. In addition, several other methods are briefly described and explained where such a direct link is not possible, but which are likely to be encountered by neuropsychologists in their clinical work.

2 The clinical neurological examination

The full clinical neurological assessment includes taking a history, observing the patient's behaviour, and carrying out a formal neurological examination of his/her motor, sensory, and reflex functions. A brief mental status examination also comprises part of this assessment. In about two-thirds of cases, this clinical information alone will enable the neurologist to make a correct anatomical diagnosis regarding the localization of the lesion, and a pathological diagnosis as to the nature of the underlying disease.

2.1 History

Taking the patient's history provides us with important clues about the nature of the disease, and also the patient's ability to cope with it. In addition to listening to the patient's account, the following kinds of questions need to be asked.

- What is the precise description (quality) of the complaints?
- Where are they localized?
- When did they first start?
- How did they start, suddenly or gradually?
- What course have they taken?
- Which situations trigger or relieve them?
- What treatment has been tried?

In conditions that affect the patient's cognitive functions temporarily (such as epilepsy) or continuously (such as dementia), it is necessary to get a relative's or partner's history of the patient.

2.2 Observation of the patient's behaviour

The observation of the patient's spontaneous behaviour comprises the way he/she walks, moves, and talks. Important criteria include the following.

- Level of alertness. Sleepiness is called *somnolence* when it is mild and *stupor* when it is more severe. *Coma* is enduring complete loss of consciousness.
- Speed of movements and speech. Unusual slowness of movement is called *bradykinesia*.
- Involuntary movements. *Tremor* is a rhythmic shaking of the limbs, the head, or, rarely, the whole body. Depending on the underlying disease, it can be most pronounced in rest, in holding the limbs outstretched, or during active movements.

- *Dystonia, dyskinesia, chorea,* and *athetosis* are different types of involuntary movements that are not rhythmic.
- Speech. *Aphasia* is the disturbed production and/or understanding of language; *dysarthria* is a defect in articulation, making the speech slurred.
- Structuring of the patient's account of his problems.
- Social appropriateness.

2.3 Neurological assessment

The neurological examination usually starts with the head and assessment of the 12 cranial nerves and then proceeds to the motor functions, sensations, and reflexes of the limbs and trunk. It should also include a brief mental status examination.

2.3.1 The 12 cranial nerves

The 12 cranial nerves relay motor functions, senses, and reflexes of the head.

- Motor functions:
  —facial expression: weakness of facial muscles is called *facial palsy*;
  —gaze: disturbed control of eye movements can lead to double vision or *nystagmus* (rhythmic movements of the eyes);
  —speaking (see Section 2.2);
  —swallowing: disturbed swallowing can cause choking;
  —turning of the head.
- Senses:
  —vision: blindness is called *amaurosis*; a loss of half the visual field within one or both eyes is called *hemianopia*;
  —smell: loss of smell is called *anosmia*;
  —taste: loss of taste is called *ageusia*;
  —hearing: reduced hearing is called *hypacusis*, deafness is called *anacusis*;
  —feeling: see Section 2.3.3;
- The vestibular system in the inner ear senses the position and movements of the head and therefore plays an important part in maintaining equilibrium.
- Reflexes. The most widely used reflex is the light reflex of the pupils.

2.3.2 Motor functions of the body

- Muscle power. The maximum power of each muscle group is described on a scale from 0 (no muscle contraction) to 5 (full power) according to the Medical Research Council. Muscle weakness is called *paresis* or *paralysis*; complete loss of force is called *plegia*. *Hemiparesis* is weakness of one side of the body, *paraparesis* weakness of both legs, and *tetraparesis* or *quadriparesis* weakness of all four limbs.
- Coordination. The dexterity of both coarse and fine movements is tested by the finger–nose test (touching his/her own nose with his/her index finger) and the

shin–heel–test (moving the heel to the opposite knee and along the shin). Clumsiness in these tests is called *ataxia*.

◆ Muscle tone. Increased tone can be either *spasticity* or *rigor*, reduced tone is called *flaccid*.

◆ Posture and gait. Observe whether the patient stands straight or bent, secure or insecure, and whether the movements seem clumsy (*ataxic*) or asymmetrical.

2.3.3 Sensation

The sensory modalities are:

◆ touch;

◆ pain;

◆ temperature;

◆ vibration;

◆ position of limbs.

Reduction of sensation is called *hypaesthesia*, complete loss *anaesthesia*. The feeling of pins and needles is called *paraesthesia*.

2.3.4 Reflexes

The most commonly tested reflexes are the biceps and triceps reflexes in the arms and the knee jerk and the ankle jerk in the legs. Note whether the reflexes are unusually weak or brisk, whether there are side differences, or differences between the reflexes of the arms and those of the legs.

Pathological reflexes indicate a lesion within the central nervous system. The *Babinski reflex* is the most widely used, whereby scratching of the outer side of the foot sole causes a dorsal extension (upward movement) of the big toe.

2.3.5 Cognitive functions

Every patient with known or suspected brain injury or disease should have a brief mental status examination. This detects signs of attentional, memory, or constructional deficits, aphasia, apraxia, agnosia, neglect, or executive dysfunction. This assessment falls under the term *cognitive neurology* (in the UK) or *behavioral neurology* (in the USA). A full neuropsychological examination will then provide a more detailed analysis of the nature and extent of the patient's cognitive deficits.

3 Laboratory examinations

3.1 Computerized tomography (CT)

Computerized tomography uses the extent of absorption of X-rays to demonstrate pathological changes in the body.

In a CT scanner, X-rays are transmitted through the head from different sides, and their strength measured by detectors on the opposite side. The X-rays' weakening (absorption) during the passage through the head depends on the density of the different

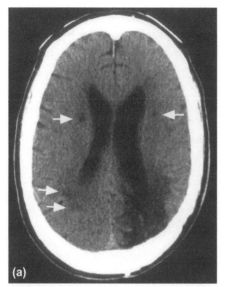 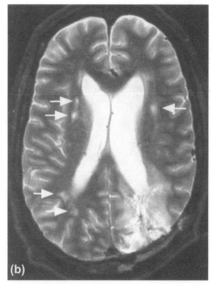

Fig. 42.1 Brain (a) CT and (b) MRI scans of a 57-year-old man 4 months after an ischaemic stroke in the right occipital lobe. He suffered from left hemianopia and hemineglect as well as other visuospatial deficits. There are additional small subcortical infarcts (arrows) that the MRI with its higher resolution shows more clearly than the CT scan.

tissues within and around the brain. The information from these different projections is transformed by a computer into a series of two-dimensional pictures that show air as black, bone as white, and brain tissue in different shades of grey (Fig. 42.1(a)).

The main criteria for analysing CT scans are:

- *Hypodense* areas which are darker than the surrounding tissue. These indicate ischaemic infarctions, oedema, inflammation, or certain tumours.

- *Hyperdense* areas which are lighter than the surrounding tissue. These indicate a fresh bleeding, calcification, or certain tumours.

- Size of the ventricles. An increase in size indicates either hydrocephalus or brain atrophy; a decrease in size indicates brain oedema (swelling of the brain).

- Shape and width of gyri and sulci of the cortical surface. Widened sulci and shrunken gyri indicate brain atrophy; swollen gyri with disappearing sulci indicate brain oedema.

Contrast enhancement can be achieved by intravenous injection of iodide-containing substances. This emphasizes natural and pathological blood vessels, and also areas of disrupted blood–brain barrier, such as infarctions after 2–3 days, abscesses, and some tumours.

The relevance of CT in the context of clinical neuropsychology lies in its ability to depict the anatomical structure of the brain and associated pathologies (Fig. 42.2). These pathologies can be related to findings of neuropsychological deficits. For instance, a patient's expressive aphasia (see Chapter 13) can be explained by the CT finding of a

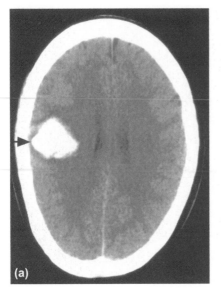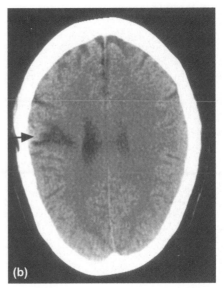

Fig. 42.2 Brain CT scans of a 32-year-old woman who suffered a left hemisphere haemorrhagic stroke (arrows) from an arteriovenous malformation (AVM). She had expressive aphasia and a right hemiparesis. (a) The CT on the day of the stroke shows fresh blood as hyperdense (white) areas. The AVM is not visible here, but was surgically removed after 3 weeks. (b) On the CT scan 8 months later, the blood is completely resorbed, and the resulting brain lesion shows up as hypodense (dark).

stroke involving Broca's area, and another patient's left hemineglect (see Chapter 5) may correspond to a right parietal tumour. The spatial resolution of CT is approximately 2 mm, which means that anatomical structures or pathological processes have to be at least that big to be detected. CT does not assess the functioning of the brain or its parts.

3.2 **Magnetic resonance imaging (MRI)**

MRI uses the magnetic properties of hydrogen protons (H^+) in brain tissue to generate images of the brain. Hydrogen protons constantly rotate ('spin') and therefore act as electrical dipoles. The MRI scanner creates a powerful magnetic field that forces all these protons into a single direction. Their direction is briefly diverted by short electromagnetic impulses and, when they return to their previous state, they emit high-frequency radiation ('echo') that can be measured by the MRI scanner. The characteristic of each proton's echo is influenced by the tissue immediately surrounding it, which allows the computer to generate high-resolution pictures of the different parts of the brain. These images look similar to those of CT, but show in much more detail pathological processes such as ischaemic infarctions (Fig. 42.1(b)), bleedings, inflammation, tumours, pathological blood vessels, hydrocephalus, brain oedema, or atrophy (see Section 3.1). Small lesions that are missed by CT, such as areas of inflammation in multiple sclerosis, can be demonstrated precisely in MRI.

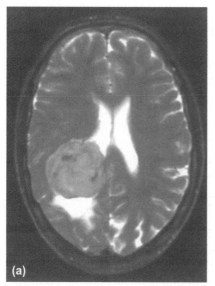 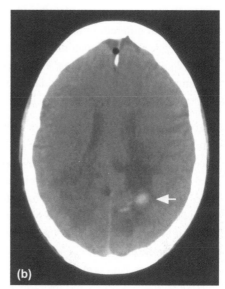

Fig. 42.3 Brain scans of a 46-year-old woman with a meningioma in the left lateral ventricle. (a) MRI scan before the operation. (b) CT scan 7 days after surgical removal of the tumour. The right hemisphere was chosen as the surgical access route in order to spare speech-related brain areas. Note the blood in this region (arrow). After the operation, the patient has moderate left-sided hemineglect and verbal and nonverbal memory deficits but no disorder of speech.

Just as with CT, MRI can be used to examine any part of the body, and the main use of MRI is the depiction of anatomical structures and pathological processes of the brain (Fig. 42.3). The spatial resolution of MRI is better than that of CT, approximately 1 mm. Like CT, MRI does not give us information about the functioning of the brain. Due to the use of a strong magnet, people with pacemakers or with metal implants in their brain or inner ears must not be examined with MRI.

3.3 Functional MRI (fMRI)

Functional MRI is not a method used in routine clinical practice, but a method of brain research that shows in which brain areas the blood flow increases while the subject performs a certain activity. It achieves this by making use of the different magnetic properties of oxygenated haemoglobin and deoxygenated haemoglobin in the bloodstream. An increased blood flow in a certain brain area is interpreted as a sign of increased activity in this area. In contrast to MRI itself, fMRI allows us to deduce the functioning of different brain areas.

3.4 Single-photon emission computer tomography (SPECT) and positron emission tomography (PET)

Both SPECT and PET use radioactive substances ('tracers') that are either injected into the person's bloodstream or inhaled, and are taken up preferentially into those parts of the brain which are most active. SPECT and PET therefore provide images of the blood flow and activity of different brain areas. They are, however, much less suited than MRI and CT to provide a detailed anatomical picture of the brain. Both methods are rarely used in clinical routine, e.g. in situations where a patient is suspected of having a mild ischaemia or traumatic brain injury that could not be detected with CT or MRI scanning.

3.4.1 SPECT

SPECT uses radioactive technetium (^{99m}Tc-HMPAO (hexamethyl propyleneamine oxime)), iodine (^{123}I-IMP (inosine 5′-phosphate)), or ^{133}xenon as its radioactive tracers. During their radioactive decay, they emit photons (γ-quanta), which are measured by one of many γ-cameras which are arranged in a circle around the person's head. From the distribution patterns of the measured γ-quanta, the regional cerebral blood flow (rCBF) in the different parts of the brain can be estimated. The spatial resolution of SPECT is 1–2 cm and the temporal resolution is 30 minutes.

An alternative use of SPECT lies in the use of radioactive tracers that bind specifically to certain receptors. An example of this is the use of ^{123}I-benzamide (IBZM) which binds to D_2 dopamine receptors and therefore provides us with information about the density of these receptors in subjects with (suspected) Parkinson's disease or related conditions.

3.4.2 PET

PET uses radioactive oxygen (H_2^{15}O), glucose (^{18}F-deoxyglucose), carbon (^{11}C), or nitrogen (^{13}N) as tracers. They are much more unstable than the tracers used in SPECT and emit positrons during their radioactive decay. When one of these positrons collides with a nearby electron, 2 photons (γ-quanta) are released that travel in precisely the opposite direction to each other. Simultaneous measurement of these photons by two γ-cameras on opposite sides of the head ('coincidence measurement') gives information about their source which is more precise than that provided by SPECT. With PET, rCBF and regional cerebral metabolic rate (rCMR) can be estimated. The spatial resolution of PET is 0.5–1 cm and the temporal resolution approximately 2 minutes.

Like SPECT, PET allows for receptor-binding studies and has been used to examine D_2 dopamine receptors, benzodiazepine receptors, serotonin receptors, and opiate receptors. Because of the fast decay of the tracers used in PET, this method depends on a nearby cyclotron to provide the radioactive substances. PET is not used in clinical routine, but as a method of brain research.

3.5 Angiography

Angiography or arteriography uses conventional X-ray examination after the injection of iodine-containing contrast substance to visualize the arteries and veins. In neurology, one is mostly interested in the arteries and veins of the brain or, sometimes, the spinal cord. Angiography is most useful in showing:

◆ stenosis (narrowing) of an artery;

◆ occlusion of an artery or vein;

- ◆ aneurysm: a bulging of an artery by a weakness of the artery wall;
- ◆ arteriovenous malformation or angioma: a tangle of pathological blood vessels;
- ◆ pathological vessels in a brain tumour.

3.6 Electroencephalography (EEG)

This method measures the electrical activity of the cerebral cortex with electrodes that are placed on the scalp (Fig. 42.4(b)).

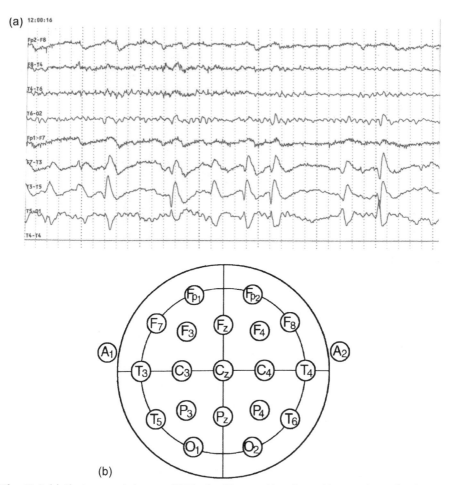

Fig. 42.4 (a) Electroencephalogram (EEG) of a 29-year-old patient with recurring epileptic seizures. The upper four traces demonstrate a normal alpha rhythm over the right hemisphere. The fifth trace is from the frontal part of the left hemisphere and is also normal. The lower three traces are from the posterior part of the left hemisphere and show spike-wave complexes, indicative of an epileptogenic focus in the left temporo-occipital region. (b) The positioning of the EEG electrodes on the skull.

The neurons generate action potentials that spread across the axons and dendrites, and the multitude of action potentials of the cortical neurons adds up to electrical field potentials that can be measured. These field potentials show regular rhythms that are classified as:

- beta, 14–30 Hz;
- alpha, 8–13 Hz;
- theta, 4–7 Hz;
- delta, 1–3 Hz.

These rhythms are probably caused by synchronization of the cortical activity mediated by the thalamus. In rest with the eyes closed, alpha is the predominant rhythm in the healthy adult. During sleep, the slower frequencies become more prominent and sleep-specific wave-forms appear: sleep spindles, vertex sharp transients, and K-complexes.

The EEG gives indications for pathological processes in the brain if the following patterns are found:

- General slowing of the EEG with diffuse theta- and delta-activity occurs in degenerative diseases such as Alzheimer's disease, intoxication, and metabolic encephalopathy (e.g. in liver or kidney dysfunction). In the latter case, the EEG activity can sometimes take the shape of 'triphasic waves' with high amplitude and delta frequency.
- Frontal intermittent rhythmic delta activity (FIRDA) is mainly found in lesions of deep brain structures such as the thalamus.
- Focal changes of rhythm or shape of the EEG waves (e.g. only left parietal) are a sign of an underlying pathological process such as stroke, traumatic brain injury, or brain tumour.
- Epileptic activity is indicated by rhythmic slow waves of unusually high amplitude or by 'sharp waves' that have a pointed rather than sinusoid shape (Fig. 42.4(a)). 'Sharp/slow wave complexes', which show a sharp wave immediately followed by a high-amplitude delta wave, are regarded as proof of epilepsy.

Searching for signs of epileptic activity is by far the most important use of EEG. However, even patients with proven epilepsy can have normal EEG recordings between seizures (inter-ictal EEG). A normal EEG therefore does not exclude epilepsy. If there is sufficient clinical evidence, either a sleep EEG after a wakeful night or a 24-hour EEG recording can then sometimes provide the signs of epileptic activity.

3.7 Evoked responses

Evoked responses are electrical potentials that are recorded from the scalp surface as a response to an external stimulus. They give us information about the functioning of sensory pathways within the nervous system. Visual, auditory, or somatosensory stimuli can be used, and they have in common that hundreds of consecutive stimuli are applied before a reliable evoked response can be measured. The evoked responses consist of a series of waves. The latencies, amplitudes, and shapes of these waves are altered when a sensory system is damaged and therefore allow inferences as to the part of the sensory system that is dysfunctional. A special case are motor-evoked potentials induced by transcranial magnetic stimulation, which are used to examine the functioning of the motor pathways.

- Visual evoked responses (VER) use a flickering draughtboard (checkerboard) for the patient to watch, and they are recorded occipitally over the visual cortical areas.
- Brainstem auditory evoked responses (BAER) are recorded over the mastoid or from the earlobe while the patient listens to click stimuli through headphones.
- Somatosensory evoked responses (SSER) are recorded after stimulation of the median nerve, tibial nerve, peroneal nerve, trigeminal nerve, or pudendal nerve. In addition to recordings from the scalp over the corresponding somatosensory cortical areas, SSER can also be recorded over the cervical spinal cord.
- Motor-evoked potentials (MEP): this method uses electromagnetic impulses to the motor cortex through the scalp (transcranial magnetic stimulation) to elicit electrical potentials in certain target muscles. Their amplitude, shape, and latency give information about the functioning of the motor pathways.

3.8 Event-related potentials (ERPs)

Unlike the evoked responses, which document the reaction of primary cortical areas to an external stimulus, event-related potentials record the responses of secondary cortical areas that occur slightly later. The ERPs are therefore considered to represent cognitive processes such as focusing of attention, detection of a stimulus, and reacting to an unexpected stimulus. The most commonly analysed ERPs are:

- P 300: a positive potential with its maximum 300 milliseconds after the stimulus, it can be found during tasks in which the subject is required to watch (or listen to) a series of identical stimuli and recognize occasionally interspersed different stimuli.
- N 400: in a task in which the subject reads or listens to sentences, an unexpected word that does not fit into the semantic context and therefore violates expectation is followed by a negative potential 400 milliseconds later.

In spite of intensive research, the precise meaning of the different ERPs is still unclear. They are therefore not commonly used in routine clinical practice.

3.9 Doppler ultrasound

Doppler ultrasound is used to detect a *stenosis* (narrowing) of an artery that leads blood to the brain: the internal carotid artery or the vertebral artery. A probe is pressed on to the skin above one of these arteries in the neck area. It emits ultrasound, which is bounced back from the blood cells and recorded by the same probe. The character of the returning ultrasound signal depends on the speed of the flow of blood cells. This makes it possible to determine where in the underlying artery the speed of the blood-stream is increased, which is an indication of a stenosis in this area. With transcranial Doppler ultrasound, it is even possible to measure the speed of the bloodstream in intracranial arteries, particularly the middle cerebral artery. The finding of a stenosis indicates that the blood supply to a part of the brain may be compromised.

3.10 Cerebrospinal fluid (CSF)

CSF is usually collected by lumbar puncture between the 3rd and 4th or between the 4th and 5th lumbar vertebrae. The analysis of the CSF helps in the diagnosis of the following conditions.

- Hydrocephalus: the hydrostatic CSF pressure is increased.

- Subarachnoid haemorrhage: the CSF is tainted with blood.

- Inflammation (meningitis or encephalitis): the amount of protein and the number of leukocytes in the CSF are increased. Multiple sclerosis is characterized by oligoclonal bands, with an increase of only a few types of immunoglobulines.

- Tumours: pathological tumour cells can sometimes be found in the CSF.

Selective references

Bradley, W.G., Daroff, R.B., Fenichel, G.M., and Marsden, C.M. (eds.) (2000). *Neurology in clinical practice*. Butterworth Heinemann, Oxford.

Donaghy, M. (ed.) (2001). *Brain's diseases of the nervous system*. Oxford University Press, Oxford.

Gilman, S. (1999). *Clinical examination of the nervous system*. McGraw-Hill, London.

Lee, S.H., Rao, K.C., and Zimmermann, R.A. (1996). *Cranial and spinal MRI and CT*. McGraw-Hill.

Misulis, K.E. (1997). *Essentials of clinical neurophysiology*. Butterworth-Heinemann, Oxford.

Strub, R.L. and Black, W. (1999). *The mental status examination in neurology*. F.A. Davis.

Chapter 43

Neuropsychological deficits within the World Health Organization's model of illness (ICIDH-2)

Derick T. Wade

1 Introduction

Rehabilitation practice needs a conceptual model or framework in which to work. In the past many health professions developed or employed their own model, some explicitly (e.g. Roper's model of nursing), but most less so (e.g. the so-called medical model and the so-called psychosocial model). One advance over the last 20 years has been the growing awareness and acceptance, in research practice at least, of the World Health Organization's (WHO) model of illness embodied in the original International Classification of Impairments, Disabilities, and Handicaps (ICIDH) and more recently revised, expanded, and renamed (as the International Classification of Functioning or ICF) but still referred to as the ICIDH-2 model (Wade and de Jong 2000).

Although widely known in some circles, this model of illness is not always fully understood or used by other health professionals. The WHO's ICIDH is not without controversy and there exist differences of opinion about how certain deficits should be classified. In particular, many clinicians have difficulty placing cognitive difficulties within the WHO's ICIDH-2 model. This appendix provides a possible framework.

The basic ICIDH-2 is shown in Table 43.1 with a revised version in Table 43.2 and Fig. 43.1. This is a slightly revised version that acknowledges that there are subjective (personal to the patient) and objective (observed by outside observers) aspects of most illness (Wade 2001). In addition this version includes pathology (i.e. disease) that is not covered in the ICF, since disease is already covered in the WHO's International Classification of Disease (ICD-10). Finally, the framework includes some acknowledgement of the concept of quality of life (Post *et al.* 1999). Otherwise, the model is essentially the same as the ICIDH-2.

The framework is intended to be used when considering and describing problems faced by patients with brain damage (including cognitive deficits) and provides a common and consistent language between medical and paramedical professionals. Patients

Table 43.1 The WHO's ICIDH-2 framework

Level of description: Term	Level of illness	
	Synonym	**Comment**
Pathology	Disease/diagnosis	Refers to abnormalities or changes in the structure and/or function of an *organ* or *organ system*
Impairment	Symptoms/signs	Refers to abnormalities or changes in the structure and/or function of the *whole body* set in a *personal context*
Activity (was *disability*)	Function/ observed behaviour	Refers to abnormalities, changes, or restrictions in the interaction between a person and his/her environment or *physical context* (i.e. changes in the *quality* or *quantity of behaviour*)
Participation (was *handicap*)	Social positions/ roles	Refers to changes, limitation, or abnormalities in the position of the person in their *social context*

Contextual factors		
Domain	**Examples**	**Comment**
Personal	Previous illness	Primarily refers to attitudes, beliefs, and expectations, often arising from previous experience of illness in self or others, but also to personal characteristics
Physical	House, local shops, carers	Primarily refers to local physical structurers but also includes people as carers (not as social partners)
Social	Laws, friends, family	Primarily refers to legal and local cultural setting, including expectations of important others

seen by clinical neuropsychologists will often (but not necessarily) have an underlying pathology such as frontal lobe infarction (stroke), diffuse axonal injury (after head injury), or degeneration in specific neuronal groups (e.g. Huntington's disease).

2 Impairments, disabilities, and handicaps

2.1 Impairments

Abnormal structure or function of the brain (i.e. abnormal neuroanatomy and/or neurophysiology) should be recognized as one cause of impairment to cognitive skills or functions. Emotional disturbance is another potent cause and often a contributing factor. Some patients may have many cognitive impairments such as:

♦ reduced initiation;

♦ reduced ability to recall and/or lay down new memories;

♦ reducing learning;

♦ increased distractability;

Table 43.2 Expanded model of illness

System	Experience/location	
	Subjective/internal	Objective/external
Level of illness		
Person's organ: pathology	Disease: label attached by person, usually on basis of belief	Diagnosis: label attached by others, usually on basis of investigation
Person's body: impairment	Symptoms: somatic sensation, experienced moods, thoughts, etc.	Signs: observable abnormalities (absence or change), explicit or implicit
Person in environment: behaviour	Perceived ability: what person feels they can do, and feeling about quality of performance	Disability/activities: What others note that person does do; quantification of that performance
Person in society: roles	Role satisfaction: person's judgement (valuation) of their own role performance (what and how well)	Handicap/participation: judgement (valuation) of important others (local culture) on role performance (what and how well)
Context of illness		
Internal, personal context	Personality: person's beliefs, attitudes, expectations, goals, etc.	Past history: observed/recorded behaviour prior to and early on in this illness
External, physical context	Salience: person's attitudes towards specific people, locations, etc.	Resources: description of physical (buildings, equipment, etc.) and personal (carers, etc.) resources available
External/social context	Local culture: the people and organizations important to person and their culture; especially family and people in same accommodation	Society: the society lived in and the laws, duties and responsibilities expected from and the rights of members of that society
Totality of illness		
Quality of life: summation of effects	Happiness: person's assessment of and reaction to achievement of or failure to reach important goals *and* sense of being a worthwhile person	Status: society's judgement on success in life; material possessions

- inability to shift attention to the left side of space;
- inability to use language, etc.

It is difficult to construct a comprehensive framework to encompass all possible cognitive impairments. More importantly, it is crucial to remember that almost all apparent cognitive impairments are extrapolated psychological constructs, largely derived to explain constrained and naturalistic observed behaviour. As pointed out by Halligan and Marshall (1992), there is, for example, no single brain centre or naturally occurring entity that corresponds to the clinically well established neuropsychological constructs of neglect or aphasia. Both represent constructs employed *post hoc* by clinicians

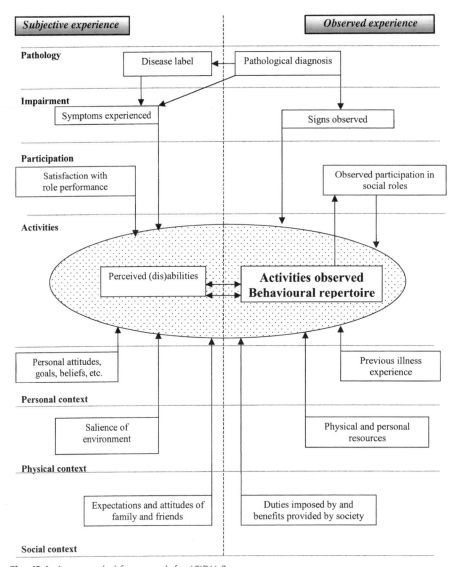

Fig. 43.1 An expanded framework for ICIDH-2.

and researchers to refer to specific deficits observed to occur in spatial awareness and language production after right and left brain damage, respectively.

2.2 Disability

Patients may suffer some limitation on or change in the quality of their behaviour (disability or alteration in or limitation of their activities). This can cover anything from maintaining continence through personal activities such as dressing and washing to complex activities such as working, shopping, or participating in conversations. The changes in activities may arise from several different underlying impairments, often in combination. The nature and extent of changes in these activities is greatly influenced by the particular person's physical, personal, and social context (see Section 3).

Some activities of daily living are more likely to be affected by cognitive impairments, but few if any are exclusively and only due to cognitive impairment. Hence it is important to recognize that there are *no* cognitive disabilities, only disabilities that may be attributable to cognitive impairments that are typically demonstrated on clinical or experimental tests.

2.3 **Handicap**

In illness, patients may experience a change in or limitation on their participation within society, once known as a change at the level of handicap. As for disability, cognitive impairments may be a contributing and, indeed, major factor, but there are no exclusively cognitive handicaps.

3 **The relevance of context**

All patients live within a context that is important for understanding and interpreting the significance of the acquired impairments.

- They have a *personal* context (experiences, beliefs, expectations, attitudes, response styles, etc.). This personal context might be altered by cognitive impairments (but probably less than we expect!). Personal context certainly influences the relationship between cognitive impairment and the resultant disability and handicap.

- Patients also have a *physical* context. The complexity of the environment might well have an influence on how much effect cognitive impairments have and vice versa. For example, an overstimulating environment with complex perceptual demands might lead to aggression in someone with marked cognitive impairments, whereas a well structured environment might help someone.

- Patients have a *social* context. Again this might influence the effect of cognitive impairment. For example, a predictable, stable social context might ameliorate the effects of impaired planning and initiation.

To provide a specific example, a patient might have a subarachnoid haemorrhage (primary pathology) with secondary frontal lobe infarction (secondary pathology) leading to impairment in planning, initiation, and self-awareness (cognitive impairments). In the context of work as a manager in a hospital (social and physical contexts) the person might fail in activities such as chairing meetings or organizing duty rosters, but, at home, in the context of wife and daughter (social and personal contexts), the person might not show any problems and be able to help with such activities as washing dishes. However, if the person's husband fell ill, she might not be able to look after the house.

Table 43.3 Rehabilitation interventions—some examples

Level (term)	Intervention	Comment
Level of illness		
Organ (pathology)	◆ Prevent disease ◆ Reverse or remove pathology ◆ Replace lost physiological function (e.g. insulin) ◆ Give information and advice	Important to know pathology for prognosis and likely impairments; cure often not possible *NB.* Pathology is not always present in an illness
Person (impairment)	◆ Prevent occurrence or worsening of impairment ◆ Reverse or improve impaired skill ◆ Replace lost skill or part with external or internal aid	May use therapy, drugs, orthoses, prostheses, surgery, etc.; may learn technique to overcome loss *NB.* Impairment may improve secondary to functional practice
Person in environment (activities)	◆ Prevent patient learning abnormal behaviours ◆ Teach how to undertake activities in presence of immutable impairments ◆ Practise activities, advising on risks, techniques, etc.	Involves altering behaviour in one way or another. Will often also involve changing the environment. May involve changing patient's goals or goals of others *NB.* This takes time and depends upon learning
Person in society (participation)	◆ Prevent loss of social contacts and roles ◆ Help identify new roles and how to develop them ◆ Ensure patient has opportunities to develop new or maintain old roles	Will almost always involve other people. May involve change in accommodation. For most people work is a central role *NB.* This takes a long time
Context of illness		
Personal context	◆ Prevent development of maladaptive beliefs and expectations ◆ Alter beliefs and expectations if necessary, usually through giving information and psychological therapy	Beliefs and expectations are major determinants of behaviour, but consequences of behaviour may also affect beliefs and expectations
Physical context	◆ Avoid loss of familiar environment if possible ◆ Adjust environment physically, including providing support from other people	Could include environmental control equipment, mobility aids, housing adaptations, etc.
Social context	◆ Adjust or help patient find new social context or help adapt to new social context	Usually strongly linked to accommodation and work
Totality of illness		
Quality of life	◆ Full rehabilitation	

4 Implications for treatment

Treatments can focus on several components and are not mutually exclusive (see Table 43.3), but typically take the form of one of the following four types.

♦ Some treatments attempt to directly *reduce the impairment*, usually through repetitive practice of the assumed cognitive domain. Usually, this involves a structured set of activities *that are thought to need good function in the impaired domain*. Examples within the area of cognitive deficits are the programmes that are supposed to reduce neglect or improve memory.

♦ Other treatments focus more on *improving the functional activities* that are affected, again through repeated practice in the specific activities affected. For example, someone with neglect might practise dressing or cooking until able to achieve these activities safely and independently, without the practice being targeted at the assumed impairment.

♦ Yet other treatments may try to *alter the context*, e.g. through providing external prompts and cues (post-it notes, alarms) or through ensuring a predictable routine through the day. This may involve other people. Many patients with persistent cognitive impairments are best helped in this way.

♦ Lastly, one may try to *alter expectations and beliefs*, and to find alternative roles and ways of participating in society.

This analysis emphasized that there is no separate cognitive rehabilitation. There is rehabilitation for people with cognitive impairments, rehabilitation that might include trying to reduce the impairment itself but that will include many other interventions. It is also worth noting that much of all rehabilitation involves altering behaviour, a process that depends upon learning, which is a cognitive skill or function. Thus, all rehabilitation is cognitive. It is not surprising, therefore, that patients with neurological disease are perhaps the most difficult to rehabilitate. The very organ and skill needed to succeed in rehabilitation (i.e. the brain and an ability to learn and adapt) are themselves damaged, which often slows the process.

Selective references

Halligan, P.W. and Marshall, J.C. (1992). Left visuo-spatial neglect: a meaningless entity? *Cortex* 28 (4), 525–35.

Post, M.W.M., de Witte, L.P., and Schrijvers, A.J.P. (1999). Quality of life and the ICIDH: towards an integrated conceptual model for rehabilitation outcomes research. *Clin. Rehabil.* 13, 5–15.

Wade, D.T. (2001). Disability, rehabilitation and spinal injury. In *Brain's diseases of the nervous system* (ed. M. Donaghy), pp. 185–209. Oxford University Press, Oxford.

Wade, D.T. and de Jong, B. (2000). Recent advances in rehabilitation. *Br. Med. J.* 320, 1385–8.

Chapter 44

The internet and clinical neuropsychology

Vaughan Bell

1 Introduction

The internet is the single largest and most diverse resource available to clinical neuropsychologists and remains a powerful ally for any patient-focused practitioner. It is useful not only because it provides convenient access to a vast array of clinical and scientific information but also because it allows disparate individuals to widen the informal networks that provide the bedrock of the mutual cooperation and education that characterize contemporary clinical science. (See Al-Shahi *et al.* 2002.)

This silver lining does not however, come without an accompanying cloud and, as with any clinical tool, there are practical and ethical issues that have to be addressed. Whilst no clinician would dream of using a novel practice without fully understanding its implications, it is not unusual for even the most accomplished of clinical scientists to understand only enough of the internet to facilitate its use without being able to address these issues. This inevitably leads at best to wasted time and frustration, and at worst to serious implications for the welfare of patients (Alejandro *et al.* 2000).

This chapter aims to provide practical advice so that time on the internet can be used effectively, whilst giving an outline of the additional ethical considerations that internet communication presents.

2 E-mail communication and etiquette

E-mail has always been the *lingua franca* of internet communication by virtue of its ubiquitous nature and flexibility. The utility of a system that allows electronic messages to be delivered to an individual, usually within minutes and regardless of their physical location, would seem to be self-evident. See Table 44.1 for an explanation of common e-mail and internet terms and abbreviations.

As Smith and Senior (2001) have noted, e-mail is becoming the preferred method of communication for the psychologist, and clinical neuropsychologists will undoubtedly find this facility as useful, if not more so, than any other e-mail user. For this reason it is important that clinicians should be fully aware of the facilities, pitfalls, and customs that accompany e-mail communication.

Table 44.1 Glossary of abbreviations

Abbreviation	Name	Definition
ADSL	Asynchronous digital subscriber line	• A broadband telecommunication technology
ARPA	Advanced Research Projects Agency	• The central research and development organisation of the US Department of Defense
bps	Bits per second	• The standard rating of speed of data flow
CGI	Common gateway interface	• A means of generating dynamic content from a database on the WWW
DNS	Domain name system	• A means to translate host names into IP addresses
eTOC	Electronic table of contents	• An emailed table of contents of an online journal
FTP	File transfer protocol	• A means to exchange files between servers over a network
GIF	Graphics interchange format	• A compressed image format using minimal memory, best for block images
HTML	Hypertext markup language	• The principal programming language used to write pages on the WWW
HTTP	Hypertext transfer protocol	• The communication protocol used by servers to send files to browsers
ISDN	Integrated services digital network	• Digital telephone connections delivering broadband internet access
ISP	Internet service provider	• An intermediary company that connects a user to the internet
IP address	Internet protocol address	• One of a potential 4.2 billion 32 bit numbers in dotted decimal notation identifying a computer on the internet
JPEG	Joint Photographic Expert Group	• A compressed image format using minimal memory, best for shaded photographic images
LAN	Local area network	• A network serving a small geographical area, which permits faster transmission speeds. Versus MAN and WAN
MAN	Metropolitan area network	• A network in a geographical area larger than a LAN but smaller than a WAN
Modem	Modulator/demodulator	• Converts digital to analogue signals and back, to enable computers to communicate over a telephone line

Table 44.1 Continued

Abbreviation	Name	Definition
MPEG	Moving Picture Expert Group	• The digital format encoding video images, displayed by dedicated software
NeLH	National electronic Library for Health	• A digital library for NHS staff in the UK
PDF	Portable document format	• A universal electronic document format that enables the style and layout of text and images to appear identical to the printed page
PGP	Pretty good privacy	• Freely available encryption software
POP	Point of presence	• Types of servers that convey email
RDF	Resource description framework	• An infrastructure that enables the exchange of metadata
SHTTP	Secure hypertext transfer protocol	• A communications protocol for financial exchanges over the internet
SMTP	Simple mail transfer protocol	• A communications protocol for regulating traffic between mail servers
SSL	Secure sockets layer	• A communications protocol for transmitting private documents via the internet
TCP/IP	Transmission control protocol/internet protocol	• The universal communication protocol used by the internet to transmit packets of data
URL	Uniform resource locator	• The unique address of a file accessible over the internet (Fig 2)
W3C	World Wide Web Consortium	• A forum for information, commerce, communication, and collective understanding of the WWW
WAN	Wide area network	• A network in a geographical area larger than a LAN and a MAN
WWW	World wide web	• A global collection of interconnected servers, whose contents are viewed through a browser
XML	Extensible markup language	• A universal format for structured documents and data on the WWW

With permission from *JNNP* by Al-Shahi *et al.* (2002): 73, pp. 619–28.

2.1 One-to-one email communication

As with any sort of communication, messages must be appropriate to their recipient and content and style may differ accordingly. However, there are several ways of using the medium to its best advantage for the benefit of both parties.

2.1.1 Write clearly and provide context

Whilst an email may be perfectly understandable in the context of an ongoing dialogue, when read some months or even weeks later it may make little sense. This may not be such an issue for informal communication but exchanges concerning issues of importance may be referred back to frequently in clinical settings.

One simple way of doing this is to use context quoting, where the *relevant* section of the received e-mail is quoted with the response added below, thus:

> > I still haven't found the amnesia paper I was after.

> Not to worry, I found a copy and will post it to you.

This allows your reply to be concise whilst maintaining context and avoiding the unnecessary bulk of including the whole of the previous e-mail.

2.1.2 Use the lowest common denominator

Plain text is preferable to any form of embellishment that an e-mail program may provide, such as sending HTML mail (creating and sending e-mail as web pages). Everyone on the internet can read plain text e-mail. Not everyone may be able to read any additional features that may be added. Even if you know that the person you are writing to can read your special format of e-mail, this might prevent someone else from reading it if it gets forwarded on, as is often the case in the team environments that clinical neuropsychologists commonly work in.

2.1.3 Attachments must be appropriate

Whilst many pages of plain text will still only take seconds to download on the slowest internet connection, attaching a file can greatly increase download time. It is good practice to ask whether a person wishes to receive an attachment if it exceeds 500k in size. When sending an attachment, state its size and type clearly, as this may not always be obvious to the recipient (e.g. 'the attached paper is a 240k Microsoft Word 97 file').

2.1.4 Remember that e-mail is not written speech

Due to the nature of text-based communication many of the subtleties of face-to-face communication are easily lost, leading to a message being misinterpreted. Particular caution must be taken when using sarcasm, humour, or ambiguous statements. Similarly, short functional replies may be interpreted as showing irritation. Sentences or phrases can be emphasized or softened by the use of punctuation such as asterisks ('I really must *stress* this point') or by using emoticons or 'smileys' to indicate the emotional context of a statement. Excessive use of emoticons is considered a little gauche and most people stick to simplified versions such as ':)' to indicate positive emotion, e.g.

I really enjoyed your talk :)

or ':(' to indicate a negative emotion

That's the third time this week :(

2.2 One-to-many e-mail communications

Discussion lists, where e-mail is used to continue an ongoing dialogue with a group of people, can be a source of practical help, support, and inspiration as well as a distraction and annoyance. One enquiring e-mail to a group of similarly focused professionals can be worth many hours searching through databases or on the phone, and such lists may also serve as a source of news and announcements and as a way of forming informal associations that can lead to valuable collaborations. Internet discussion lists are, however, notorious for bringing out the worst in people, not least because e-mail can so easily be misinterpreted, but also because it is often difficult to fathom the unwritten rules of the group without accidentally violating them.

Simple guidelines (colloquially called 'netiquette') have been formulated to facilitate group interaction in internet discussion groups and include the points covered in our discussion for one-to-one e-mail communication, with a few additions and alterations.

2.2.1 Attachments should not be sent to a discussion list

Such lists may involve hundreds of subscribers, many of whom will not appreciate having to receive a large file that may only be of interest to a minority. If you have a file you wish to disseminate, either ask who wishes to receive it and mail it to them personally or, if possible, upload it to a web site and post the location so subscribers can download it at their leisure.

2.2.2 Watch who you are replying to

Additional recipients can be included in an e-mail and by clicking the 'Reply' button you may inadvertently reply to them all. Similarly, if you wish to respond to a public e-mail privately, make sure you are doing so and not accidentally mailing the whole list. Sending a personal e-mail to a public list can be a cause of embarrassment or, in a clinical environment, a potential breach of confidentiality.

2.2.3 Group e-mails should be of group benefit

Discussion lists are measured by their signal-to-noise ratio. Lots of irrelevant chatter and 'content-free' contributions encourage an overall decrease in useful interaction and cause genuinely interested people to unsubscribe. That's not to say you necessarily always have to stick exactly to the list topic, but signal-heavy content is usually much preferred. In some cases, the discussion list will be moderated so irrelevant messages will not reach the mailing list at all.

2.2.4 Don't fan the flames

'Flaming' or the descent into vitriolic argument seems to be a fact of life on internet discussion lists. Clinical practice is, for most practitioners, a passionate interest and is likely to cause heated debate. Whilst it may seem a little patronizing to remind competent professionals that other list members should be treated with respect, I have yet to find a discussion list where this has not happened at least once. Such heated exchanges are usually the result of a perceived but unintended slight, or when the participants do not realize that their exchange has gone beyond an informative debate of general interest into petty pedantry.

3 Using the internet (see Fig. 44.1 for simplified schema)

The worldwide web has two major advantages for clinical neuropsychologists.

◆ It allows the targeted retrieval of relevant clinical and scientific information

◆ It allows information to be easily disseminated with the burden of acquisition placed upon the retriever. Documents, pictures, video or any other sort of digital information need only to be placed on the web, and their existence flagged so that interested parties can access them, all without further intervention from the author.

3.1 Information retrieval

The most useful skill in searching the web for relevant information is not fishing out the gold but filtering out the rubbish. Search engines use entered keywords to identify pages that contain those words somewhere on the page, and hence the best strategy is often not to use words that best describe what you want to find, but to use words that are most likely to appear on pages containing the information you require. For example, searching the web using the keyword 'amnesia' brings up lots of irrelevant information as it is often used as a catchy name for everything from nightclubs to novels. However, a similar search using the keywords 'memory loss' returns lots of highly relevant references.

Humans are inevitably better at evaluating small amounts of information for relevancy than are computers, so another useful technique is to use search engines to narrow the field or to give leads. In fields such as clinical neuropsychology where the sources of information may be limited, it is often the case that you may find yourself searching for pages that will then point you to the information you are eventually hoping to find. For example, if I wanted to find information about the notional conference 'Neuropsychology and the internet' entering these terms may produce a great numberl of irrelevant results, either because there may be many pages containing these words that have nothing to do with the conference I wish to find, or because the conference web pages are either non-existent, or have not been catalogued by the search engines' databases. A preferred approach may be to search using the keywords 'neuropsychology

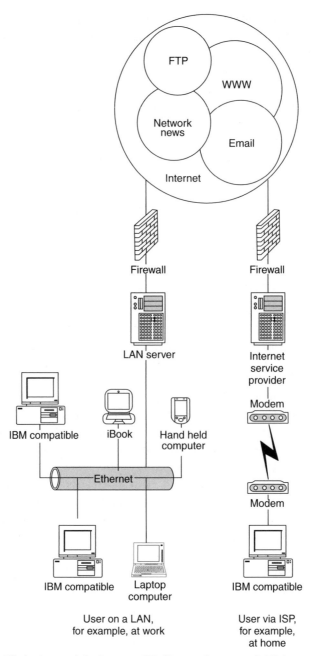

Fig. 44.1 Simplified schema of the internet. FTP, file transfer protocol; ISP, internet service provider; LAN, local area network; WWW, world wide web. With permission from the JNNP by Al-Sharhi *et al.* (2002); 73, pp. 619–28.

conferences' to find a page that lists conferences relevant to neuropsychologists (of which there are many) and look for a listing made by an ever reliable human.

Some search engines, and many online databases may allow searches to be made specific by searching for an exact phrase, or by using terms such as AND, OR, and NOT. The use of such terms is beyond the scope of this particular chapter but almost all facilities that allow such searches have online help and guides in their use.

It is worth noting that there is more to effective searching than being familiar with the tools. The internet can be thought of as a town. Whilst you may be perfectly competent at buying items in a shop, it is your knowledge of the town that makes this ability useful. Similarly, spending time to overview the general internet resources available to clinical neuropsychologists is often useful for the same reason that general theoretical overviews are useful in any science. Whilst you may not have the information to hand, at least you know the best place to go and find it, saving you valuable time and frustration along the way.

3.2 Publishing information on the web

Internet publishing can, in principle, simplify a great deal of the information distribution problem. Attendees can download notes from your talk and colleagues can retrieve minutes of meetings and important documentation such as ethics forms and other administrative templates. You can do the same without having to chase after the person with the keys to the right filing cabinet.

In practice, it is a lot more difficult, largely because the easy to use click-and-go tools are not yet available for web publishing as they are for web searching. To publish effectively on the web you either need to put some time and effort into learning the necessary steps or, if working in a suitable institution, have the support of suitably skilled computer or internet technicians.

It is unnecessary to outline all the required steps here, both because they will vary wildly depending on the web page hosting arrangements available (institution's own/commercial services/free services) and because high-quality easy-to-understand guides are regularly published in internet magazines and provided by web-hosting companies, who often have support lines to aid in technical issues. As with most technology issues, the initial curve is the hardest to climb but once completed, web publishing can be as painless as sending an e-mail.

Some desirable features may or may not be available and it might be worth checking if you feel these might be necessary. Such features may include:

- password protection for areas or particular documents within your web site;
- large amounts of storage space, particularly if you wish to disseminate video data;
- the ability to run interactive programs, if you wish to make use of certain types of online questionnaires and data collection.

When creating public web pages, you may wish to consider some of the aspects that allow pages to be successfully found via search engines, such as including your own keywords and all the relevant names if a theory, concept, or object has alternative naming conventions. Similarly, you may use your own experience of what is pleasant to read and navigate when designing your layout or consult the growing range of books that attempt to explain good web page design to non-computer professionals.

3.3 Effective use of internet software

There are two main problems which may affect a useful internet work session. The first is poor design or broken technology on the remote web site or resource, the second is inefficient use of web browser software.

Frequently, there is little a user can do about remote web site failures or errors, frustrating as they might be. It is however, often worth sending the site administrator a short email pointing out the problem you have encountered. System administrators tend to be somewhat overburdened and are unable to spend vast amounts of time checking every nook and cranny of a complex web site to make sure it still works after every alteration. A polite email pointing out an error in the site is often useful for them, and may mean your required information is fixed within a matter of hours. On a less positive note, technically competent people (especially the overworked ones who are contacted out of the blue), tend to attribute problems to stupidity in the first instance and stop investigating a reported problem (rightly or wrongly) at the first sign that a user might not understand the technology. Less confident users may wish to quickly check with a more experienced colleague that their problem is genuinely with the web site, and not their usage of the software, to increase the chances of a helpful response.

One alternative solution to missing or broken pages is to make use of internet search engines. If you click on a link which leads nowhere, or a web address you have been given does not work, try typing the title of the page into a search engine. If the page has moved, the search engine may have catalogued its new location. Another useful feature, pioneered by the search engine Google (www.google.com) is a system which stores copies of all the pages it knows about. Even if a page has been deleted from its original location, Google may still have a copy in its cache. Simply search for the page normally, and click the 'Cached' link to see the saved version. A web site called the Way Back Machine (www.archive.org), solely exists for this purpose and has archives of web pages stretching back some years. It is also worth remembering that such archives are kept by third parties if you are considering putting personal or sensitive information on the web. You may be able to remove your own web pages, but will not be able to remove the same information from external archives.

The problem of inefficient web browser use can greatly affect the speed and ease of an internet work session. In the early days of the web, browsers were fairly small and lightweight. They had only limited functionality as web sites were relatively unsophisticated. More recently, due to the demands of newer web site technology, increased multimedia usage and (it has to be said) poor design, browsers have obtained a reputation for being slow, buggy, and monolithic. Whilst this situation is gradually improving, a good grasp of how to maximize browser performance may save you a great deal of time and hair-loss.

There are some good practices that apply to almost all computer software you will use. First, it is important to get a good overview of the software, a good habit is to read through all the main menus and familiarize yourself with the options before you start using any new piece of software. This will give you an instant overview of the package's functionality, and will also make any additional documentation (like the electronic help files) much more cognisant. Secondly, try and load or enable only the software, features or options that you need. If you feel competent in software configuration, experiment and see which options improve your usage. Often there are many like-minded users on the internet, some of which kindly publish their pearls of wisdom. A web search using the name of your software package and the word 'optimisation' (or 'optimization' to retrieve pages using the alternative spelling) as key words will often give you a wealth of information. An excellent review article by Al-Shahu *et al.* (2002) has lots of useful pointers in this regard, and the Table 44.2 is derived from their paper.

4 Ethics of internet communication

The use of internet communication by clinical neuropsychologists causes some novel ethical dilemmas because of two major considerations:

* the *privacy* implications of using the internet and internet software (notorious for their lack of adequate security) for information that you may be legally and ethically bound to keep confidential;

* the issue of *copyright* and its use to restrict the dissemination of information that could aid the treatment of patients or education of clinicians, when such dissemination can be conducted for near zero cost when conducted via the internet.

4.1 Internet security and confidentiality

The idea that a patient's medical information should only be available to people directly involved in their medical care, and that it is the carer's responsibility to maintain this confidentiality is a core value in the health-care system. It will perhaps come as a surprise to many clinicians that sending information over the internet is as confidential as discussing a patient's details on a crowded bus. It may be true that no one is interested but that does not change the fact that the information is available to many people to whom the patient has not consented access.

With easily available software, any person can intercept and store all of the unencrypted information on your local network without being detected. Government agencies routinely intercept internet traffic and, while this may not be considered a major concern for the majority of patients, it must be noted that in the recent case of

Table 44.2 Strategies to enhance use of the internet browser

Maintain software

- Use the latest version of your browser (determine which version you are using under the 'Help' menu, 'About' in Windows, or Apple menu 'About'on the Macintosh).
- Check for new browser software monthly for the latest security patches.
- Use the latest versions of free software to view multimedia content

    (e.g.) Adobe Acrobat Reader (www.adobe.com/products/acrobat)

    Shockwave (www.macromedia.com/shockwave)

    QuickTime (www.quicktime.com)

    RealPlayer (www.real.com)

- Install virus protection software and keep it up to date (www.symantec.com, www.nai.com, www.zonelabs.com).

Shorten the time you spend on line

- For downloading large amounts of data, use the internet before global use rises (between midnight and noon in Europe).
- If available, use mirror sites (exact copies of web sites) located in, or close to, your own country.
- If the web site allows it, select text-only or low bandwidth options and omit multimedia content if the bandwidth of your connection is low.
- If network response is sluggish, open pages in their own windows (for relevant menu, right click in Windows, click and hold on the Macintosh) and continue working or browsing other pages, and return to them in a few minutes.

Minimize memory use

- Choose to install only the components of the browser that are essential to you (a full installation can consume many megabytes of disk space).
- Close down browser windows and applications you are no longer using.
- Optimize the size of your cache or 'Temporary Internet Files' folder.

Customize your browser

- Set your browser's home page to a blank page (about:blank) or the web site you use the most.
- Organise your 'Favorites' or 'Bookmarks' into folders.
- Set your preferred font type and size (under 'Text Size' on the 'View' menu)
- Maximize the viewable area in your browser by removing the explorer bar and customising toolbars to show only the functions you use (as small icons).
- Use the appropriate default programs for sending email, etc., from your browser.

Take short cuts

- When typing web addresses, omit 'http://', as your browser will automatically append it.
- Use copy and paste functions to transfer web addresses between documents and browser.
- Right click (Windows) or click and hold (Macintosh) with your mouse to save images, sounds, or videos from a web site to your hard drive.
- If a web site cannot be found with the web address you have entered use a search engine to see if it is available at an alternative location.
- Learn the shortcut keys that allow you to directly type in a web address without having to click on the location bar.

General Augusto Pinochet's extradition from the UK, the decision rested on a neuropsychology assessment of his mental fitness. Whilst not all such ethical dilemmas might be as dramatic, each patient should be able to rely on the confidentiality of their clinical records or related information, including when they are communicated via the internet.

Similarly, much common internet software is susceptible to viruses that can also breach such confidentiality agreements. In the case of one particular virus that exploits vulnerabilities in popular e-mail software, a document is randomly selected and mailed to everyone in a user's address book. This author has personally received a confidential case report that got mailed by this virus to a *public mailing list* that happened to be listed in the infected user's e-mail address book.

One way of assuming responsibility for clinical confidentiality is to ensure that adequate advice is taken on the implications of using particular software and taking precautions to prevent unhappy accidents, such as running up-to-date antivirus software. In the case of internet communication the use of encryption software to scramble the contents of messages so that only the intended recipient can decrypt or unscramble the potentially sensitive information is currently the best method to ensure private communication.

Encryption software is, unfortunately, still scarcely used, and not as user-friendly as it could be. However, this is rapidly changing and it is becoming accessible to motivated individuals willing to spend a little time learning the ropes. Any clinical neuropsychologists who are provided with their internet access by an employer or institution should push for encryption to be common practice rather than the exception and take good advice from competent computer professionals on suitable software for this purpose.

4.2 Electronic publishing

The debate over the ownership of scientific literature has recently become particularly salient, largely because the traditional role of publishers as the cogwheels of journal distribution is becoming increasingly redundant as the internet becomes the preferred method for information dissemination. Since information can be distributed across the internet for near zero cost, questions have been raised about the ethics of using copyright to restrict information that could be used for the benefit of the patient and society at large (Bachrach *et al.* 1998).

However, whilst no one would doubt the benefits of peer review in scientific and clinical research, doubts have been raised about the possible decline in quality that may occur if copyright for clinical and scientific journals is abolished (Bloom 1998).

Clinical neuropsychologists may also face similar dilemmas when producing standardized neuropsychological tests. The question of whether it is ethical to cede copyright to a publisher who may charge large sums of money for a copy of a potentially beneficial clinical test is a thorny issue. For some tests (such as the Block Design subscale of the Wechsler Adult Intelligence Scale) that may require specifically prepared materials that cannot be simply provided as digital templates, it would seem that a third-party publisher may be the best method of effective distribution. Many neuro-psychological tests are, however, produced by publically funded neuropsychologists and can easily be distributed as digital copies to appropriate recipients. Many would argue that to restrict and charge for clinical tests that may be used directly in a patient's care, or in valuable clinical research when a near zero cost distribution method is available, could be considered a unethical or, at the very least, obstructive.

5 Internet resources

A static list of internet resources is likely to become increasingly obsolete as time goes on. However, these have been chosen as useful and reliable resources and may provide a starting point for the creation of your own internet resource list.

5.1 General internet resources (see also Al-Shahi *et al.* 2002)

- **Google.** The most popular and arguably the best general internet search engine.
  http://www.google.com

- **Google and Yahoo groups.** Two discussion-list hosting sites, that both have established e-mail discussion lists and allow creation of custom lists for free.
  http://groups.google.com
  http://groups.yahoo.com

- **Netiquette and Good Internet Practice Guidelines.**
  http://www.faqs.org/rfcs/rfc1855.html

5.2 General neuropsychology resources

- **Neuropsychology.co.uk.** Excellent, frequently updated site with links to conference and neuroscience-specific search tools.
  http://www.neuropsychology.co.uk

- **PsychCrawler.** Psychology-specific internet search engine.
  http://www.psychcrawler.com/

- **NeuroGuide.** Neuroscience-specific search engine.
  http://www.neuroguide.com/

- **The Whole Brain Atlas.** Comprehensive atlas of neuroimaged human brain structures, showing both normal structure and neuropathology. Has extensive interactive features to aid navigation and study.
  http://www.med.harvard.edu/AANLIB/home.html

5.3 Sites to support evidence-based health care and research

- **PubMed.** Free web-based access to the Medline Literature Database.
  http://www.ncbi.nlm.nih.gov/PubMed/

- **CliniWeb.** An index and table of contents to clinical information on the world-wide web

  http://www.ohsu.edu/cliniweb/

- **OMNI.** Free access to a searchable catalogue of health and medicine internet sites.

  http://omni.ac.uk/

- **BioMail.** Free journal contents alerting service that allows custom searches to be regularly conducted on the PubMed database, and the results e-mailed directly to you.

  http://www.biomail.org

- **Highwire Press.** Archive of full-text journals that provide unrestricted free access.

  http://highwire.stanford.edu/

- **Free Medical Journals.** Archive of full-text clinical and medical journals that provide free unrestricted access.

  http://www.freemedicaljournals.com/

5.4 Relevant associations and societies on the web

- **British Psychological Society – Division of Neuropsychology.** UK section of BPS designed to promote the professional development of clinical neuropsychology. Arrange meetings and training course and seeks to encourage research in the field.

  http://www.bps.org.uk/sub-syst/DON/index.cfm

- **British Neuropsychological Society.** UK neuropsychological association that organizes regular high-quality talks and conferences throughout the year. Includes archive of past abstracts and programmes for forthcoming events.

  http://www.hop.man.ac.uk/bns/

- **Headway.** Website of head injury support organization providing information and support for head injury patients and their friends and family.

  http://www.headway.org.uk/

- **National Institute of Neurological Disorders and Stroke** (NINDS). American website that has comprehensive resources on brain disease and pathology as well as regularly updated relevant news and contacts sections.

  http://www.ninds.nih.gov/

- **Division 40 (Clinical Neuropsychology) of the American Psychological Association.** is a scientific and professional grouping of the APA active in developing and promoting professional training and education.

  http://www.div40.org/

- **National Academy of Neuropsychology.** Has plenty of professional information including online training materials, news and updated list of neuropsychology e-mail discussion lists.

  http://nanonline.org/

- ◆ **British Neuropsychiatric Association.** This group comprises psychiatrists, psychologists, and neurologists and provides for cross-disciplining discussion of the resting to brain function and behaviour.

  http://freespace.virgin.net/bnpa.website/

- ◆ **Public Library of Science.** Organization aiming to make scientific literature and journal articles freely available over the internet.

  http://www.publiclibraryofscience.org/

Selective references

Alejandro, R., Jadad, R., Haynes, B., Hunt, D., and Browman, G.P. (2000). The Internet and evidence-based decision-making: a needed synergy for efficient knowledge management in health care. *Can. Med. Assoc. J.* **162** (3), 362–5.

Al-Shahi, R., Sadler, M., Rees, G. and Bateman, D. (2002). Review: the internet. *Journal of Neurology, Neurosurgery and Psychiatry*, 73, 619–28.

Bachrach S. *et al.* (1998). Intellectual property: who should own scientific papers? *Science* **281** (5382), 1459–60.

Bloom, F. (1998). The rightness of copyright [editorial]. *Science* **281** (5382), 1451.

Laporte, R. and Hibbitts, B. (1996). Rights, wrongs and journals in the age of cyberspace. *British Medical Journal*, 313, 1609–12.

Smith, M.A. and Senior, C. (2001). The internet and clinical psychology: a general review of the implications, *Clinical Psychology Review*, 21 (1), 129–36.

Stone, J. and Sharpe, M. (2003). Internet resources for psychiatry and neuropsychiatry *J. Neurol. Neurosurg. Psychiatry* 74; 10–12.

Index